Atlas of Trichoscopy

Lidia Rudnicka • Malgorzata Olszewska
Adriana Rakowska
Editors

Atlas of Trichoscopy

Dermoscopy in Hair and Scalp Disease

Springer

Editors
Lidia Rudnicka
Faculty of Health Sciences
Medical University of Warsaw
Poland

Department of Dermatology
CSK MSW
Warsaw
Poland

Malgorzata Olszewska
Department of Dermatology
Medical University of Warsaw
Warsaw
Poland

Adriana Rakowska
Department of Dermatology
CSK MSW
Warsaw
Poland

ISBN 978-1-4471-7008-2 ISBN 978-1-4471-4486-1 (eBook)
DOI 10.1007/978-1-4471-4486-1
Springer London Heidelberg New York Dordrecht

Printed on acid-free paper

Springer is part of Springer Science+Business Media (www.springer.com)

Preface

This is a book for beginners as well as for those who perform trichoscopy in their everyday practice. It is written by trichoscopy enthusiasts, and I am sure dermatologists who learn this method will begin to love it, just as we do.

I use trichoscopy in my daily clinical practice, just as radiologists use ultrasonography or cardiologists make use of electrocardiograms. A world without trichoscopy is difficult for me to imagine. I could not agree more with the statement of Antonella Tosti that diagnosing hair and scalp disorders without trichoscopy is a professional practice gap.

It is difficult to establish when trichoscopy was born. Was it the 1993 publication by Steven Kossard and Sam Zagarella, who described the dermoscopic white dots in cicatricial alopecia? Was it the 2004 article by Giuseppe Micali's group, who showed that videodermatoscopy enhances diagnostic capability in hair loss? Was it the initial work of the dermatologists from Italy, Japan, and Poland who developed the first standards, diagnostic criteria, and algorithms? Or was it the moment when trichoscopy received its name, in 2006?

Whatever the date, trichoscopy is still in its childhood, and there is still much to learn in the great field of hair and scalp disorders. Recent years have brought multiple results from original studies, new case descriptions, and analytic reviews, as well as know-how derived from unpublished but widely shared experience. Also, as I write these words, trichoscopic knowledge is developing rapidly worldwide. I am sure readers of this book will make their own, new discoveries, and I encourage everyone to share their experience with others in this developing field of knowledge. If you have any suggestions or questions regarding this book, feel free to drop me an e-mail (lidia.rudnicka@euderm.eu).

I hope this atlas will help you in your daily practice. Keeping in mind that we find only what we look for, I hope this book helps you define what you are seeking in the field of hair and scalp diseases.

Lidia Rudnicka

Acknowledgments

We thank our families for their support, our colleagues for their help, and all the dermatologists in the world who encouraged us to write this book for their inspiration.

Lidia Rudnicka
Malgorzata Olszewska
Adriana Rakowska

Contents

Contributors

Leonardo Spagnol Abraham Department of Hair Diseases, Instituto de Dermatologia Prof. Rubem David Azulayl, Rio de Janeiro, Brazil

Alexandre Abramavicus Department of Dermatology, Unit of Skin Tumors, São Paulo Hospital, São Paulo, Brazil

Giuseppe Albertini Dermatology and Skin Cancer Unit, Arcispedale Santa Maria Nuova IRCCS, Reggio Emilia, Italy

Giuseppe Argenziano Dermatology and Skin Cancer Unit, Arcispedale Santa Maria Nuova IRCCS, Reggio Emilia, Italy

Barbara Borkowska Department of Dermatology, CSK MSW, Warsaw, Poland

Joanna Czuwara Department of Dermatology, CSK MSW, Warsaw, Poland

Franco Dinotta Dermatology Clinic, University of Catania, Catania, Italy

Bruna Duque-Estrada Department of Dermatology, Instituto de Dermatologia Prof. Rubem David Azulayl, Rio de Janeiro, Brazil

Shigeki Inui Department of Regenerative Dermatology, Osaka University School of Medicine, Yamadaoka Suita-shi, Osaka, Japan

Agnieszka Kardynal Department of Dermatology, CSK MSW, Warsaw, Poland

Elzbieta Kowalska-Oledzka Department of Dermatology, CSK MSW, Warsaw, Poland

Marta Kurzeja Department of Dermatology, CSK MSW, Warsaw, Poland

Francesco Lacarrubba Dermatology Clinic, University of Catania, Catania, Italy

Malgorzata Lukomska Department of Dermatology, CSK MSW, Warsaw, Poland

Malgorzata Maj Department of Dermatology, CSK MSW, Warsaw, Poland

Magdalena Majsterek Department of Dermatology, CSK MSW, Warsaw, Poland

Giuseppe Micali, M.D. Dermatology Clinic, University of Catania, Catania, Italy

Mariya Miteva Department of Dermatology and Cutaneous Surgery, University of Miami Health System, Miami, FL, USA

Elvira Moscarella Department of Dermatology, University of Modena and Reggio Emilia, Modena, Italy

Malgorzata Olszewska Department of Dermatology, Medical University of Warsaw, Warsaw, Poland

Ana Maria Costa Pinheiro Department of Internal Medicine, Hospital Universitario de Brasilia, Brasilia, Brazil

Adriana Rakowska Department of Dermatology, CSK MSW, Warsaw, Poland

Ewa Ring Department of Dermatology, CSK MSW, Warsaw, Poland

Alfredo Rossi Medicina Interna e Specialità Mediche Sapienza, University of Rome, Rome, Italy

Lidia Rudnicka Faculty of Health Sciences, Medical University of Warsaw, Poland

Department of Dermatology, CSK MSW, Warsaw, Poland

Magdalena Rusek Department of Dermatology, CSK MSW, Warsaw, Poland

Justyna Sicinska Department of Dermatology, CSK MSW, Warsaw, Poland

Monika Slowinska Department of Dermatology, CSK MSW, Warsaw, Poland

Catherine Stefanato Department of Dermatopathology, St. John's Institute of Dermatology, St. Thomas' Hospital, London, UK

Jacek C. Szepietowski Department of Dermatology, Venereology, and Allergology, Medical University (University Hospital), Wroclaw, Poland

Elzbieta Szymanska Department of Dermatology, CSK MSW, Warsaw, Poland

Antonella Tosti Department of Dermatology and Cutaneous Surgery, University of Miami Health System, Miami, FL, USA

Ralph M. Trüeb Center for Dermatology and Hair Diseases, Wallisellen, Switzerland

Irena Walecka Department of Dermatology, CSK MSW, Warsaw, Poland

Olga Warszawik-Hendzel Department of Dermatology, CSK MSW, Warsaw, Poland

Iris Zalaudek Department of Dermatology, Medical University of Graz, Graz, Austria

Part I

Introduction

Introduction

1

Lidia Rudnicka, Magdalena Rusek,
and Barbara Borkowska

Abstract
Trichoscopy may be performed with any dermoscope. This chapter focuses on the features of different types of dermoscopes, such as handheld dermoscopes, basic digital dermoscopes, dermoscopic accessories for the iPhone, and advanced digital dermoscopes (videodermoscopes). Basic information is provided on performing trichoscopy.

Keywords
Dermoscopes • Gray hair • Hair colorization • Hair washing • Immersion fluid • Magnification
Nonpolarized light • Polarized light • Videodermoscope

Any handheld dermoscope may be used to perform trichoscopy. Digital dermoscopes (videodermoscopes) also may be used. These have the advantages of easier photography and a higher magnification but are time consuming and expensive.

Among handheld dermoscopes, there are devices that require immersion fluid and those that use polarized light to cancel out reflections from the stratum corneum. Polarized light dermoscopes may have a contact or noncontact lens. Devices that combine contact and noncontact attributes (hybrid dermoscopes) also are available. The choice of a particular device is a matter of individual preference.

Results of studies addressing the differences among these three types of dermoscopes (nonpolarized light, polarized light, and noncontact polarized light) in skin cancer indicate that keratotic structures are visualized better in nonpolarized light, whereas blood vessels are seen best with noncontact polarized light dermoscopes [1, 2]. Considering that most published trichoscopic images have been taken with nonpolarized light, this type of dermoscope may appear slightly more beneficial than polarized light dermoscopes for learning trichoscopy.

Most handheld dermoscopes allow one to observe the skin surface at a 10-fold magnification, whereas digital dermoscopes have working magnifications from 20- to 100-fold and higher. Lower magnifications have the benefit of providing a better overview of a large scalp area, whereas higher magnifications allow visualization of fine details. Most images in this atlas were taken at a 20- or 70-fold magnification (FotoFinder 2 dermoscope; FotoFinder Systems GmbH, Bad Birnbach, Germany).

Trichoscopy differs from skin cancer dermoscopy, among others, in the large area that needs to be examined. In diffuse hair loss, the frontal and occipital areas should be investigated. In cases of focal alopecia, the hairless plaque and hair-bearing margin should be examined. In some diseases, additional evaluation of the eyebrows may be informative.

When using a contact dermoscope, the roll-on technique of applying the lens to the scalp surface allows the best image analysis. In this technique, one edge of the lens is placed against the scalp surface at an approximately 45° angle, then the lens is "rolled" until the whole lens is in contact with the

L. Rudnicka (✉)
Faculty of Health Sciences, Medical University of Warsaw, Poland

Department of Dermatology, CSK MSW,
Woloska 137, Warsaw 02-502, Poland
e-mail: lidia.rudnicka@euderm.eu

M. Rusek • B. Borkowska
Department of Dermatology, CSK MSW,
Warsaw, Poland

L. Rudnicka et al. (eds.), *Atlas of Trichoscopy*,
DOI 10.1007/978-1-4471-4486-1_1, © Springer-Verlag London 2012

skin surface [3]. This technique allows detailed visualization of the structures when applying different amounts of pressure. When immersion fluid is used, this technique also allows one to squeeze out air inclusions (bubbles).

Nonpolarized light dermoscopes require immersion fluid (alcoholic, aqueous, or oily). Various types of immersion fluids exist: alcohol solutions, aqueous solutions, gels, and oils [3, 4]. Our preference is to use an alcoholic skin disinfection solution (e.g., 70 % ethanol), because it evaporates rapidly from the skin surface and has antibacterial properties. Aqueous solutions include distilled water and saline (0.9 % sodium chloride). Gels are most convenient for convex surfaces and when visualization of blood vessels under low lens pressure is required. Oils are not used in trichoscopy. Nonpolarized dermoscopes also may be used without immersion fluid [5]. This method, called "dry trichoscopy," allows better visualization of perifollicular scaling.

Hair washing generally does not influence trichoscopic results. Hair colorization also does not hinder trichoscopic analysis; it may even be beneficial for analyzing hair shaft structure and evaluating hair thickness in persons with light blond or gray hairshaft structure abnormality (pili torti).

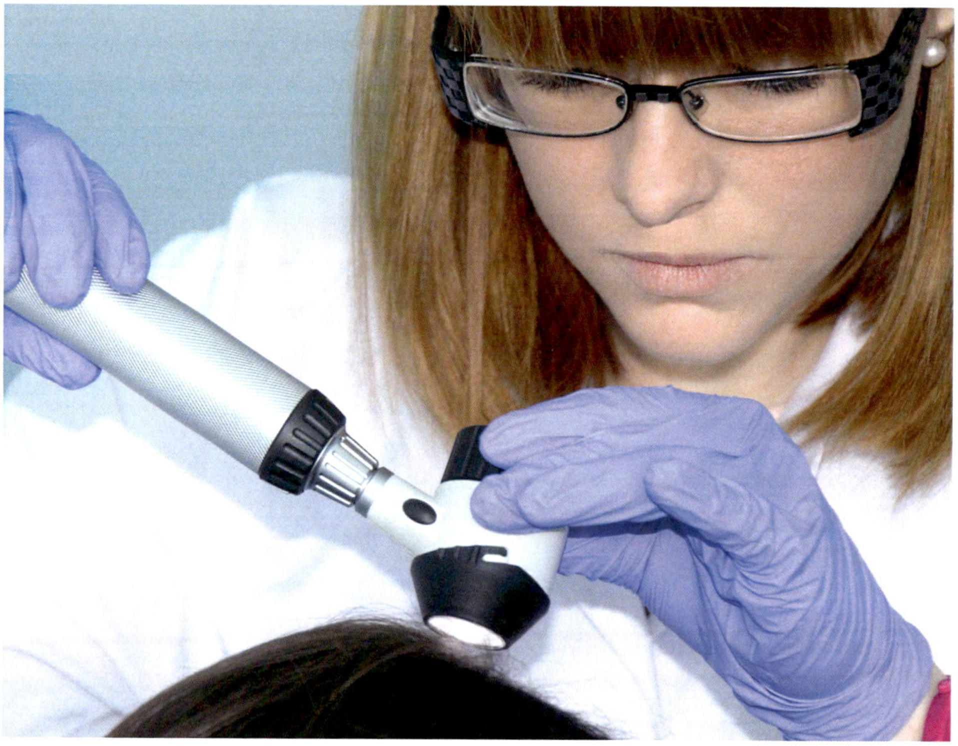

Fig. 1.1 **Dr. Borkowska performing trichoscopy with a handheld dermoscope**. Any handheld dermoscope may be used to perform trichoscopy. It does not require any additional lenses or parts. You may use your dermoscope just as you would for diagnosing melanoma

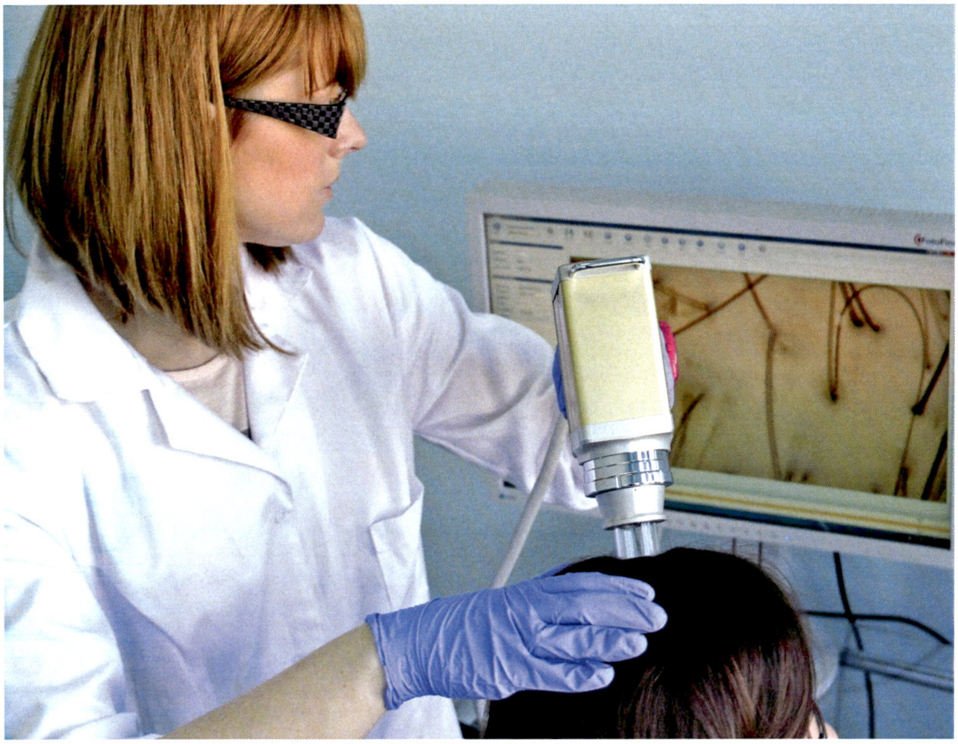

Fig. 1.2 Dr. Borkowska performing trichoscopy with a digital dermoscope (**videodermoscope**). A digital dermoscope (videodermoscope) has the benefit of better working comfort, higher magnification, and easy photography. It is, however, more time consuming and expensive. Thus, it rarely is used in clinical practice. The old term *videodermoscopy* refers to dermoscopy performed with a digital dermoscope

a

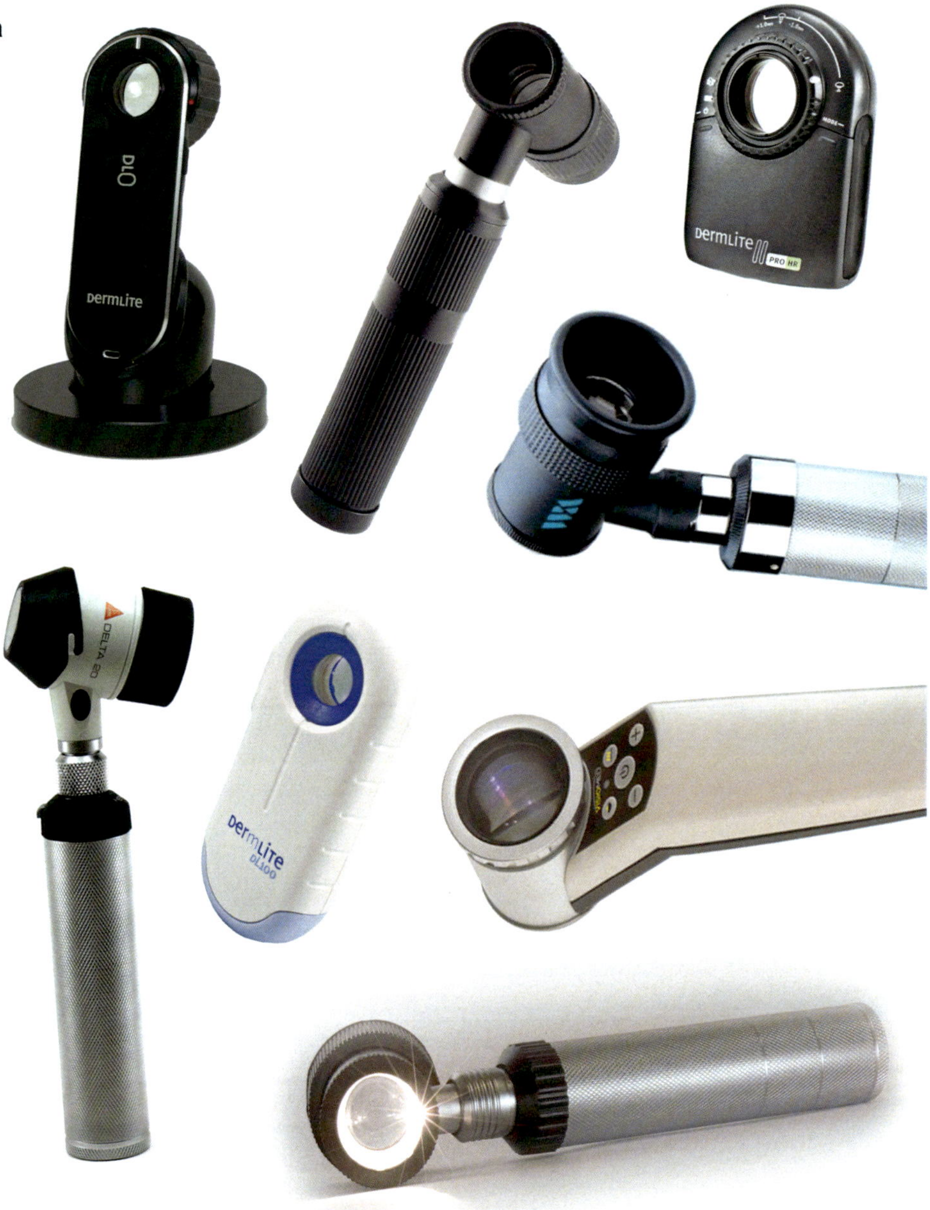

Fig. 1.3 Examples of equipment that may be used to perform trichoscopy. Trichoscopy may be performed with (**a**) handheld dermoscopes, (**b**) basic digital dermoscopes and photographic equipment, or (**c**) advanced digital dermoscopes. Handheld dermoscopes may be divided into three groups: contact dermoscopes, polarized light contact dermoscopes, and polarized light noncontact dermoscopes. Also available are handheld dermoscopes that work in either the contact or noncontact mode; these are known as hybrid dermoscopes. Which device to choose is a matter of individual preference; there is no preferred type of dermoscope for performing hair and scalp examinations. The standard magnification of handheld dermoscopes is ×10; the cost varies between about US $700 and US $1,800 (**a**). New devices on the market include simplified digital dermoscopes that may be connected to a computer (e.g., via USB) and kits allowing one to connect selected handheld dermoscopes to a regular photo camera or to an iPhone 4/4S. They are a good solution for dermatologists who like to take trichoscopic photographs in their daily practice. The usual magnification is ×10 to ×80, depending on the device. Although higher magnifications may be possible, they usually are not sufficiently supported by the light source of the equipment currently available. The price of these devices varies between US $400 and US $2,000 (not including the computer, camera, or iPhone) (**b**). The large, expensive digital dermoscopes (videodermoscopes) allow one to take high-magnification, high-quality photographs. The price of these devices varies significantly, depending on the presence or absence of software, which is not necessary for trichoscopy. Most companies now offer these devices with laptops instead of full-size computers. This type of digital dermoscope offers multiple magnifications in the range of ×20 to ×70 (or ×100) and higher. The price varies from about US $10,000 to about US $20,000 (**c**). These images show examples of dermoscopes available on the market when we were writing this chapter (*Courtesy of* 3Gen LLC, San Juan Capistrano, CA; AnMo Electronics Corp., New Taipei City, Taiwan; Bechtold & Co, Lodz, Poland; Consultronix S.A., Krakow, Poland; Delasco Dermatologic Lab & Supply, Inc, Council Bluffs, IA; Derma Medical Systems GmbH, Vienna, Austria; DermoScan GmbH, Regensburg, Germany; FotoFinder Systems GmbH; Medit Inc., Winnipeg, MB, Canada; IDCP B.V., Naarden, The Netherlands; Schuco International Ltd., London, UK.)

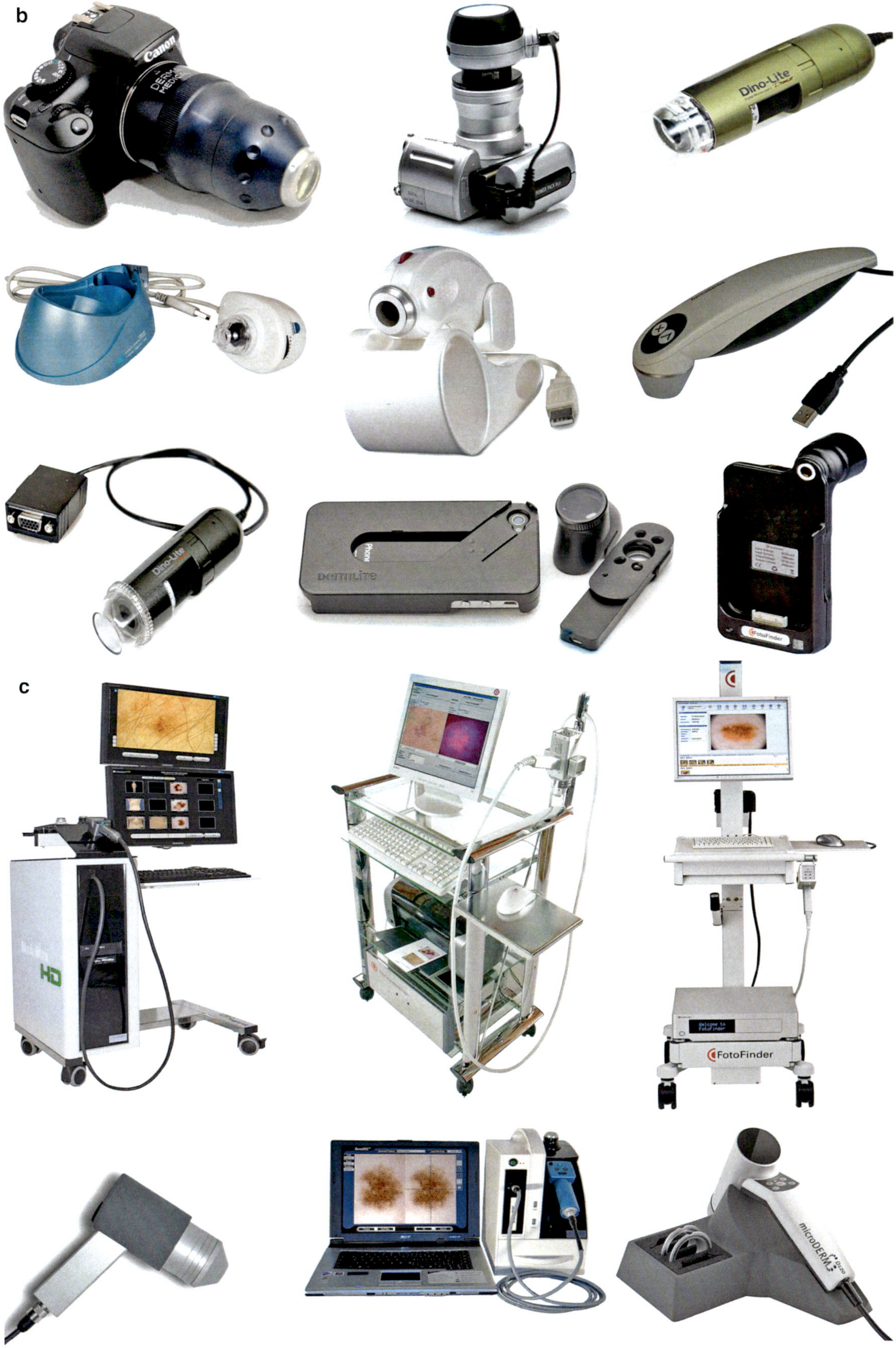

Fig. 1.3 (continued)

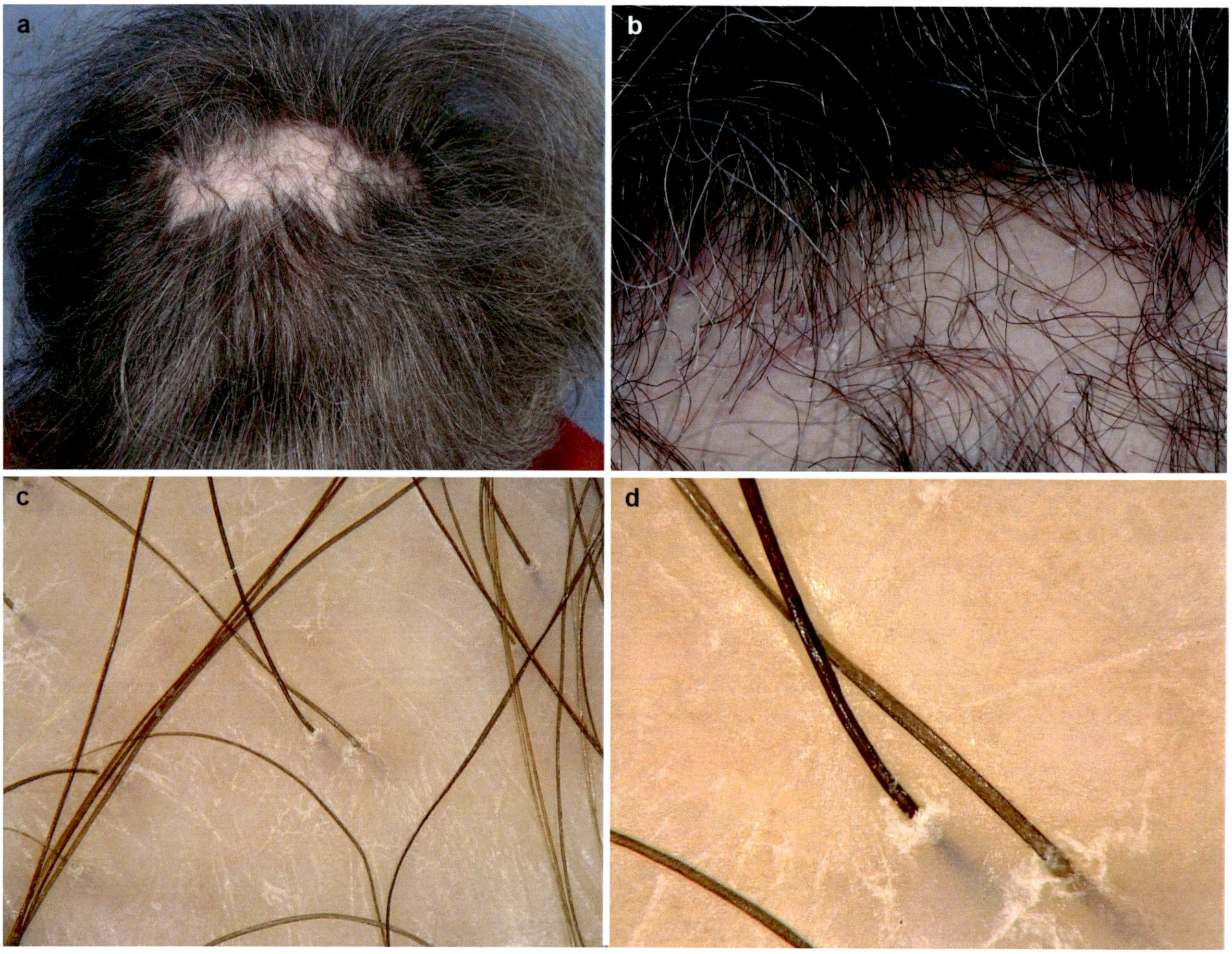

Fig. 1.4 **A dermoscope is not a loupe**. Obviously, trichoscopy is not comparable with evaluation of hair with a magnifying glass, as some may think. Trichoscopy brings detailed analysis of the hair and scalp into new dimensions. These images show the same patient with cicatricial alopecia visualized by (**a**) clinical evaluation, (**b**) a magnifying glass, (**c**) a handheld dermoscope, and (**d**) a digital, high-magnification dermoscope. *Panels* c and d show details of perifollicular scaling, the skin surface structure, and a hair shaft structure abnormality (pili torti)

References

1. Liebman TN, Jaimes-Lopez N, Balagula Y, Rabinovitz HS, Wang SQ, Dusza SW, et al. Dermoscopic features of basal cell carcinomas: differences in appearance under non-polarized and polarized light. Dermatol Surg. 2012;38(3):392–9.
2. Benvenuto-Andrade C, Dusza SW, Agero AL, Scope A, Rajadhyaksha M, Halpern AC, et al. Differences between polarized light dermoscopy and immersion contact dermoscopy for the evaluation of skin lesions. Arch Dermatol. 2007;143(3):329–38.
3. Gewirtzman AJ, Saurat JH, Braun RP. An evaluation of dermoscopy fluids and application techniques. Br J Dermatol. 2003;149(1):59–63.
4. Tasli L, Oguz O. The role of various immersion liquids at digital dermoscopy in structural analysis. Indian J Dermatol Venereol Leprol. 2011;77(1):110.
5. Inui S, Nakajima T, Itami S. Dry dermoscopy in clinical treatment of alopecia areata. J Dermatol. 2007;34(9):635–9.

Part II

Trichoscopic Structures and Patterns

Hair Shafts

2

Lidia Rudnicka, Adriana Rakowska, Malgorzata Olszewska, Monika Slowinska, Joanna Czuwara, Magdalena Rusek, and Ana Maria Costa Pinheiro

Abstract

Normal hair shafts are uniform in thickness and color. Trichoscopy allows detection of several hair shaft abnormalities, including various types of fractured hairs, hairs with narrowings, hairs with node-like structures, twisted or curled hairs, hairs with bands, and short hairs. In this chapter, we propose a classification of hair shaft abnormalities that may be detected by trichoscopy.

Keywords

Block hairs • Broom hairs • Coiled hairs • Comma hairs • Corkscrew hairs • Exclamation mark hairs • Flame hairs • Hair casts • Hair shafts • i-Hairs • Medulla • Monilethrix • Morse code–like hairs • Pigtail hairs • Pili annulati • Pili torti • Regrowing hairs • Tapered hairs Trichoptilosis • Trichoschisis • Trichorrhexis invaginata • Trichorrhexis nodosa • Tulip hairs Vellus hairs • Woolly hairs • Z-hairs • Zigzag hairs

Most hairs viewed on trichoscopy are normal terminal hairs that are more than 55 μm wide and are uniform in thickness and color [1, 2]. Hair shaft thickness may be roughly estimated with a handheld dermoscope (thin, normal, thick). Many videodermoscopes include software allowing a detailed assessment of hair shaft thickness in micrometers. Although precise measurement of hair shaft thickness is not essential for diagnosis, it may be useful for monitoring treatment efficacy and in clinical trials. In normal hair shafts, trichoscopy allows visualization of the medulla, which is classified as continuous, interrupted, fragmented, or absent [3]. The trichoscopic impression of the "fragmented" medulla is in fact a thick medulla separated by a thin medulla, which is not visible on trichoscopy. The thickness or presence of a medulla is believed to have no influence on hair shaft properties [3]. Up to about 10 % of normal human scalp hairs are vellus hairs, defined as hypopigmented, nonmedullated hairs less than 30 μm thick and less than 2–3 mm long [1, 2]. An increased proportion of vellus hairs is characteristic of male and female androgenetic alopecia, in which vellus hairs replace terminal ones during the process of hair follicle miniaturization [4, 5]. A high percentage of vellus and intermediate hairs contributes to increased hair shaft thickness heterogeneity, a hallmark of androgenetic alopecia [4, 6]. Vellus hairs must be differentiated from new, regrowing hairs, which are short and thin but differ from vellus hairs by not being hypopigmented and by their firm appearance and pointed end.

Various hair shaft structure abnormalities may be evaluated by trichoscopy. Exclamation mark hairs are characteristic of

L. Rudnicka (✉)
Faculty of Health Sciences, Medical University of Warsaw, Poland

Department of Dermatology, CSK MSW, Woloska 137, Warsaw 02-502, Poland
e-mail: lidia.rudnicka@euderm.eu

A. Rakowska • M. Slowinska • J. Czuwara • M. Rusek
Department of Dermatology, CSK MSW, Warsaw, Poland

M. Olszewska
Department of Dermatology, Medical University of Warsaw, Warsaw, Poland

A.M.C. Pinheiro
Department of Internal Medicine, Hospital Universitario de Brasilia, Brasilia, Brazil

L. Rudnicka et al. (eds.), *Atlas of Trichoscopy*,
DOI 10.1007/978-1-4471-4486-1_2, © Springer-Verlag London 2012

(but not specific for) alopecia areata. Trichoscopy allows visualization of exclamation mark hairs that are 1–2 mm long. Thus, some authors refer to these structures as "micro–exclamation mark" hairs [7]. On the other end of the spectrum are very long exclamation mark hairs emerging from follicles that are only partially struck by alopecia areata, becoming thinner as they grow. Terms used to describe such hairs are *tapered hairs* and *coudability hairs*, from the French word *coude* [8, 9].

Slowinska et al. [10] described comma hairs (short bent hairs) as a specific feature of tinea capitis. In later studies, corkscrew hairs [11, 12] and zigzag hairs, or Z-hairs [13], were identified as other characteristic features of tinea capitis.

Most genetic hair shaft dystrophies, such as monilethrix, trichorrhexis invaginata, trichorrhexis nodosa, pili torti, and pili annulati [14], may be diagnosed by trichoscopy [15].

Another feature that may be evaluated by trichoscopy is the number of hairs in one follicular unit; usually one to three hairs emerge from one follicular opening [1, 16]. The percentage of follicular units with only one emerging hair shaft is less than 30 % in healthy individuals and may be decreased in various types of hair loss, especially telogen effluvium and androgenetic alopecia.

In this chapter, we propose a classification of hair shaft abnormalities that may be detected by trichoscopy. This classification partly corresponds to comparable observations on light microscopy [14, 17, 18].

Table 2.1 Classification of hair shaft abnormalities in trichoscopy

1. **Fractured hairs**
Trichoptilosis
Trichoschisis/trichoclasis
Irregular fractures caused by mechanical force
Golf tee hairs (trichorrhexis invaginata)
2. **Narrowings**
Monilethrix
Monilethrix-like congenital hypotrichosis
Monilethrix-like hairs (Pohl-Pinkus constriction)
Pseudomonilethrix
Tapered hairs
Exclamation mark hairs
3. **Node-like appearance**
Trichonodosis
Trichorrhexis nodosa
Bamboo hairs (trichorrhexis invaginata)
Hair casts
4. **Curls and twists**
Pigtail hairs (circular or oval)
Coiled hairs
Comma hairs
Corkscrew hairs
Z-hairs (zigzag hairs)
Pili torti
Woolly hairs
5. **Bands**
Interrupted medulla
Continuous medulla
Pili annulati
Interrupted (Morse code–like) hairs
6. **Short hairs**
Upright regrowing
Vellus hairs
Dark lines
Tulip hairs
Block hairs
i-Hairs
Broom hairs
Broom fibers
Flame hairs

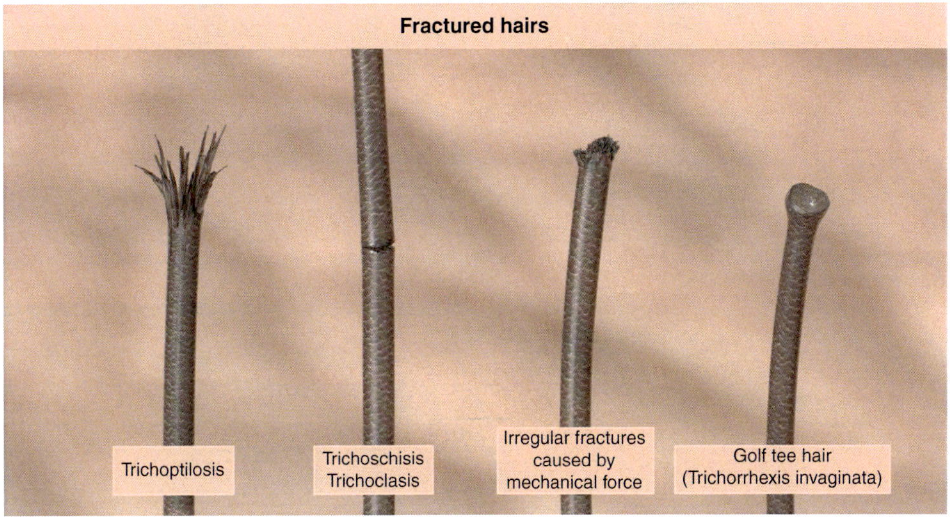

Fig. 2.1 **Hair shaft fractures observed on trichoscopy** (*Graphic by* Dr. Wawrzyniec Podrzucki, *Journal of Dermatological Case Reports* [JDCR])

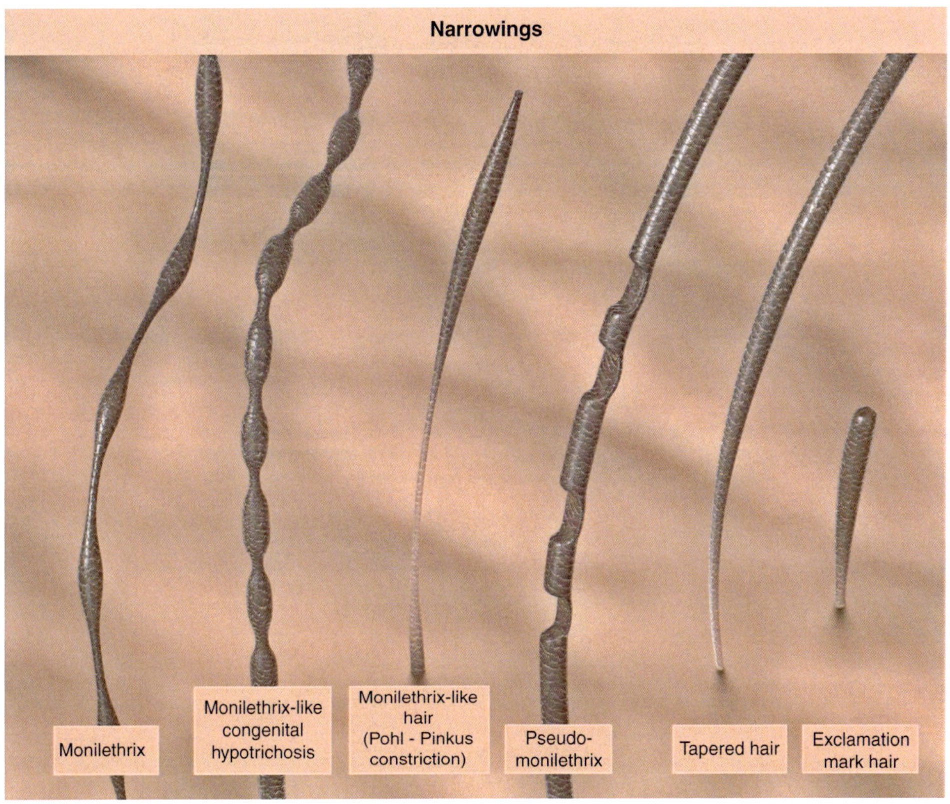

Fig. 2.2 **Hair shaft narrowings observed on trichoscopy** (*Graphic by* Dr. Wawrzyniec Podrzucki, *courtesy of* JDCR)

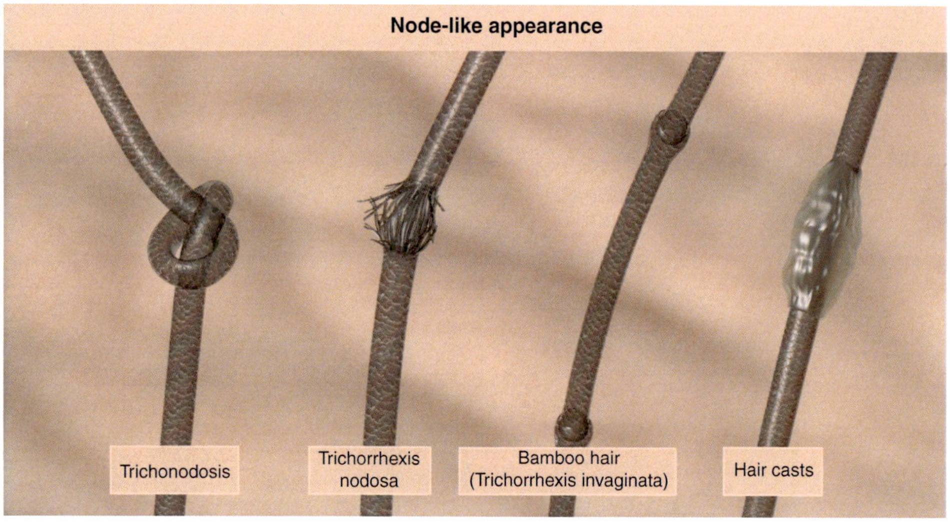

Fig. 2.3 **Hair shafts with a node-like appearance on trichoscopy** (*Graphic by* Dr. Wawrzyniec Podrzucki, *courtesy of* JDCR)

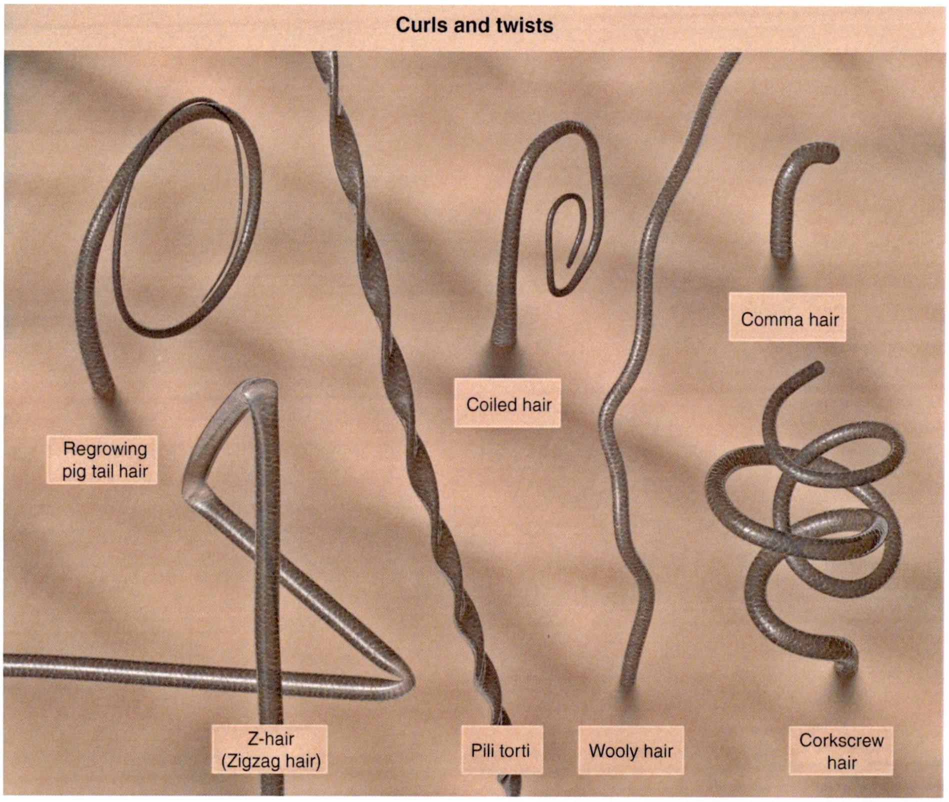

Fig. 2.4 **Twisted and curled hair shafts observed on trichoscopy** (*Graphic by* Dr. Wawrzyniec Podrzucki, *courtesy of* JDCR)

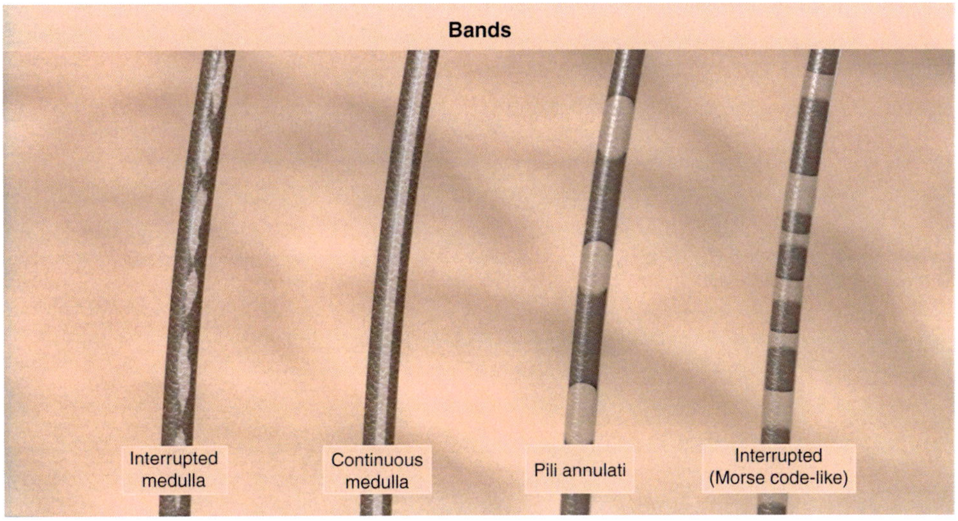

Fig. 2.5 **Hair shafts with bands on trichoscopy** (*Graphic by* Dr. Wawrzyniec Podrzucki, *courtesy of* JDCR)

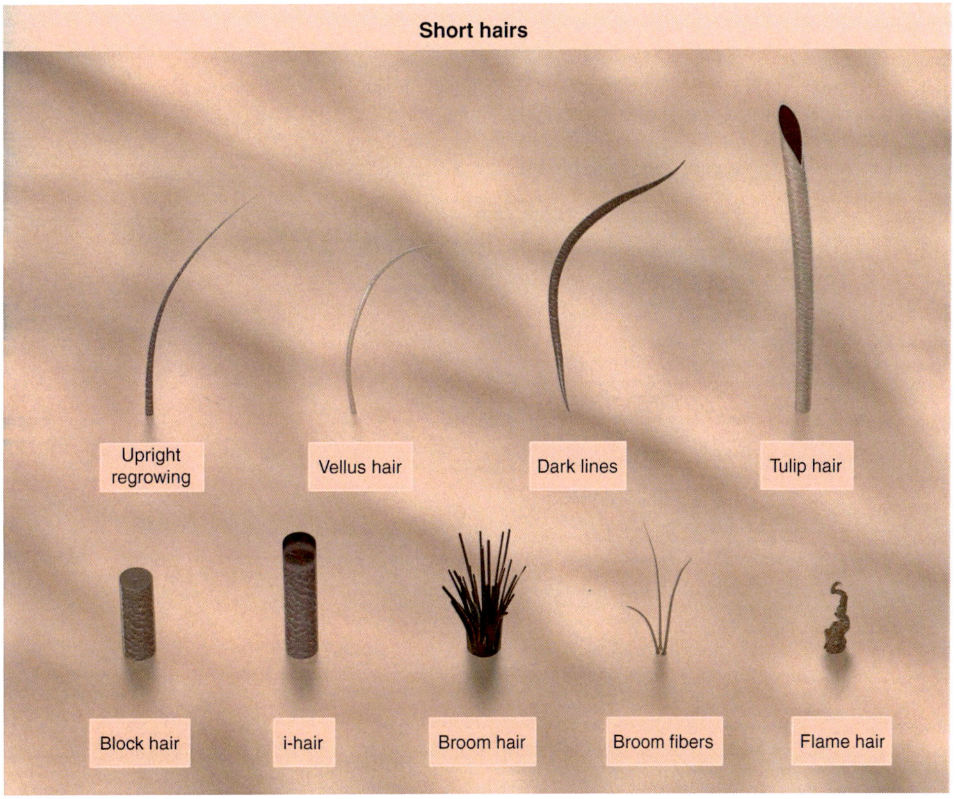

Fig. 2.6 **Short hair shafts on trichoscopy** (*Graphic by* Dr. Wawrzyniec Podrzucki, *courtesy of* JDCR)

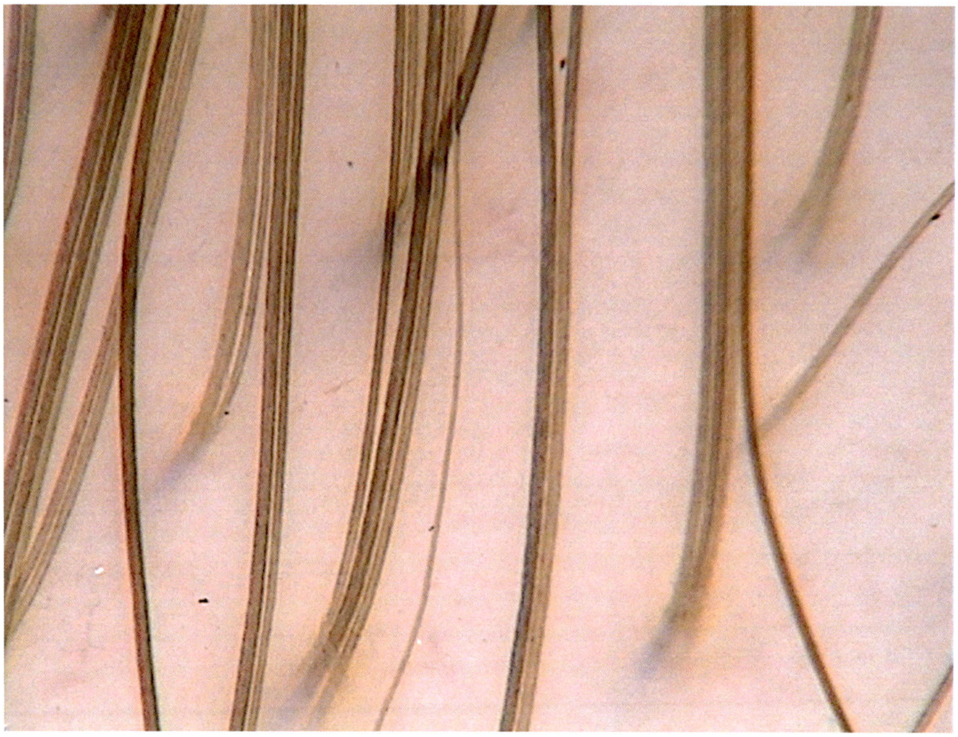

Fig. 2.7 **Normal terminal hairs**. In a healthy person, a hair shaft is uniform in thickness and color throughout its length. Normal hairs are more than 55 μm thick [1], but there may be variability in thickness among different populations as well as in an individual person (*see also* Fig. 2.9). The concomitant presence of hair shafts that differ from one another in color is a normal finding in graying persons. In children and young adults, the simultaneous presence of dark and gray hairs is rare and may be indicative of vitiligo, ectodermal syndrome, or premature graying of different causes [19]. Dark hair shafts usually are visualized better on trichoscopy compared with light blond and gray hairs. Using dry trichoscopy or videodermoscopy with higher magnification may enhance the visibility of light-colored hairs. Shown here is a normal trichoscopic image from a Central European female with dark blond hair (×70)

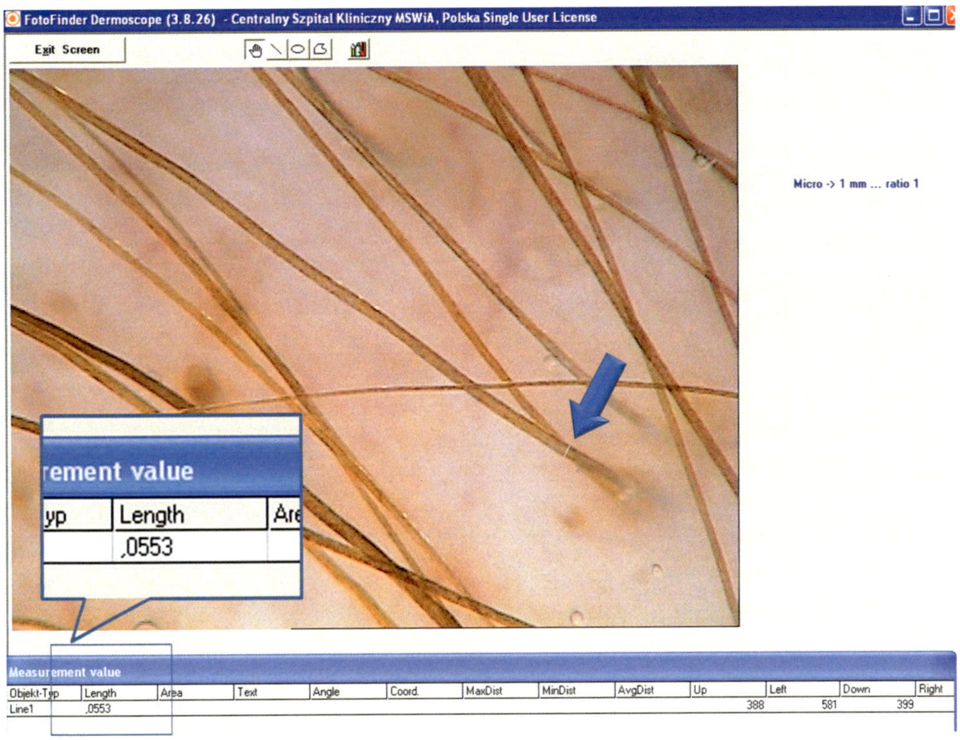

Fig. 2.8 **Measuring hair shaft thickness**. Hair shaft thickness may be roughly estimated with a handheld dermoscope based on the examiner's experience (thin, intermediate, or thick). Some videodermoscopes have software that allows precise assessment of hair shaft thickness in micrometers. Shown here is a screen shot from an evaluation of hair shaft thickness with FotoFinder Dermoscope II, model 2008 (FotoFinder Systems GmbH, Bad Birnbach, Germany). The *arrow* points to a hair shaft whose thickness was measured (*white line*). This hair shaft is 55.3 μm thick (*box*). In clinical practice, we evaluate hair shaft thickness mainly for the purpose of monitoring treatment efficacy in androgenetic alopecia. It is also a useful tool for research and clinical trials. According to the method by Rakowska et al. [1], we assess the average thickness of about 20 hair shafts in the frontal area, 20 in the parietal area, and 20 in the occipital area. The 2011 FotoFinder Dermoscope model does not have this option

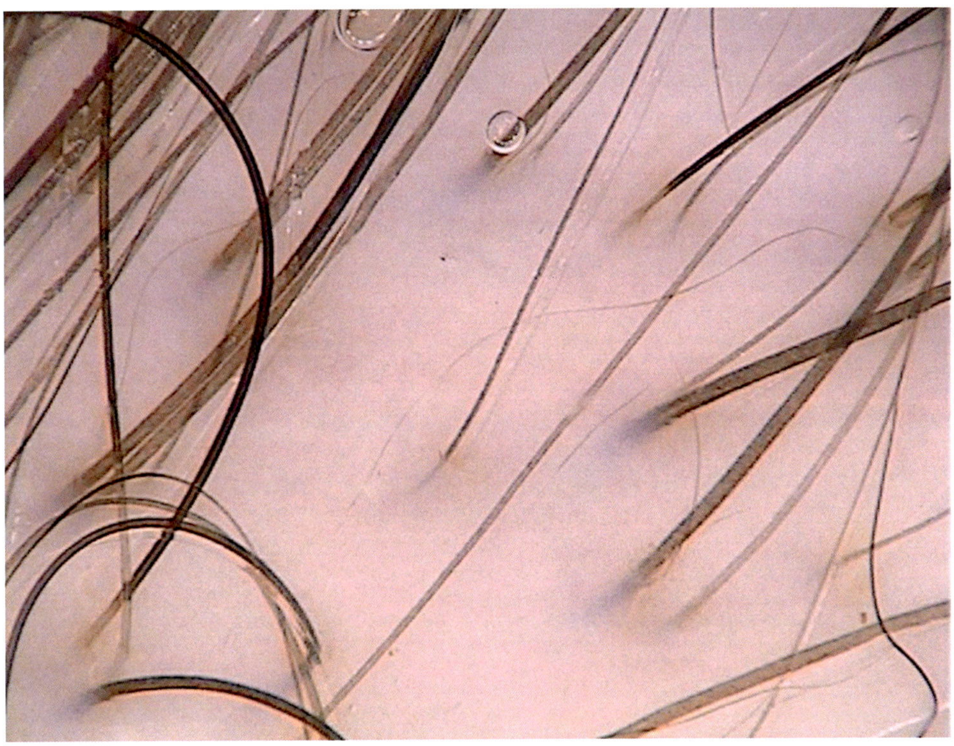

Fig. 2.9 **Heterogeneity in hair shaft thickness in female androgenetic alopecia**. The concomitant presence of thick, intermediate, thin, and vellus hairs results from unsynchronized miniaturization of hair follicles and is a hallmark of androgenetic alopecia. This feature is the same in male and female androgenetic alopecia. An increased percentage of thin and vellus hairs in areas that are otherwise normal may indicate a subclinical stage of androgenetic alopecia (×70)

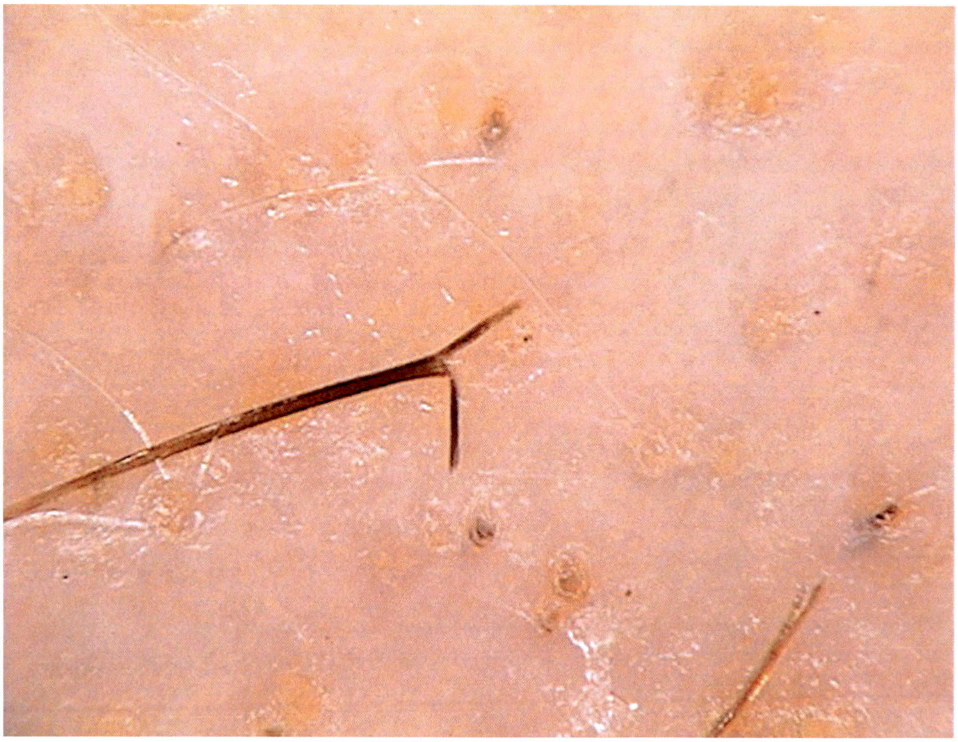

Fig. 2.10 **Trichoptilosis in alopecia areata**. The term *trichoptilosis* refers to the longitudinal splitting of the distal end of the hair shaft. This feature can be assessed easily by trichoscopy but is not pathognomic for any alopecia type. It may be observed in healthy individuals (×70)

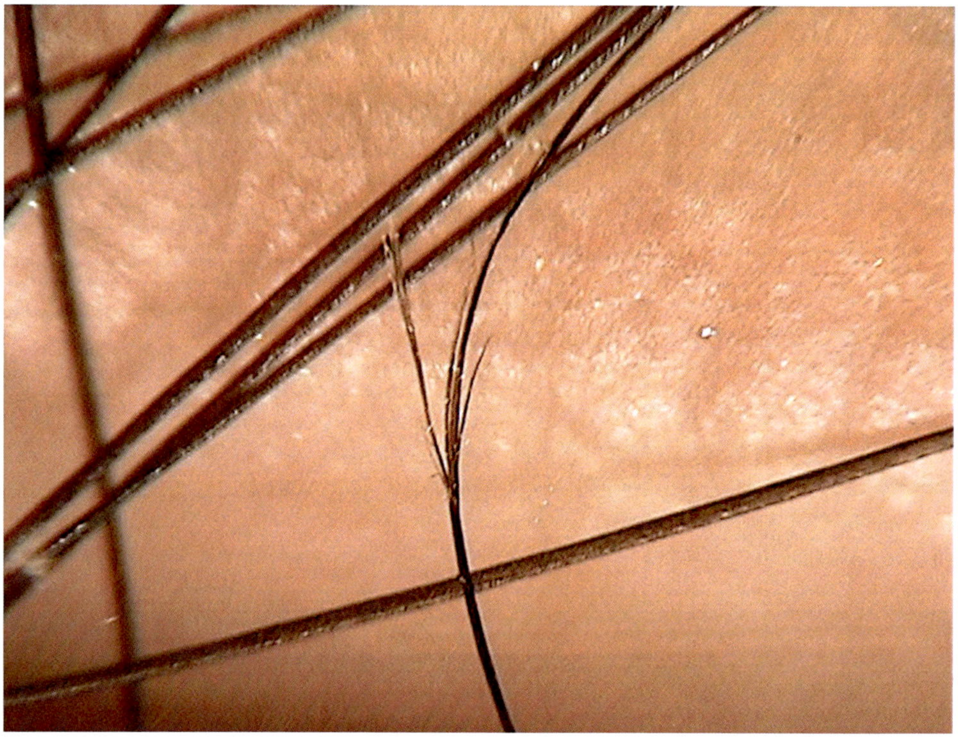

Fig. 2.11 **Trichoptilosis caused by a hairstyling procedure**. This image shows a long longitudinal break caused by a hairstyling procedure. Trichoptilosis is a symptom of hair shaft damage ("hair weathering") that may be caused by hair-damaging environmental factors and cosmetic procedures (×70)

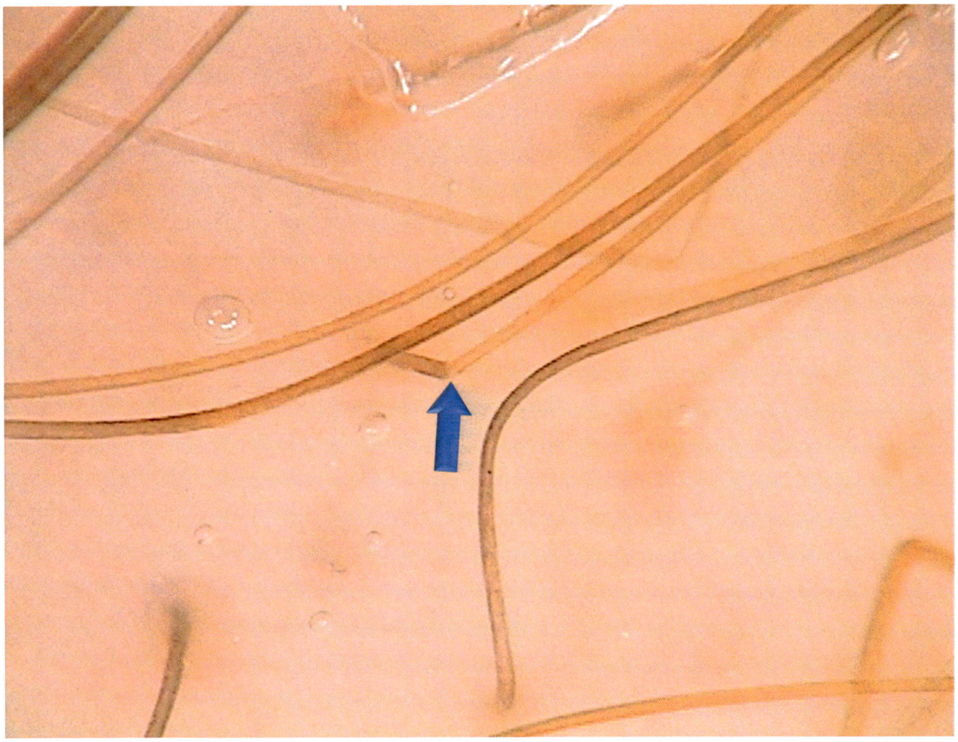

Fig. 2.12 Trichoclasis in alopecia areata. Trichoclasis is a clean transverse fracture across the hair shaft (*arrow*). It may develop secondary to conditions that weaken the hair. Idiopathic trichoschisis also has been described. This image shows a hair shaft with a clean transverse fracture, bound only by an intact cuticle. Some authors use the terms *trichoschisis* and *trichoclasia* interchangeably; others indicate that in trichoschisis there is a localized absence of the cuticle at the fracture site, whereas in trichoclasia the cuticle is intact (×70)

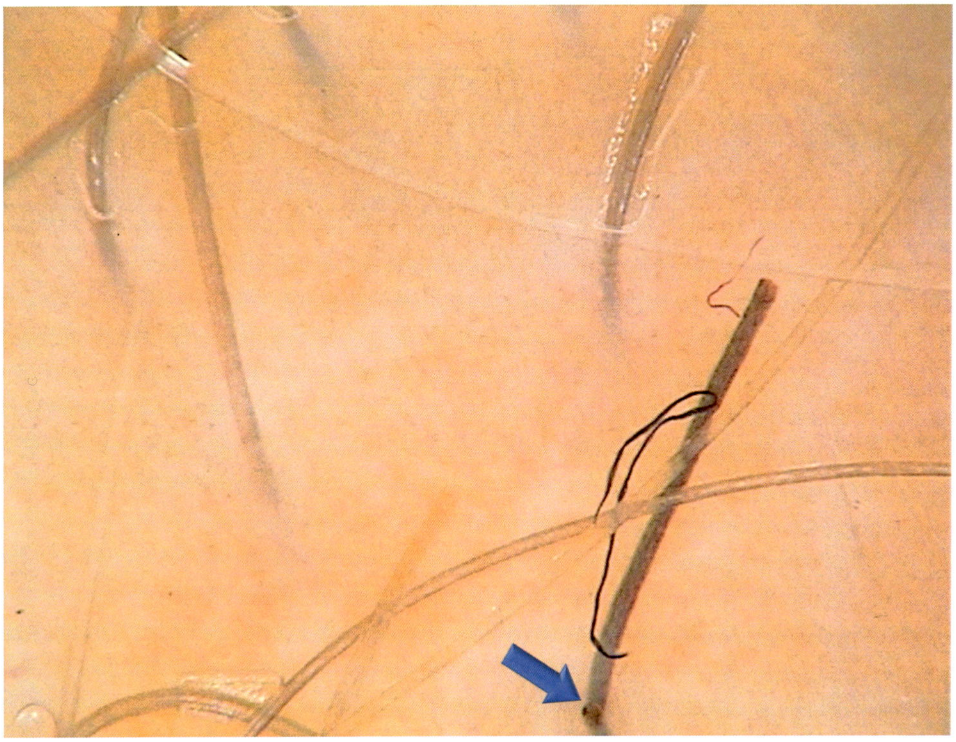

Fig. 2.13 Trichoschisis in trichothiodystrophy. The clean transverse fracture across the hair shaft (*arrow*) results from absence of the hair shaft cuticle in the affected area. Trichoschisis is a common finding in trichothiodystrophy. Trichothiodystrophy is a rare autosomal recessive disorder characterized by sulfur-deficient brittle hair and multisystem abnormalities (×70)

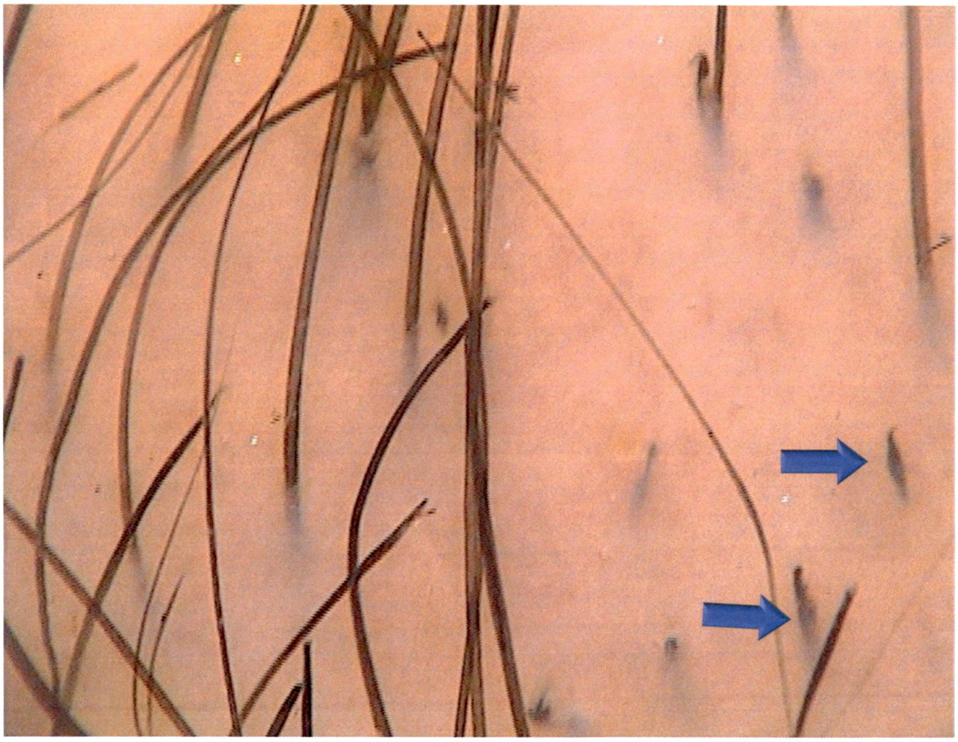

Fig. 2.14 Broken hairs in trichotillomania. This image shows multiple hairs broken by mechanical force in a patient with trichotillomania (*arrows*). The hair shafts have an irregular, ragged distal end, which differs from the regularly split ends in trichoptilosis (also seen in this image). Hairs are broken at different levels above the scalp. A similar image may be observed in traction alopecia, which may be indistinguishable from trichotillomania on trichoscopy. Broken hairs also may be observed in conditions that significantly weaken the hair shafts, such as alopecia areata. In contrast to trichotillomania, in alopecia areata hairs are usually fractured at the same level above the scalp. The length of broken hair shafts in alopecia areata corresponds to hair growth during the period between the onset of increased disease activity and the moment of examination (×70)

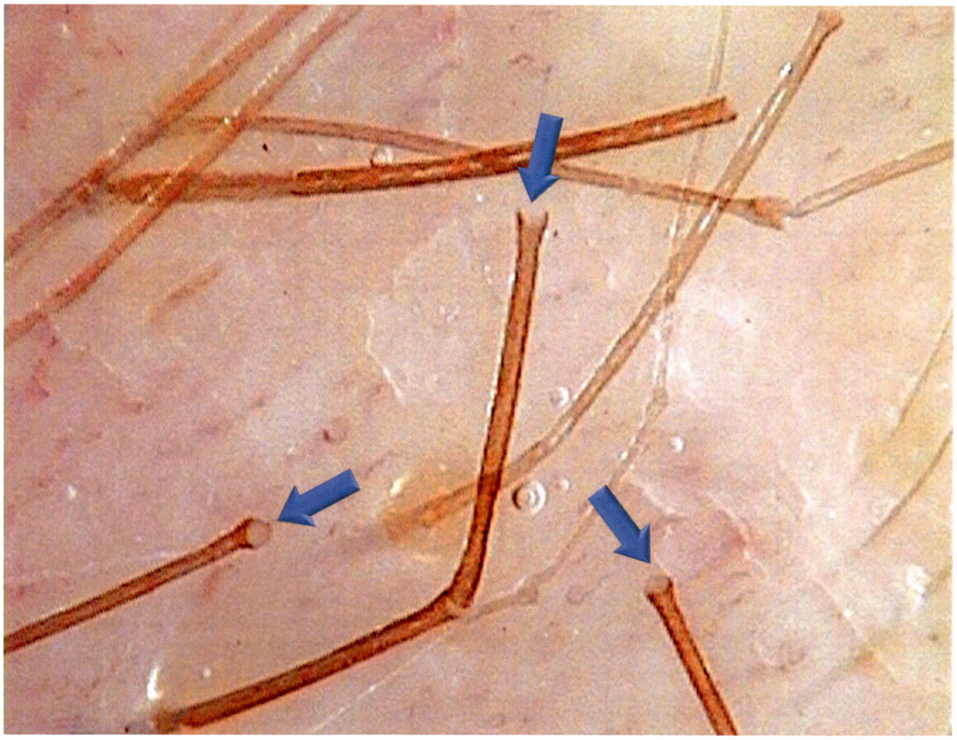

Fig. 2.15 Golf tee hairs in Netherton's syndrome. In trichorrhexis invaginata, the hair shaft telescopes into itself. The proximal part of the abnormality is concave, whereas the distal end is convex (bulging). When the hair shaft breaks at the site of this abnormality, the distal end of the broken hair will have a concave, cupped appearance (*arrows*), which is called "golf tee" hair because it reassembles the plastic tee used to support a golf ball [20]. In the absence of typical bamboo hairs, trichorrhexis invaginata may be diagnosed based on the presence of golf tee hairs only (×70)

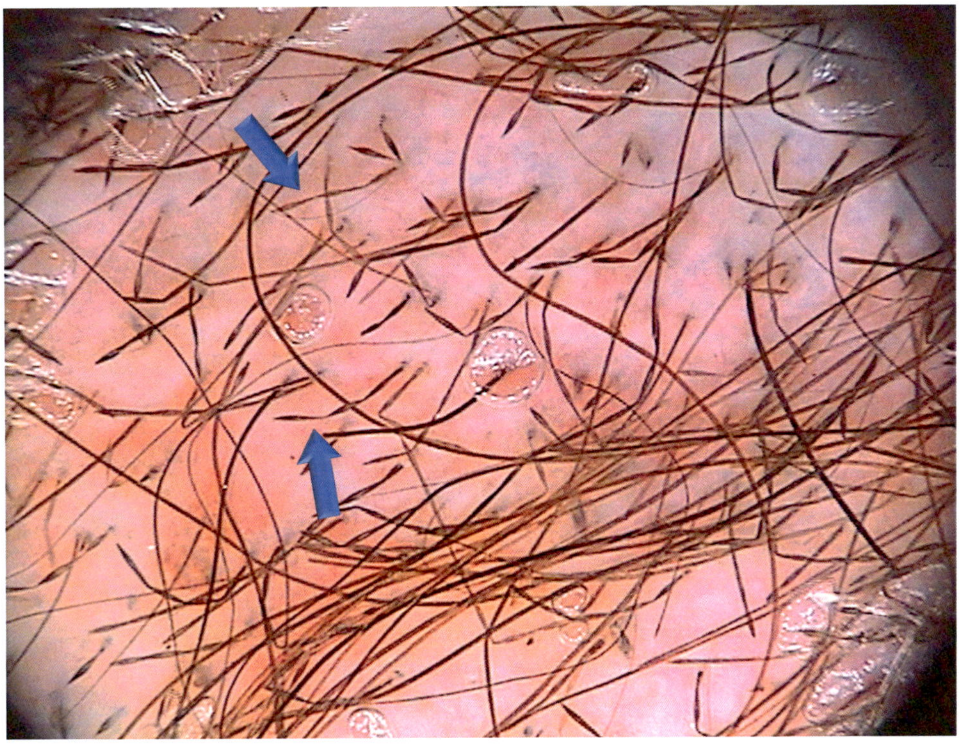

Fig. 2.16 Monilethrix. Typical regularly distributed nodes and internodes are visible within the hair shafts (*arrows*). These nodes correspond to normal hair shaft thickness, whereas the internodes are narrowings. Hair shafts are bent in different directions and tend to fracture at constriction points (×20)

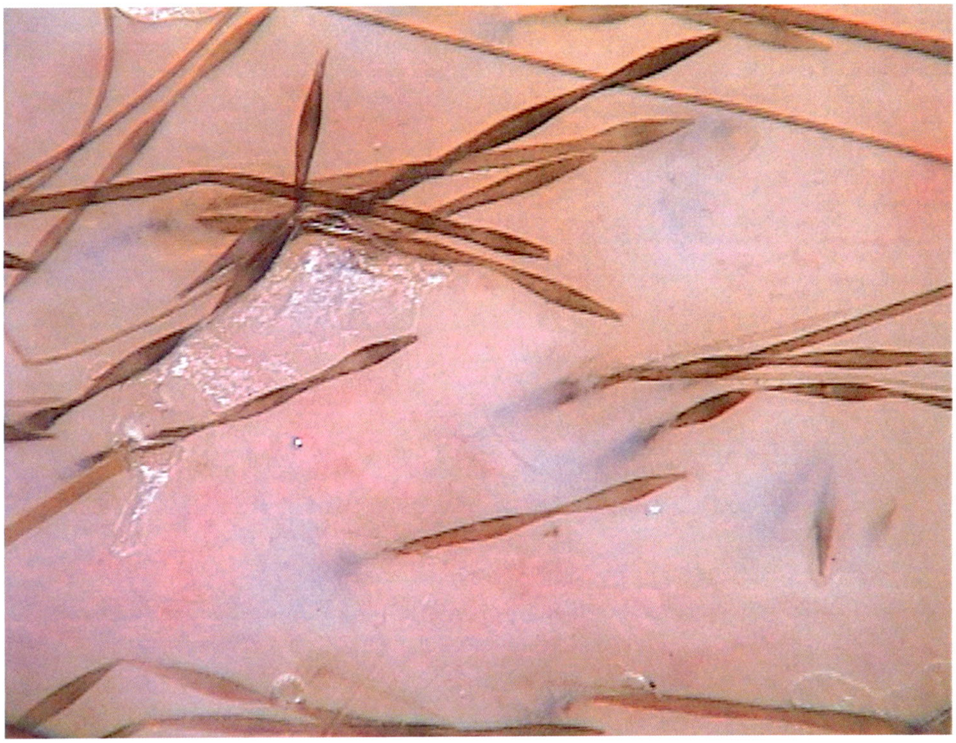

Fig. 2.17 Typical monilethrix hairs with regularly distributed nodes and internodes. In this image, almost all the hair shafts show the abnormality. Usually, only a small proportion of hairs is affected. In patients with only a few monilethrix hairs, this abnormality is most likely to be found in the occipital and parietal areas. Eyelashes rarely are involved (×70)

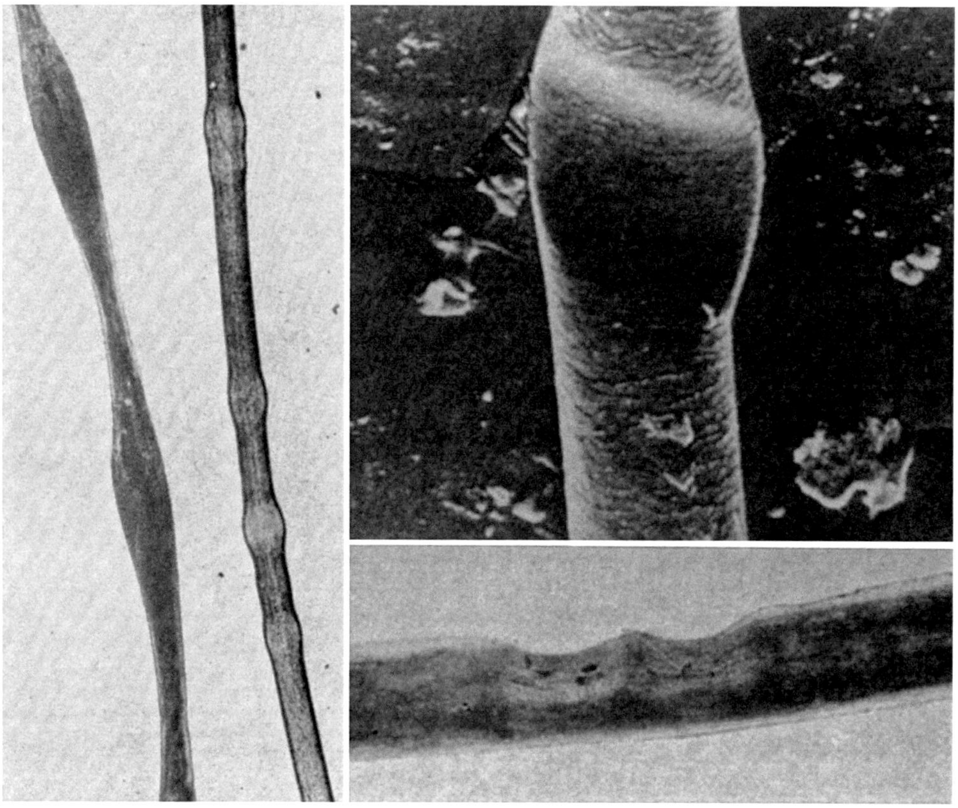

Fig. 2.18 Pseudomonilethrix. This image is reproduced from an initial description of the disease observed by Bentley-Phillips et al. [18] in four families from Durban, South Africa. It shows light microscopy of two hair shafts, one with regularly distributed constrictions in monilethrix, and one with irregular nodules in pseudomonilethrix (*left*). The disease differs from monilethrix in that nodes appear thicker than the normal hair shaft and internodes are as thick as a normal hair shaft. The authors showed that this is an optical illusion. Detailed analysis by scanning electron microscopy (*upper right*) and light microscopy (*lower right*) revealed rectangular indentations on one side of the hair shaft. These rectangular indentations in pseudomonilethrix must be differentiated from irregular fusiform narrowing (Pohl-Pinkus constrictions) observed in monilethrix-like hairs following chemotherapy or resulting from the variable course of a chronic disease such as alopecia areata. In a retrospective analysis including more than one million trichoscopic photographs, we did not find this abnormality in our patients (*Image reprinted from* Phillips et al. [18]; *with permission*)

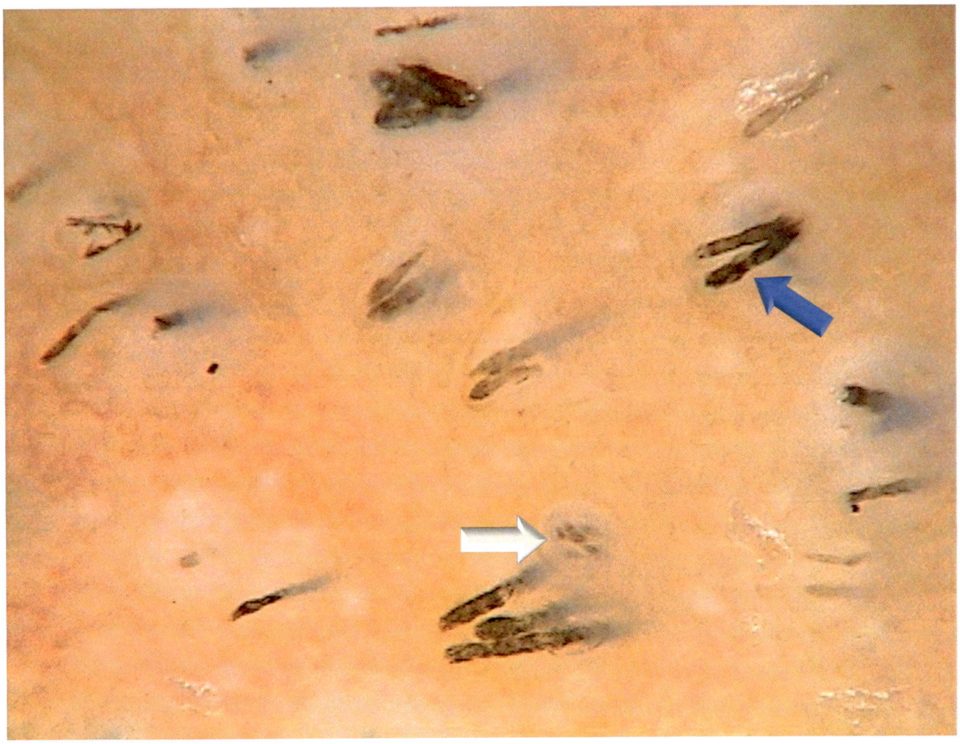

Fig. 2.19 Monilethrix-like congenital hypotrichosis. In monilethrix-like congenital hypotrichosis, the spaces between narrowings are very short (*white arrow*) and are almost invisible in thicker hairs (*blue arrow*). Hairs have a very high tendency to break at the site of the internodes; thus clinically, hair loss is more severe in this condition than in monilethrix (×70)

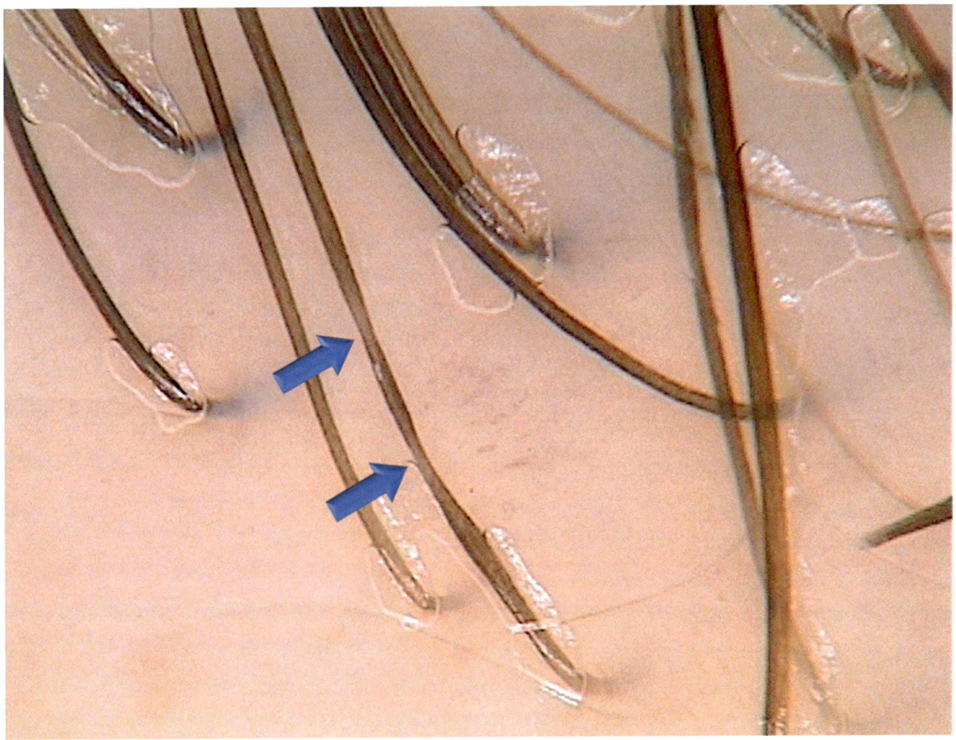

Fig. 2.20 Monilethrix-like hairs in alopecia areata. Irregular hair shaft constrictions (Pohl-Pinkus constrictions; *arrows*) may be observed in various chronic, acquired, and congenital diseases. This abnormality is observed in alopecia areata, cicatricial alopecias, and localized hereditary hypotrichosis, as well as after chemotherapy or interferon alfa-2c therapy. Shown here is a monilethrix-like hair in a patient with alopecia areata (×70)

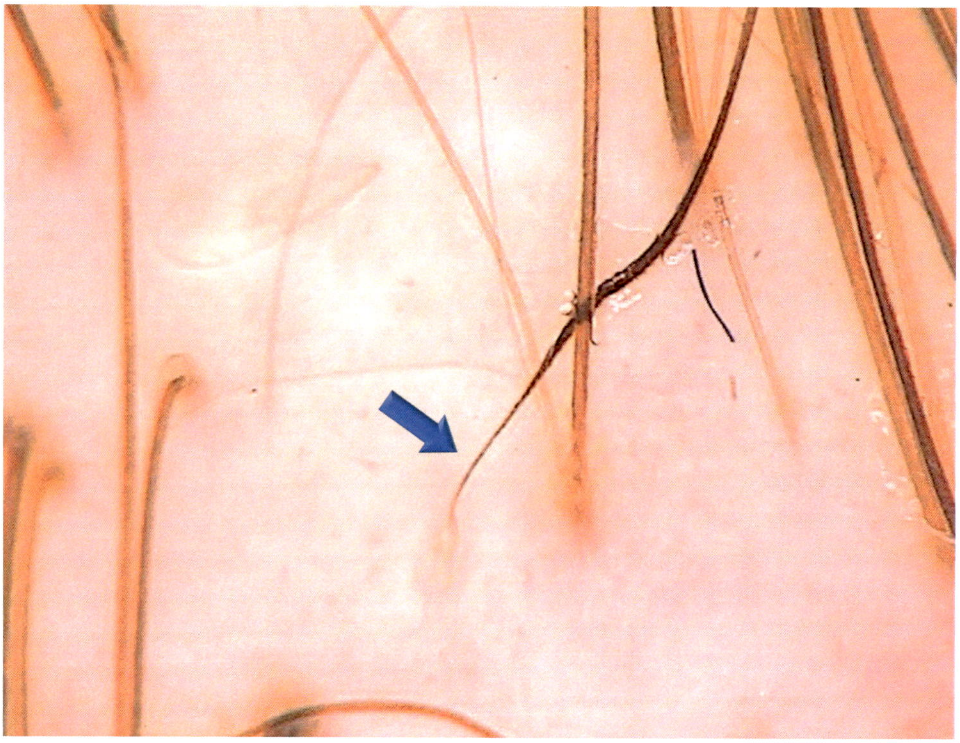

Fig. 2.21 Tapered hairs. Tapered hairs are best described as very long exclamation mark hairs (*arrow*). They are most characteristic for alopecia areata and emerge from follicles that are only partially affected by the disease. As the hair grows, these hairs slowly become thinner with increasing disease activity. A tapered hair corresponds to a very long Pohl-Pinkus constriction. Technically, hairs that are thin at the proximal end and become normal distally are called *tapered hairs* when the hair is longer than one dermoscopic field of view (×70)

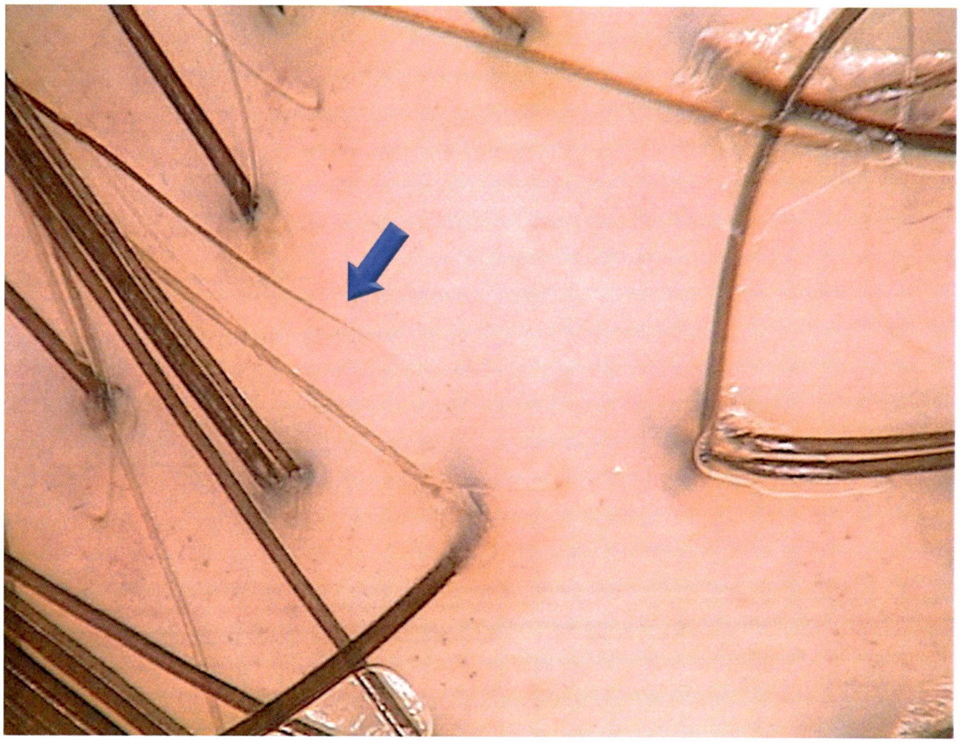

Fig. 2.22 Tapered hairs in alopecia areata. Tapered hairs are thin at the proximal end (*arrow*). In some cases, they become so thin that follicular openings cannot be seen on trichoscopy. Tapered hairs are seen commonly in alopecia areata but are not pathognomonic for the disease (×70)

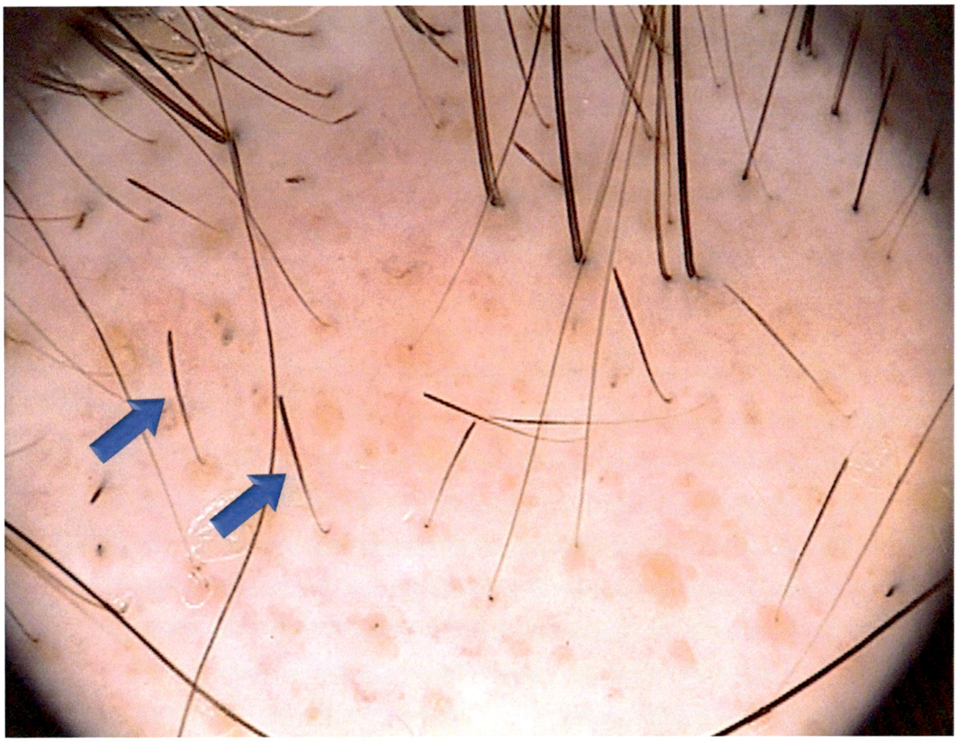

Fig. 2.23 Exclamation mark hairs in alopecia areata. The term *exclamation mark hairs* refers to short hairs that are thin and hypopigmented at the proximal end and thicker and darker at the distal end (*arrows*). Trichoscopy allows visualization of exclamation mark hairs shorter than 1–2 mm (micro–exclamation mark hairs). Exclamation mark hairs are most characteristic of, but not specific for, alopecia areata. Also shown are black dots and regularly distributed yellow dots, a hallmark of alopecia areata (×20)

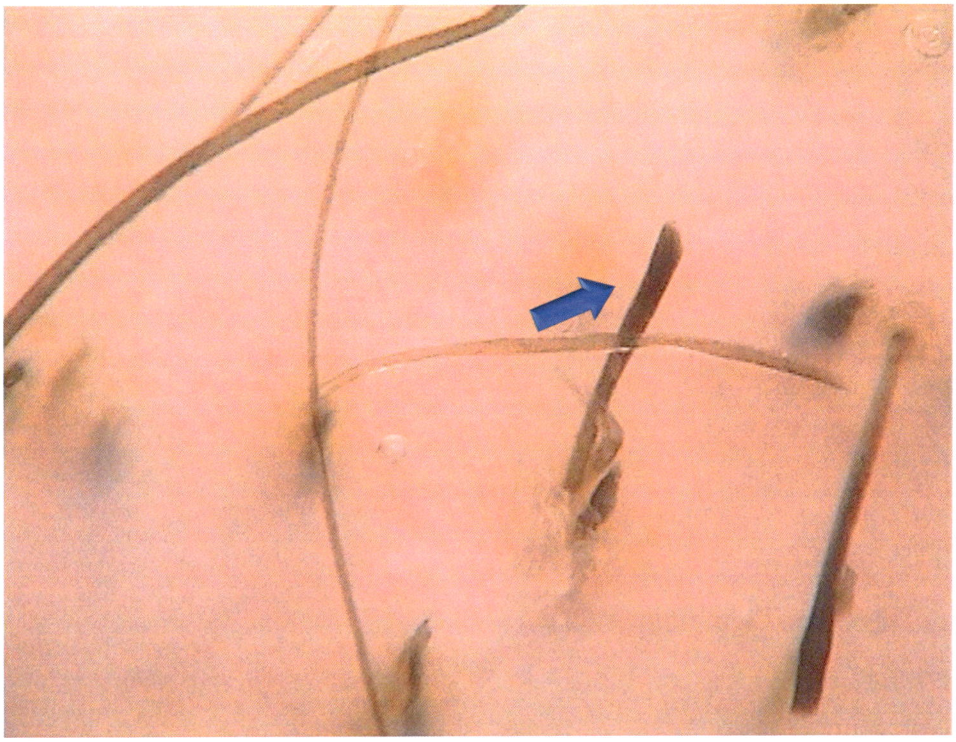

Fig. 2.24 Exclamation mark hairs in trichotillomania. Exclamation mark hairs may lead to a misdiagnosis of alopecia areata because they are commonly believed to be pathognomonic for alopecia areata. This image shows exclamation mark hairs (*arrow*) in a patient with trichotillomania. A study using light microscopy showed that most exclamation mark hairs in patients with alopecia areata have frayed distal ends, whereas most exclamation mark hairs from trichotillomania patients have blunt distal ends [21]. This difference is not observed on trichoscopy. Our experience shows that exclamation mark hairs in alopecia areata tend to have a hypopigmented proximal end and a pointed distal end, whereas most exclamation mark hairs in trichotillomania have a dark proximal end and a flat distal end. The differentiation may be especially problematic in patients with coexisting alopecia areata and trichotillomania (×70)

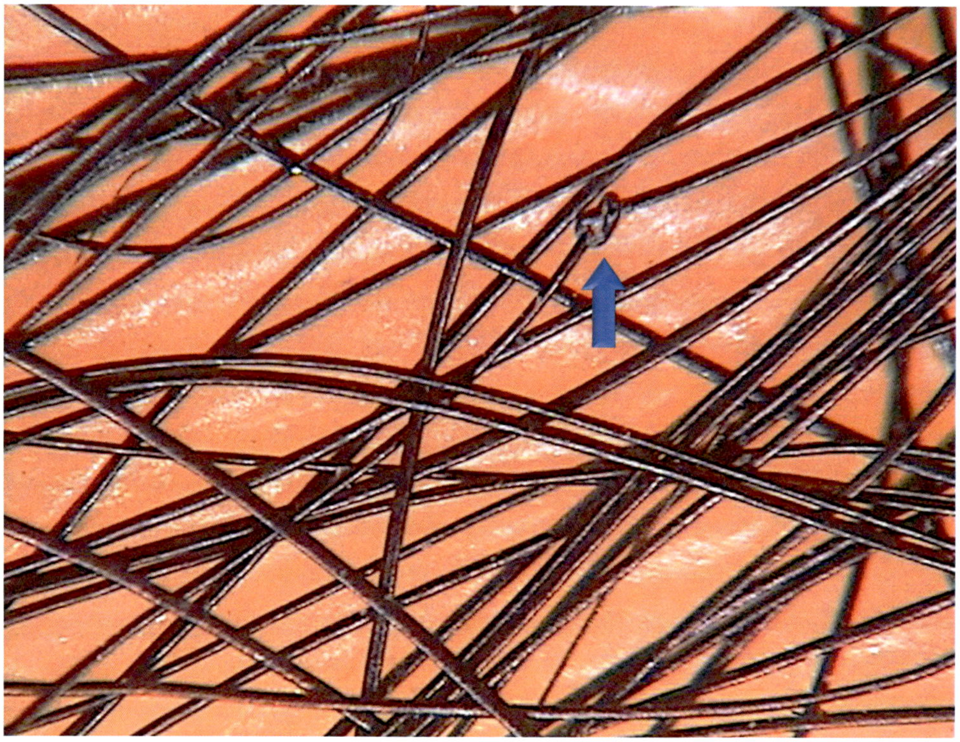

Fig. 2.25 Trichonodosis. Trichonodosis (hair knotting) is an acquired, transient condition in which a single or double knot occurs in the hair shaft (*arrow*), either spontaneously or in response to scratching. It is observed in patients with short, curly hair. Trichonodosis is usually an incidental finding of little clinical significance (×70)

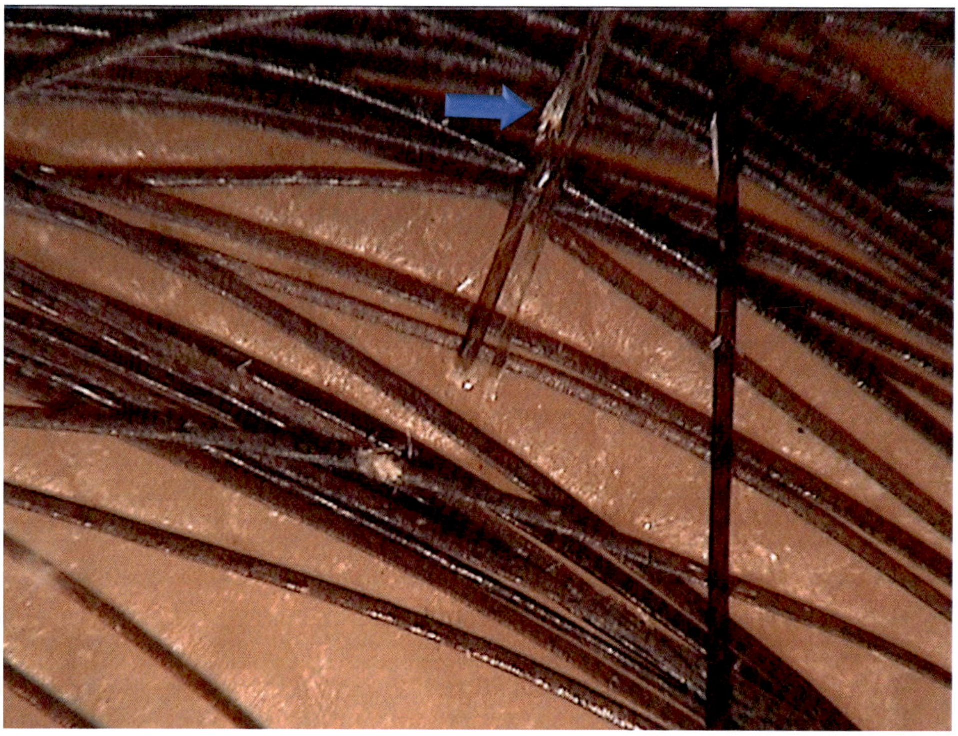

Fig. 2.26 Trichorrhexis nodosa. In trichorrhexis nodosa, the hair develops a restricted area in which the shaft splits longitudinally into numerous small fibers. The outer fibers bulge outward, causing a segmental increase in hair diameter. Trichoscopy may give slightly different images depending on magnification and technique. At high magnifications and in dry trichoscopy, as in this image, the split hair shaft appears as two white brushes aligned in opposition (*arrow*). At low magnifications, trichoscopy shows nodular thickenings along the hair shaft. These thickenings appear light in the darker hair shaft (×70)

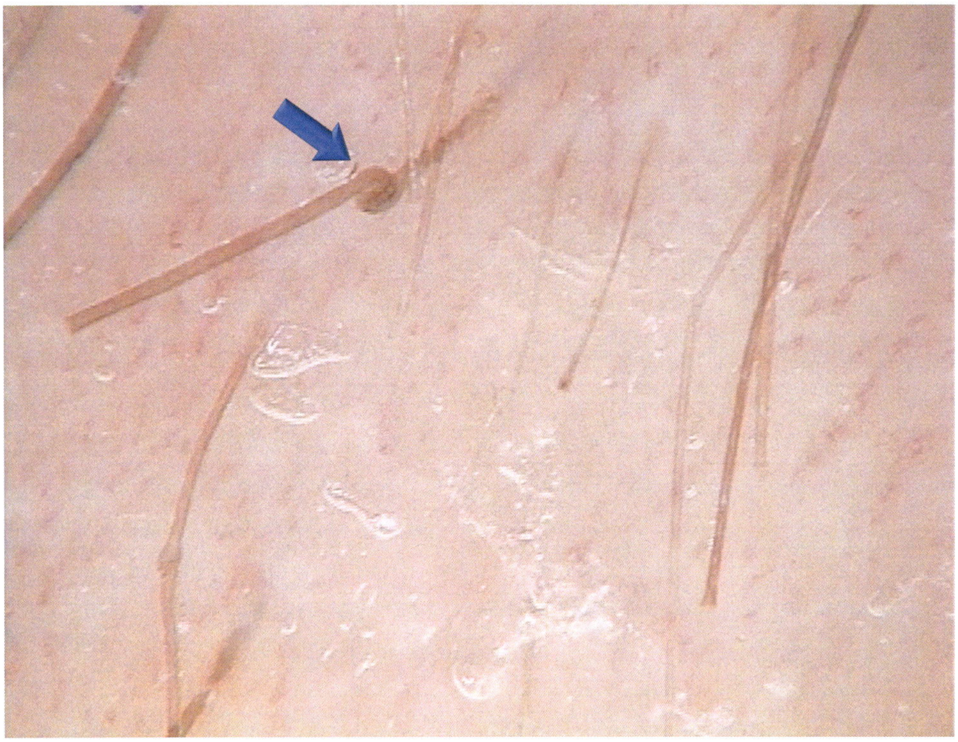

Fig. 2.27 Bamboo hair in Netherton's syndrome. Bamboo hairs are a manifestation of trichorrhexis invaginata, a hallmark of Netherton's syndrome. In trichorrhexis invaginata, the hair shaft telescopes into itself (*arrow*). The proximal part of the abnormality is concave, whereas the distal end is convex (bulging). This produces a nodular swelling along the hair shaft with a "ball in a cup" appearance. The presence of many of these nodes along the hair shaft gives it the appearance of a bamboo tree (×70)

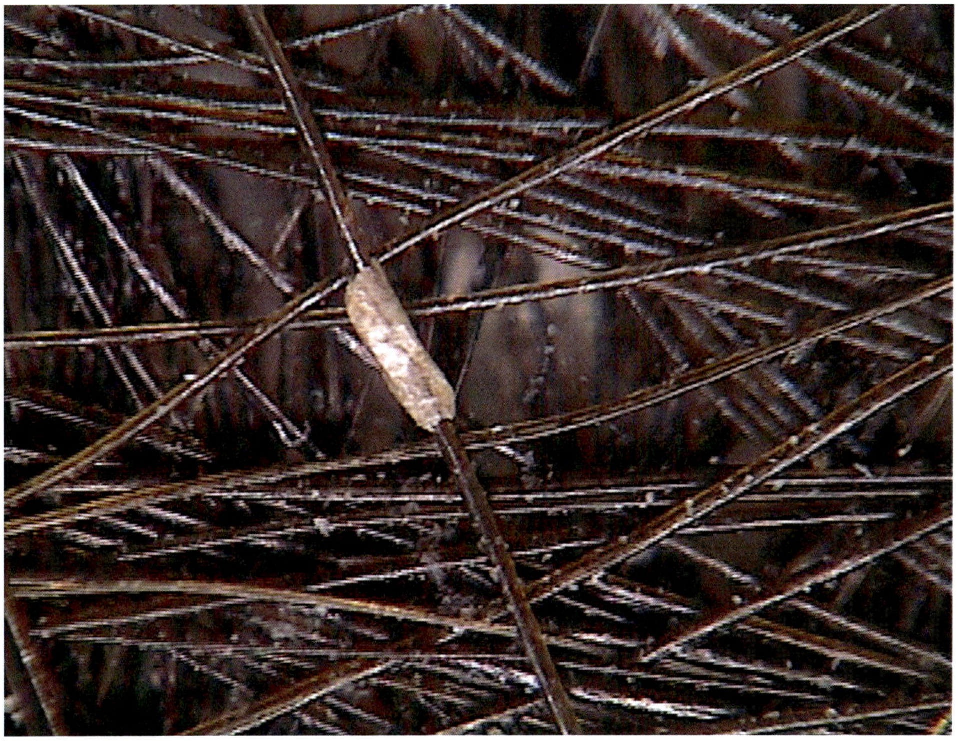

Fig. 2.28 Hair cast in lichen planopilaris. Hair casts (peripilar keratin casts) are firm, white, freely movable tubular masses that encircle the hair shafts. Historically, these also were called "pseudonits," because macroscopic evaluation of these structures may lead to an erroneous diagnosis of pediculosis capitis. Hair casts may be a secondary phenomenon in the course of psoriasis, seborrheic dermatitis, or lichen planopilaris. Idiopathic hair casts may be observed in healthy individuals. This image shows a hair cast in a patient with active lichen planopilaris (×70)

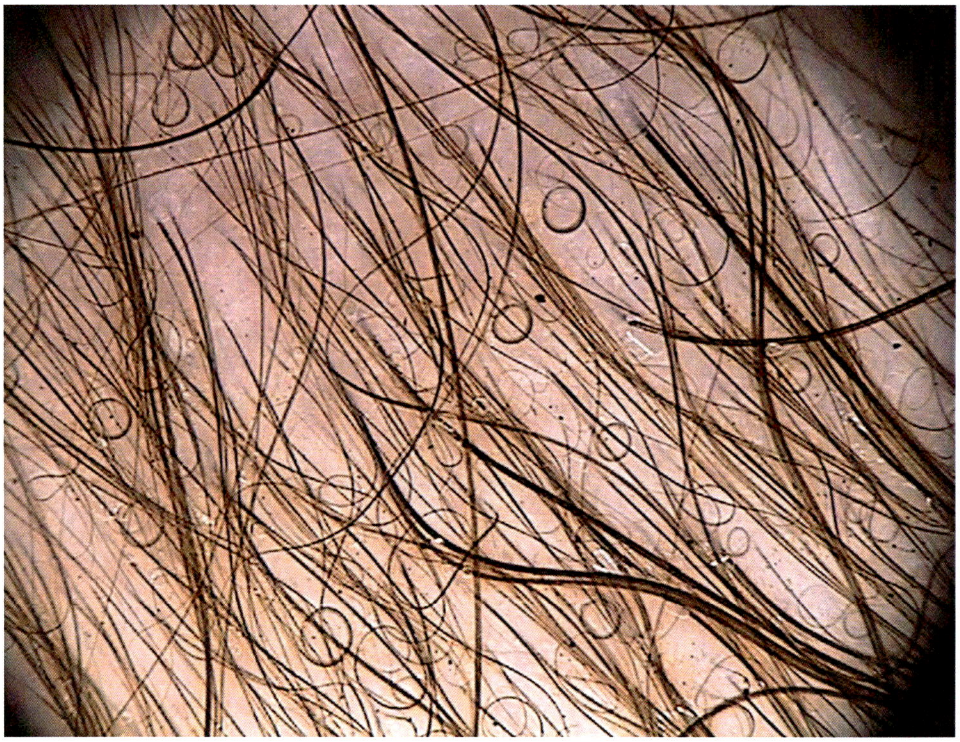

Fig. 2.29 Pigtail hairs in alopecia areata. Regrowing pigtail hairs are short, regularly twisted hairs with tapered ends and resemble a pig's tail. They may be circular or oval. Shown here is a trichoscopic image from a patient with alopecia areata with unusual hair regrowth due to hair cycle synchronization after intralesional triamcinolone injections. Solitary regrowing pigtail hairs also may be observed in cicatricial alopecia (×20)

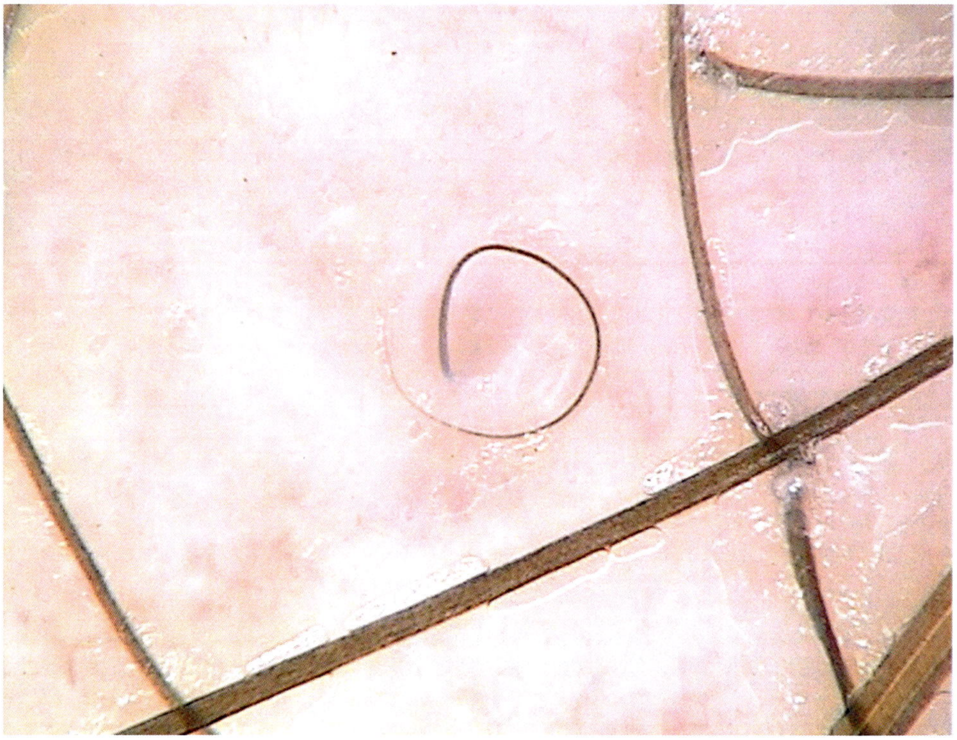

Fig. 2.30 Pigtail hair in lichen planopilaris. Regrowing pigtail hairs most probably result from rapid hair regrowth, before full recovery of the hair follicle. Although most characteristic for alopecia areata, regrowing pigtail hairs also may be present in cicatricial alopecia. This image shows a regrowing pigtail hair in a patient with lichen planopilaris. The hairs are regularly twisted and have tapered (pinpoint) distal ends. In this regard, they differ from irregular coiled hairs (×70)

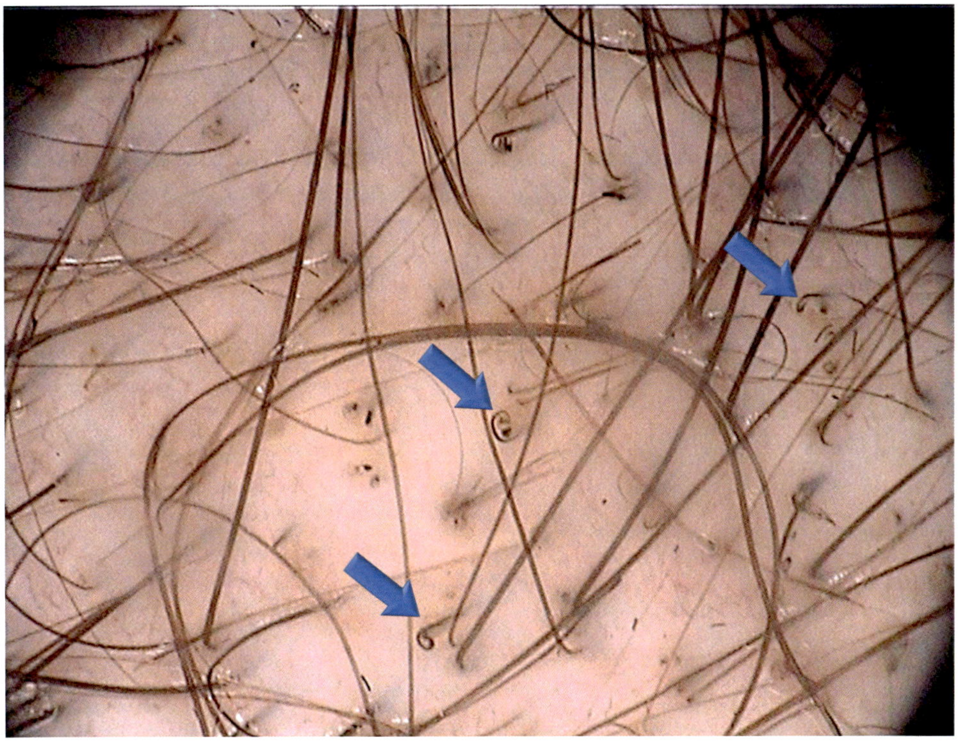

Fig. 2.31 Coiled hairs in trichotillomania. Irregularly coiled hairs observed in trichotillomania develop as a result of hair-pulling tension force. After fracturing, the remaining part of the hair coils irregularly at the fracture site (*arrows*). The appearance of the coiled hair depends on the tension, pulling direction, length of the remaining hair, and hair growth after the moment of pulling. In patients with multiple coiled hairs, this will result in each coiled hair having a different appearance (×20)

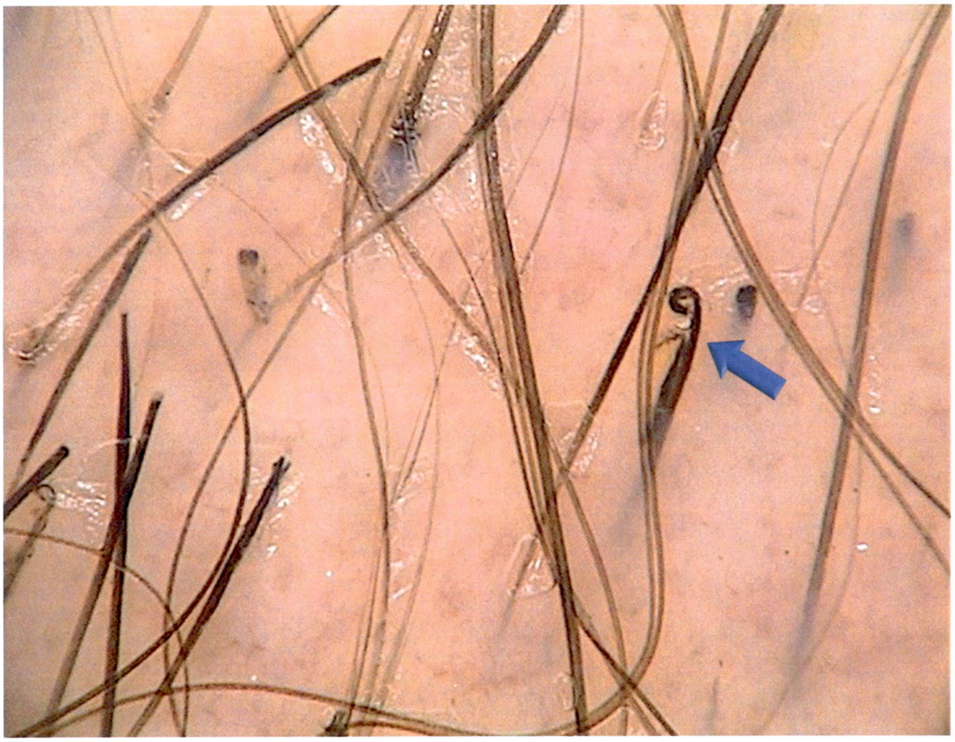

Fig. 2.32 Coiled hairs in trichotillomania. Irregular coiled hairs are most typical of trichotillomania but also may be present in small numbers in patients with traction alopecia and in healthy individuals as a result of hair pulling during hairstyling procedures. The fractured, irregular coiled hairs differ from regrowing pigtail hairs in their irregular, oval appearance and blunt end. Occasionally, they may have a hook-like appearance (*arrow*; ×70)

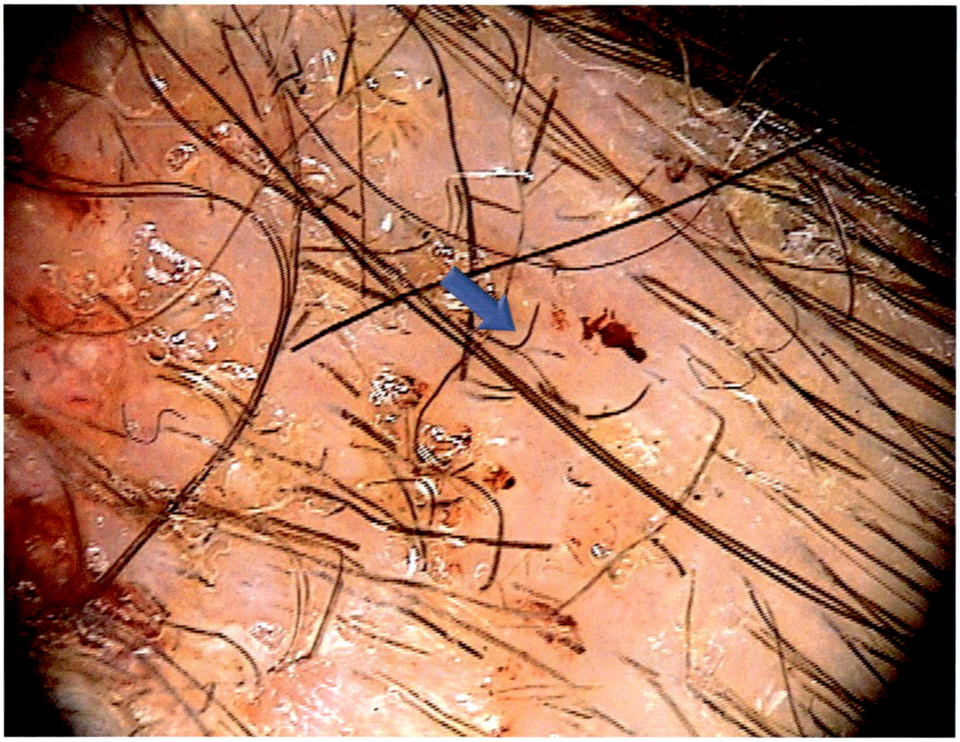

Fig. 2.33 Comma hairs in tinea capitis. These short comma-like hairs are characterized by homogeneous thickness and pigmentation of the hair shaft and a sharp diagonal end (*arrow*). As first described by Slowinska et al. [10], the presence of multiple comma hairs in focal alopecia is pathognomonic for tinea capitis. Single hairs that curl into a comma-like structure occasionally may be observed in healthy individuals with very short hair and during hair regrowth in alopecia areata (×20)

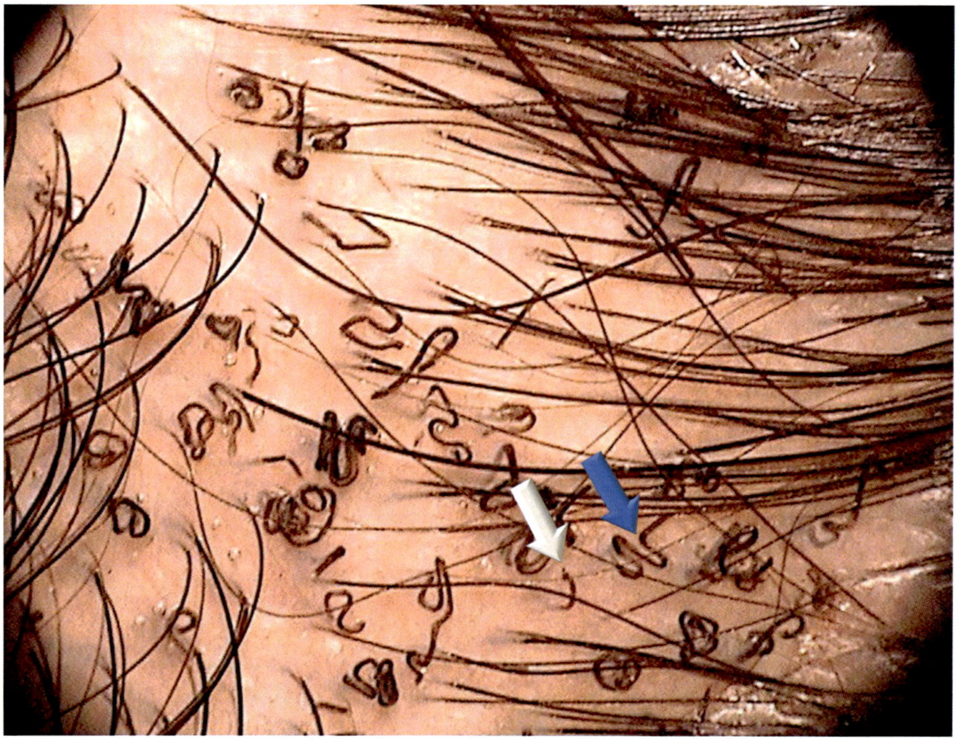

Fig. 2.34 Corkscrew hairs in tinea capitis. Hairs curling into corkscrew structures were first identified in a black child with tinea capitis in France and described by Hughes et al. [12]. Our experience shows that corkscrew hairs (*blue arrow*) are a hallmark of tinea capitis in patients of all skin phototypes. However, the curls are more common and more prominent in patients with dark skin phototypes. These corkscrew hairs should not be confused with those observed on light microscopy in children with ectodermal dysplasia [22–24]. Comma hairs (*white arrow*) often coexist with corkscrew hairs. They are shorter and show less curling than corkscrew hairs (×20)

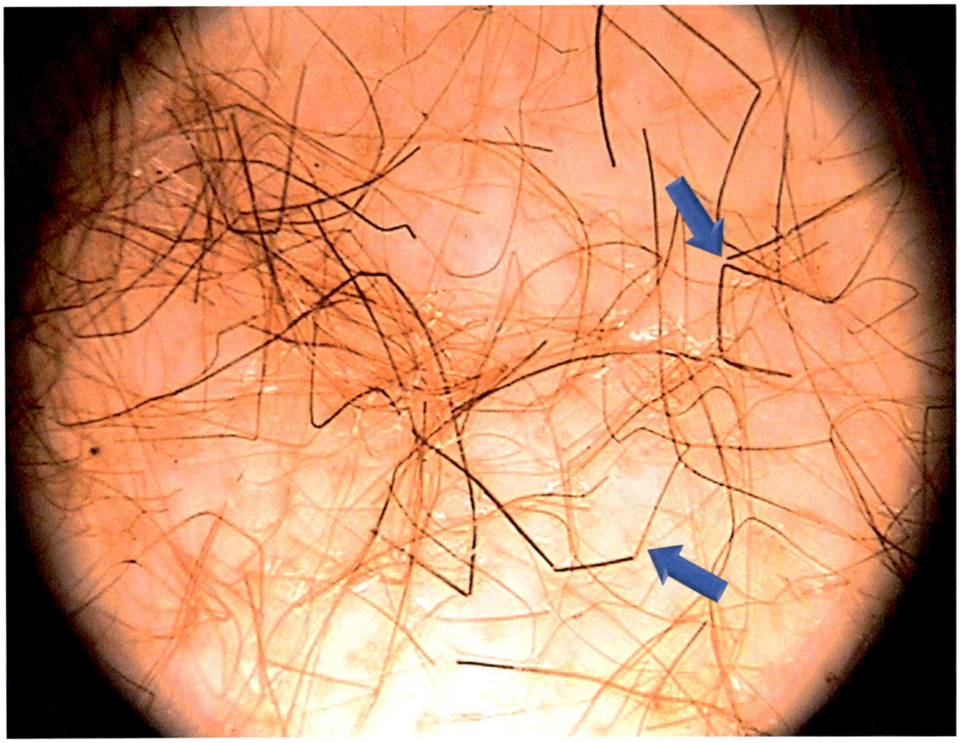

Fig. 2.35 Zigzag hairs in tinea capitis. Hairs that form zigzag structures (also called Z-hairs; *arrows*) are observed in tinea capitis, alopecia areata, trichorrhexis nodosa, and other diseases that cause focal weakening of the hair shaft [13]. They are not pathognomonic for tinea capitis (×20)

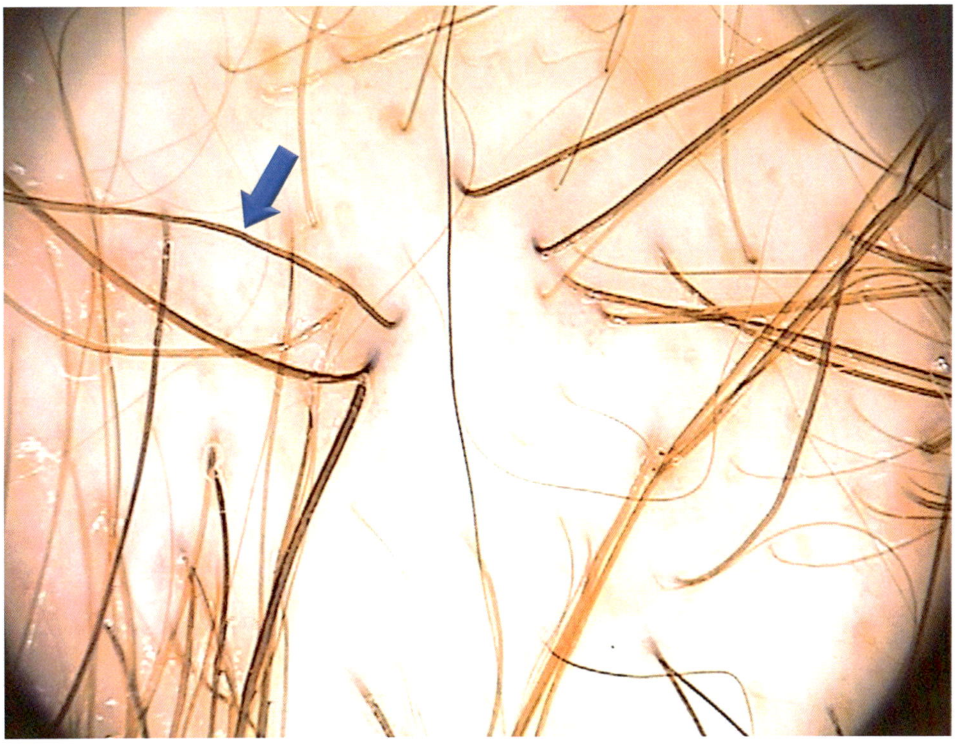

Fig. 2.36 Pili torti. In pili torti, the affected hair is flattened and twisted on its own axis at irregular intervals, usually at a 180° angle (*arrow*). Pili torti has numerous causes, both inherited and acquired. See Chap. 11 for details (×20)

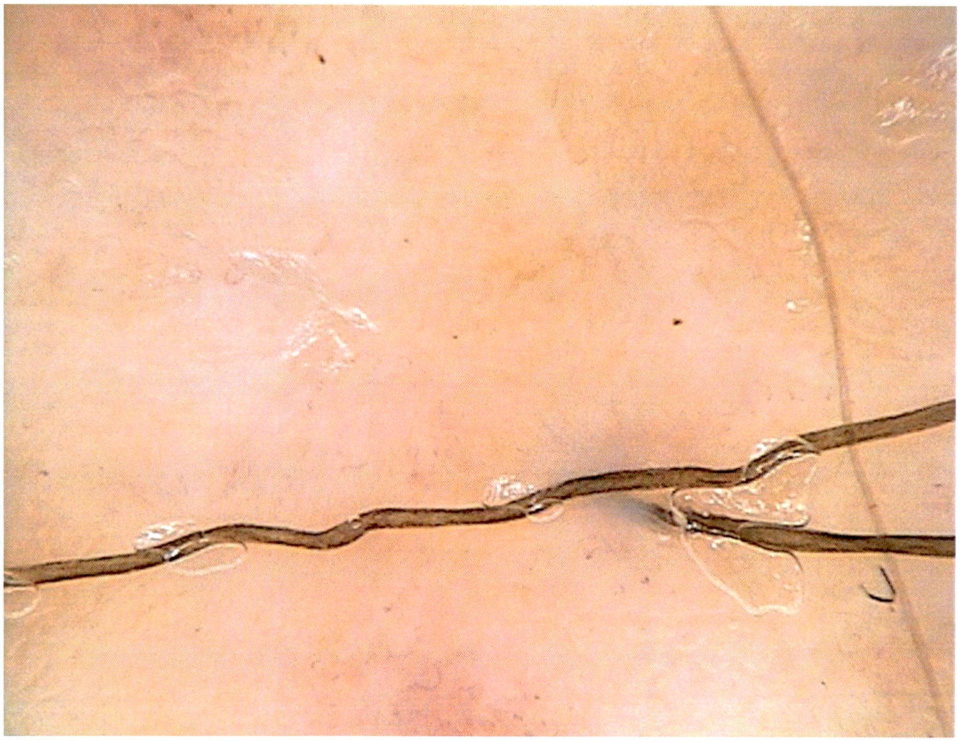

Fig. 2.37 **Woolly hair**. The term *woolly hair* refers to an abnormal variant of hair with tightly coiled curls. The hairs are often thin and hypopigmented. Three variants of woolly hair have been distinguished based on clinical and light microscopic investigation: local woolly hair nevus and two generalized variants, autosomal dominant hereditary woolly hair and autosomal recessive familial woolly hair. Trichoscopy has revealed that hairs fulfilling the definition of *woolly hairs* are more common than previously reported (×70)

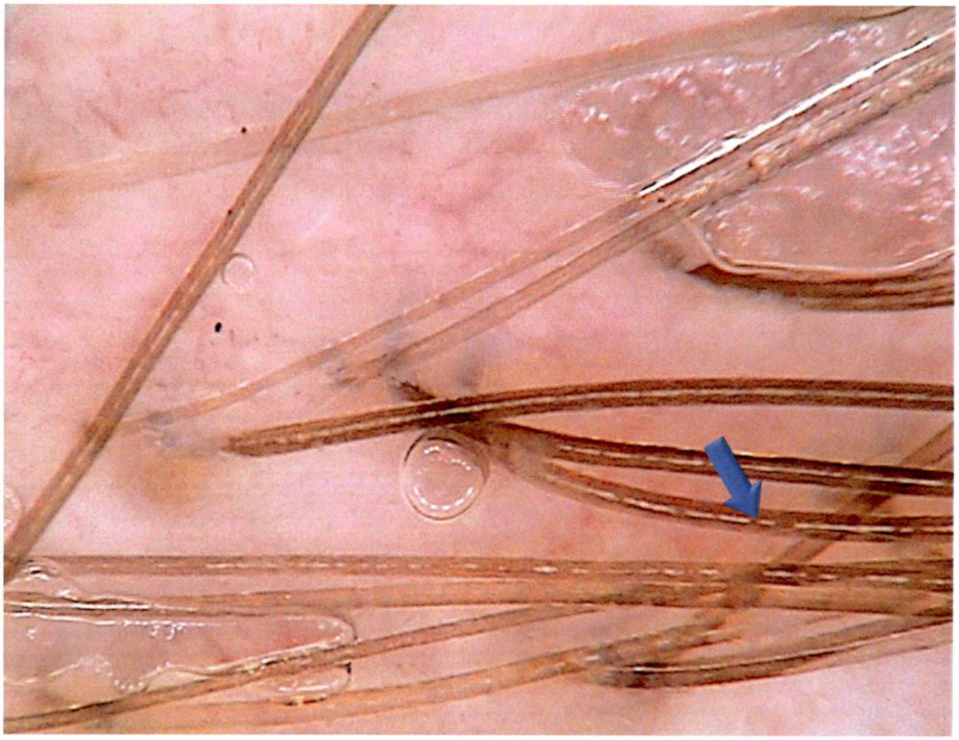

Fig. 2.38 **Interrupted and fragmented medulla in a normal hair shaft**. In normal hair shafts, trichoscopy allows visualization of the medulla, which appears as a longitudinal white band along the midpart of the hair shaft. The medulla may be continuous, interrupted, fragmented, or absent [3]. The trichoscopic impression of the "fragmented" medulla (*arrow*) is in fact a thick medulla intercalated with a thin medulla, which is not visible on trichoscopy. The thickness or presence of the medulla is believed to have no influence on hair shaft properties (×70)

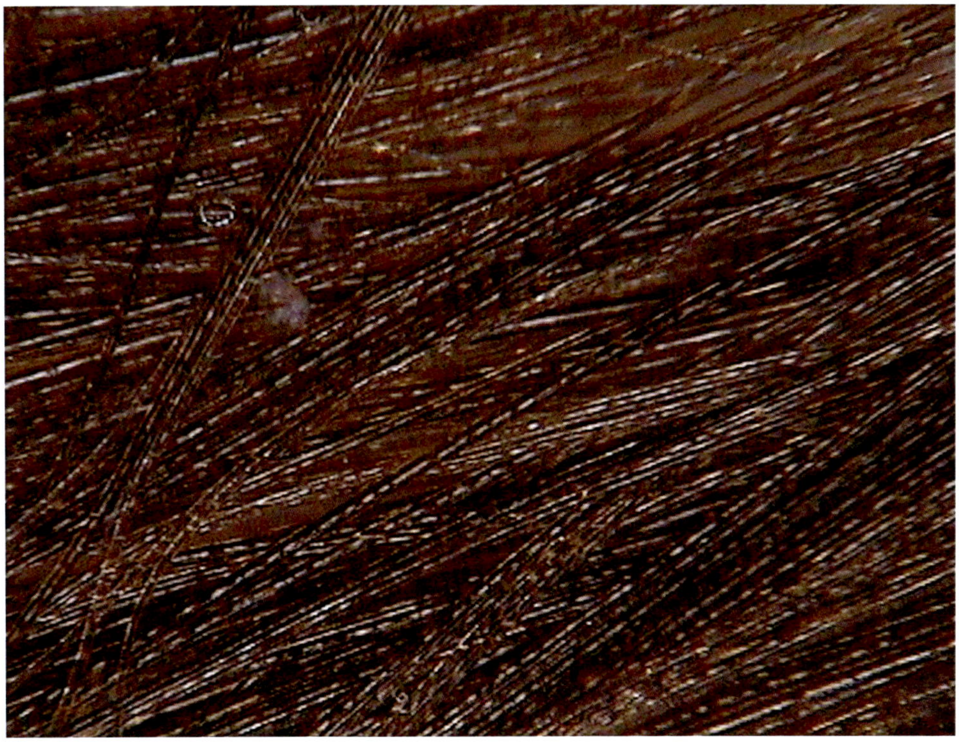

Fig. 2.39 Interrupted and fragmented medulla in a normal hair shaft. All the hair shafts in this image have an interrupted white line in their midpart. An interrupted medulla may be differentiated from pili annulati in that it covers less than 50 % of the hair shaft thickness (×50)

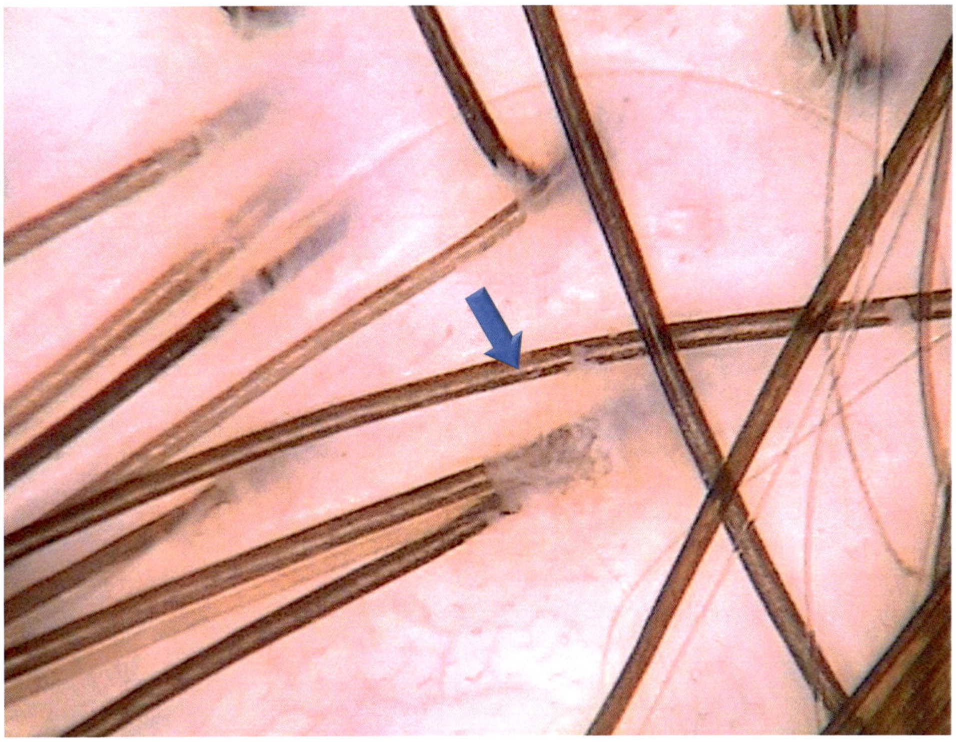

Fig. 2.40 Continuous medulla in normal hair shafts. Thick terminal hairs often have a continuous medulla, which is a white midline thinner than 50 % of the hair shaft thickness (*arrow*). A continuous medulla is observed most commonly in the Asian population (×70)

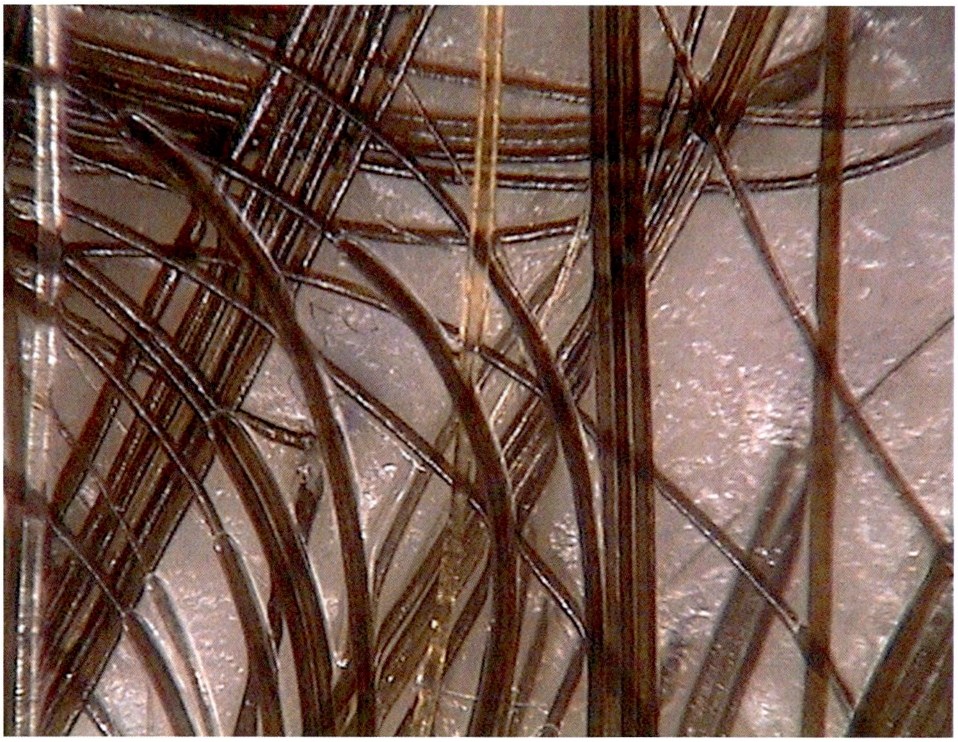

Fig. 2.41 Absent medulla in normal hair shafts. Note that in this image, most of the hair shafts are uniform in color and no medulla is visible. This also is in normal range (×70)

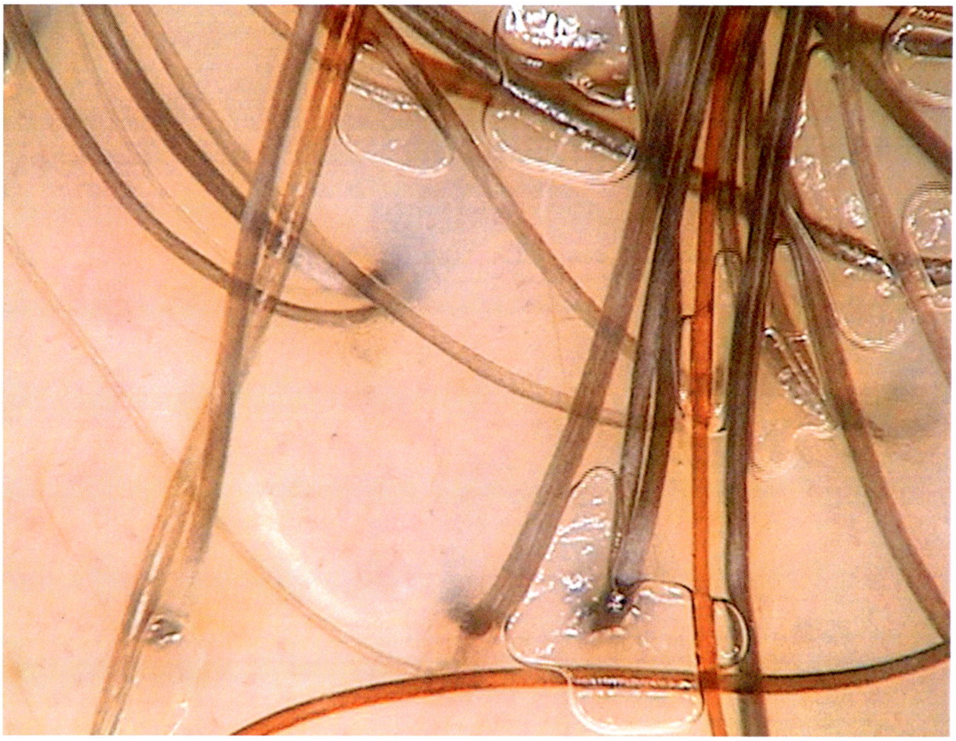

Fig. 2.42 Hair shafts with light whitish bands in pili annulati. Note that these bands are nearly the width of a hair and their borders are not clear-cut, which differentiates white bands in pili annulati from an interrupted medulla (×70)

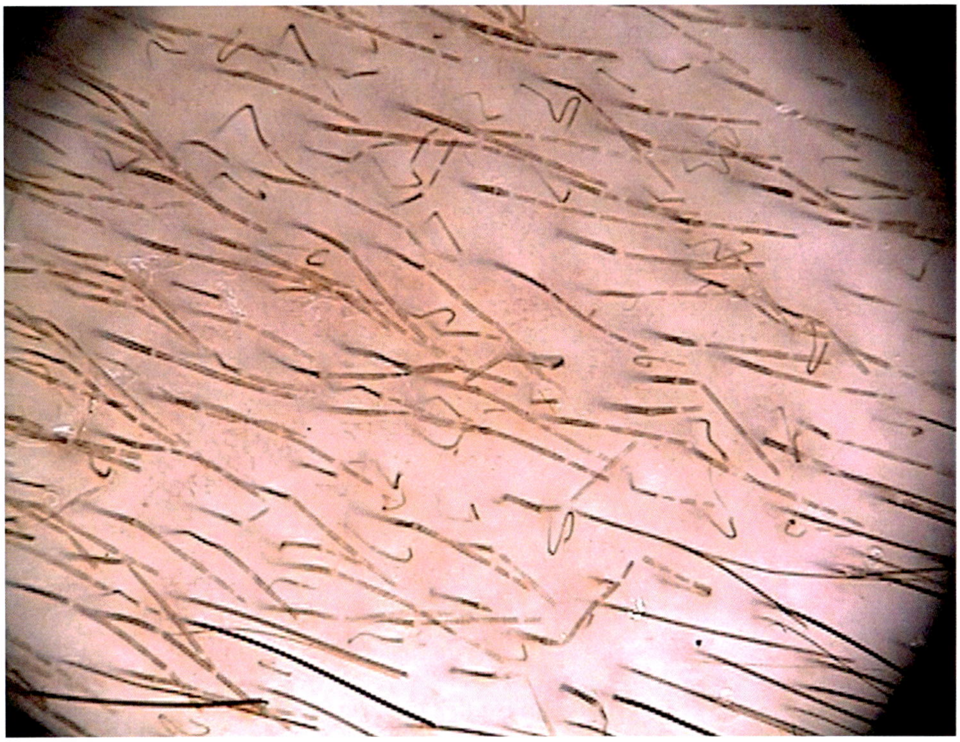

Fig. 2.43 Interrupted hairs in tinea capitis. Interrupted hairs (Morse code–like hairs) with multiple thin white bands across the hair shaft were first observed in our patients with tinea capitis due to *Microsporum canis* and described by Rudnicka et al. [13]. The specificity of this finding is a subject for further investigation (×20)

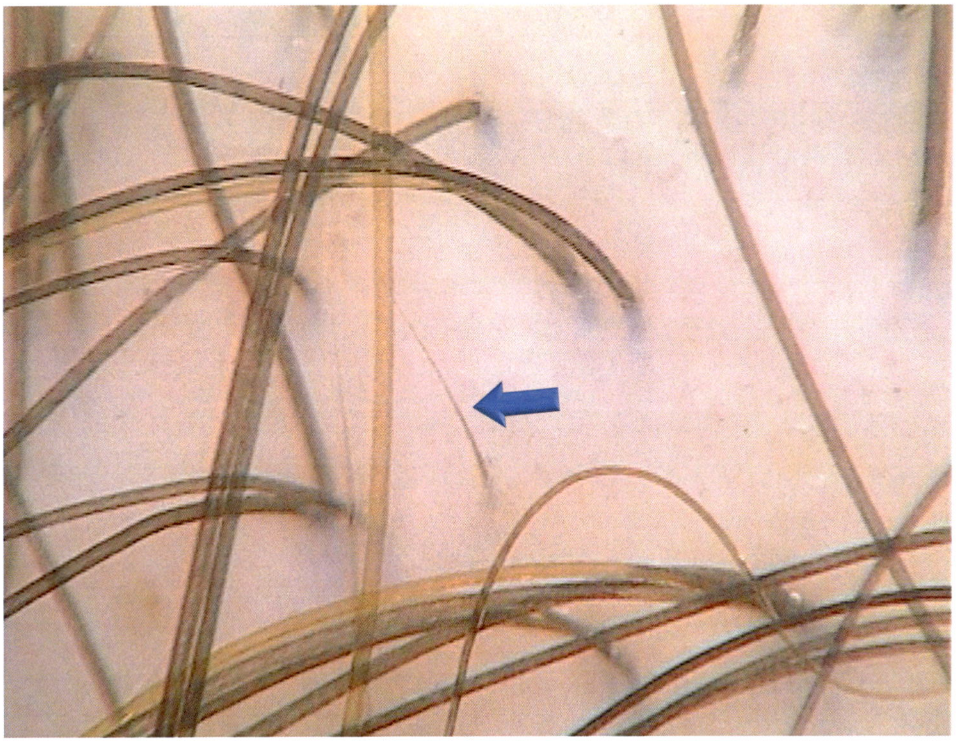

Fig. 2.44 Upright regrowing hair in a healthy individual. New, upright regrowing hairs are a sign of hair regrowth in healthy individuals. The presence of multiple upright regrowing hairs is characteristic of the hair regrowth phase in telogen effluvium but also may be observed in other types of noncicatricial alopecia. These hairs look different from the delicate, thin, vellus hairs seen in androgenetic alopecia. Note the tapered end and continuous hair shaft thickening toward the follicular opening (*arrow*; ×70)

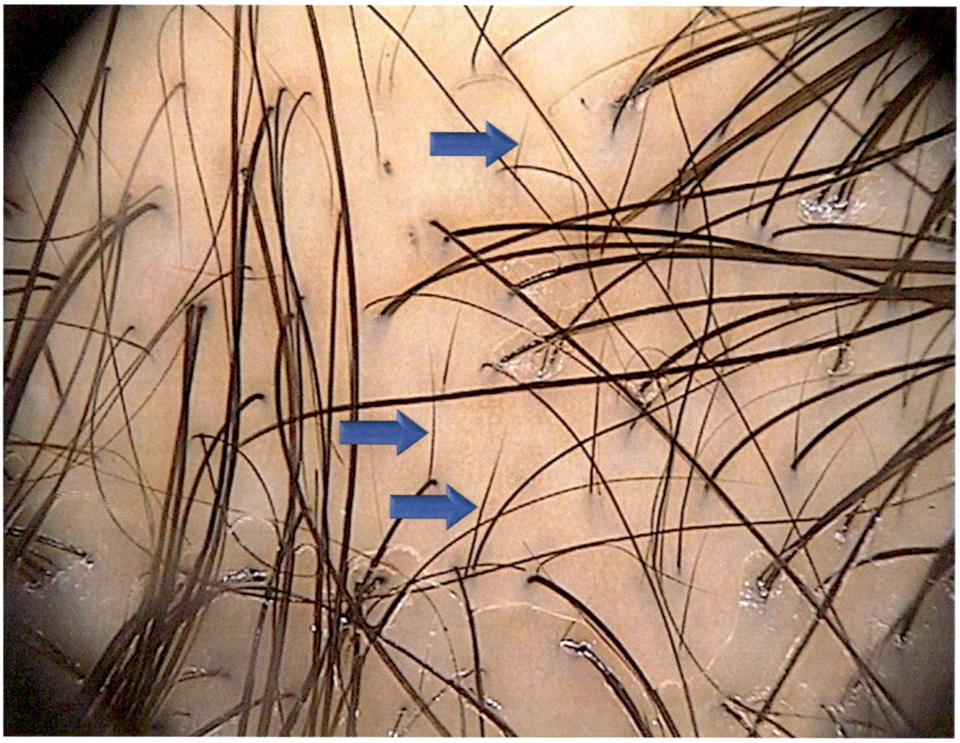

Fig. 2.45 Upright regrowing hairs in telogen effluvium. The presence of multiple upright regrowing hairs (*arrows*) is the effect of hair cycle synchronization and the simultaneous regrowth of hairs. This is one of the most characteristic (but not specific) trichoscopic features of telogen effluvium (×20)

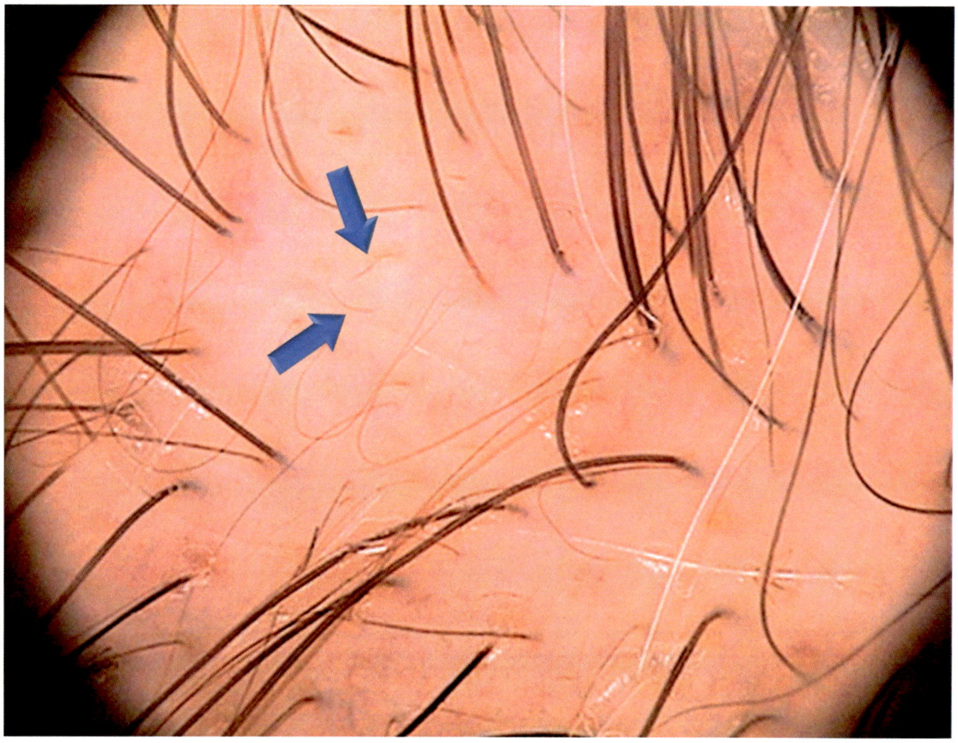

Fig. 2.46 Vellus hairs in androgenetic alopecia. In this image, almost 30 % of the hair shafts are vellus hairs (*arrows*). These hairs are hypopigmented, nonmedullated, less than 30 μm thick, and less than 3 mm long. They are delicate, thin, and short. Up to about 10 % of normal human scalp hairs are vellus hairs. An increased proportion of vellus hairs is characteristic of male and female androgenetic alopecia (×20)

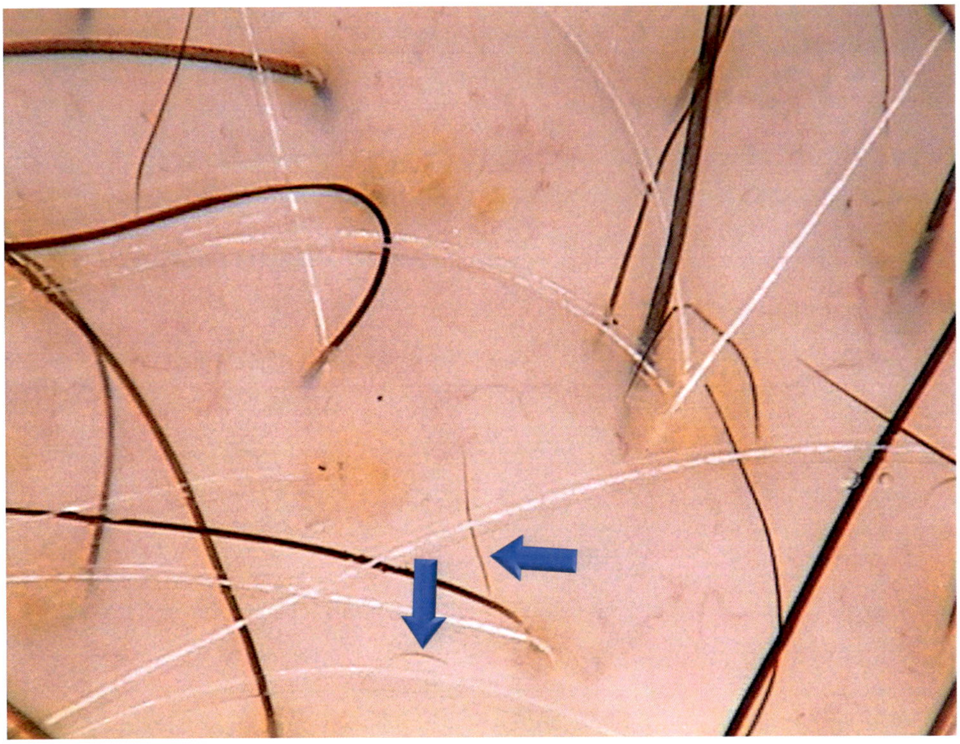

Fig. 2.47 Dark lines. Dark lines are hairs that are thin and short but very dark (*arrows*). Occasionally, they are darker than the patient's natural hair color. Their characteristic feature is that it is difficult to determine at which end of the hair the follicle is located. Dark lines are present in noncicatricial alopecia, most commonly alopecia areata incognita (×70)

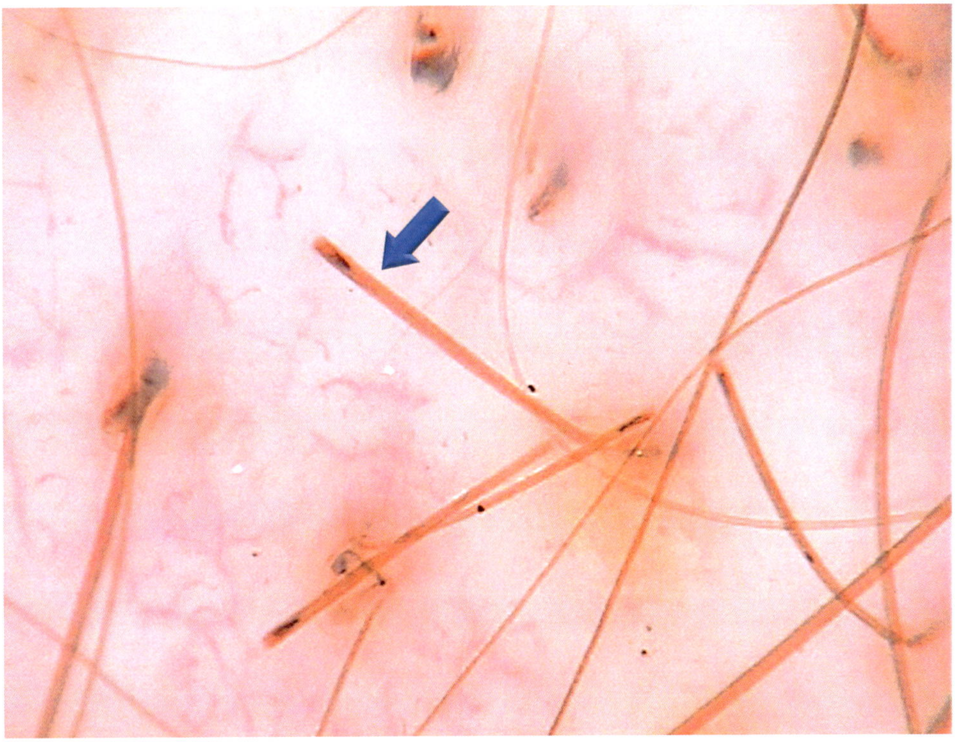

Fig. 2.48 Tulip hairs in trichotillomania. Tulip hairs tend to be slightly thinner at the base than at the distal end and show a tulip leaf–like hyperpigmentation at the distal end (*arrow*). These short hairs are seen in patients with trichotillomania and alopecia areata (×70)

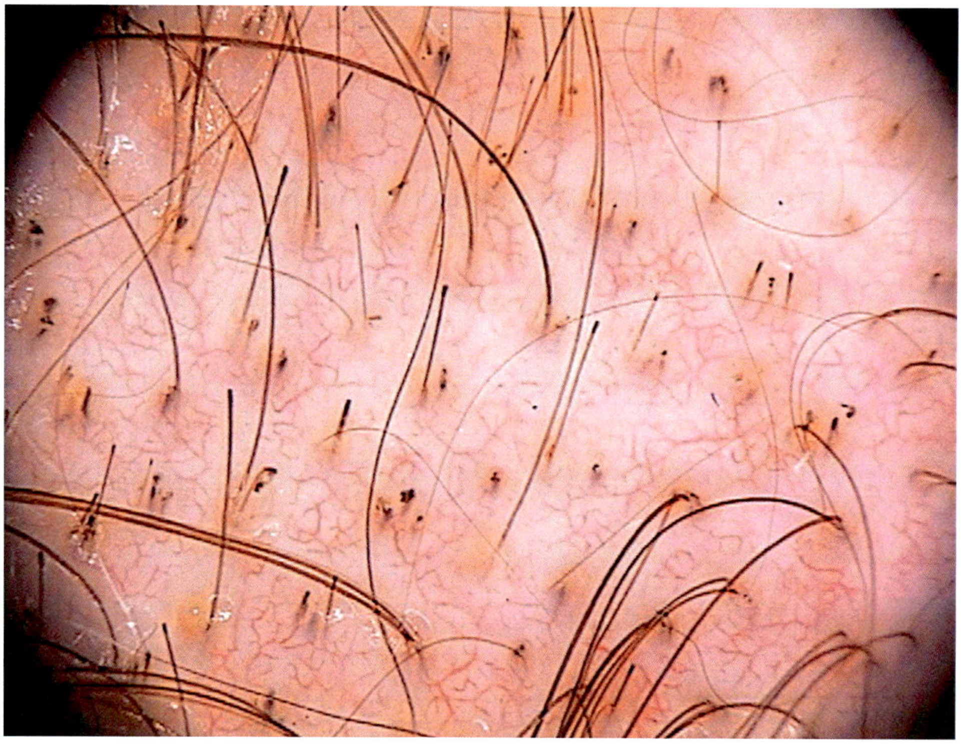

Fig. 2.49 Tulip hairs in trichotillomania. At low magnification, tulip hairs appear as light-colored hair shafts with dark distal ends. They most likely correspond to broken hairs with a diagonal fracture surface and a cuticle detached at the distal end. Tulip hairs are characteristic of, but not pathognomonic for, trichotillomania (×20)

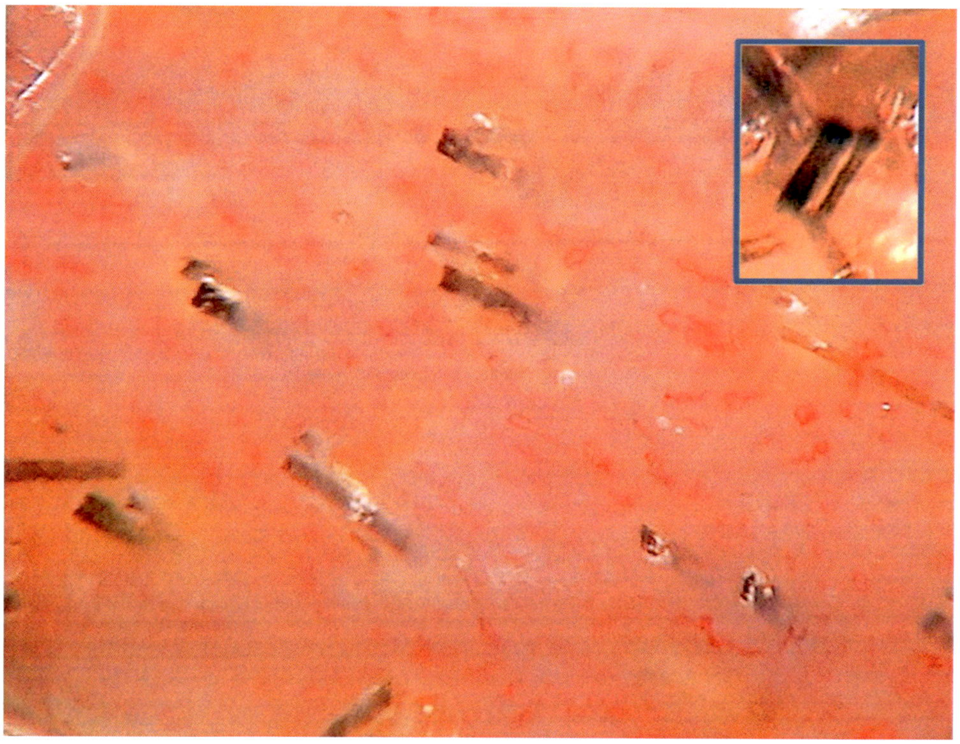

Fig. 2.50 Hair blocks and i-hairs in tinea capitis. Hair blocks are very short hairs with a horizontal distal end. This image shows block hairs in tinea capitis; however, block hairs are a common finding that may be associated with several acquired diseases. i-Hairs (*inset*) are block hairs with an accented dark distal end (×70)

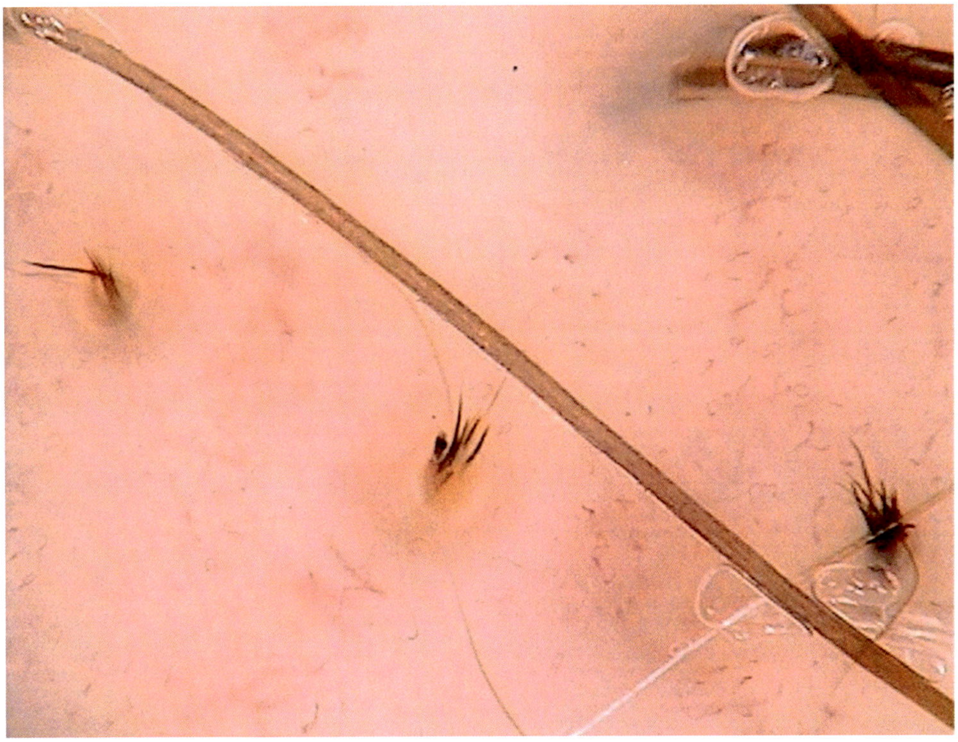

Fig. 2.51 Broom hairs in cicatricial alopecia. We suggest the common term *broom hair* for all abnormalities associated with a few or more linear, short, thin, dark hairs emerging from one follicular opening [13]. Only some of these abnormalities may correspond to trichostasis spinulosa [25], which is usually associated with facial hairs. This picture reveals a few of these follicular units in a female patient with cicatricial alopecia (×70)

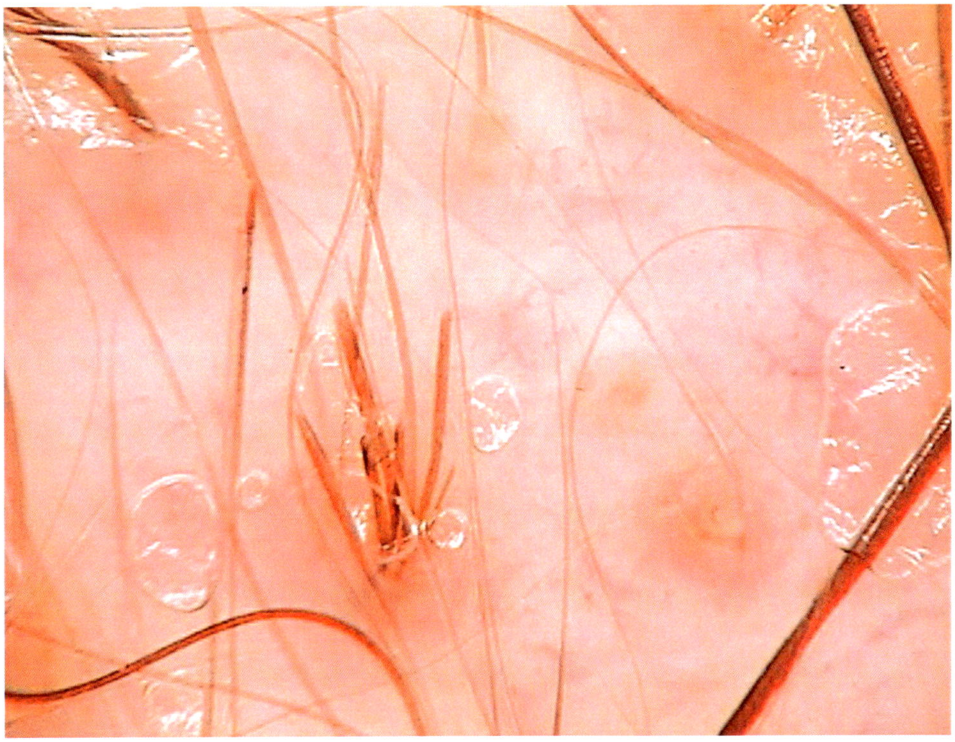

Fig. 2.52 Broom hairs in noncicatricial alopecia. This image shows a different manifestation of broom hairs in a patient with trichotillomania. These are multiple short full-thickness hairs emerging from one follicular unit in a patient who otherwise has long hair (×70)

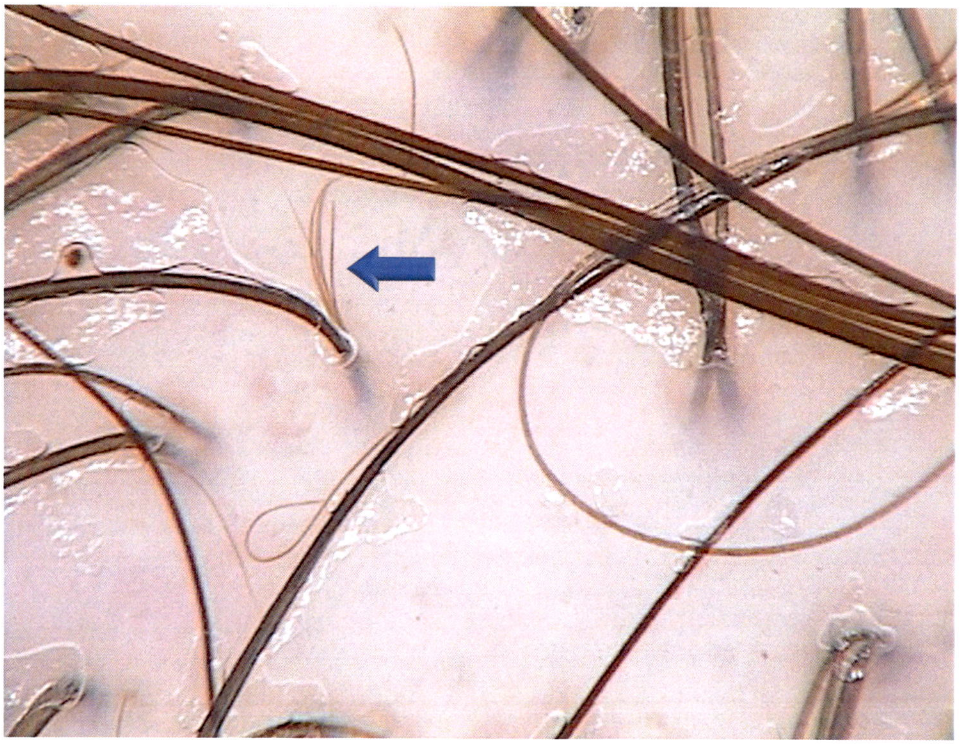

Fig. 2.53 Broom hairs. Broom hair–like structures (broom fibers; *arrow*) may be observed in different entities, both cicatricial and noncicatricial. Most likely, they reflect different pathologic mechanisms and histopathologies (×70)

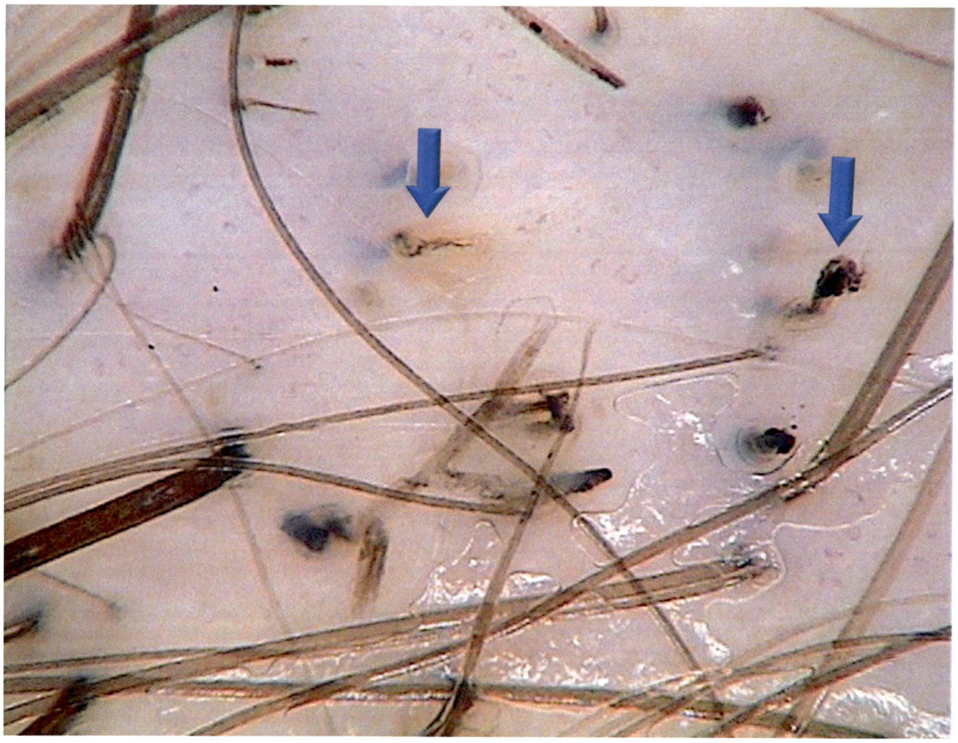

Fig. 2.54 Flame hairs in trichotillomania. Flame-like hairs (*arrows*) are residues from recently pulled hairs and are observed most commonly in active trichotillomania [13]. We have not observed flame hairs in other diseases (×70)

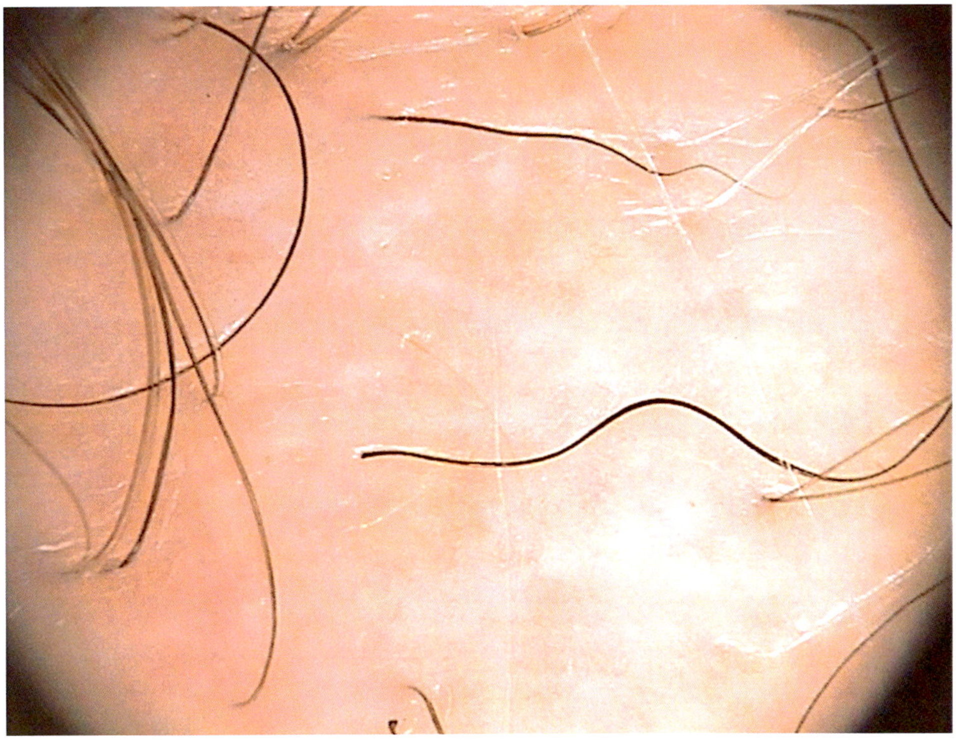

Fig. 2.55 Acquired hair shaft dystrophy in cicatricial alopecia. The most common reason for this condition is perifollicular fibrosis. Before a follicle is completely destroyed, it produces various types of dystrophic hair shafts. They usually emerge in whitish or milky red areas with a decreased number of hair follicles (×20)

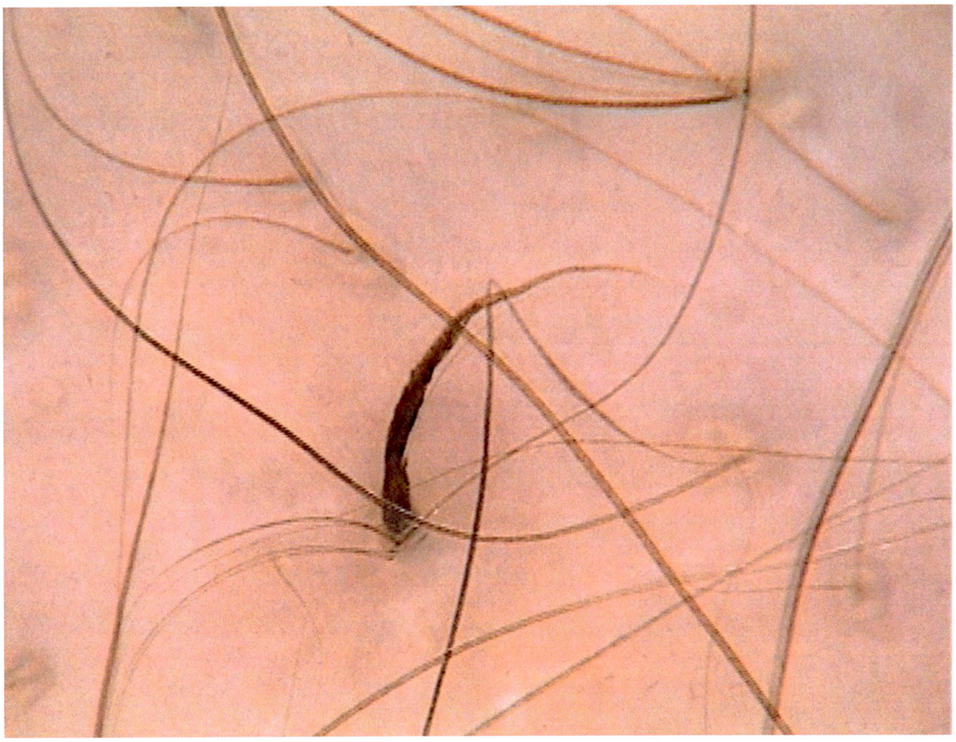

Fig. 2.56 Acquired hair shaft dystrophy in cicatricial alopecia. This image shows another example of acquired hair shaft dystrophy in a patient with cicatricial alopecia. The hair is short and very thick compared with other hairs in this patient with dissecting cellulitis (×70)

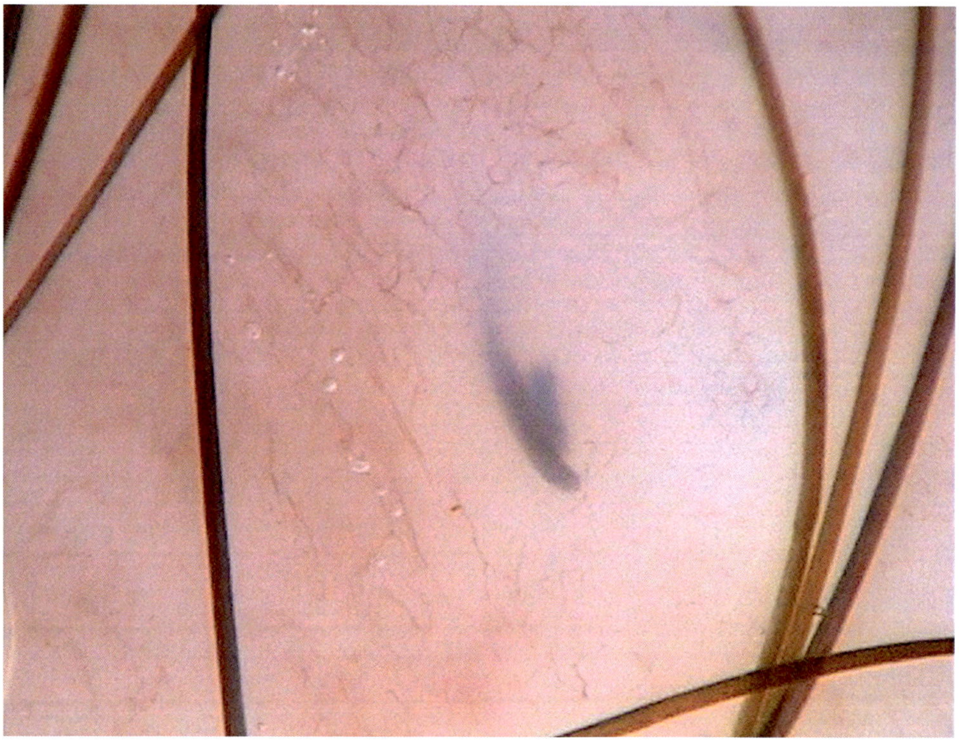

Fig. 2.57 Ingrowing scalp hair in cicatricial alopecia. Dermatologists have evaluated ingrowing scalp hairs much less often than ingrowing eyelashes (trichiasis) [26] and ingrowing facial hairs (pseudofolliculitis barbae) [27]. Trichoscopy allows visualization of ingrowing scalp hairs; they usually are U-shaped and are observed more commonly in cicatricial than noncicatricial alopecia (×70)

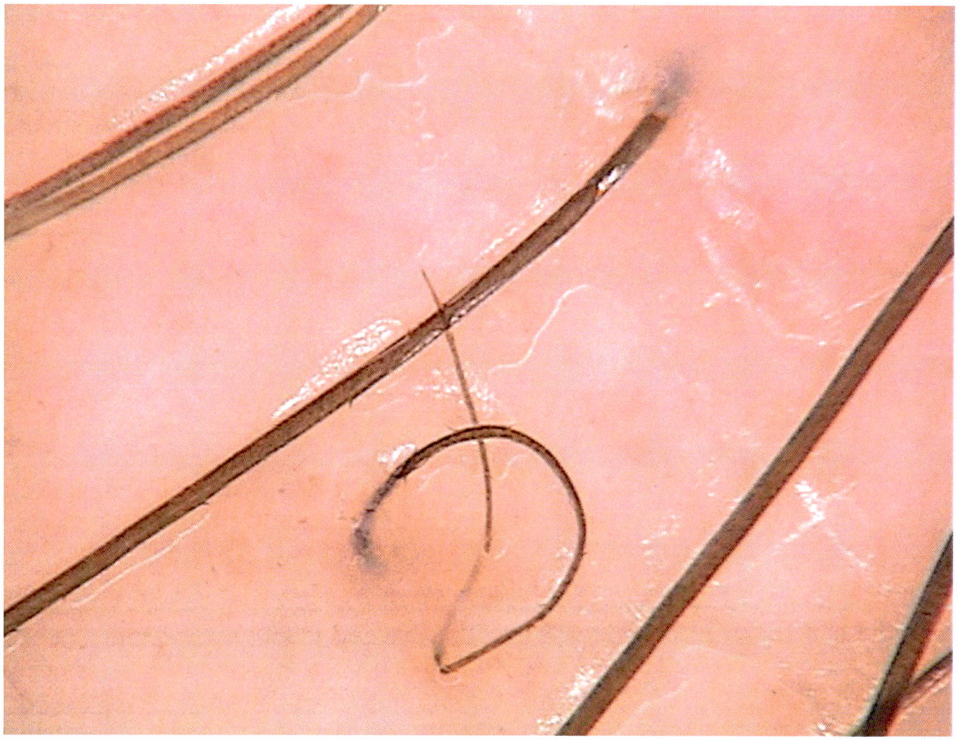

Fig. 2.58 Ingrowing scalp hairs in cicatricial alopecia. The image shows an ingrowing scalp hair curling, then penetrating the epidermis. An inflammatory reaction is visible at the site of the ingrowing hair. This indicates possible subjective discomfort for the patient as a result of ingrowing scalp hairs (×70)

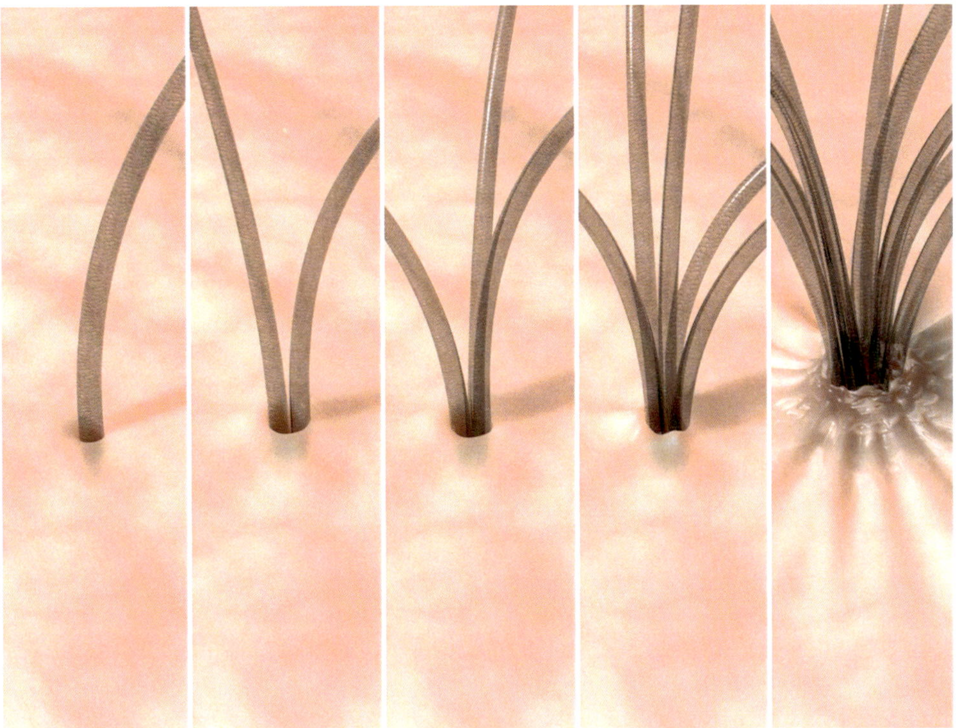

Fig. 2.59 **Number of hairs emerging from one follicular unit**. Usually, two to three hairs emerge from one follicular unit. Occasionally, four emerging hairs may be found, but this is more common in patients with dark skin phototypes than in Caucasians. The percentage of follicular units with only one emerging hair shaft is usually less than 30 % in healthy individuals. The number of hair shafts emerging from one follicular unit is *decreased* in various types of hair loss, especially telogen effluvium and androgenetic alopecia. The number of hairs in one follicular unit is *increased* in tufted folliculitis. The tufts may be small, with five to seven hairs; small tufts may be observed in inflammatory diseases such as tinea capitis and lichen planopilaris. Large tufts of ten or more hairs are characteristic of folliculitis decalvans; these tufts usually are walled by a wide, hyperkeratotic, scaly hair follicle opening (*Graphic by* Dr. Wawrzyniec Podrzucki)

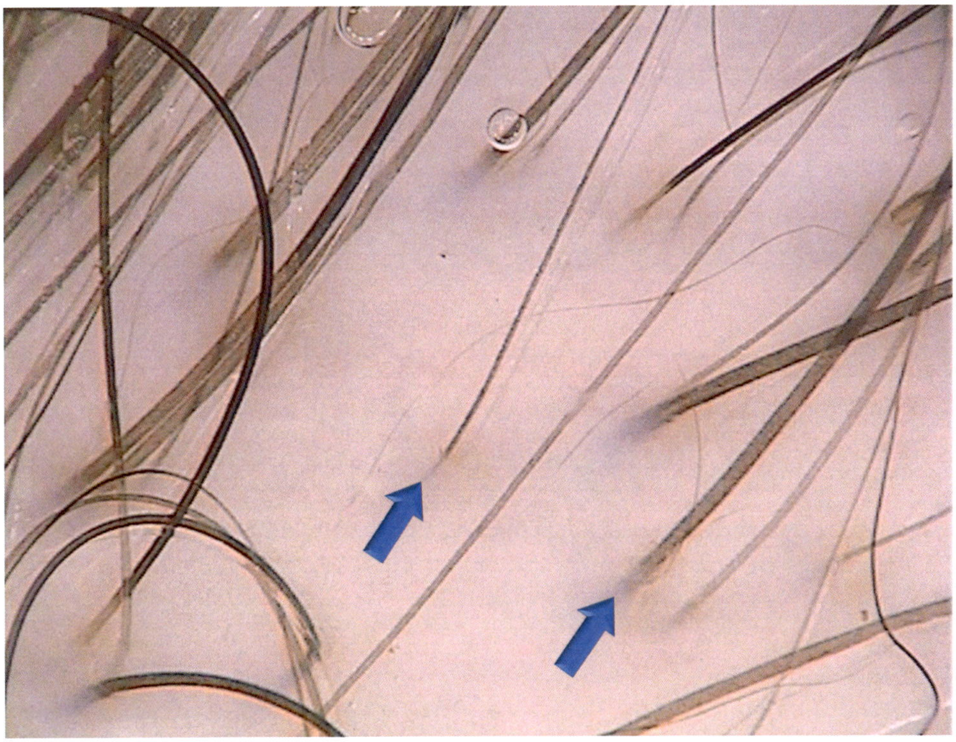

Fig. 2.60 **One hair per follicular unit in androgenetic alopecia**. In this trichoscopic image of a 42-year-old woman with female androgenetic alopecia, only one hair shaft emerges from most follicular units (single-hair units; *arrows*; ×70)

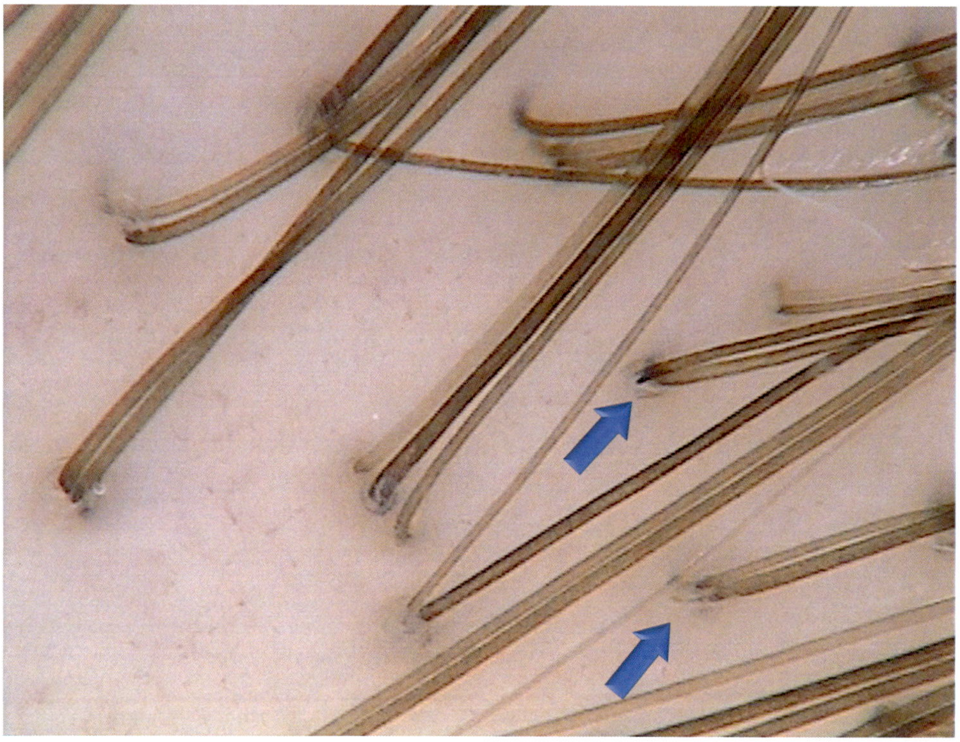

Fig. 2.61 Two hairs per follicular unit in a healthy individual. The number of hairs in a follicular unit varies from one to three in healthy persons. Shown is a trichoscopic image of a healthy person's scalp, in which two hairs emerge from most follicular units (two-hair units; *arrows*; ×70)

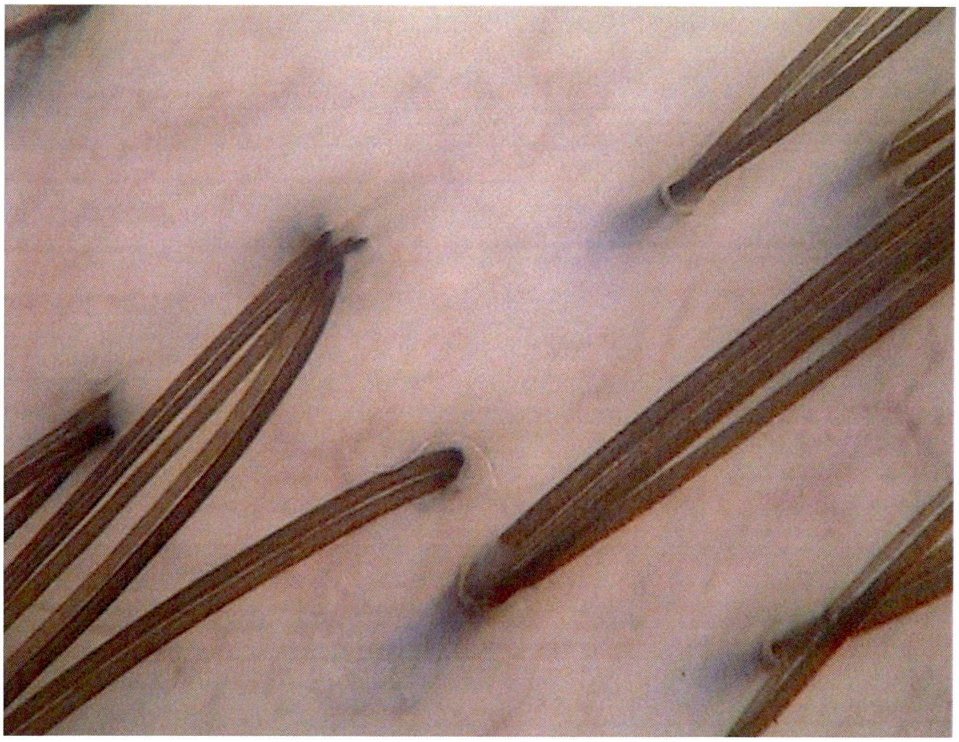

Fig. 2.62 Small hair tufts in lichen planopilaris. In this 56-year-old woman with lichen planopilaris, trichoscopy shows tufts of five to seven hairs. Some authors may consider this number borderline normal (×70)

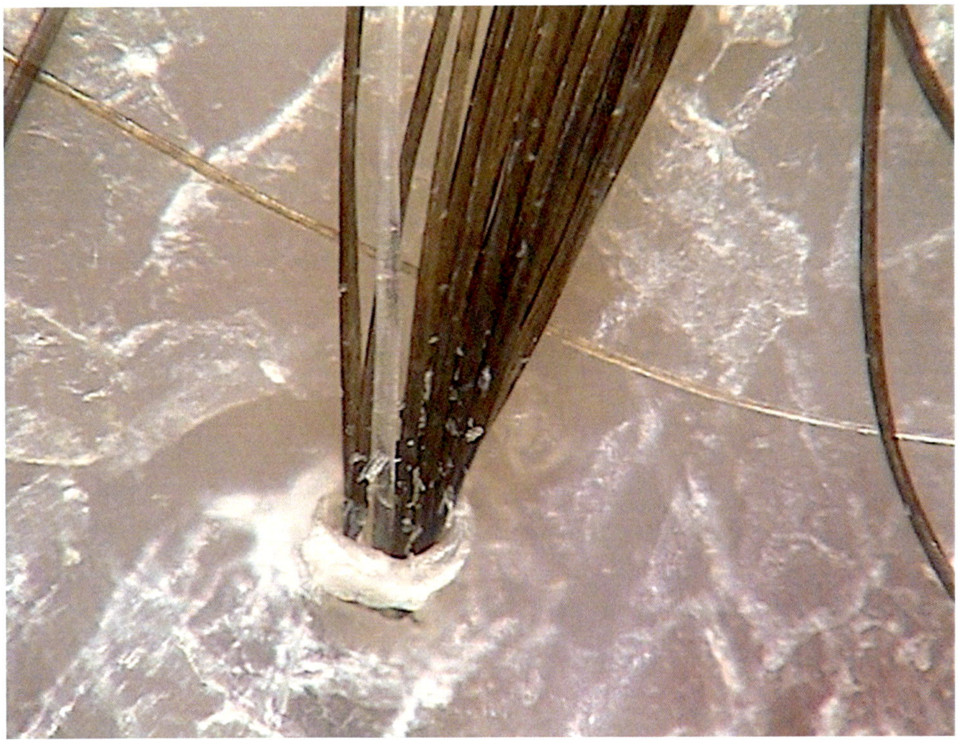

Fig. 2.63 Tufted hairs in folliculitis decalvans. Shown is a tuft containing more than 20 hairs in a 33-year-old man with folliculitis decalvans. The hair tuft is walled by a widened, hyperkeratotic, scaly hair follicle opening. Adjacent to this hair follicle opening is an area of scarring alopecia, with a complete loss of follicles (×70)

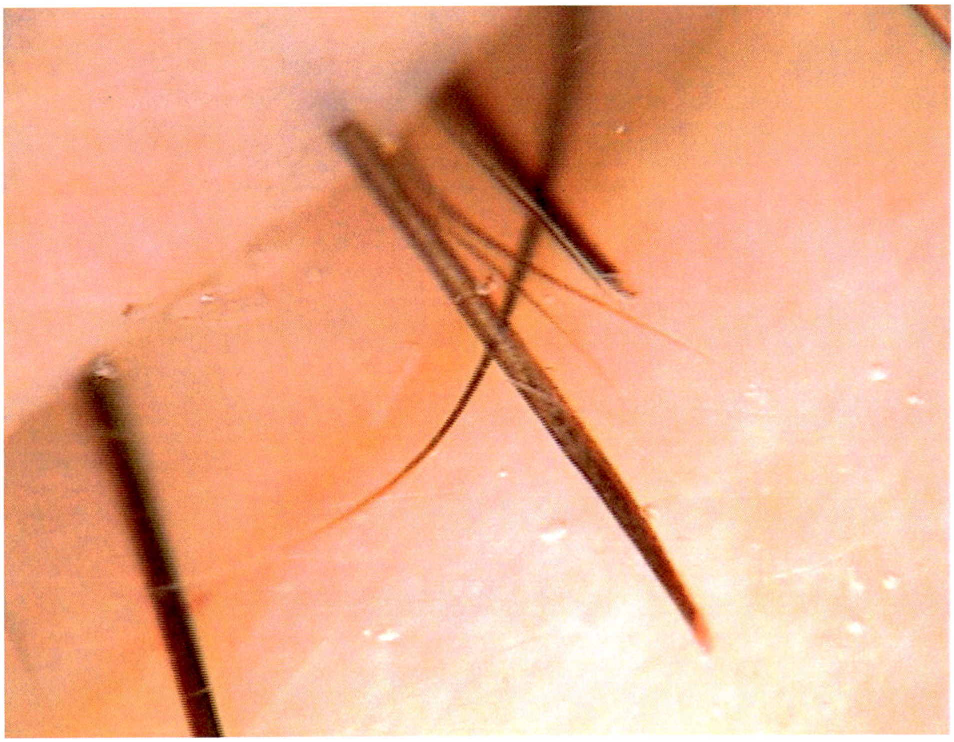

Fig. 2.64 Eyelashes. Eyebrows, eyelashes, and other body hair also may be evaluated with trichoscopy. Abnormalities evaluated trichoscopically thus far are described in the respective chapters. Shown here is a typical trichoscopic image of eyelashes. Trichoscopy was performed with 0.9 % NaCl as an immersion fluid. Special caution must be used in evaluating eyelashes to avoid touching the eye with the dermoscope lens (×70)

References

1. Rakowska A. Trichoscopy (hair and scalp videodermoscopy) in the healthy female. Method standardization and norms for measurable parameters. J Dermatol Case Rep. 2009;3(1):14–9.
2. Vogt A, McElwee KJ, Blume-Peytavi U. Biology of the hair follicle. In: Blume-Peytavi U, Tosti A, Whiting D, Trüeb R, editors. Hair; from basic science to clinical application. Berlin: Springer; 2008. p. 1–22.
3. Wagner R, Joekes I. Hair medulla morphology and mechanical properties. J Cosmet Sci. 2007;58(4):359–68.
4. Inui S, Nakajima T, Itami S. Scalp dermoscopy of androgenetic alopecia in Asian people. J Dermatol. 2009;36(2):82–5.
5. Van Neste D. Natural scalp hair regression in preclinical stages of male androgenetic alopecia and its reversal by finasteride. Skin Pharmacol Physiol. 2006;19(3):168–76.
6. Rakowska A, Slowinska M, Kowalska-Oledzka E, Olszewska M, Rudnicka L. Dermoscopy in female androgenic alopecia: method standardization and diagnostic criteria. Int J Trichol. 2009;1(2):123–30.
7. Rudnicka L, Olszewska M, Rakowska A, Kowalska-Oledzka E, Slowinska M. Trichoscopy: a new method for diagnosing hair loss. J Drugs Dermatol. 2008;7(7):651–4.
8. Shuster S. The coudability sign of alopecia areata: the real story. Clin Exp Dermatol. 2011;36(5):554–5.
9. Inui S, Nakajima T, Itami S. Coudability hairs: a revisited sign of alopecia areata assessed by trichoscopy. Clin Exp Dermatol. 2010; 35(4):361–5.
10. Slowinska M, Rudnicka L, Schwartz RA, Kowalska-Oledzka E, Rakowska A, Sicinska J, et al. Comma hairs: a dermatoscopic marker for tinea capitis: a rapid diagnostic method. J Am Acad Dermatol. 2008;59(5 Suppl):S77–9.
11. Sandoval AB, Ortiz JA, Rodriguez JM, Vargas AG, Quintero DG. Dermoscopic pattern in tinea capitis [in Spanish]. Rev Iberoam Micol. 2010;27(3):151–2.
12. Hughes R, Chiaverini C, Bahadoran P, Lacour JP. Corkscrew hair: a new dermoscopic sign for diagnosis of tinea capitis in black children. Arch Dermatol. 2011;147(3):355–6.
13. Rudnicka L, Olszewska M, Rakowska A, Slowinska M. Trichoscopy update 2011. J Dermatol Case Rep. 2011;5(4):82–8.
14. Adya KA, Inamadar AC, Palit A, Shivanna R, Deshmukh NS. Light microscopy of the hair: a simple tool to "untangle" hair disorders. Int J Trichol. 2011;3(1):46–56.
15. Rakowska A, Slowinska M, Kowalska-Oledzka E, Rudnicka L. Trichoscopy in genetic hair shaft abnormalities. J Dermatol Case Rep. 2008;2(2):14–20.
16. Yazdabadi A, Magee J, Harrison S, Sinclair R. The Ludwig pattern of androgenetic alopecia is due to a hierarchy of androgen sensitivity within follicular units that leads to selective miniaturization and a reduction in the number of terminal hairs per follicular unit. Br J Dermatol. 2008;159(6):1300–2.
17. Bentley-Phillips B, Bayles MA. A previously undescribed hereditary hair anomaly (pseudo-monilethrix). Br J Dermatol. 1973;89(2): 159–67.
18. Phillips BB, Bayles MA, Grace HJ. Pseudo-monilethrix: further family studies. Humangenetik. 1974;25(4):331–7.
19. Trueb RM. Pharmacologic interventions in aging hair. Clin Interv Aging. 2006;1(2):121–9.
20. de Berker DA, Paige DG, Ferguson DJ, Dawber RP. Golf tee hairs in Netherton disease. Pediatr Dermatol. 1995;12(1):7–11.
21. Ihm CW, Han JH. Diagnostic value of exclamation mark hairs. Dermatology. 1993;186(2):99–102.
22. Abramovits-Ackerman W, Bustos T, Simosa-Leon V, Fernandez L, Ramella M. Cutaneous findings in a new syndrome of autosomal recessive ectodermal dysplasia with corkscrew hairs. J Am Acad Dermatol. 1992;27(6 Pt 1):917–21.
23. Trueb R, Burg G, Bottani A, Schinzel A. Ectodermal dysplasia with corkscrew hairs: observation of probable autosomal dominant tricho-odonto-onychodysplasia with syndactyly. J Am Acad Dermatol. 1994;30(2 Pt 1):289–90.
24. Argenziano G, Monsurro MR, Pazienza R, Delfino M. A case of probable autosomal recessive ectodermal dysplasia with corkscrew hairs and mental retardation in a family with tuberous sclerosis. J Am Acad Dermatol. 1998;38(2 Pt 2):344–8.
25. Pozo L, Bowling J, Perrett CM, Bull R, Diaz-Cano SJ. Dermoscopy of trichostasis spinulosa. Arch Dermatol. 2008;144(8):1088.
26. Kirkwood BJ, Kirkwood RA. Trichiasis: characteristics and management options. Insight. 2011;36(2):5–9.
27. Chuh A, Zawar V. Epiluminescence dermatoscopy enhanced patient compliance and achieved treatment success in pseudofolliculitis barbae. Australas J Dermatol. 2006;47(1):60–2.

Hair Follicle Openings: Dots

3

Lidia Rudnicka, Malgorzata Olszewska, Adriana Rakowska, Monika Slowinska, Irena Walecka, Barbara Borkowska, and Marta Kurzeja

Abstract

The term *dots* refers to hair follicle openings seen from the perspective of a dermoscope. Black dots are residues of pigmented hairs broken or destroyed at scalp level. Yellow dots are follicular infundibula with keratotic material and/or sebum. Fibrotic white dots represent fibrosis in areas of selective follicular destruction. Pinpoint white dots are observed in patients with dark skin phototypes. They correspond to empty hair follicles or to the epidermal portion of eccrine sweat ducts. Red dots have been described in discoid lupus erythematosus. Pink to pink-brown dots are a characteristic finding in the eyebrow area of patients with frontal fibrosing alopecia.

Keywords

Alopecia areata • Alopecia areata incognita • Black dots • Cicatricial alopecia • Cutaneous lupus erythematosus • Discoid lupus erythematosus • Dissecting cellulitis • Eyebrows Lichen planopilaris • Trichomalacia • Trichotillomania • White dots • Yellow dots

The term *dots* initially was used to describe hair follicle openings seen from the perspective of a dermoscope lens. These hair follicle openings may have different features depending on the presence of hair shaft residues, follicular hyperkeratotic plugs, perifollicular fibrosis, inflammation, and other factors. Thus, terms such as *black dots*, *yellow dots*, and *white dots* were created [1]. Later studies showed that the spectrum of "dots" is wider than initially defined.

Black dots, formerly also called "cadaverized hairs," are residues of pigmented hairs broken or destroyed at scalp level [1]. They are observed in about 50 % of patients with alopecia areata and positively correlate with disease activity [2]. The presence of multiple black dots in alopecia areata is a negative prognostic factor. The histopathology of black dots in alopecia areata shows follicular damage at the level of the infundibulum, and the presence of dysmorphic hair shafts with irregular pigmentation. Black dots also are common in dissecting cellulitis, tinea capitis, chemotherapy-induced alopecia, and trichotillomania, but also may be observed incidentally in other diseases [3–5]. Black dots are not present in healthy individuals or in patients with androgenetic alopecia and telogen effluvium [6, 7].

Yellow dots are follicular infundibula with keratotic material and/or sebum [1, 4, 8]. They vary in color, shape, and size. Individual dots are uniform in color or possess an inner structure. Yellow dots usually lack hair shafts but may contain dystrophic or vellus hairs. Regularly distributed -yellow dots are present in over 60 % of patients with alopecia areata and are considered a marker of disease severity [2]. Large dark yellow to brownish yellow dots are characteristic

L. Rudnicka (✉)
Faculty of Health Sciences, Medical University of Warsaw, Poland

Department of Dermatology, CSK MSW, Woloska 137, Warsaw 02-502, Poland
e-mail: lidia.rudnicka@euderm.eu

M. Olszewska
Department of Dermatology, Medical University of Warsaw, Warsaw, Poland

A. Rakowska • M. Slowinska • I. Walecka
B. Borkowska • M. Kurzeja
Department of Dermatology, CSK MSW, Warsaw, Poland

L. Rudnicka et al. (eds.), *Atlas of Trichoscopy*,
DOI 10.1007/978-1-4471-4486-1_3, © Springer-Verlag London 2012

of discoid lupus erythematosus and correspond to wide infundibula filled with keratotic material [4]. Yellow dots also are observed in patients with androgenetic alopecia. They consist mainly of sebum, which is excreted to the scalp surface by intact sebaceous glands in the absence of terminal hairs [7]. The predominance of yellow dots in the frontal area compared with the occipital area favors the diagnosis of (female) androgenetic alopecia [7]. Yellow dots resembling large "three-dimensional (3D)" soap bubbles imposed over dark dystrophic hairs are specific for dissecting cellulitis.

There are two main variants of white dots. Fibrotic white dots represent fibrosis in areas of selective follicular destruction. These dots are observed in primary, folliculocentric cicatricial alopecia, most commonly in lichen planopilaris [1, 4]. In advanced primary scarring alopecia, white dots become confluent and form white areas lacking follicular openings. Another type of white dot is the pinpoint white dot. These white dots are observed in patients with Fitzpatrick skin phototypes IV, V, and VI [9, 10]. These small, regular white dots, occasionally with a hyperpigmented halo, correspond to empty hair follicles or to the epidermal portion of eccrine sweat ducts. They are visible on the contrasting background of the pigment network. These pinpoint white dots are observed in most diseases causing hair loss, as well as in healthy individuals.

Red dots have been described in discoid lupus erythematosus and are believed to be a positive prognostic factor indicating possible hair regrowth [11].

Regularly distributed pink to pink-brown dots are a characteristic finding in the eyebrow area of patients with frontal fibrosing alopecia. This finding also is a favorable prognostic factor because it indicates possible eyebrow regrowth.

Table 3.1 Black dots in trichoscopy

Common	Rare
Alopecia areata (acute)	Alopecia areata (long-lasting, nonactive)
Dissecting cellulitis (acute)	Dissecting cellulitis (nonactive)
Tinea capitis	Monilethrix
Trichotillomania	Chemotherapy-induced alopecia
	Aplasia cutis congenita
	Traction alopecia
	After trichogram
	After laser depilation

Table 3.2 Yellow dots in trichoscopy

Disease	Characteristics
Alopecia areata	Regularly distributed
	Small to medium size
	Keratotic plugs
	May appear rough with dry dermoscopy
Discoid lupus erythematosus	Sparse
	Large
	Keratotic plugs
	Dark yellow or yellow-brown
	Double margin may be visible at higher magnifications
Androgenetic alopecia	Irregular distribution
	Small to medium size
	Contain mainly sebum
	Predominantly present in the frontal area
	The number may decrease after intense hair washing
Dissecting cellulitis	Large
	"3D" soap bubbles imposed over dark dystrophic hairs

Table 3.3 White dots in trichoscopy

Disease	Characteristics
Fibrotic white dots	Irregular, round, oval, or polygonal, with tendency to become confluent
Cicatricial alopecia (most commonly lichen planopilaris)	Various sizes
	Present mainly close to the hair-bearing margin of a patch of alopecia
Pinpoint white dots	Small
Healthy individuals with skin phototype IV, V, or VI, or in people with sun-exposed skin	Round
	Regular
	Occasionally hyperpigmented at the border

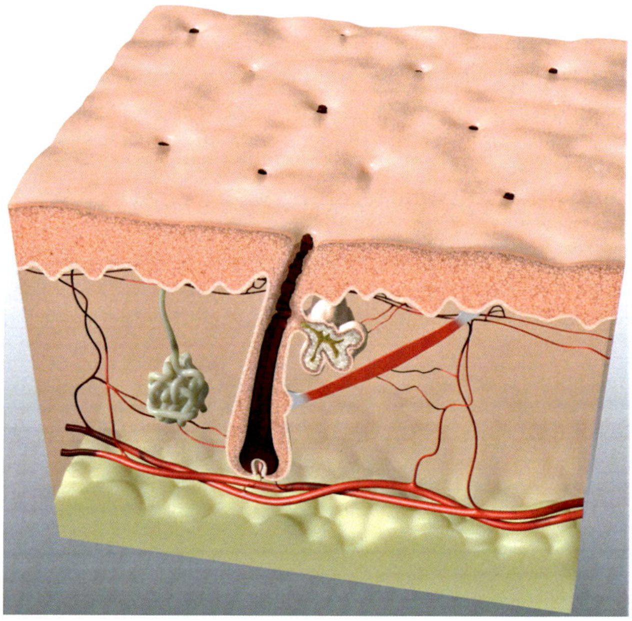

Fig. 3.1 **Black dots**. Black dots are residues of pigmented hairs broken or destroyed at scalp level. They are observed in alopecia areata, trichotillomania, traction alopecia, tinea capitis, chemotherapy-induced alopecia, and incidentally in other diseases. Black dots are not present in healthy individuals or in patients with androgenetic alopecia or telogen effluvium (*Graphic by* Dr. Wawrzyniec Podrzucki)

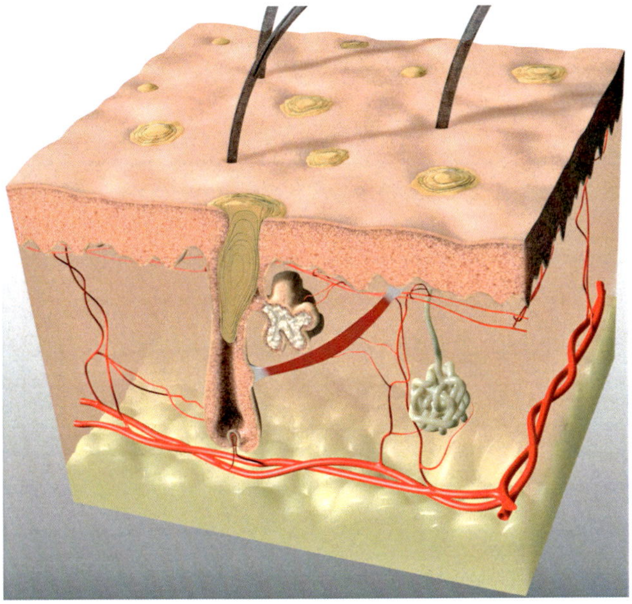

Fig. 3.2 Yellow dots (keratotic). Yellow dots result from keratotic follicular plugs in hair follicle openings. They vary in color, shape, and size. We have formulated a hypothesis [4, 7] that all yellow dots contain keratotic material and sebum. Sebum is responsible for the yellowness of these dots. The appearance of yellow dots depends on the predominance of keratotic material (keratotic yellow dot) or sebum (sebaceous yellow dot). Empty hair follicles (i.e., during the exogen phase of the normal hair cycle) may not be distinguishable from small yellow dots, because they usually contain some keratosebaceous material. The presence of multiple yellow dots or abnormally large yellow dots may be indicative of the diseases listed in Table 3.2 (*Graphic by* Dr. Wawrzyniec Podrzucki)

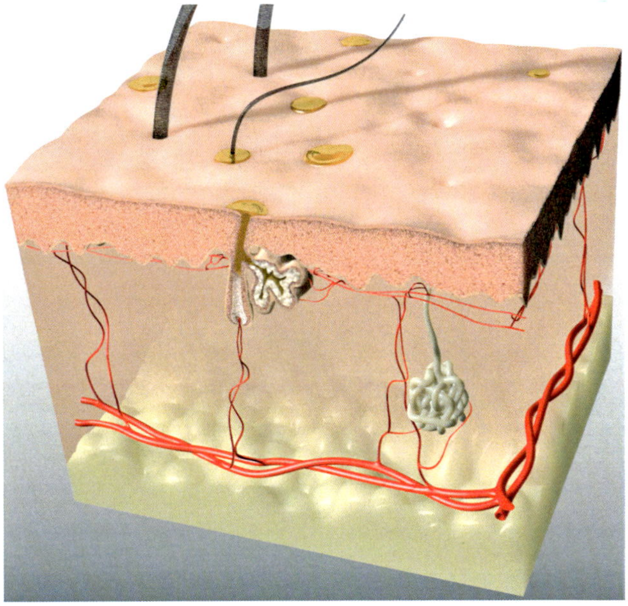

Fig. 3.3 Yellow dots (sebaceous). In androgenetic alopecia, yellow dots contain predominantly sebum mixed with variable amounts of keratotic material. To understand how these yellow dots develop, it is essential to recall that in healthy individuals, sebum is secreted from sebaceous glands along the hair shaft and remains partly attached to the hair as it grows. In androgenetic alopecia, the hair shaft is miniaturized but the sebaceous gland remains active. Sebum is secreted through the miniaturized hair follicle directly to the skin surface. Excessive sebum accumulates at the top of the hair follicle opening, forming a yellow dot. Yellow dots may contain vellus hairs (*Graphic by* Dr. Wawrzyniec Podrzucki)

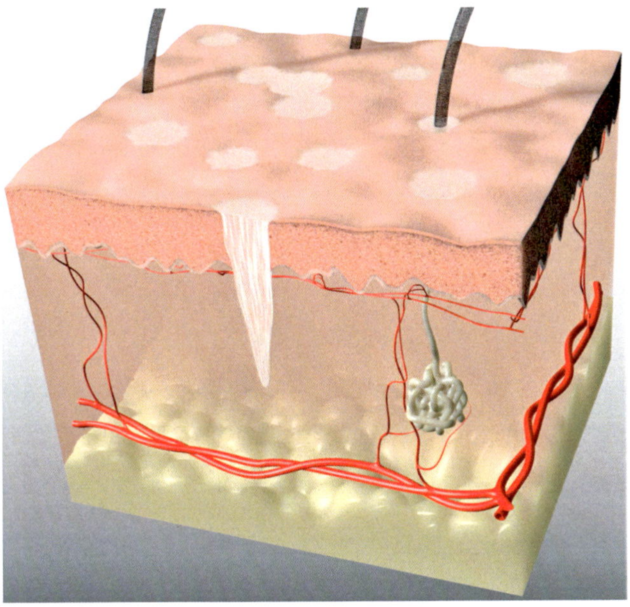

Fig. 3.4 White dots (fibrotic). Fibrotic white dots are observed most frequently in the end stage of lichen planopilaris. This is the trichoscopic manifestation of the longitudinal wedge-shaped tracts of fibrosis, which replace the hair follicles and perifollicular area destroyed by the inflammatory process. Fibrotic white dots may vary in size and shape depending on the extent of fibrosis, but they generally are significantly larger than the average hair follicle opening. White dots become confluent and form white areas of cicatricial alopecia. Some white dots may contain hair shafts, which reflect fibrosis of the perifollicular area in the pre-final stage of follicular destruction. Some authors call these dots *classic white dots* because they were described first (*Graphic by* Dr. Wawrzyniec Podrzucki)

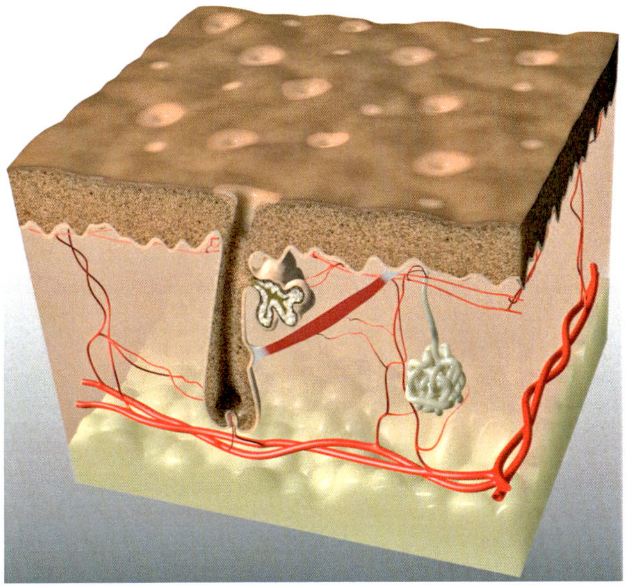

Fig. 3.5 White dots (pinpoint). Pinpoint white dots are observed on sun-exposed skin and in individuals with dark skin phototypes. They correspond to empty hair follicle openings and to the epidermal portion of eccrine sweat ducts. They are visible as white dots on the contrasting background of the pigment network. These pinpoint white dots are observed in most forms of noncicatricial hair loss and in healthy individuals. They have a very regular, circular appearance, often with slight hyperpigmentation at the periphery (*Graphic by* Dr. Wawrzyniec Podrzucki)

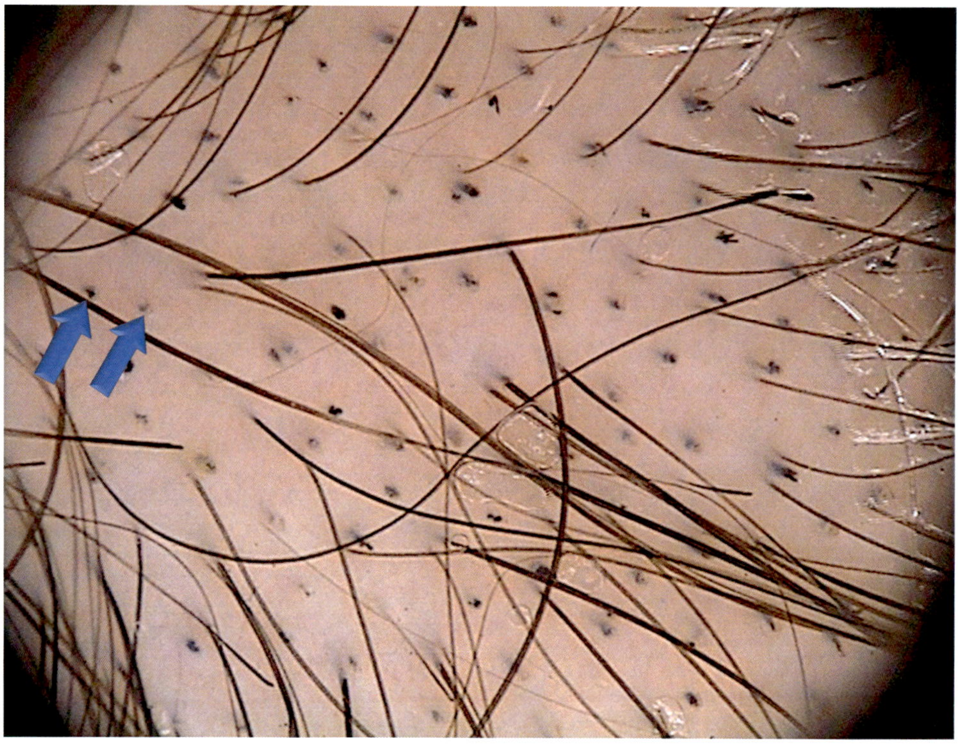

Fig. 3.6 Black dots in alopecia areata. Multiple monomorphic black dots (*arrows*) are characteristic of active alopecia areata. This feature is a negative prognostic factor indicating probable enlargement of alopecia areata patches (×20)

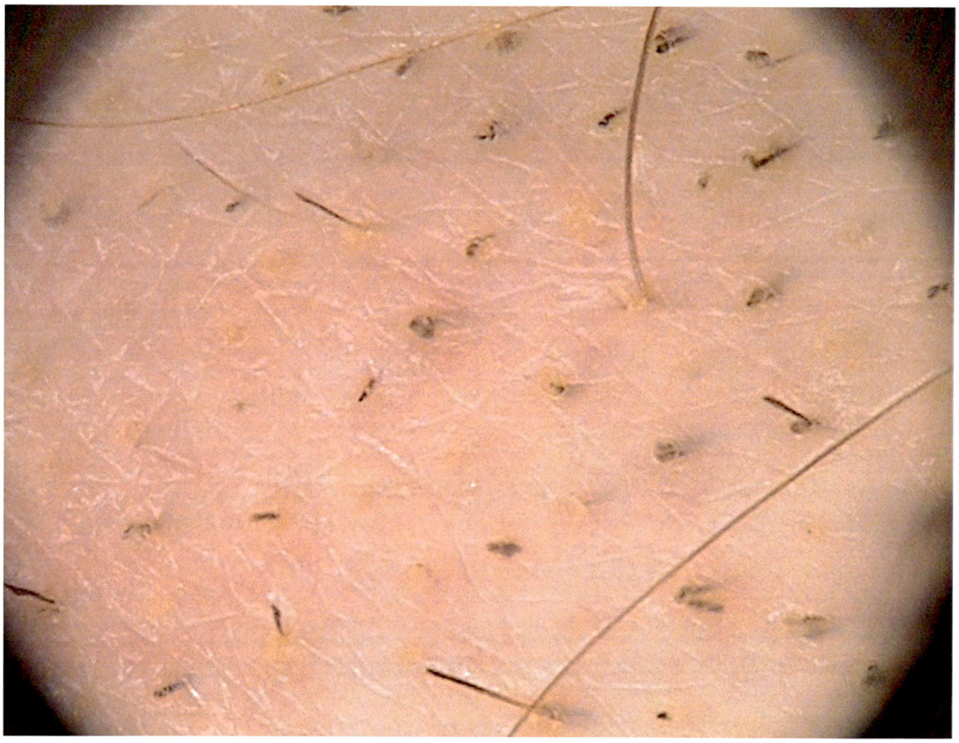

Fig. 3.7 Black dots in alopecia areata. Shown is a characteristic trichoscopic picture of long-lasting alopecia areata with a recent increase in activity. Black dots are accompanied by broken hairs, exclamation mark hairs, and multiple regularly distributed yellow dots (dry trichoscopy; ×20)

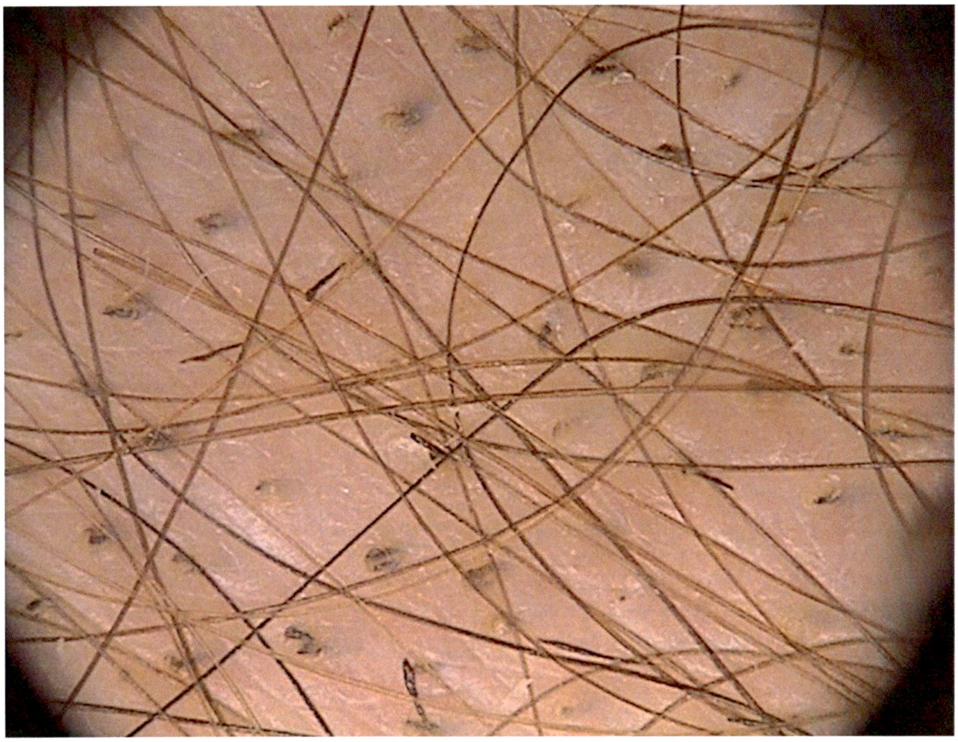

Fig. 3.8 Black dots in alopecia areata. Black dots occasionally may be seen as hair residues visible through the overlying epidermis, like most of the black dots in this image. In these cases especially, trichotillomania must be considered as a differential diagnosis (×20)

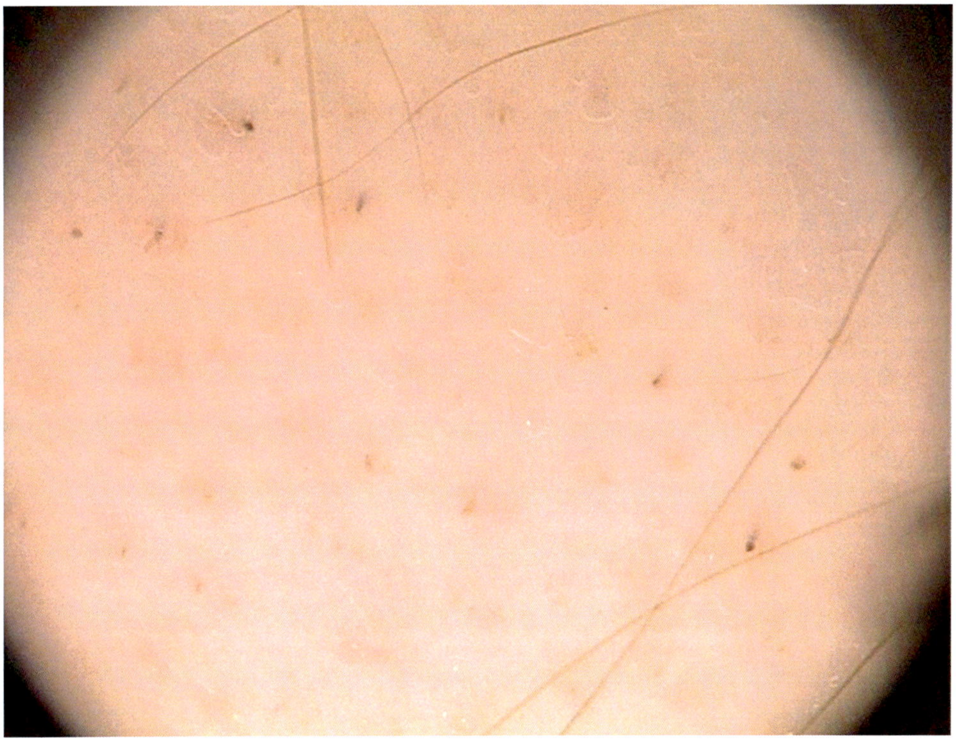

Fig. 3.9 Black dots in alopecia areata. Only a few black dots are seen in this image. The dominating feature here is the presence of yellow dots, which are most typical in nonactive, old patches of alopecia areata (×20)

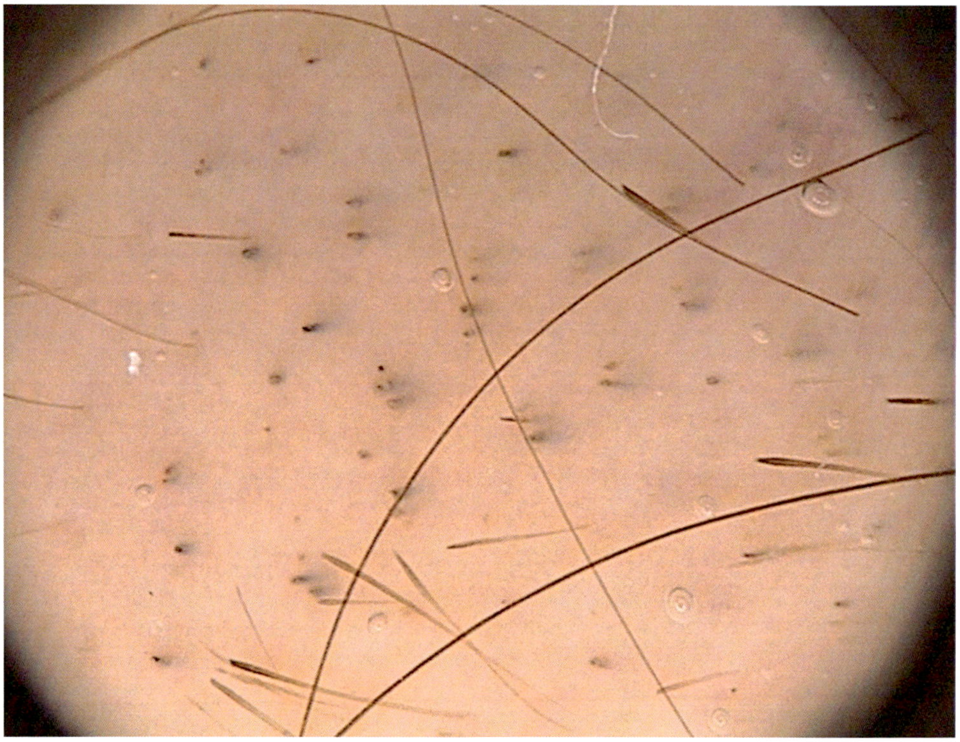

Fig. 3.10 Black dots in alopecia areata. Black dots seen together with multiple exclamation mark hairs indicate an ongoing process of active alopecia areata. The black dots are of various sizes and appear in groups of two or three, which shows that all hairs in one follicular unit are affected by the disease (×20)

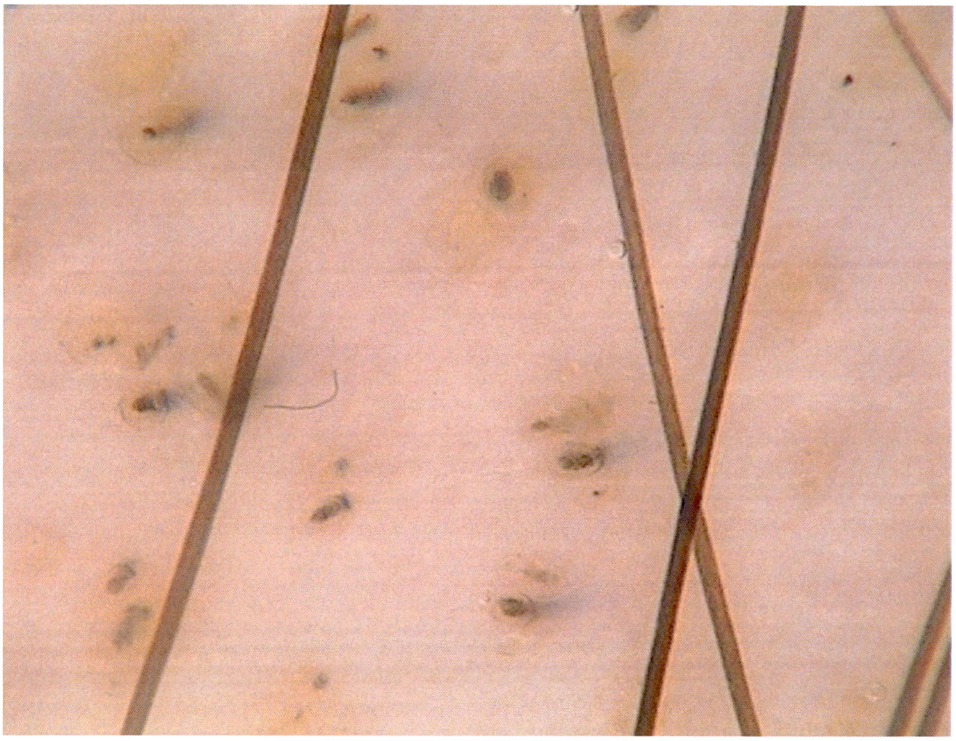

Fig. 3.11 Black dots in alopecia areata. High magnifications reveal that black dots are fragments of hairs broken at the level of the epidermis. Some of them are localized within yellow dots. Single yellow dots also are visible. Differential diagnoses in these images of multiple black dots include alopecia areata and trichotillomania. The presence of yellow dots favors the diagnosis of alopecia areata rather than trichotillomania, because yellow dots are rare in trichotillomania. Another factor contributing to the diagnosis of alopecia areata is the regular, uniform appearance of the black dots (×70)

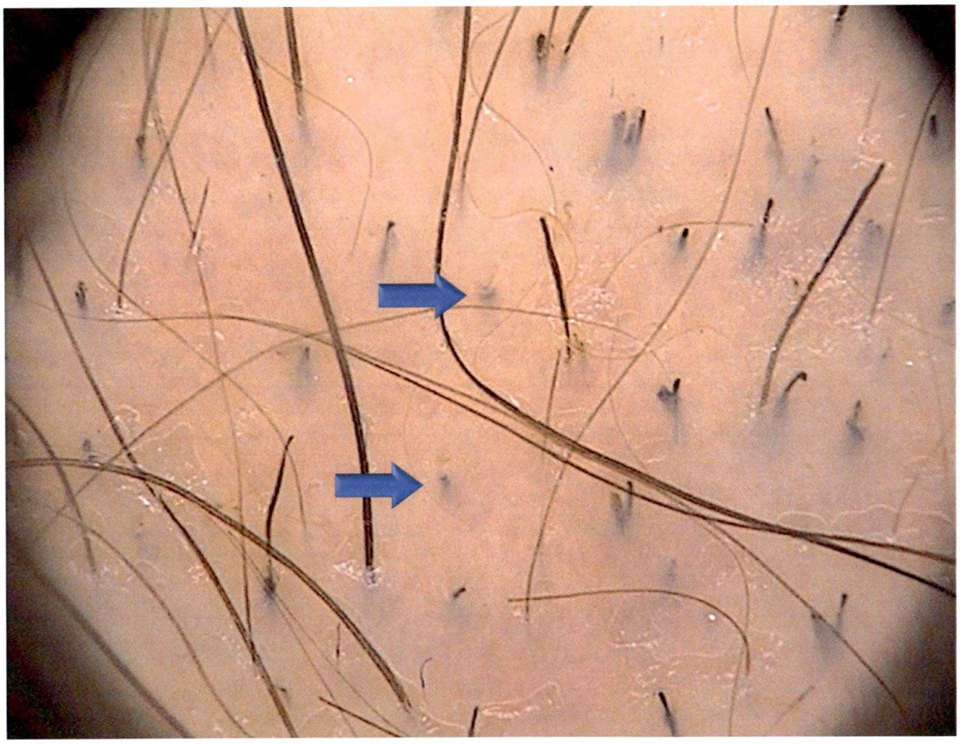

Fig. 3.12 Black dots in trichotillomania. Black dots (*arrows*) are visible in a patient with trichotillomania. Also seen are other features confirming the diagnosis: broken hairs, coiled hair, and the v-sign. This generally chaotic trichoscopic picture is one of the hallmarks of trichotillomania (×20)

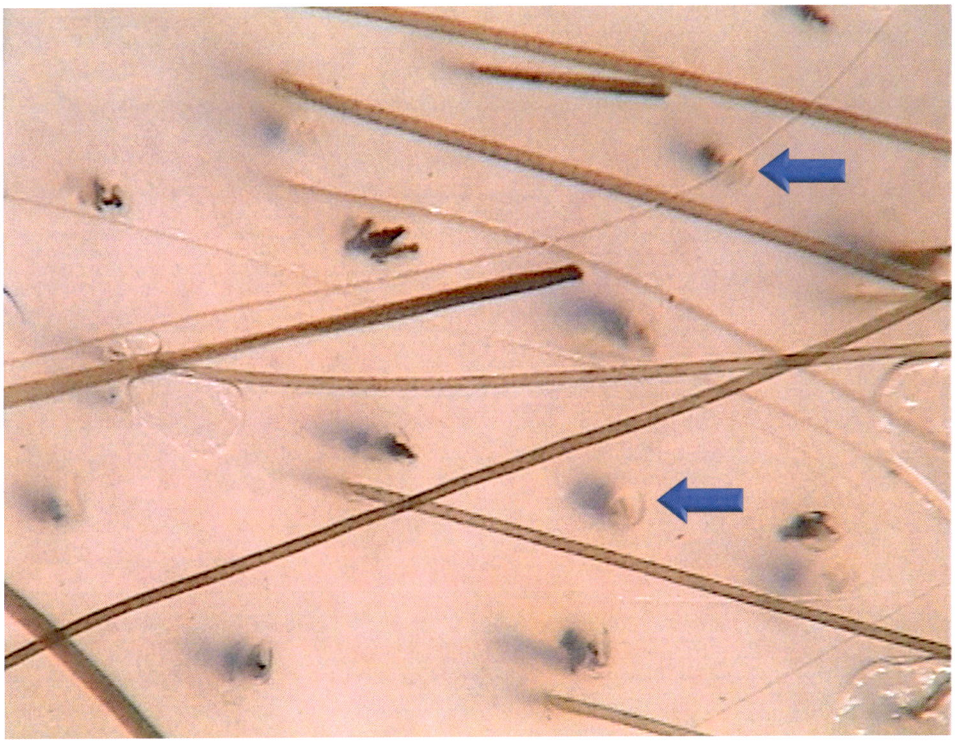

Fig. 3.13 Black dots in trichotillomania. This image reveals heterogeneity in the black dots, which is characteristic of trichotillomania rather than alopecia areata. Some black dots have a subtle translucent halo (*arrows*), which must be distinguished from yellow dots (*see* Fig. 3.11) (×70)

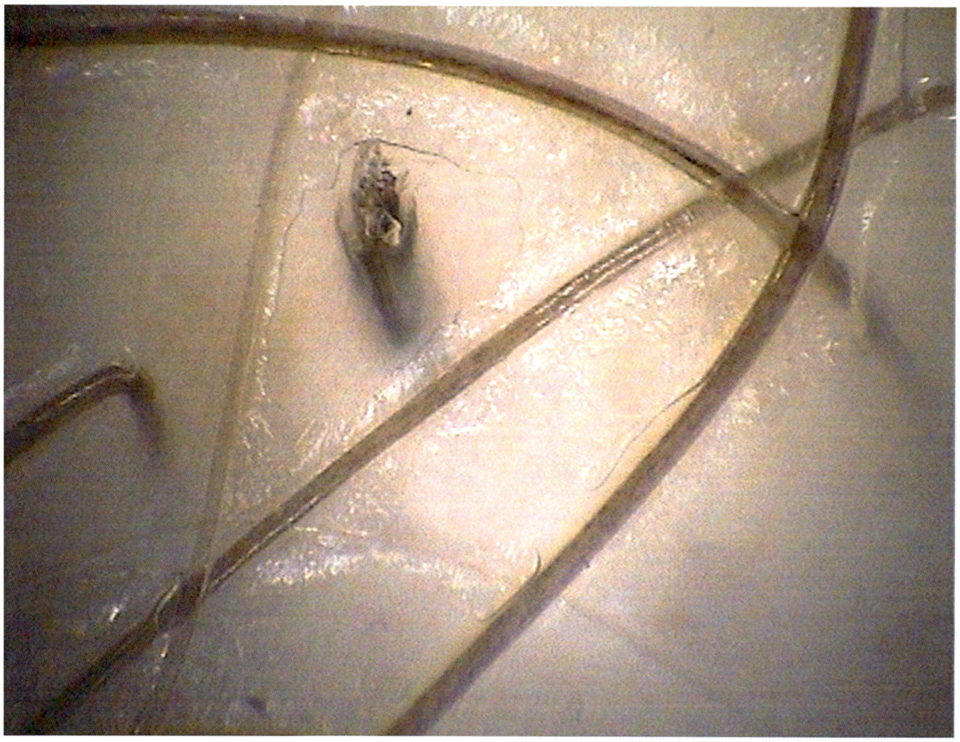

Fig. 3.14 Black dots in trichotillomania. High-magnification trichoscopy shows details of a black dot in trichotillomania. A short hair, fractured at the level of the epidermis, shows irregular, jagged split ends, which result from mechanical injury (×160)

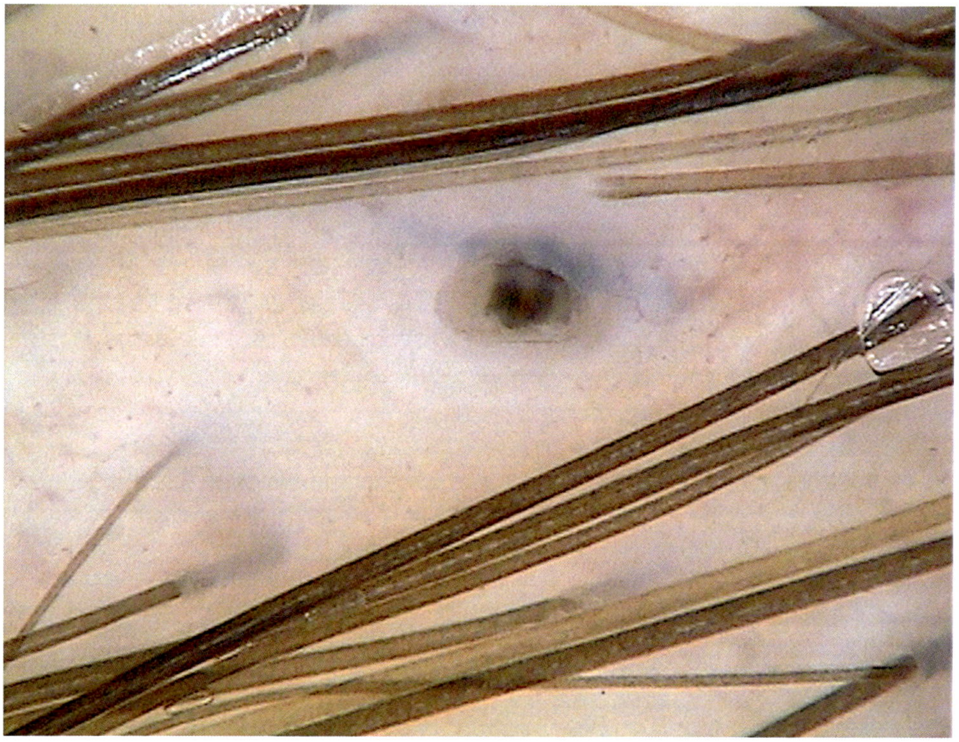

Fig. 3.15 Black dots in trichomalacia. Trichomalacia (incompletely keratinized, soft, distorted, and pigmented hair shafts) appears on trichoscopy as large, bulging black dots. Its most frequent cause is physical injury, but trichomalacia in the course of alopecia areata also has been observed [12] (×70)

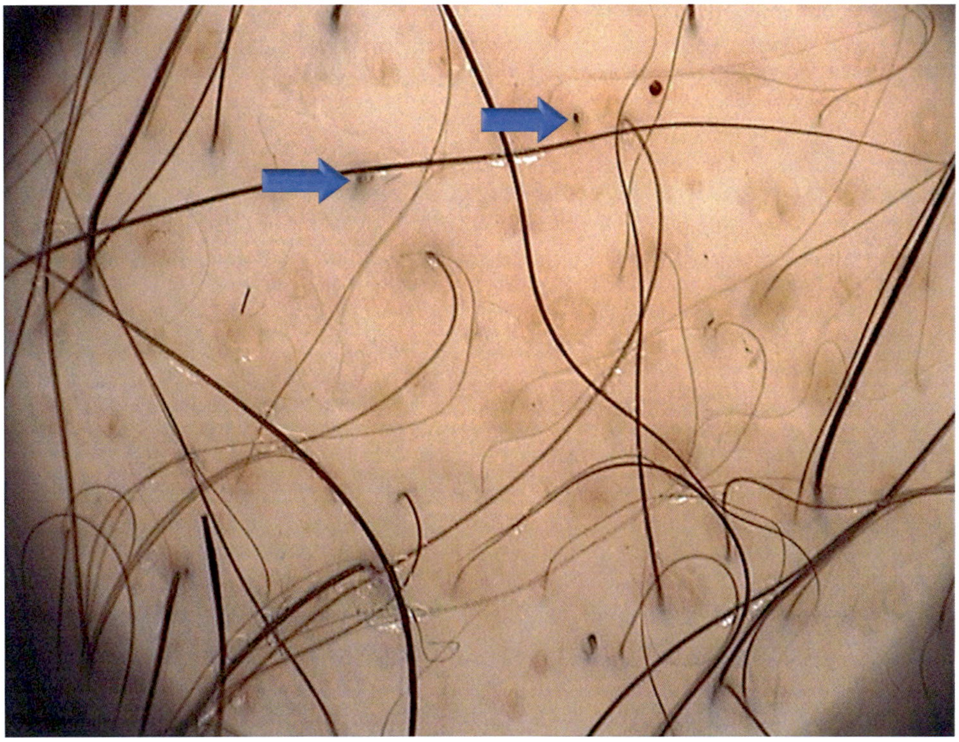

Fig. 3.16 Black dots in congenital hypotrichosis. Black dots are absent in most cases of congenital hypotrichosis. This image shows black dots (*arrows*), yellow dots, hair shaft structural abnormalities, and decreased hair density in a patient with unclassified congenital hypotrichosis (×20)

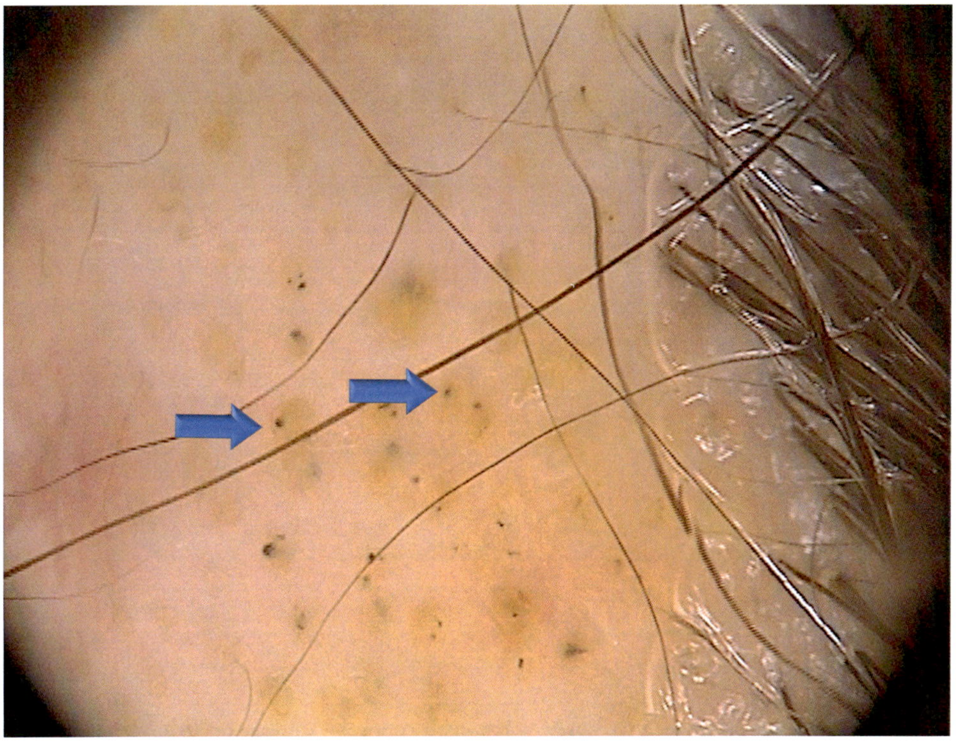

Fig. 3.17 Black dots in dissecting cellulitis. The periphery of the path of alopecia reveals multiple yellow dots with black dots inside (*arrows*). Most of these yellow dots appear as 3D soap bubbles containing hair residues (×20)

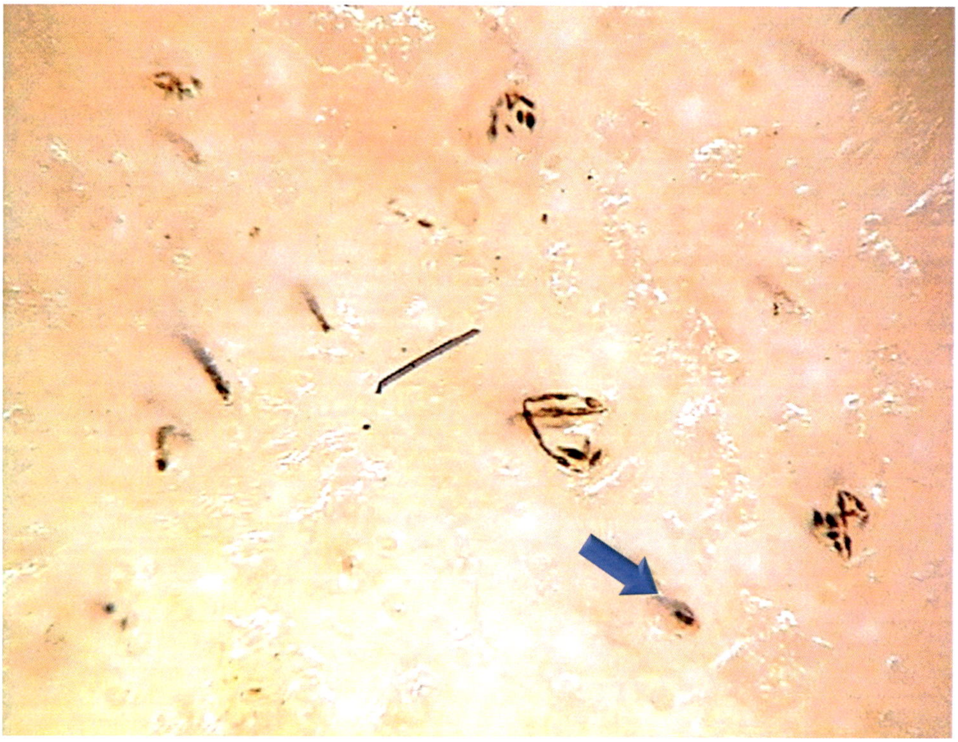

Fig. 3.18 Black dots in monilethrix and monilethrix-like congenital hypotrichosis. Black dots (*arrow*) develop in monilethrix and monilethrix-like disorders as a result of hair fractures in the internodes (constrictions), which are extremely sensitive to mechanical injury. In this patient with monilethrix-like congenital hypotrichosis, few black dots are visible. Note that the small, grouped nodes may be mistaken for black dots, especially at a lower magnification (×70)

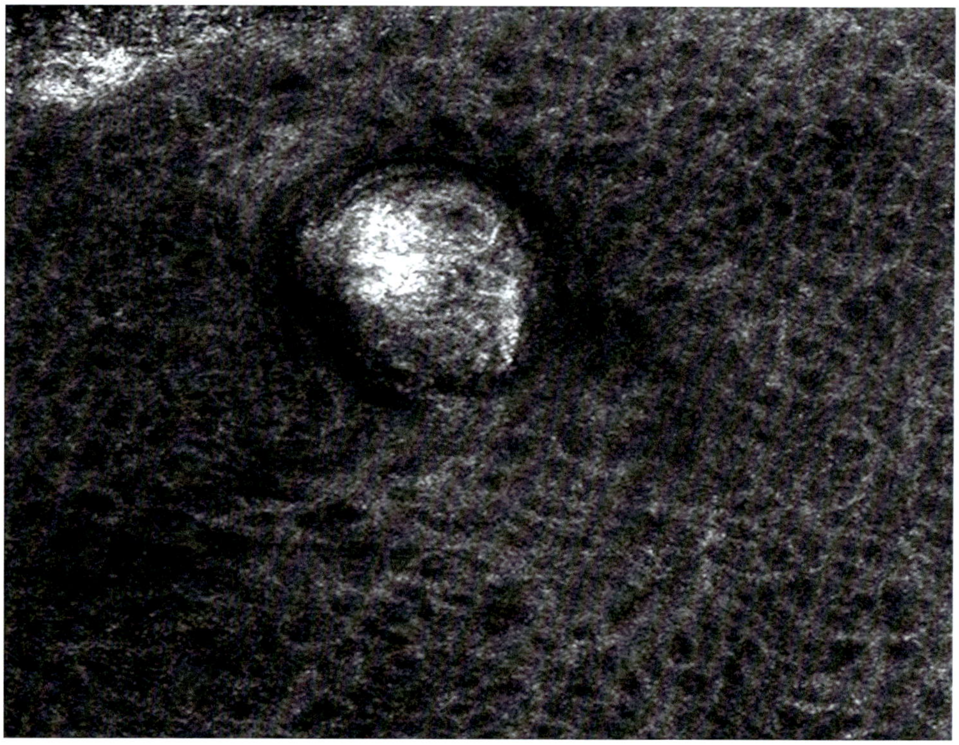

Fig. 3.19 Black dot on reflectance confocal microscopy. On reflectance confocal microscopy, black dots appear as hyperechogenic (*white*) round to oval structures that densely fill the hair follicle opening

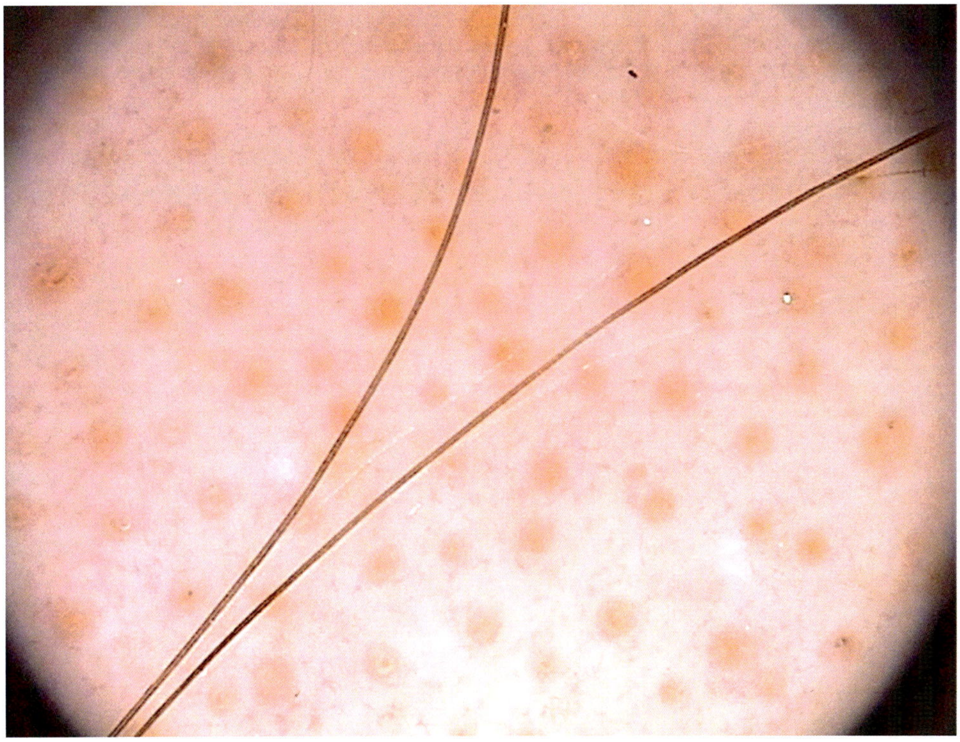

Fig. 3.20 Yellow dots in alopecia areata. This trichoscopic image reveals many yellow dots in place of follicular openings. They are regularly distributed, are homogeneous in size, and have a "double border." In some of them, residues of hair shafts are visible. This is a typical image of severe, long-lasting alopecia areata (×20)

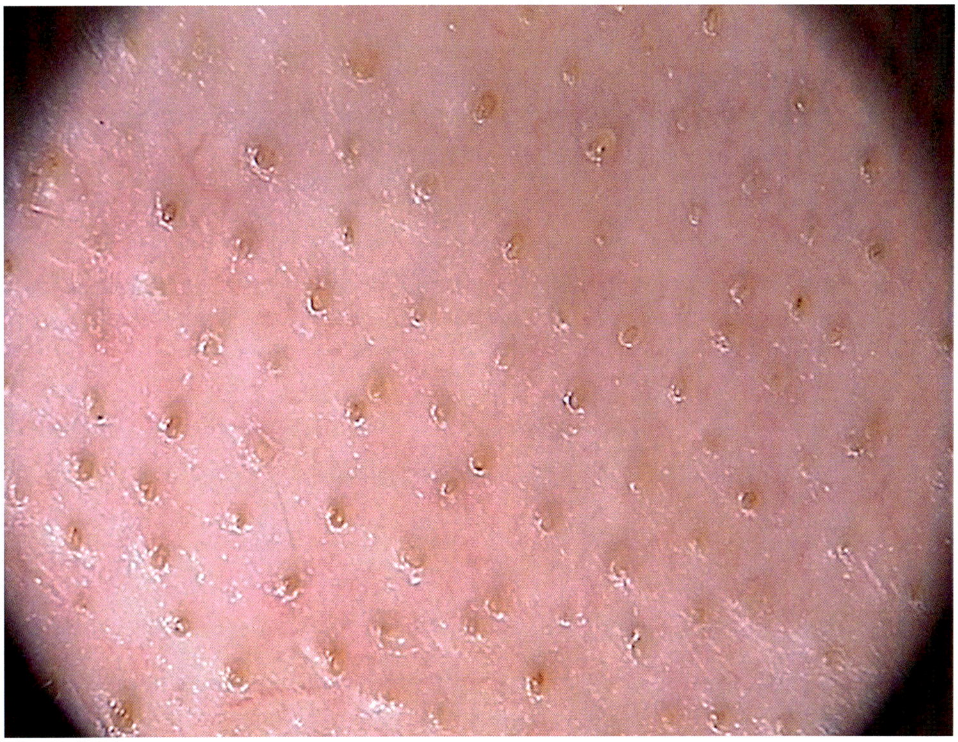

Fig. 3.21 Yellow dots in alopecia areata. Multiple regularly distributed, protruding yellow dots. The whitish halo surrounding the dots is an optical effect resulting from the use of a small amount of immersion fluid. Each yellow dot is roofed by a small air bubble that reflects light (×20)

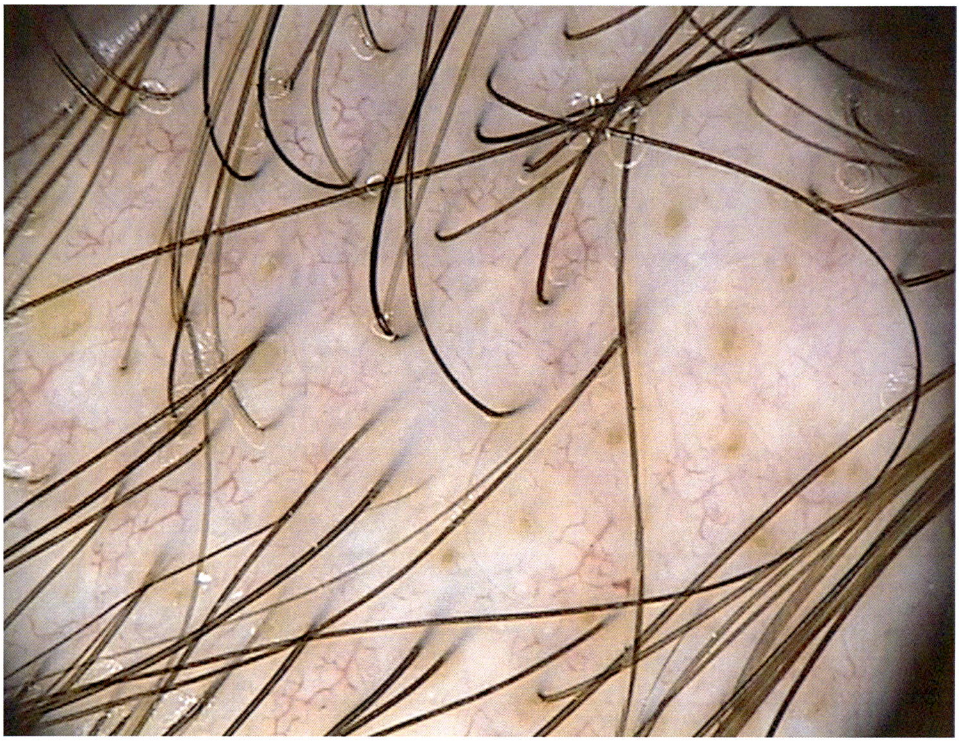

Fig. 3.22 Yellow dots in alopecia areata. Shown is a nonactive patch of alopecia areata. Between normal-looking follicular units, some yellow dots are visible. Note that the distribution of yellow dots is still comparable with that of total alopecia (*see* Fig. 3.23) (×20)

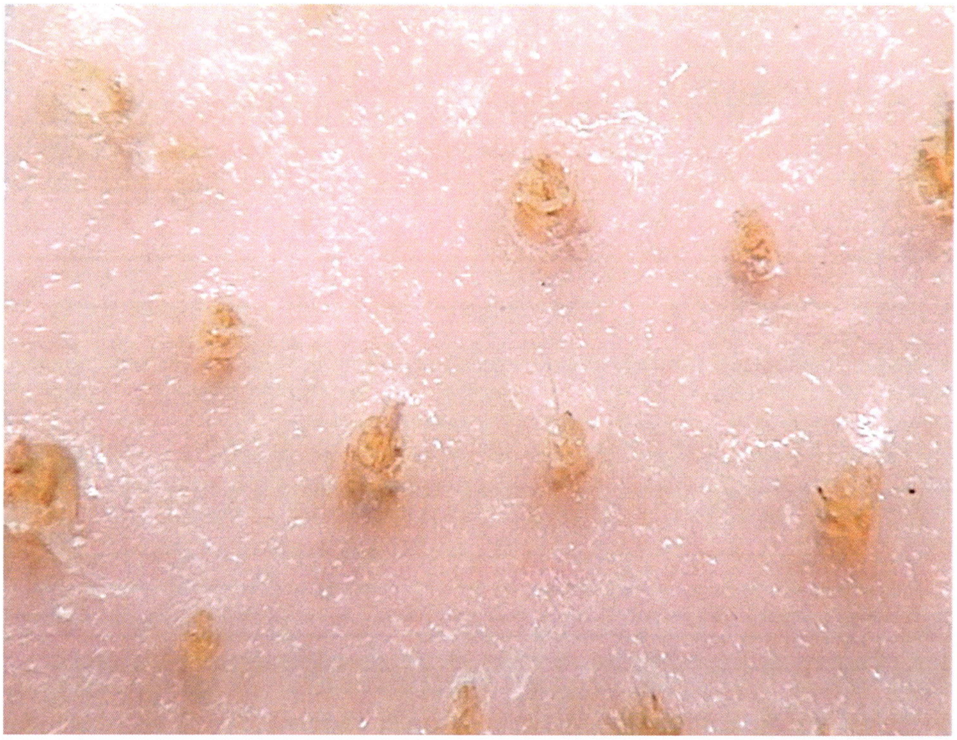

Fig. 3.23 Yellow dots in alopecia areata. This dry trichoscopic image reveals the keratotic nature of yellow dots, which cannot be observed with immersion fluid. Note the regular distribution of the keratotic yellow plugs, which corresponds to the distribution of hair follicle openings (×70)

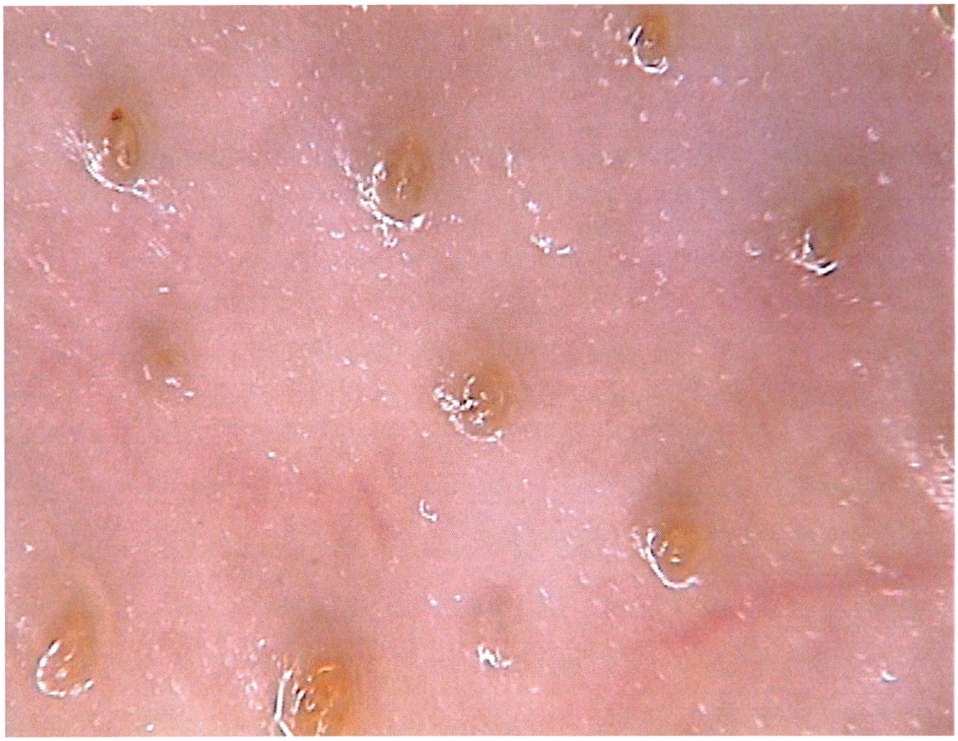

Fig. 3.24 Yellow dots in alopecia areata. This image is from the patient in Fig. 3.23. The keratotic nature of the dots cannot be appreciated. Yellow dots are visible as protruding yellow structures. White light reflection results from the air bubbles surrounding the dots (×70)

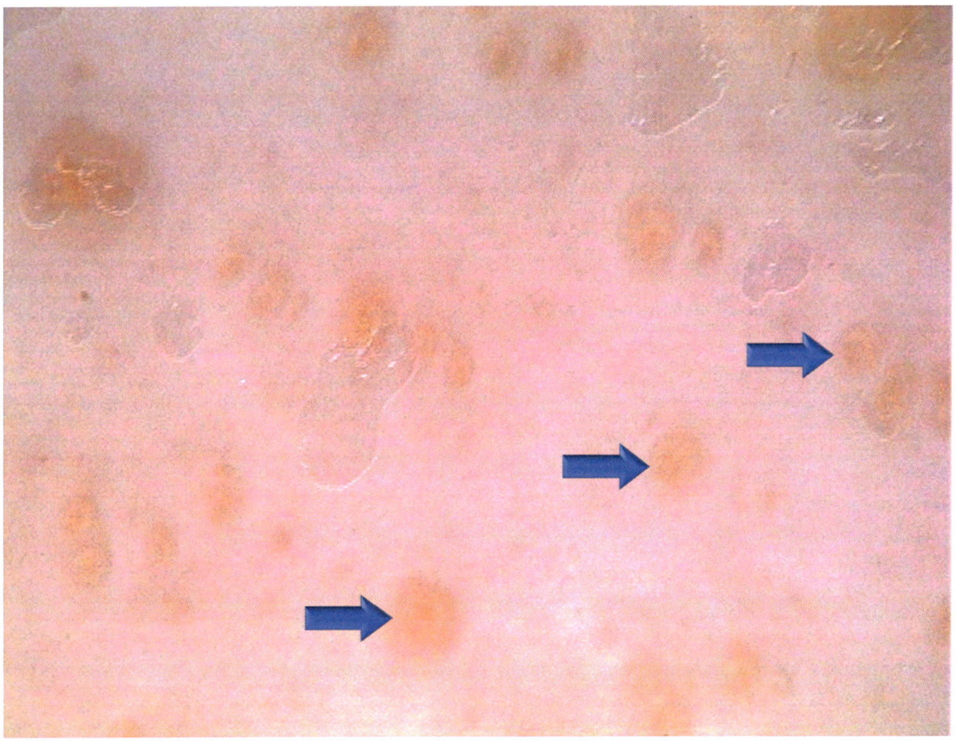

Fig. 3.25 Yellow dots in alopecia areata. Yellow dots are seen clustered into groups of two or three, corresponding to the number of hair shafts in one follicular unit. Yellow dots may show a double margin, as presented in this image (*arrows*) (×70)

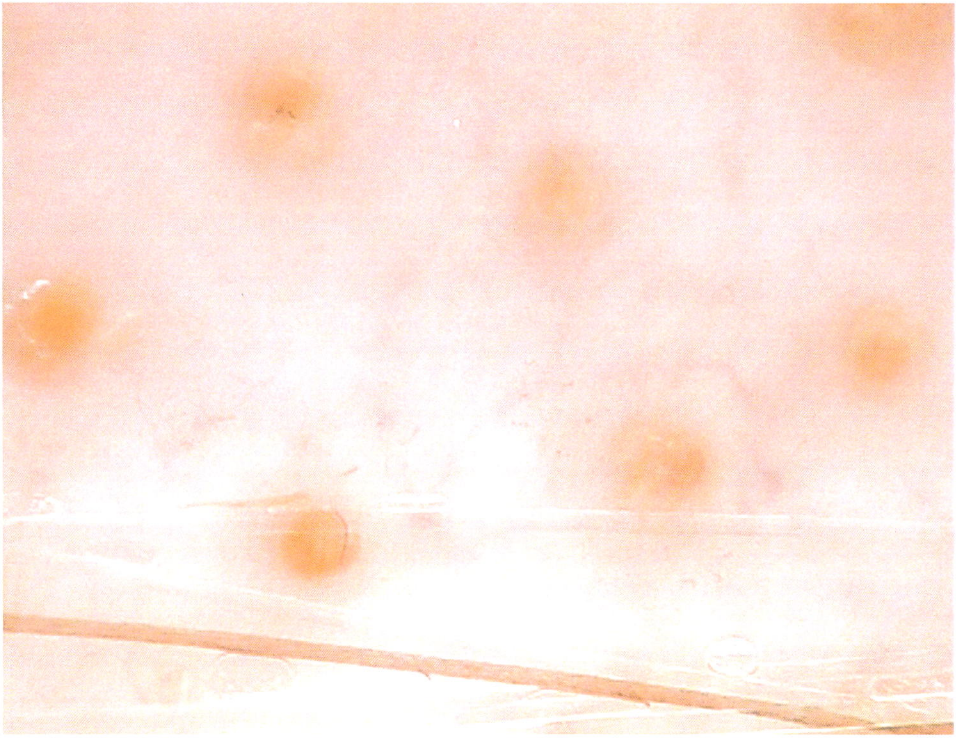

Fig. 3.26 Yellow dots in alopecia areata. The presence of yellow dots in alopecia areata is a negative prognostic factor, but it does not exclude the possibility of hair regrowth. In patients with multiple yellow dots, we apply keratolytic agents as supplementary therapy (×70)

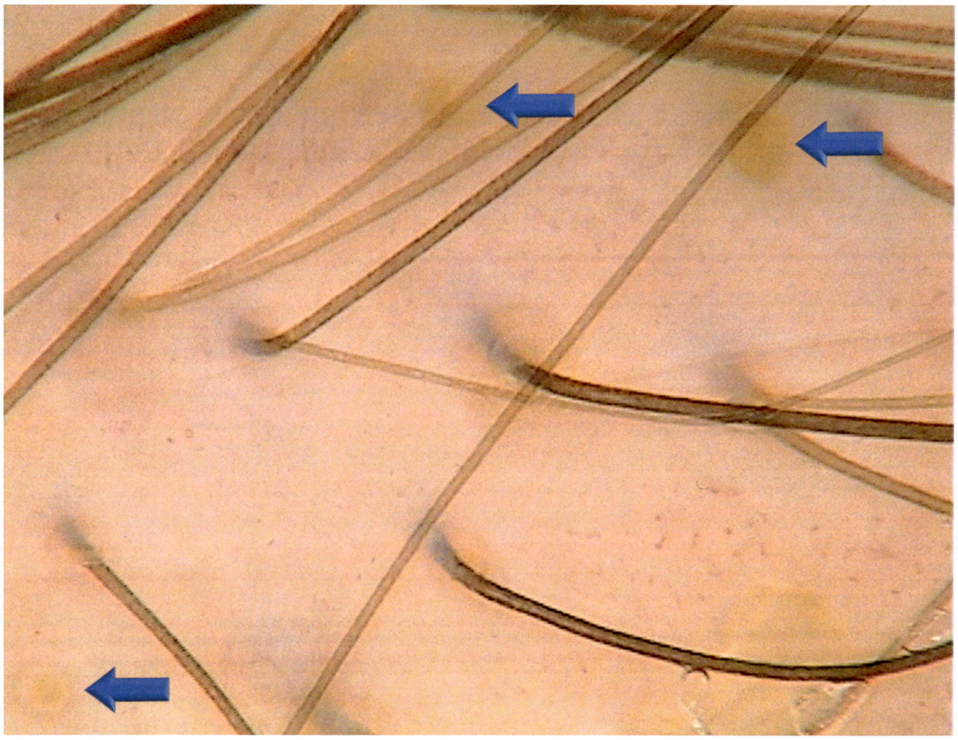

Fig. 3.27 Yellow dots in androgenetic alopecia. Yellow dots (*arrows*) are seen between follicular units in this patient with androgenetic alopecia. Yellow dots in androgenetic alopecia rarely are regularly distributed, as they are in alopecia areata. They also may differ from dots in alopecia areata by their slightly oily appearance and slightly smaller size. The oily appearance of the yellow dots is not a constant finding in androgenetic alopecia. Most yellow dots in androgenetic alopecia have a keratosebaceous appearance. In this image, additional features of androgenetic alopecia—namely, hair shaft thickness heterogeneity and a predominance of follicular units with only one hair shaft—are visible (×70)

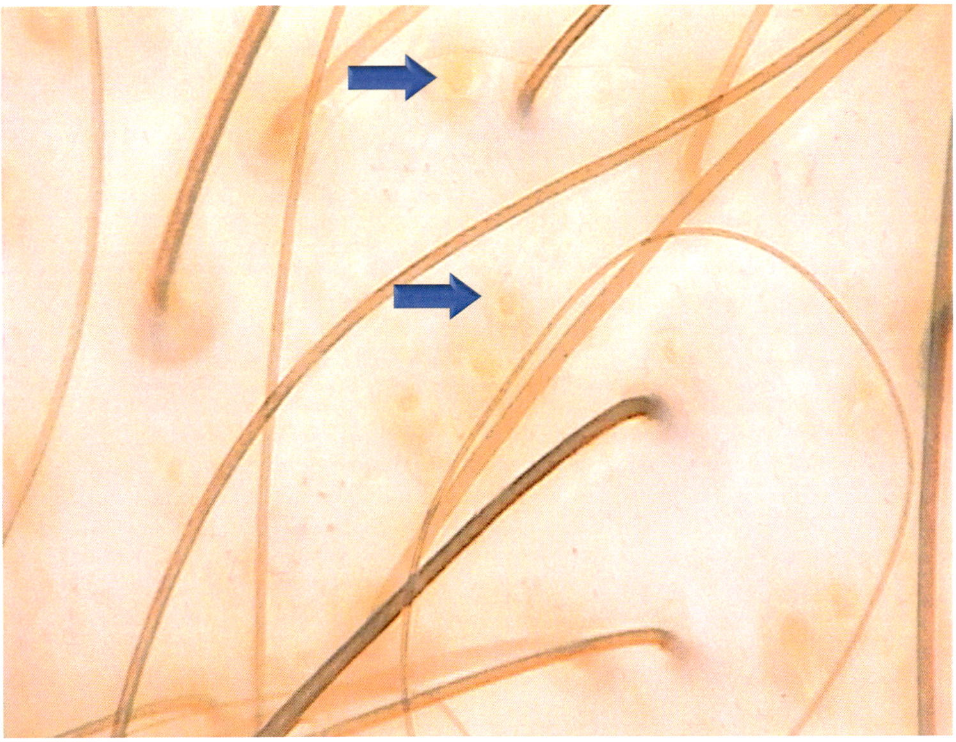

Fig. 3.28 Yellow dots in androgenetic alopecia. This image was taken from the frontal scalp area. In androgenetic alopecia, trichoscopic features of the disease are more evident in the frontal than in the occipital area [7]. Characteristically, yellow dots (*arrows*) are localized between thick terminal hairs, usually accompanied by other features of mild or moderate androgenetic alopecia. Yellow dots are observed more frequently in patients and in areas with advanced hair loss in the course of androgenetic alopecia (i.e., grade VII on the Hamilton-Norwood scale or grade III on the Ludwig scale) (×70)

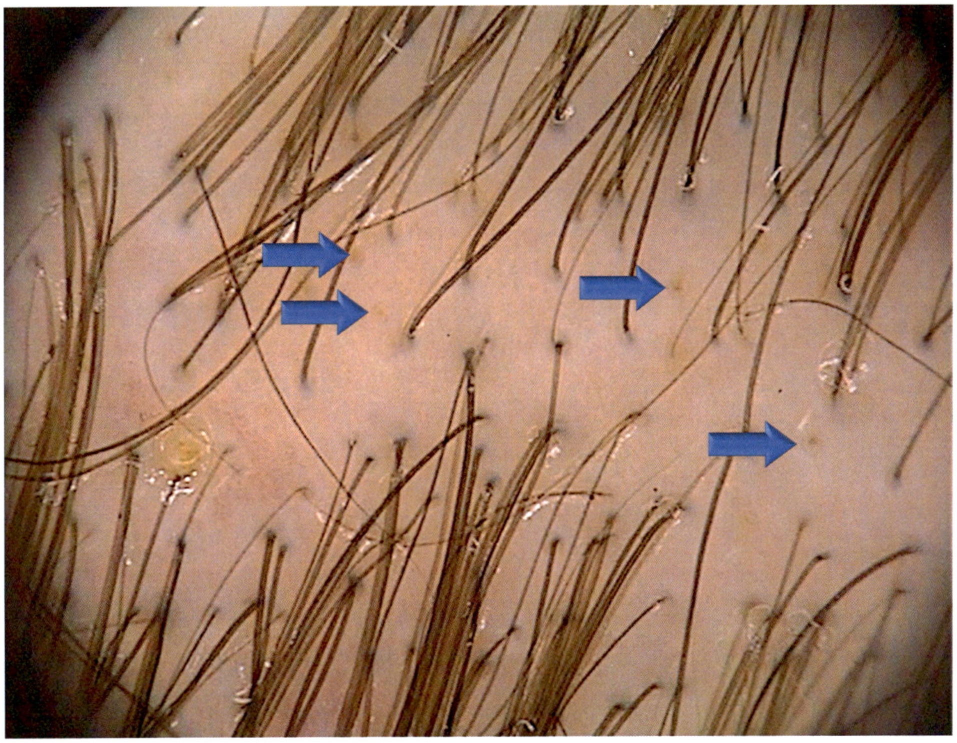

Fig. 3.29 Yellow dots in androgenetic alopecia. Yellow dots (*arrows*) differ in size, reflecting different stages of hair follicle miniaturization. In androgenetic alopecia, as in other diseases, many yellow dots have a double margin. Note the simultaneous presence of other abnormalities characteristic of androgenetic alopecia (×20)

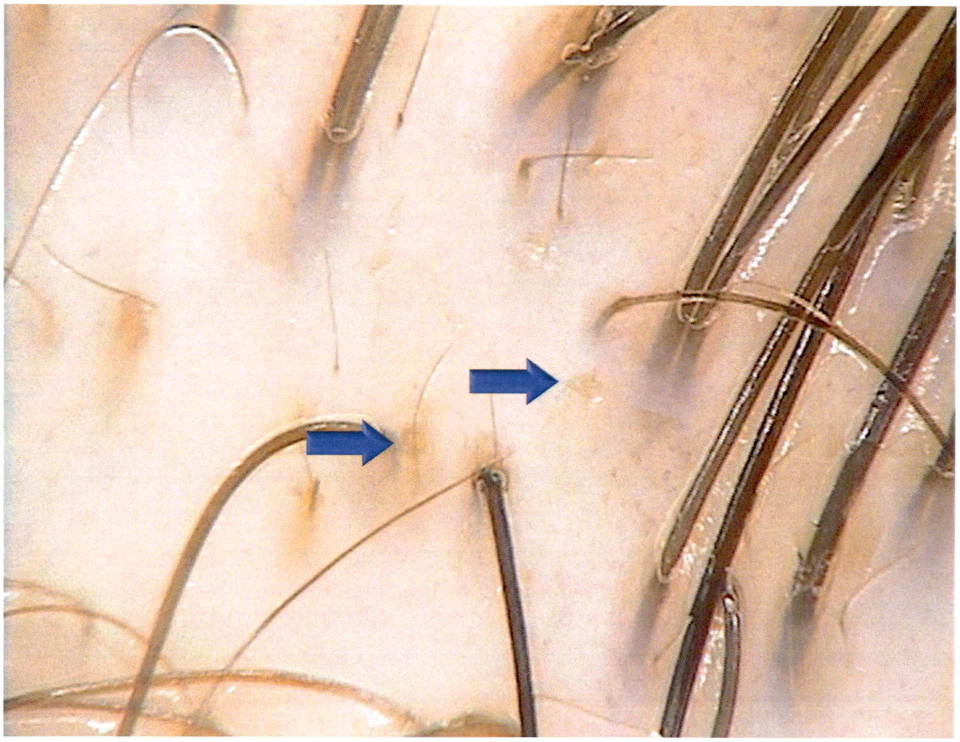

Fig. 3.30 Yellow dots in alopecia areata incognita. Yellow dots (*arrows*) are a consistent finding in alopecia areata incognita, a disease that clinically and trichoscopically shares some of the same features with alopecia areata, telogen effluvium, and androgenetic alopecia [13–15]. Note the short, thin, darkly pigmented hairs with a thicker proximal end, which rarely are observed in other diseases (×70)

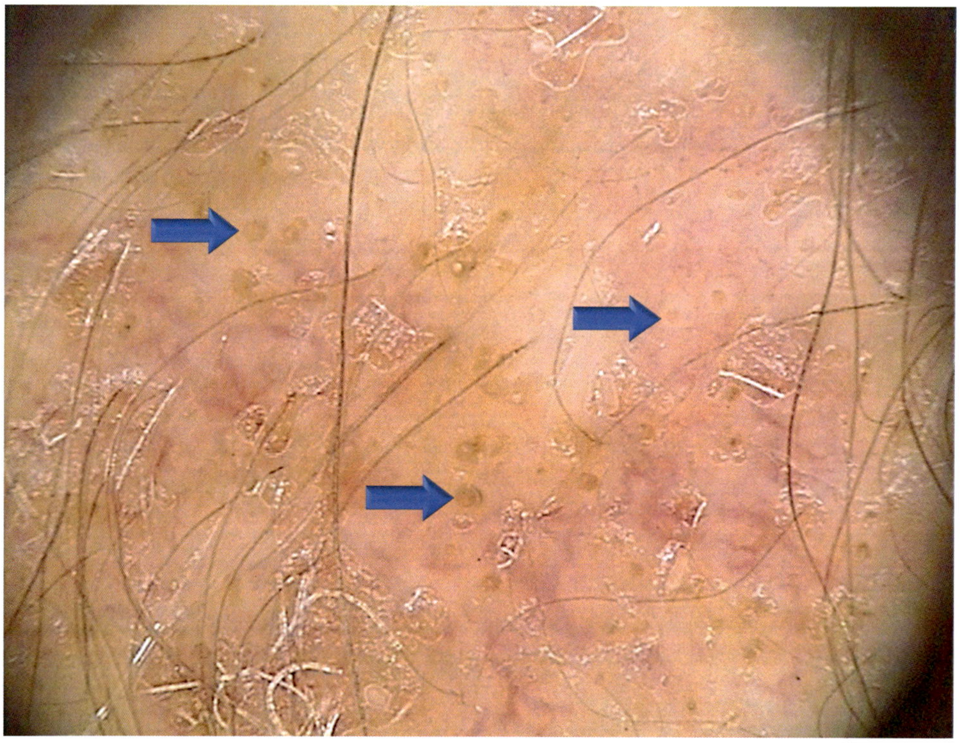

Fig. 3.31 Yellow dots in discoid lupus erythematosus. In discoid lupus erythematosus, yellow dots (*arrows*) appear firm and are significantly larger than those seen in other diseases. They have a mean diameter of 653 ± 125 μm (mean ± SD), which is significantly greater than that of yellow dots observed in alopecia areata (212 ± 66 μm) or female androgenetic alopecia (190 ± 71 μm) [4, 16]. These yellow dots correspond to follicular plugging and hyperkeratosis on histopathology (×20)

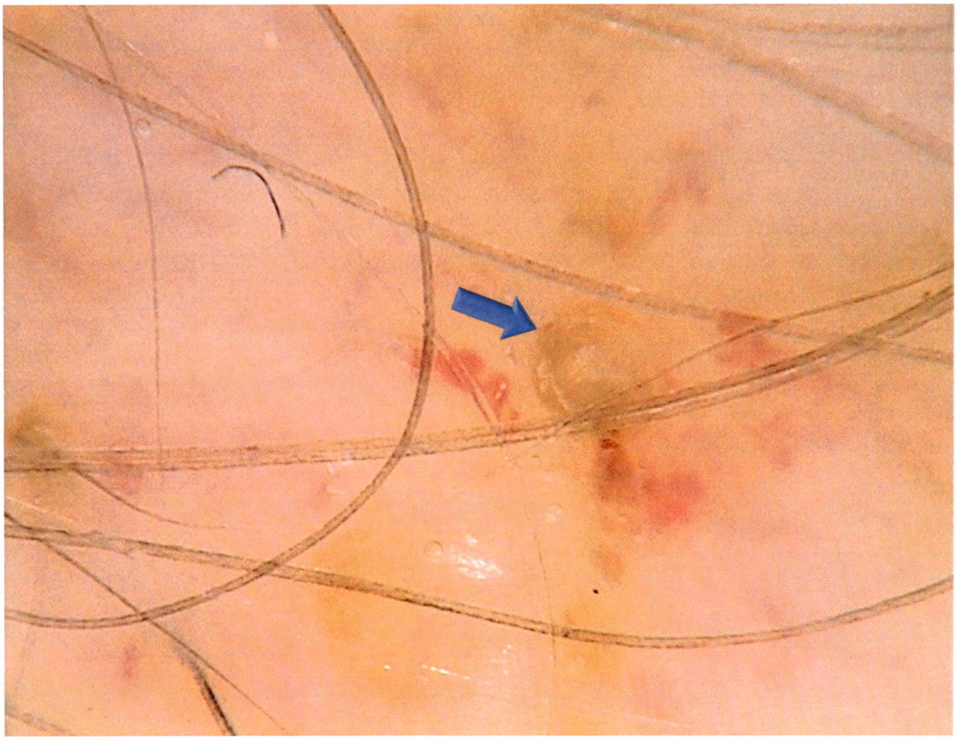

Fig. 3.32 Yellow dots in discoid lupus erythematosus. High magnification reveals a large yellow dot with a double margin and a firm, bulging appearance (*arrow*). In discoid lupus erythematosus, these dots characterize an active phase of disease. In late cicatricial lesions of discoid lupus erythematosus, the yellow dots change their character and appear faint and flat, with penetrating thin vessels (×70)

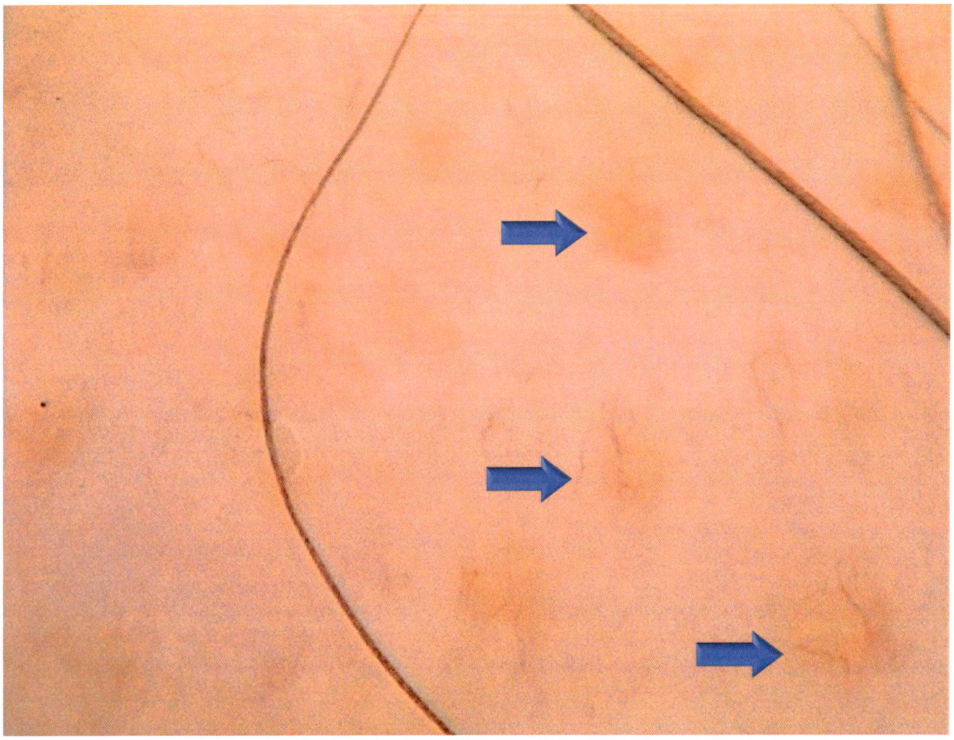

Fig. 3.33 Yellow dots in discoid lupus erythematosus. Inactive lesions of discoid lupus erythematosus show faint, flat yellow dots containing partially penetrating thin blood vessels (*arrows*). These vessels may resemble "red spiders in yellow dots" [16] (×70)

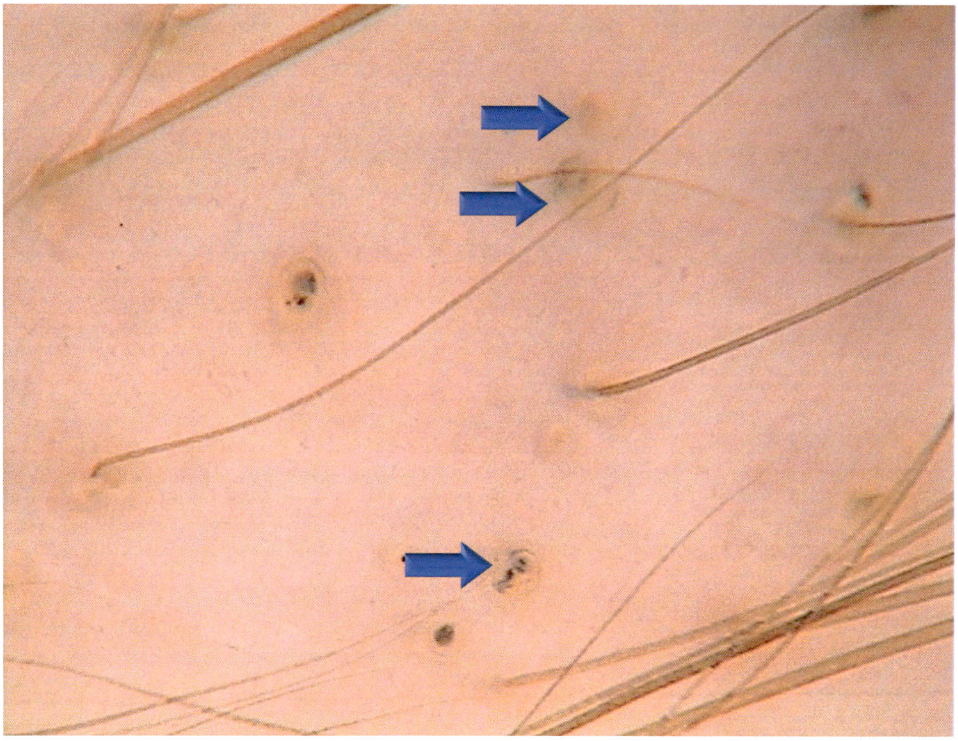

Fig. 3.34 Yellow dots in dissecting cellulitis. In active dissecting cellulitis, yellow dots are large "3D" structures resembling soap bubbles imposed over dark dystrophic hairs (*arrows*). This image also shows pinpoint vessels with a whitish halo, a common finding in dissecting cellulitis (×70)

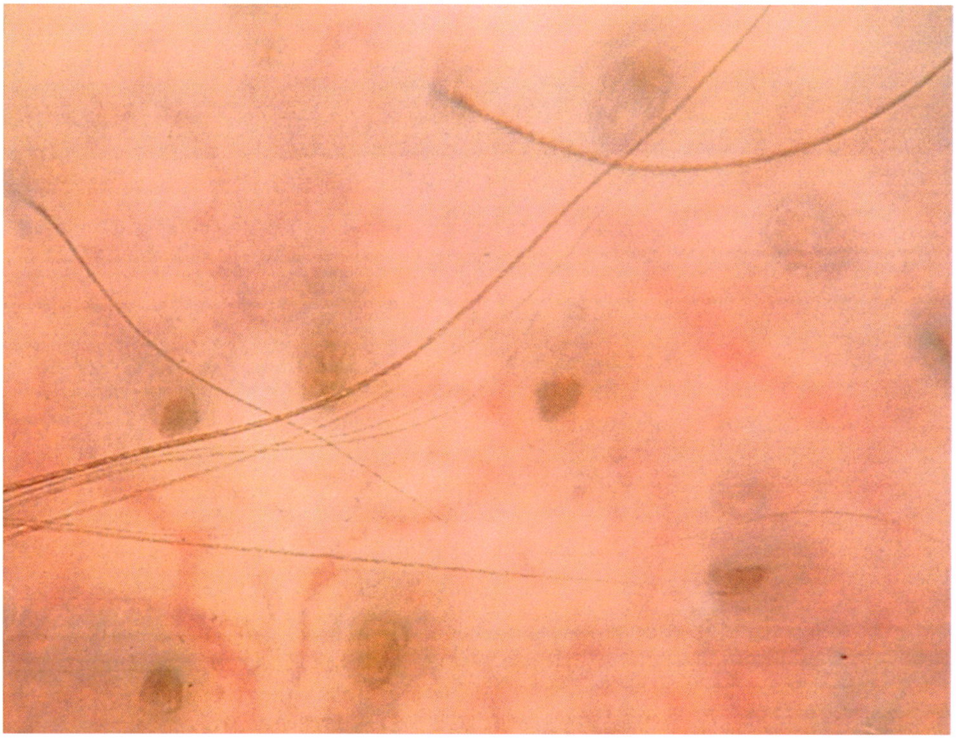

Fig. 3.35 Yellow dots in dissecting cellulitis. In long-lasting lesions of dissecting cellulitis, yellow dots become polygonal and dark yellow to brown, with a blurred halo and double margins (×70)

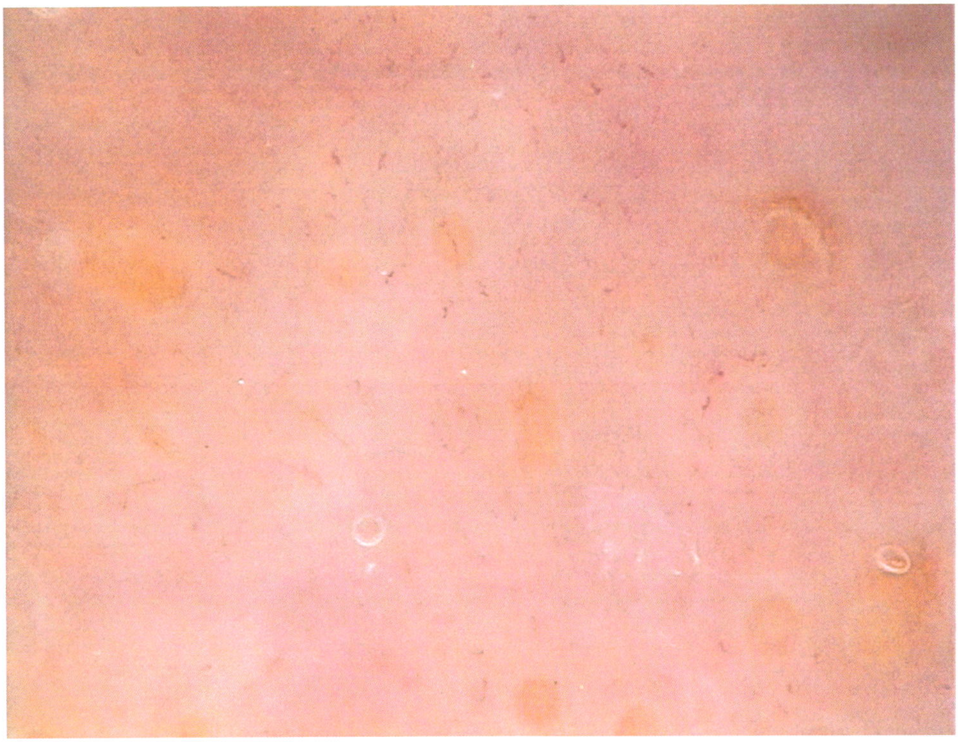

Fig. 3.36 Yellow dots in pemphigus vulgaris. Scalp involvement in pemphigus vulgaris may be associated with hair loss. This trichoscopic image was taken at direct proximity to an erosion. The yellow dots are polycyclic, with a brownish or whitish halo. Some of them appear to be detaching at the periphery (×70)

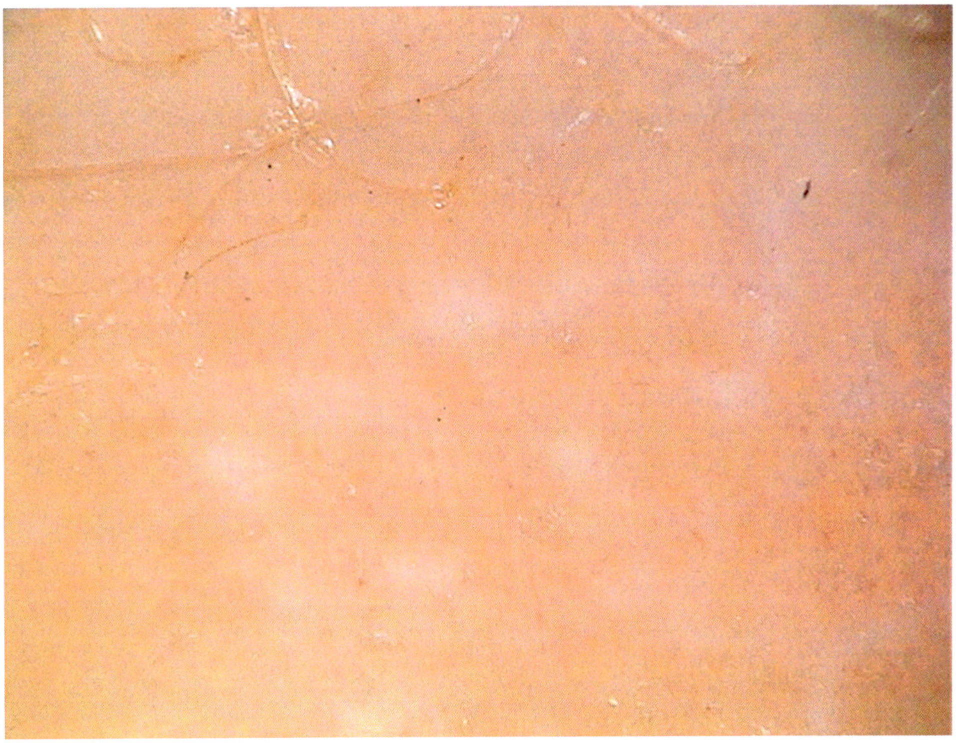

Fig. 3.37 Fibrotic white dots in cicatricial alopecia. Fibrotic white dots replace follicular openings and the perifollicular area. They may develop in every folliculocentric cicatricial alopecia, but are most common in lichen planopilaris. These white dots are large and multishaped, have blurred borders, and tend to merge into confluent white areas. The milky red color at the periphery of these dots indicates fibrosis of recent onset. Some authors refer to fibrotic white dots as *classic white dots* to emphasize that they were described first, before the first description of pinpoint white dots (×20)

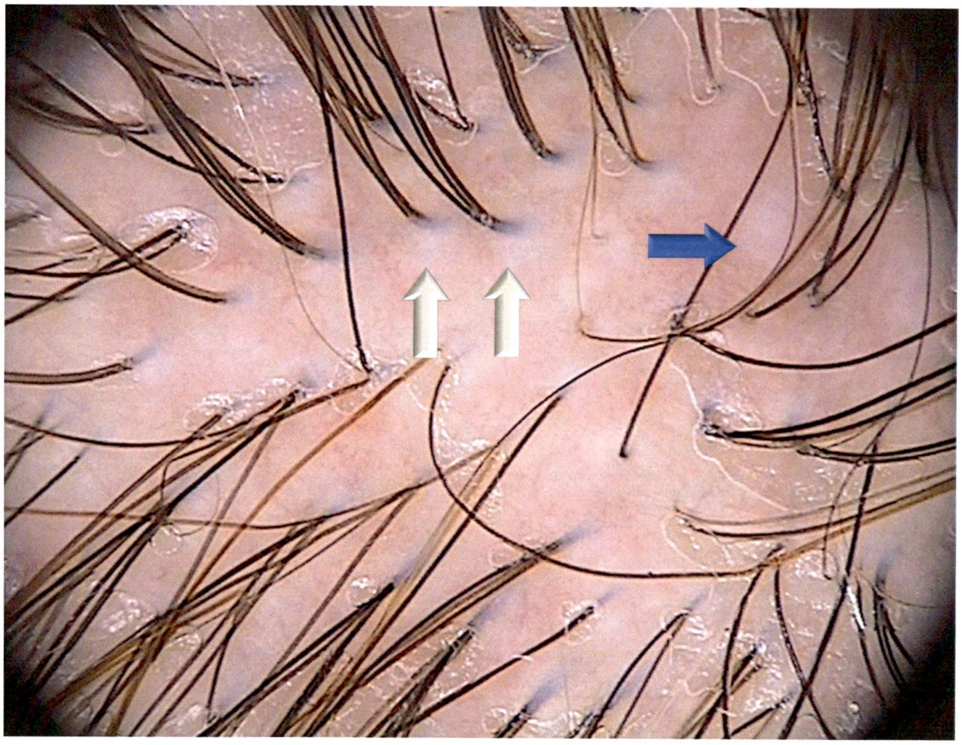

Fig. 3.38 Fibrotic white dots in cicatricial alopecia. The image shows white dots that replaced hair follicle openings (*blue arrow*). The *white arrows* point to fibrotic white dots with emerging terminal hairs, illustrating the ongoing process of perifollicular fibrosis, which eventually results in permanent cicatricial alopecia. The perifollicular fibrotic white dots should be distinguished from perifollicular scaling, which may present a similar picture on trichoscopy with immersion fluid. Perifollicular white dots may be distinguished from perifollicular scaling by dry trichoscopy. In dry trichoscopy, fibrotic perifollicular white dots appear flat and atrophic, whereas in perifollicular scaling, the scales are easily visible (×20)

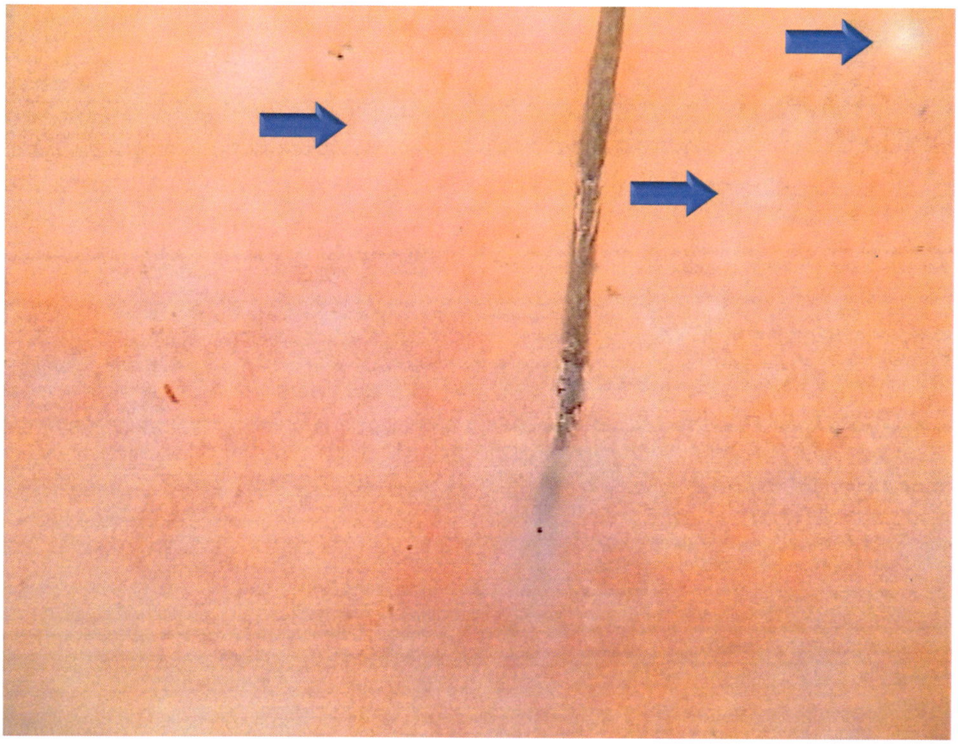

Fig. 3.39 Fibrotic white dots in cicatricial alopecia. The image shows the ongoing process of scarring in lichen planopilaris. Fibrotic white dots (*arrows*) are accompanied by a confluent white to milky red area of recent fibrosis. A single terminal hair is surrounded by a white area of fibrosis (×70)

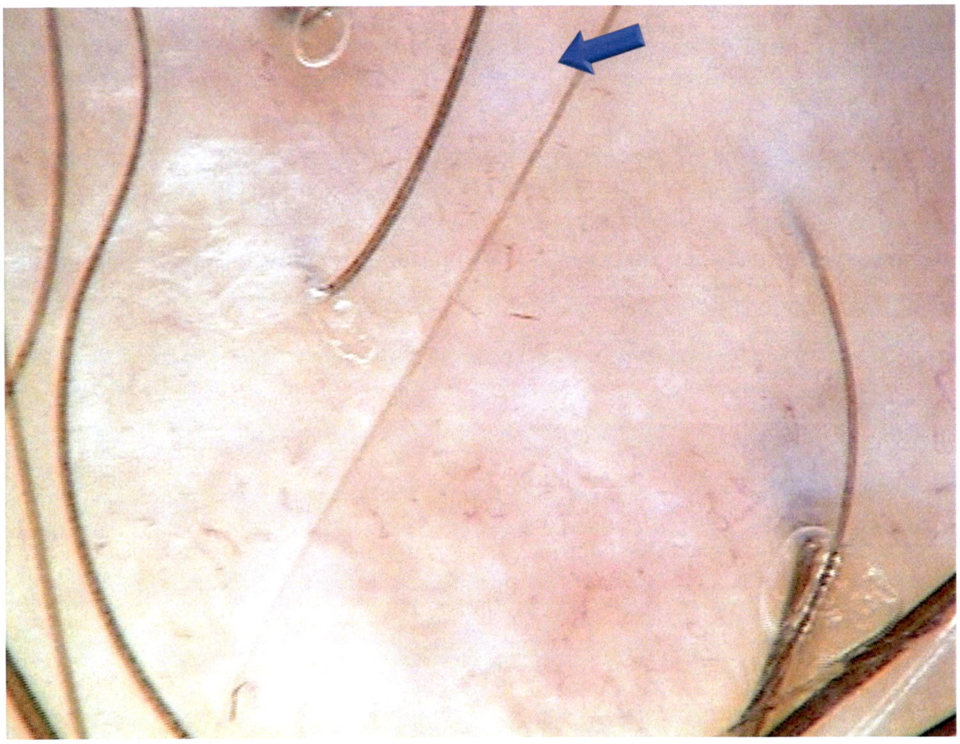

Fig. 3.40 Fibrotic white dots in cicatricial alopecia. Blurred white dots (*arrow*) in place of suspected follicular openings may be assessed. Elongated vessels are visible around the white dots and around the follicular units (×70)

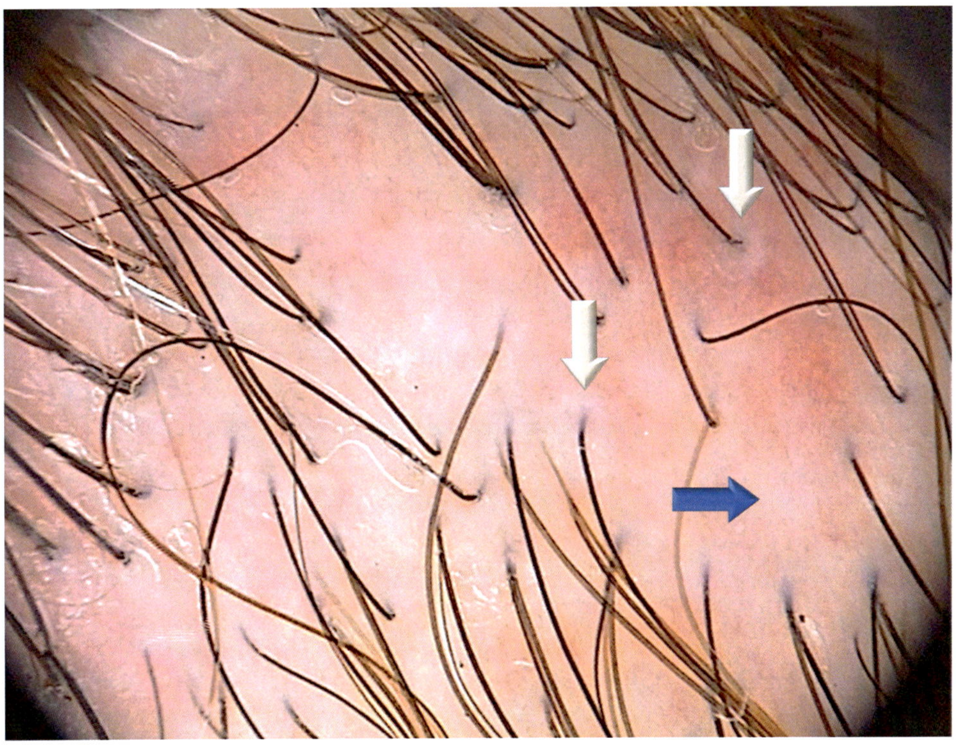

Fig. 3.41 Fibrotic white dots in cicatricial alopecia. This image shows a fibrotic white dot (*blue arrow*), which is barely visible. The dot disappears in an area of diffuse fibrosis. Other white dots, located within nonfibrotic areas, may easily be seen. Some of them still have emerging terminal hairs in their central part (*white arrows*) (×20)

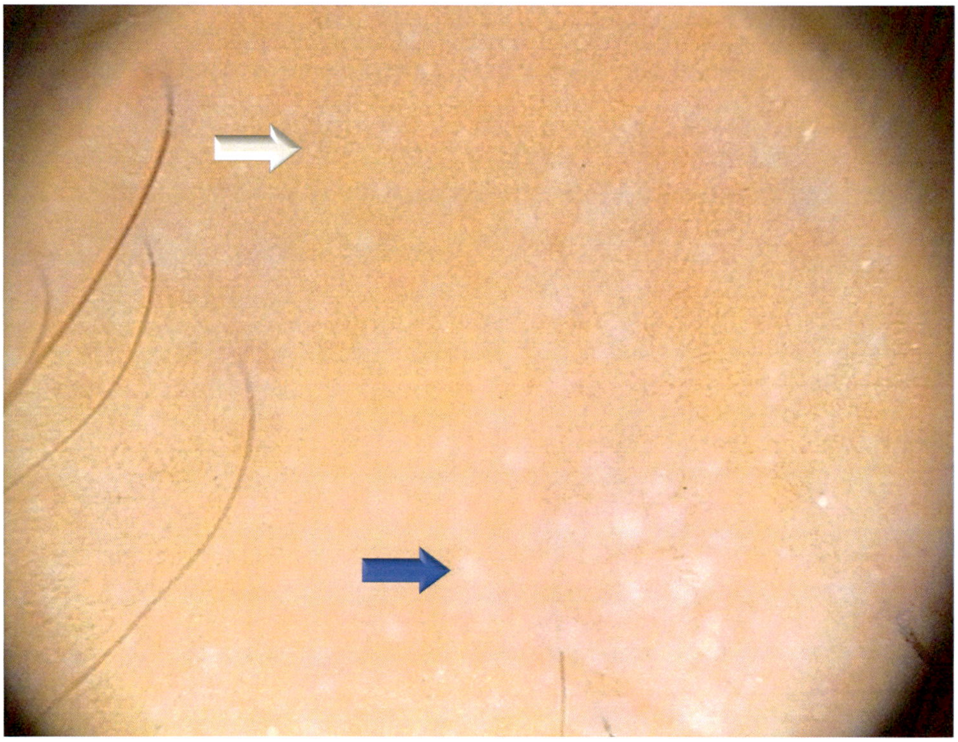

Fig. 3.42 Fibrotic white dots and pinpoint white dots. In this Caucasian male patient with long-lasting lichen planopilaris, two types of white dots are visible on sun-exposed skin. Fibrotic white dots (*blue arrow*) are large and multishaped, and tend to become confluent. Pinpoint white dots (*white arrow*) are small, round, and surrounded by the pigment network (×20)

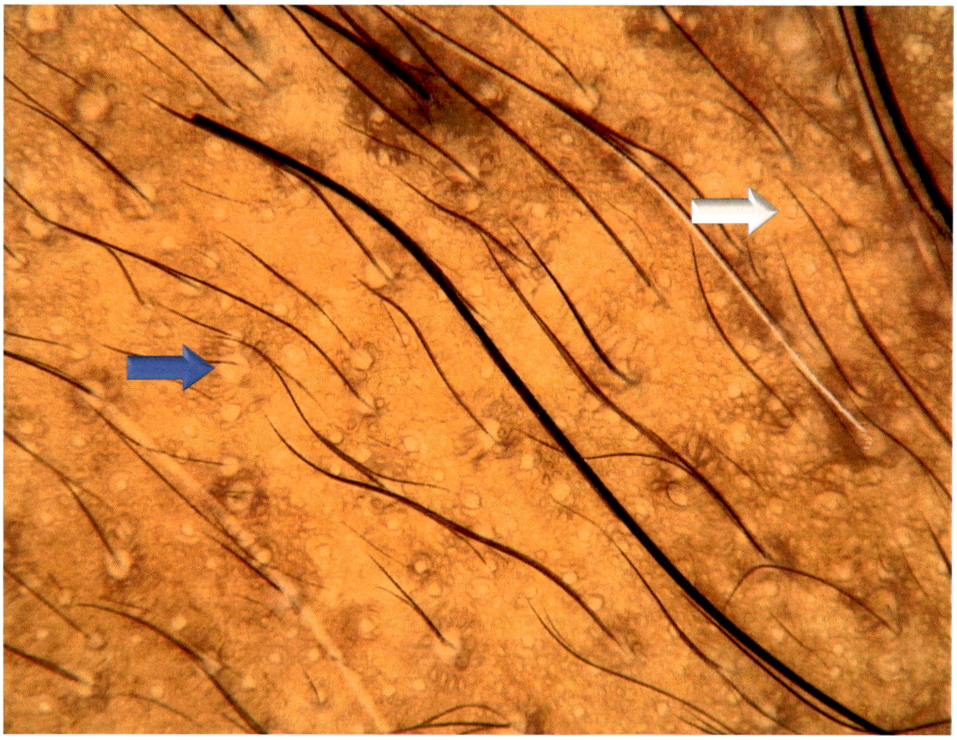

Fig. 3.43 Pinpoint white dots in a healthy individual. These pinpoint white dots are small, round, and regular. They occasionally have a hyperpigmented halo. They correspond to either normal hair follicle openings (*blue arrow*) or to the epidermal portion of eccrine sweat ducts (*white arrow*). The pinpoint white dots are visible on the contrasting background of the pigment network; therefore, they are observed in patients with Fitzpatrick skin phototypes IV, V, and VI and in lighter-skinned patients after intense sun exposure. This finding is normal and requires no medical intervention (×70)

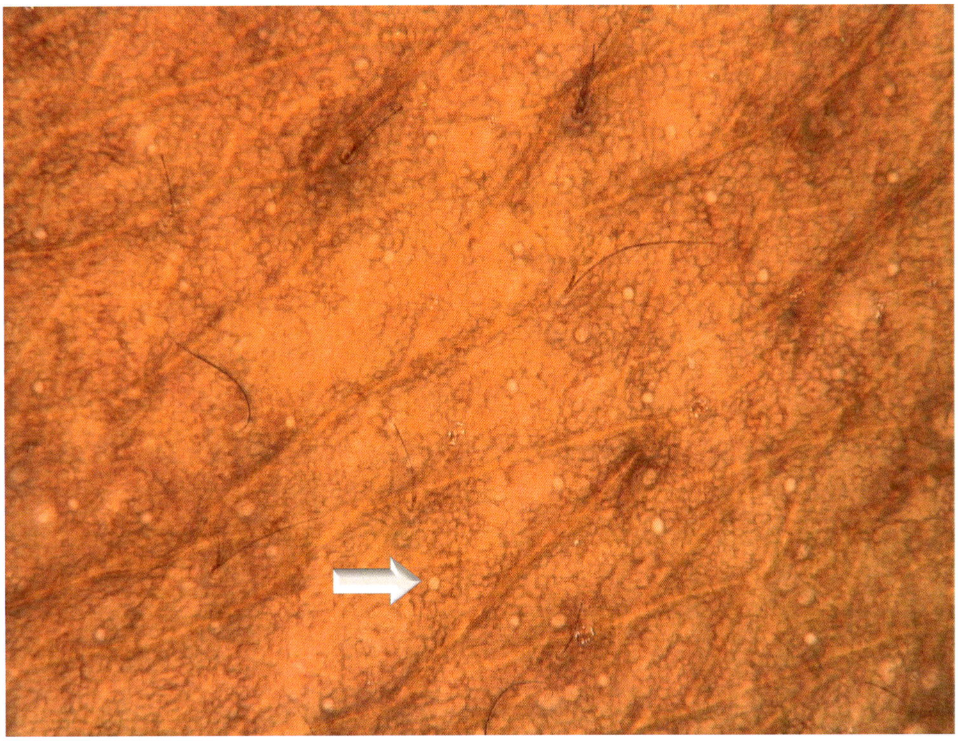

Fig. 3.44 Pinpoint white dots on glabrous skin in a healthy individual. Pinpoint white dots are small and have an ideally round, regular shape (*arrow*). These dots are present on the scalp and glabrous skin. Thus, when determining whether a trichoscopic finding is a pinpoint white dot, the skin of the face or forearms may be examined for comparison (×70)

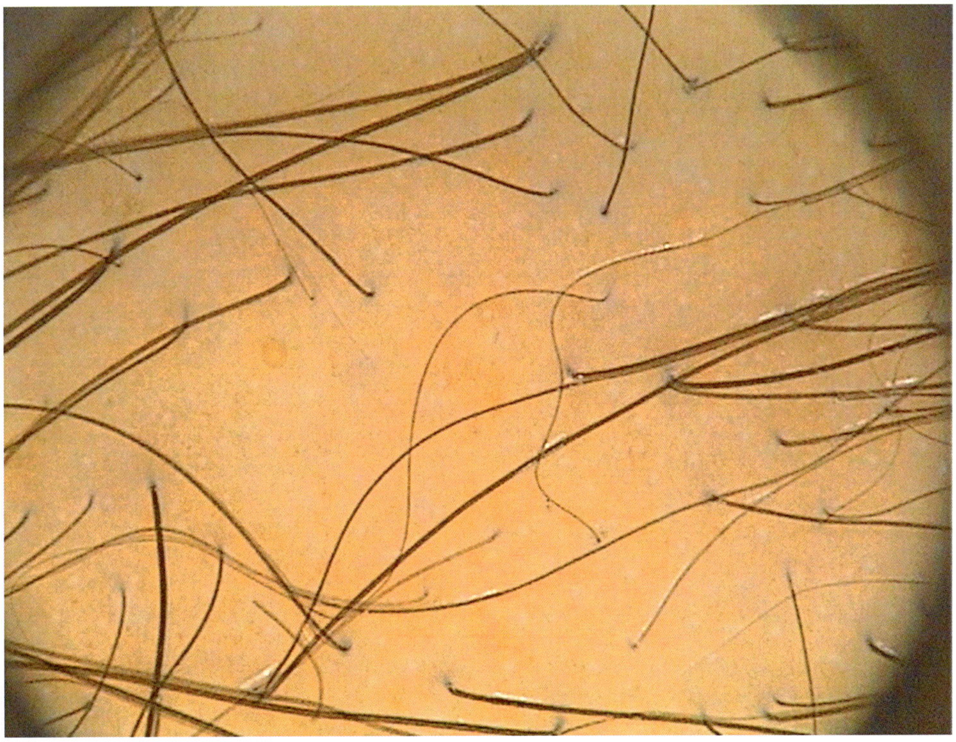

Fig. 3.45 Pinpoint white dots in androgenetic alopecia. Shown is a trichoscopic image from a male patient with androgenetic alopecia. The patient, who has skin phototype II, was examined after intense summer sun exposure. The image shows multiple pinpoint white dots, decreased hair density, and features of androgenetic alopecia. In healthy individuals with light skin phototypes, the hair protects the scalp from sun exposure and increased pigmentation. Thus, pinpoint white dots rarely are visible in healthy individuals with skin phototype I, II, or III, even after sun exposure. Decreased hair density promotes tanning of scalp skin and increases the visibility of pinpoint white dots (×20)

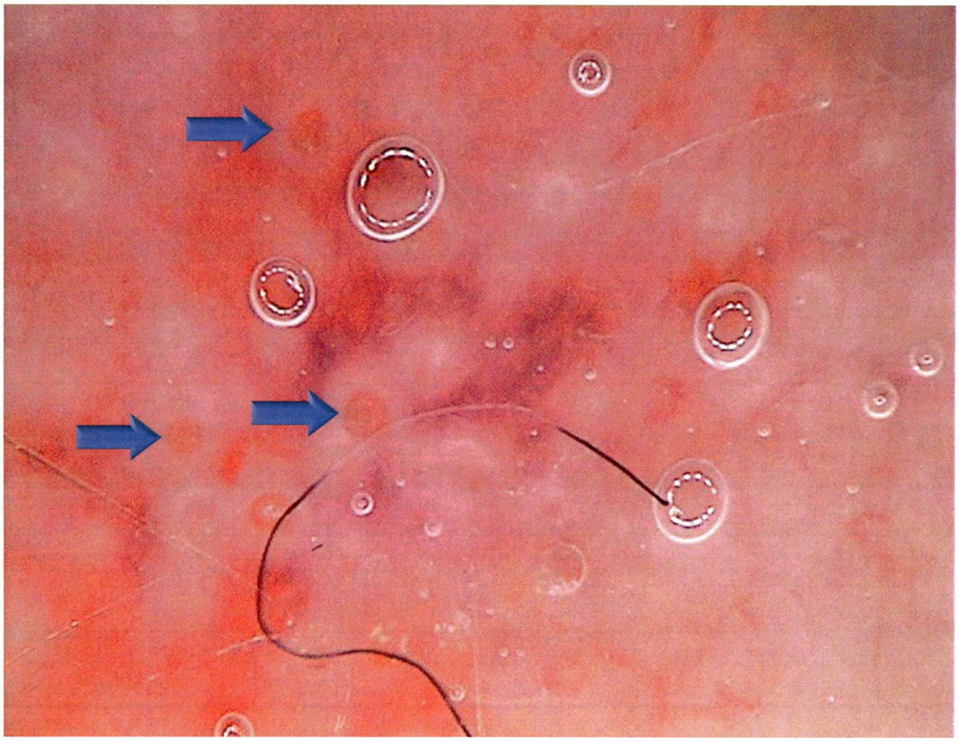

Fig. 3.46 Red dots in discoid lupus erythematosus. Follicular red dots (*arrows*) have been described in discoid lupus erythematosus and are believed to be a positive prognostic factor for possible hair regrowth. Histopathology of red dots shows enlarged infundibula surrounded by dilated vessels with red blood cell extravasation (×70)

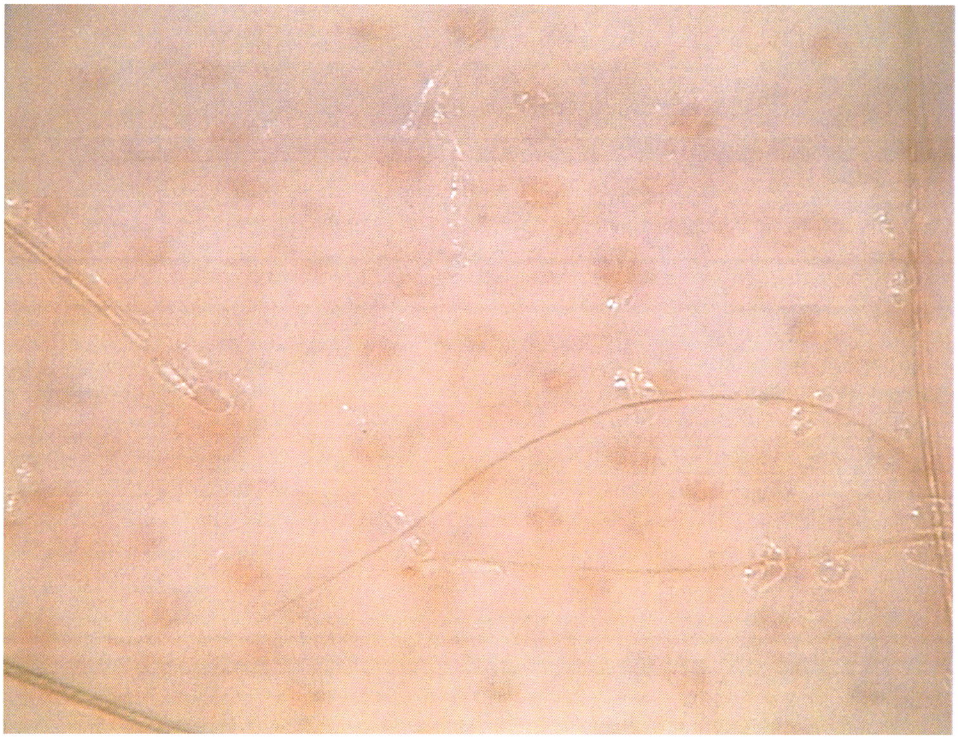

Fig. 3.47 Pink and pink-brown dots in the eyebrow area of a patient with frontal fibrosing alopecia. Loss of eyebrows in the course of frontal fibrosing alopecia is a consistent finding. However, trichoscopy of the eyebrow area exhibits features different from those observed on the scalp. In the eyebrow area, the presence of multiple regularly distributed, sharply demarcated, pink to pink-brown dots is most characteristic. In some patients, these dots have a gray tint (×70)

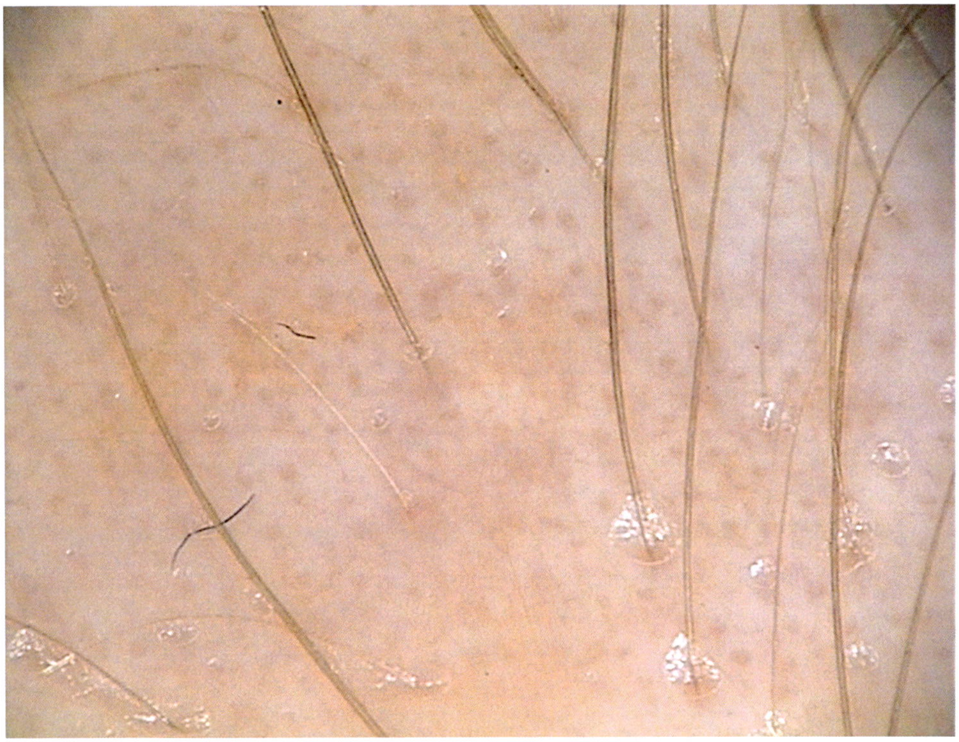

Fig. 3.48 Pink and pink-brown dots in the eyebrow area of a patient with frontal fibrosing alopecia. Trichoscopy in a female patient with frontal fibrosing alopecia of a few years' duration shows multiple pink to pink-brown dots, most of which lack hair shafts (eyebrows) and a minority of which have emerging hair shafts. Our experience shows that this type of image is a positive prognostic factor for eyebrow regrowth after adequate therapy. The diffuse brownish color in the top of the image results from coloring the eyebrows with natural henna (×70)

References

1. Ross EK, Vincenzi C, Tosti A. Videodermoscopy in the evaluation of hair and scalp disorders. J Am Acad Dermatol. 2006;55(5): 799–806.
2. Inui S, Nakajima T, Nakagawa K, Itami S. Clinical significance of dermoscopy in alopecia areata: analysis of 300 cases. Int J Dermatol. 2008;47(7):688–93.
3. Rudnicka L, Olszewska M, Rakowska A, Kowalska-Oledzka E, Slowinska M. Trichoscopy: a new method for diagnosing hair loss. J Drugs Dermatol. 2008;7(7):651–4.
4. Rudnicka L, Olszewska M, Rakowska A, Slowinska M. Trichoscopy update 2011. J Dermatol Case Rep. 2011;5(4):82–8.
5. Inui S. Trichoscopy for common hair loss diseases: algorithmic method for diagnosis. J Dermatol. 2011;38(1):71–5.
6. Rakowska A. Trichoscopy (hair and scalp videodermoscopy) in the healthy female. Method standardization and norms for measurable parameters. J Dermatol Case Rep. 2009;3(1):14–9.
7. Rakowska A, Slowinska M, Kowalska-Oledzka E, Olszewska M, Rudnicka L. Dermoscopy in female androgenic alopecia: method standardization and diagnostic criteria. Int J Trichol. 2009;1(2):123–30.
8. Lacarrubba F, Dall'Oglio F, Rita Nasca M, Micali G. Videodermatoscopy enhances diagnostic capability in some forms of hair loss. Am J Clin Dermatol. 2004;5(3):205–8.
9. de Moura LH, Duque-Estrada B, Abraham LS, Barcaui CB, Sodre CT. Dermoscopy findings of alopecia areata in an African-American patient. J Dermatol Case Rep. 2008;2(4):52–4.
10. Abraham LS, Pineiro-Maceira J, Duque-Estrada B, Barcaui CB, Sodre CT. Pinpoint white dots in the scalp: dermoscopic and histopathologic correlation. J Am Acad Dermatol. 2010;63(4): 721–2.
11. Tosti A, Torres F, Misciali C, Vincenzi C, Starace M, Miteva M, et al. Follicular red dots: a novel dermoscopic pattern observed in scalp discoid lupus erythematosus. Arch Dermatol. 2009;145(12): 1406–9.
12. Sah DE, Koo J, Price VH. Trichotillomania. Dermatol Ther. 2008;21(1):13–21.
13. Rebora A. Alopecia areata incognita. J Am Acad Dermatol. 2011;65(6):1228.
14. Tosti A, Whiting D, Iorizzo M, Pazzaglia M, Misciali C, Vincenzi C, et al. The role of scalp dermoscopy in the diagnosis of alopecia areata incognita. J Am Acad Dermatol. 2008;59(1):64–7.
15. Rakowska A, Slowinska M, Kowalska-Oledzka E, Olszewska M, Czuwara J, Rudnicka L. Alopecia areata incognita: true or false? J Am Acad Dermatol. 2009;60(1):162–3.
16. Rakowska A, Slowinska M, Kowalska-Oledzka E, Olszewska M, Rudnicka L. Trichoscopy in cicatricial alopecia. J Drugs Dermatol. 2012;11(6):753–8.

Perifollicular and Interfollicular Skin Surface

4

Lidia Rudnicka, Malgorzata Olszewska,
Adriana Rakowska, Joanna Czuwara, Justyna Sicinska,
Agnieszka Kardynal, and Olga Warszawik-Hendzel

Abstract

The perifollicular and interfollicular skin surface provides significant information that may facilitate the diagnosis of hair and scalp diseases. Abnormalities include different patterns and colors of scaling; hyperpigmentation; yellow, white, or pink-white ("strawberry ice cream"–colored) areas of skin surface; discharge; and skin hyperplasia.

Keywords

Brown areas • Classification • Extravasations • Follicular spicules • Folliculitis decalvans Hyperpigmentation • Ichthyosis • Interfollicular epidermis • Langerhans cell histiocytosis • Lichen planopilaris • Monoclonal gammopathy • Perifollicular • Pink areas • Pemphigus • Peripilar sign Psoriasis • Red areas • Scaling • Seborrheic dermatitis • Starburst hyperplasia • Strawberry ice cream areas • Tinea capitis • White areas • Yellow areas • Zoster

The perifollicular and interfollicular skin surface may be evaluated easily by trichoscopy and provides significant information that may facilitate the diagnosis of hair and scalp diseases.

A frequent finding is hyperpigmentation, which may appear in hair loss in three different patterns: honeycomb, perifollicular, and scattered interfollicular [1, 2]. Honeycomb hyperpigmentation [3] is a consistent finding in patients with Fitzpatrick skin phototypes IV, V, and VI and is frequent in lighter sun-exposed skin. Perifollicular brown coloration ("peripilar sign") corresponds to the perifollicular presence of lymphocytic infiltrates [4, 5]. This finding is common in androgenetic alopecia [6] and telogen effluvium and may be seen in up to 10 % of hair follicle openings in healthy individuals [7]. Scattered brown skin discoloration is a trichoscopic feature characteristic of discoid lupus erythematosus [8]. Reticular and globular pigmentation has been observed in Asian patients with contact dermatitis [9].

Epidermal scaling is a common finding in various inflammatory scalp diseases and in healthy individuals. A distinction between normal and abnormal is made based on scaling intensity, color, and localization. Mild diffuse scaling may be observed in healthy persons with dry skin. Moderate to severe diffuse scaling may be observed in scalp psoriasis and in seborrheic dermatitis. In psoriasis, the scales are silver white, whereas in seborrheic dermatitis they have a yellowish tint. The picture of white diffuse "scaling" with formation of white perifollicular clusters requires differential diagnosis with monoclonal gammopathy [2]. Mild perifollicular scaling is observed commonly in frontal fibrosing alopecia, but this is a nonspecific finding. Perifollicular epidermal scaling with the formation of tubular scaly structures surrounding the hair shafts is observed most frequently in lichen planopilaris and folliculitis decalvans. In folliculitis decalvans, the

L. Rudnicka (✉)
Faculty of Health Sciences,
Medical University of Warsaw, Poland

Department of Dermatology CSK MSW, Woloska 137,
Warsaw 02-502, Poland
e-mail: lidia.rudnicka@euderm.eu

M. Olszewska
Department of Dermatology, Medical University of Warsaw,
Warsaw, Poland

A. Rakowska • J. Czuwara • J. Sicinska • A. Kardynal
O. Warszawik-Hendzel
Department of Dermatology, CSK MSW, Warsaw, Poland

L. Rudnicka et al. (eds.), *Atlas of Trichoscopy*,
DOI 10.1007/978-1-4471-4486-1_4, © Springer-Verlag London 2012

purulent component will give these tubular scaly structures a yellowish tint [2, 8].

Other perifollicular and interfollicular trichoscopic symptoms include white or pink-white ("strawberry ice cream"–colored) skin surfaces devoid of hair follicles in various forms of cicatricial alopecia, amorphous yellow areas in dissecting folliculitis, and follicular pustules and starburst pattern hyperplasia in folliculitis decalvans. Artifacts may sometimes hinder interpretation of interfollicular trichoscopic findings.

We propose a classification of perifollicular and interfollicular skin surface abnormalities on trichoscopy that is based on data from the literature and on our trichoscopic experience.

Table 4.1 Classification of perifollicular and interfollicular skin surface abnormalities in trichoscopy

Scaling
Diffuse (homogenous)
White (psoriasis, discoid lupus erythematosus, allergic dermatitis, dry skin)[a]
Yellowish (seborrheic dermatitis, discoid lupus erythematosus, ichthyosis)
Perifollicular
Color of scales
White (lichen planopilaris)
Yellowish (folliculitis decalvans)
Shape of scale arrangement
Tubular (lichen planopilaris)
Tubular with collar formation (folliculitis decalvans)
Color
Brown areas
Honeycomb hyperpigmentation (common)
Perifollicular; peripilar sign (female and male androgenetic alopecia, telogen effluvium, healthy individuals)
Scattered (discoid lupus erythematosus, actinic keratosis)
White areas (cicatricial alopecia, detached epidermis, edema)
Pink, "strawberry ice cream" areas (early fibrosis in cicatricial alopecia)
Yellow areas (dissecting cellulitis, follicular pustules, bacterial infection)
Red (inflammation, extravasation, epidermal detachment, vascular abnormalities)
Discharge
Yellow and yellow red (folliculitis decalvans, bacterial infections, dissecting cellulitis, tinea capitis)
White follicular spicules (monoclonal gammopathy)
Surface structure
Starburst pattern hyperplasia (folliculitis decalvans)

[a]The most common or characteristic occurrence is shown in parentheses

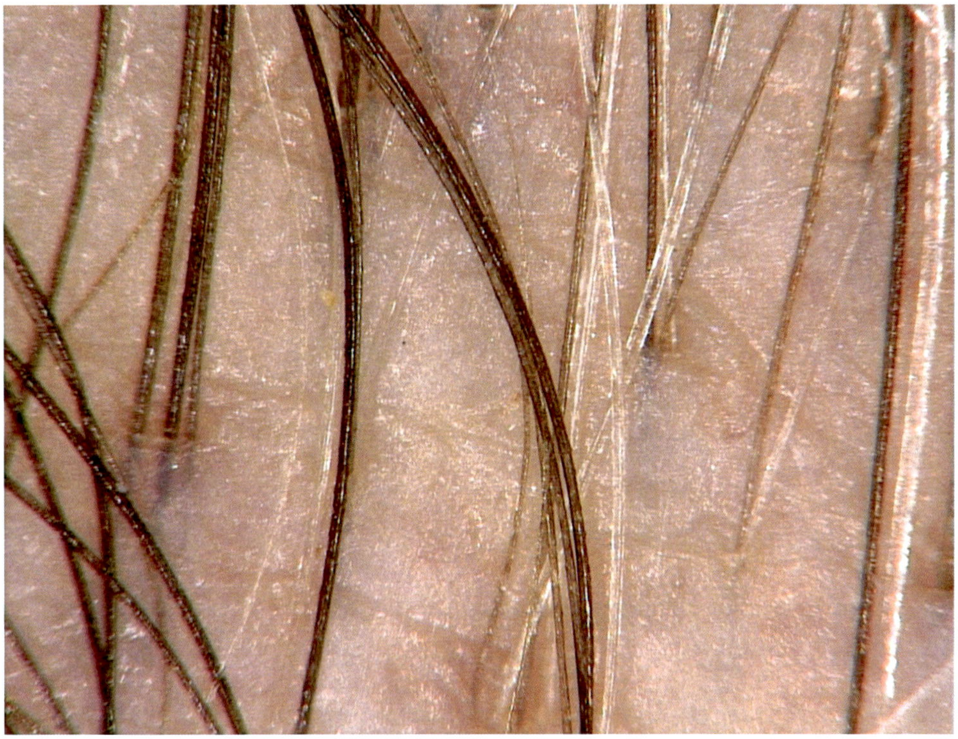

Fig. 4.1 Mild diffuse epidermal scaling in a healthy individual. This image shows mild epidermal scaling in a healthy 72-year-old man with dry skin. Similar scaling may be observed in patients who frequently use alcoholic solutions for inflammatory scalp conditions or hair loss. Scaling is seen best on dry trichoscopy. Mild scaling may not be visible when trichoscopy is performed with immersion fluid (×70)

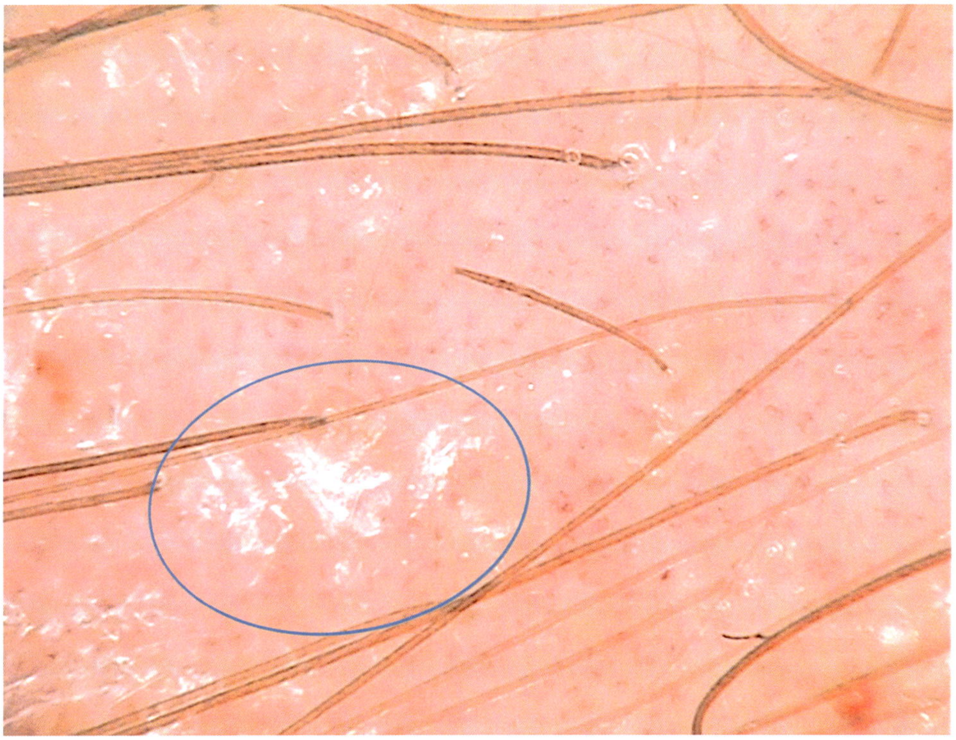

Fig. 4.2 Diffuse white scaling in psoriasis. The severity of scaling in psoriasis may vary from very mild to severe. Compared with scaling due to dry skin, the individual flakes are noticeably bigger and cumulate into white scaly areas. In psoriasis, the scales are white or silver white, which differentiates them from the yellowish scales in seborrheic dermatitis. In this patient with mild scaling (*blue ring*) in the course of psoriasis, the diagnosis may be suspected based on regularly distributed coiled blood vessels (×70)

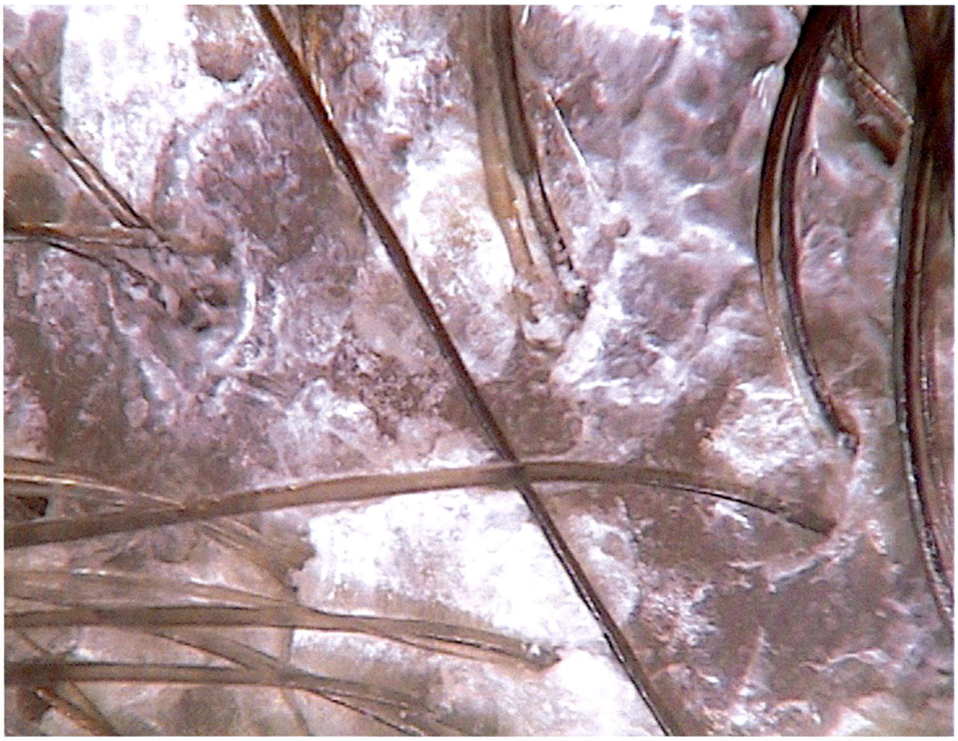

Fig. 4.3 Diffuse white scaling in psoriasis. This image shows intense white to silver-white scaling in a patient with psoriasis. The severity of scaling may be evaluated on a scale from 0 to 3 (0 = no scaling, 1 = mild scaling, 2 = moderate scaling, 3 = intense scaling). The scaling in this image would be rated 3 on this scale. Removal of scales with a keratolytic agent may be necessary to visualize the characteristic blood vessel pattern of active psoriasis (dry trichoscopy; ×70)

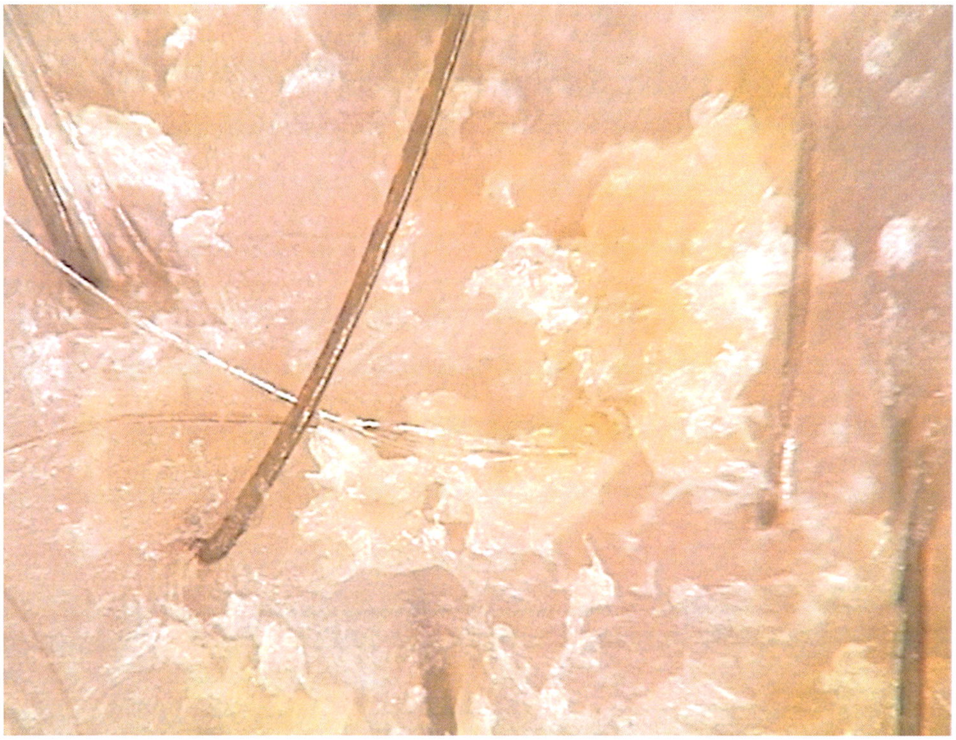

Fig. 4.4 Diffuse yellow scaling in seborrheic dermatitis. Scales in seborrheic dermatitis have a yellowish tint and do not appear as dry as psoriatic scales, even on dry trichoscopy. Scale clusters have a whitish peripheral margin. There is no tendency for perifollicular accentuation (dry trichoscopy; ×70)

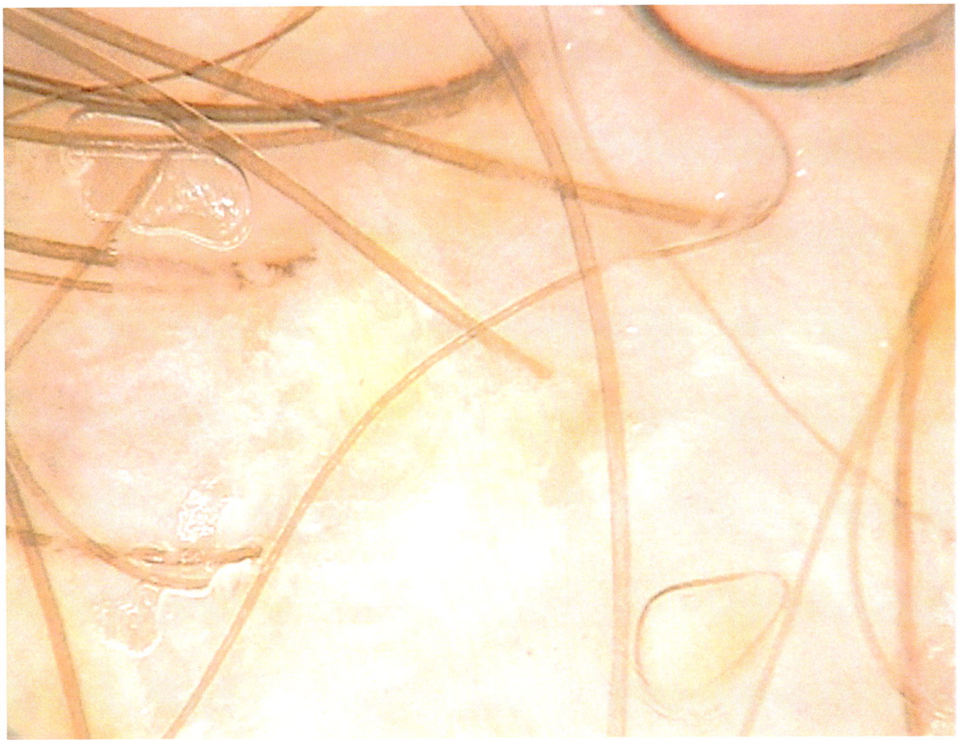

Fig. 4.5 Diffuse yellow scaling in seborrheic dermatitis. This image, obtained with immersion fluid, is from the same patient as in Fig. 4.4. Clusters of scales appear as sharp, demarcated, jagged yellow structures with a whitish peripheral margin. This appearance must be differentiated from the amorphous yellow structures of dissecting cellulitis, which appear clearly yellow and rounded at the periphery (×70)

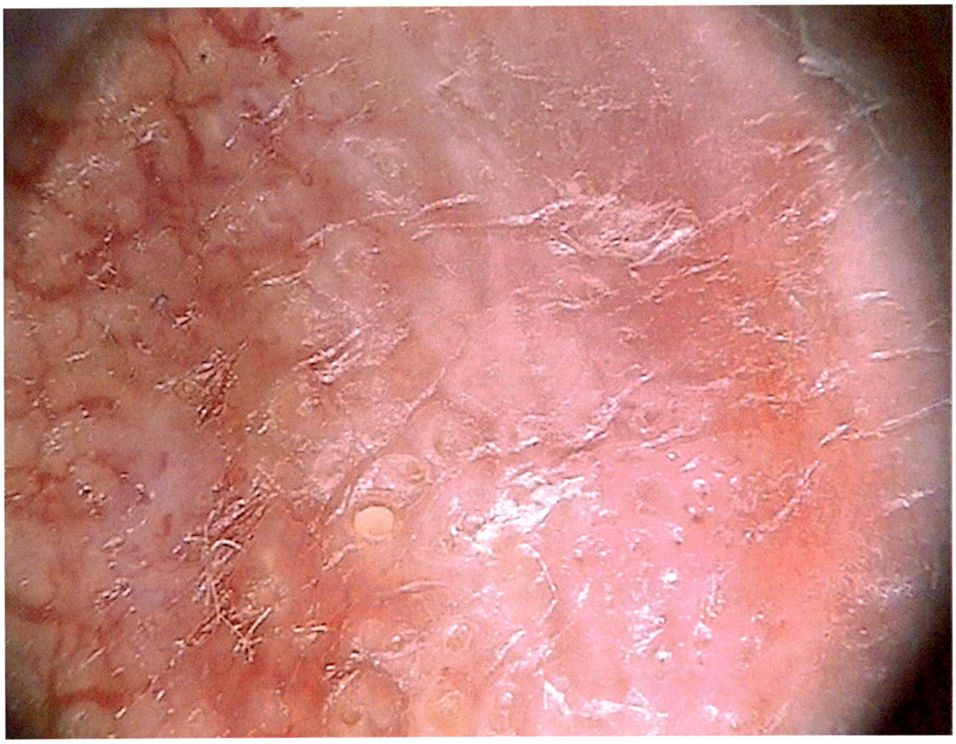

Fig. 4.6 Fine white scaling in discoid lupus erythematosus. In discoid lupus erythematosus, scaling is not a consistent finding. Scaling tends to develop in the midpart of an active lesion, preceded by thick, dilated blood vessels (*left*) and followed by fibrosis (*right*). Individual scales are small and subtle; they may be white or yellowish (dry trichoscopy; ×20)

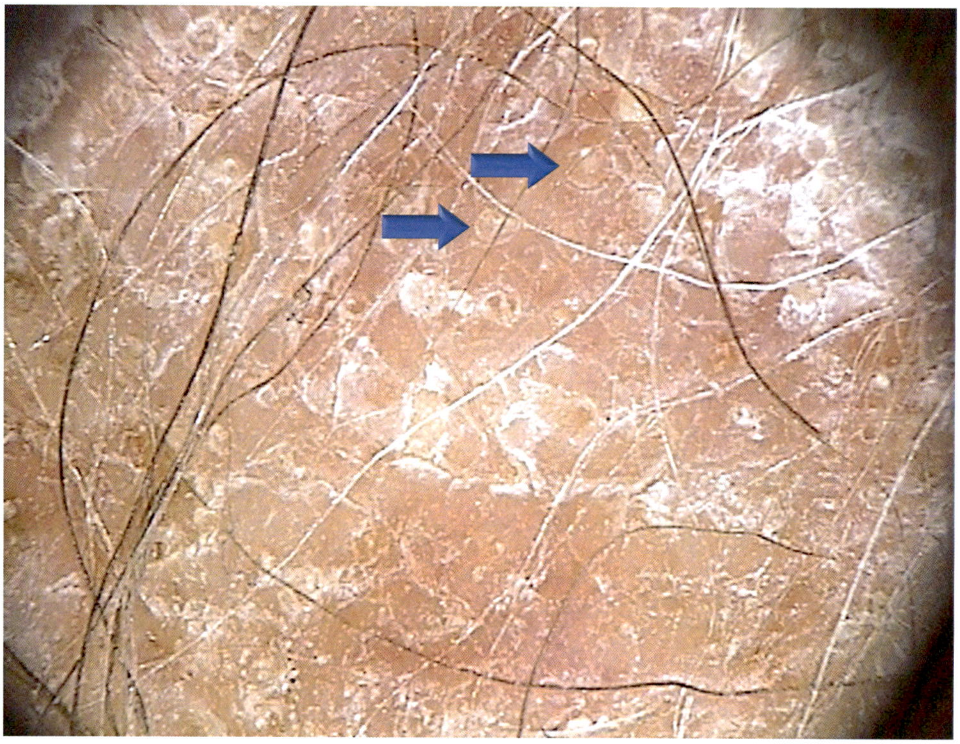

Fig. 4.7 Diffuse white and yellow scaling with follicular accentuation in discoid lupus erythematosus. Dry trichoscopy reveals fine white (*upper right*) and yellowish (*bottom left*) scaling. Note the follicular accentuation with circular shapes (*arrows*) covered by scales (dry trichoscopy; ×20)

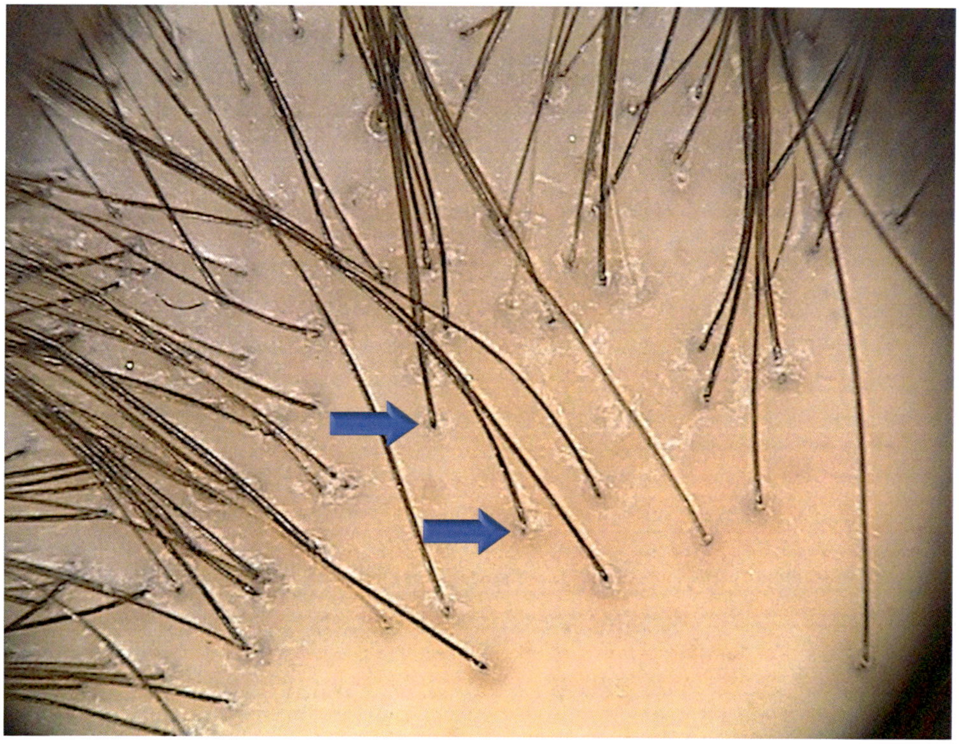

Fig. 4.8 Mild perifollicular scaling in frontal fibrosing alopecia. Mild perifollicular scaling is a nonspecific finding present in several diseases and observed occasionally in healthy individuals. This feature presents as white concentric scaling around the follicular openings (*arrows*). In frontal fibrosing alopecia, as in this image, this feature must be evaluated in the context of clinical appearance and the characteristic beige color of fibrosis (*bottom right*) (dry trichoscopy; ×20)

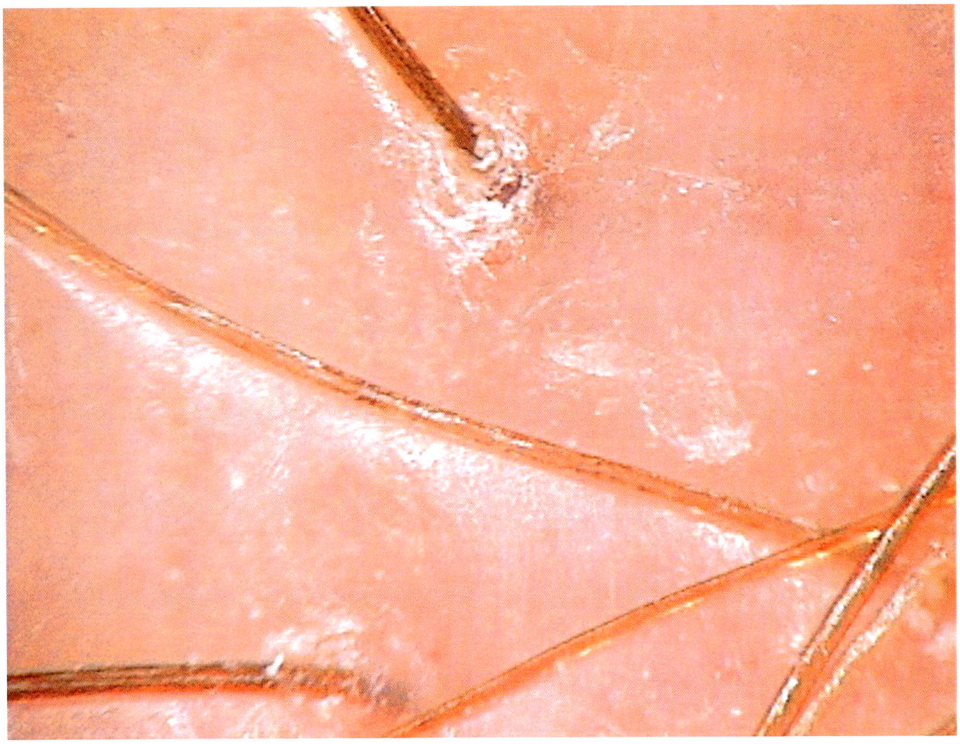

Fig. 4.9 Perifollicular scaling in lichen planopilaris. Perifollicular scaling in lichen planopilaris resembles the scaling seen in frontal fibrosing alopecia but usually is more prominent. Mild perifollicular scaling in lichen planopilaris may reflect low disease activity (dry trichoscopy; ×70)

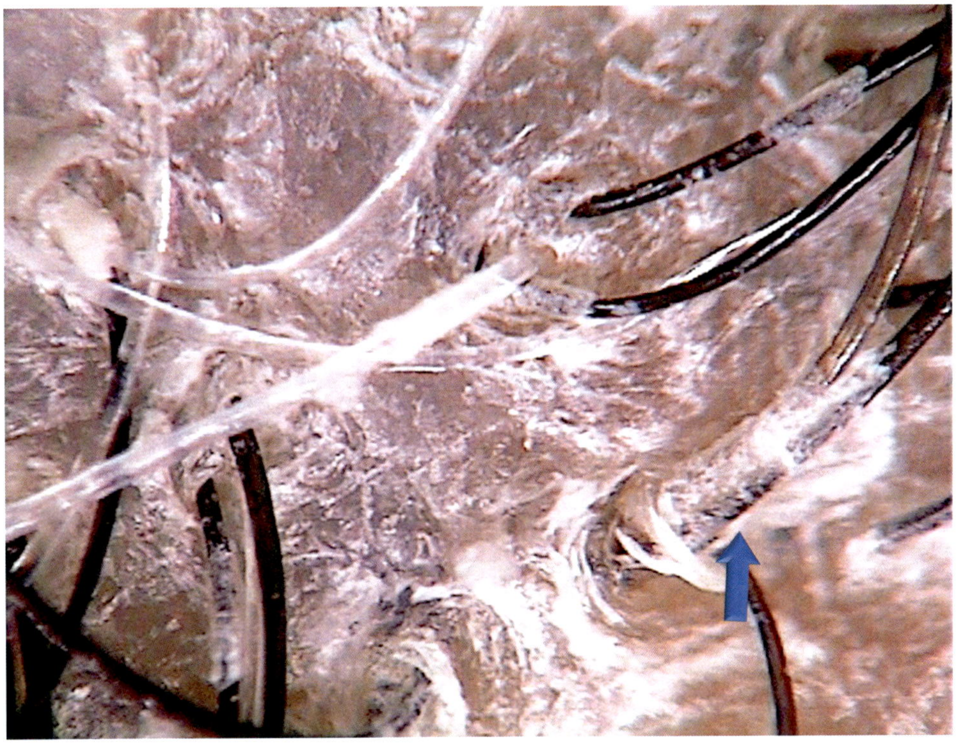

Fig. 4.10 Tubular white perifollicular scaling in lichen planopilaris. The most characteristic feature of lichen planopilaris is perifollicular scaling with formation of tubular structures surrounding the hair shafts (*arrow*). Scales migrate along the hair shaft and form a tubular structure that covers the proximal portion of the emerging hair shaft. The hair shaft may be covered by scales up to few millimeters above the scalp surface. These tubular structures may detach from the scalp surface and form hair casts, which surround the hair shaft as it grows. In lichen planopilaris, the scales are white or silver white; they may not be visible with immersion fluid (dry trichoscopy; ×70)

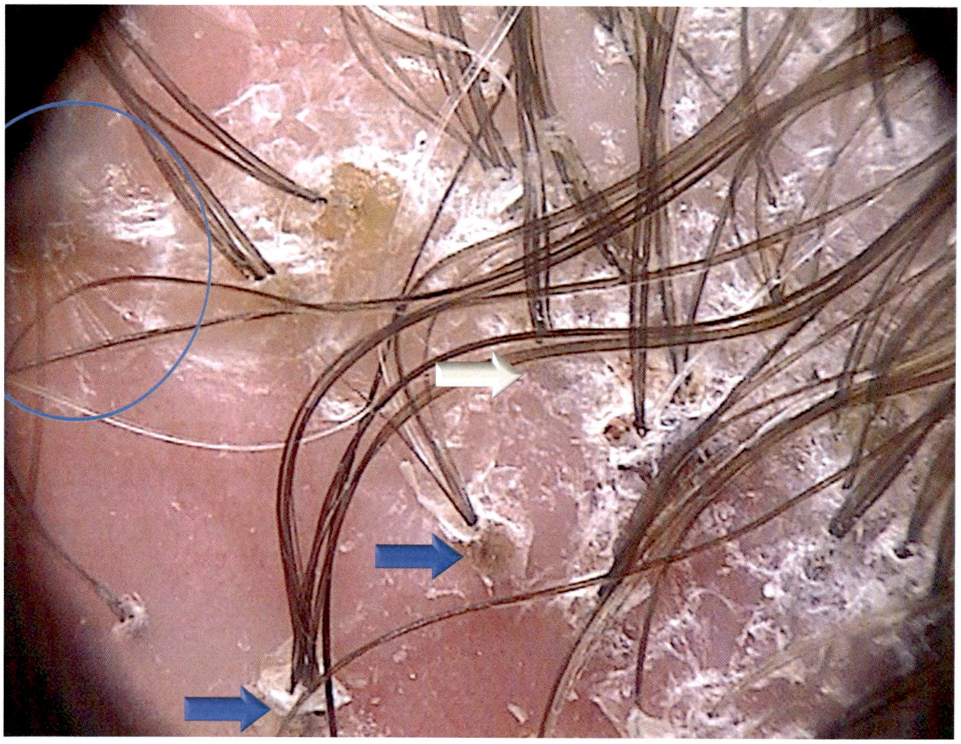

Fig. 4.11 Tubular yellowish perifollicular scaling in folliculitis decalvans. In folliculitis decalvans, as in lichen planopilaris, scales form tubular structures around the hair shaft (*blue arrows*). However, two differences compared with lichen planopilaris may be observed. First, scales tend to have a yellowish tint due to the purulent content. Second, the tubular structures are not firmly attached to the hair shaft. They unfold from the hair at the distal end and form a collar-like surface, as seen here. Another characteristic feature of folliculitis decalvans in this image is epidermal hyperplasia arranged in a starburst pattern (marked with a *blue ring*). Diffuse, homogenous scaling is also visible in this image (*white arrow*) (dry trichoscopy; ×20)

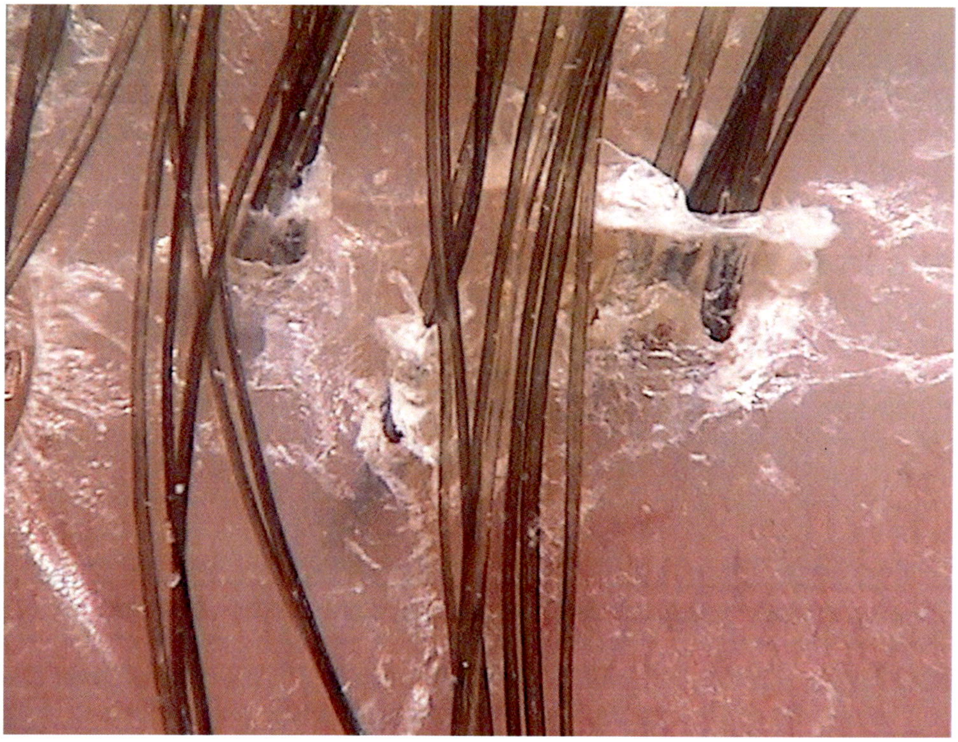

Fig. 4.12 Perifollicular scaling in folliculitis decalvans. Side view of the scaly tubular structures in folliculitis decalvans. These structures cover all hair shafts emerging from one pilosebaceous unit and unfold at the top. Prominent collar-like surfaces made of scales are visible. Note the characteristic yellowish tint of the tubular structures, epidermal hyperplasia in a starburst pattern (*left*), and pink area of fibrosis (*bottom*) (dry trichoscopy; ×70)

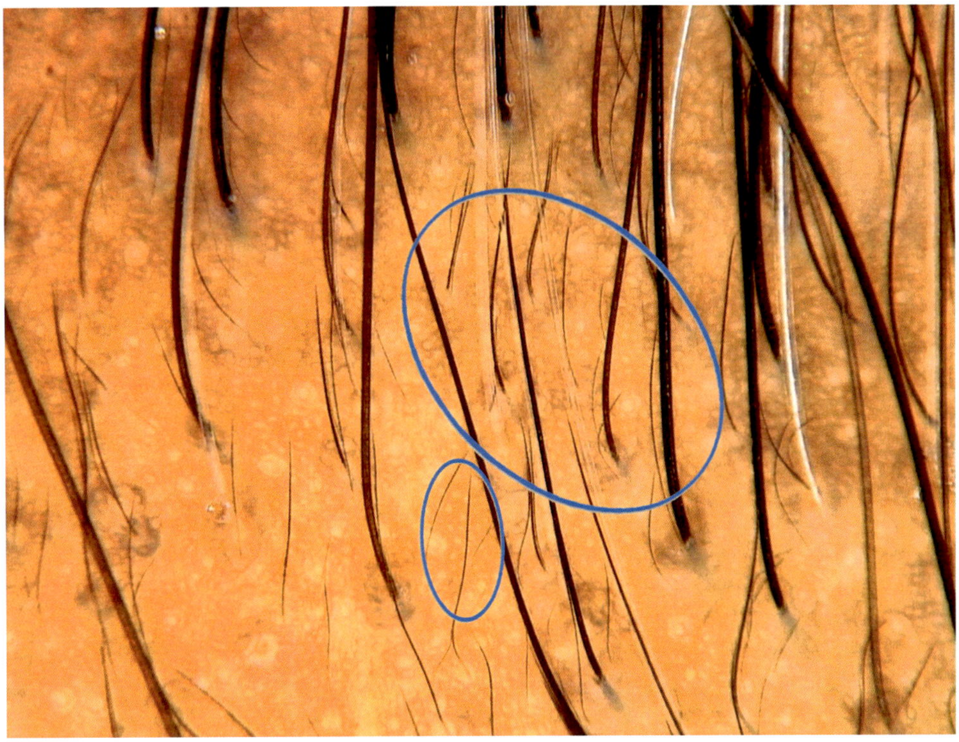

Fig. 4.13 Honeycomb pigmentation in a healthy individual with skin phototype V. Honeycomb pigmentation (*blue rings*) is a normal finding in patients with Fitzpatrick skin phototypes IV, V, and VI and is frequent on sun-exposed scalp skin in patients with noncicatricial alopecia and lighter skin. The honeycomb pattern consists of grouped, contiguous brown rings that are significantly darker than the rest of the skin surface According to Ross et al. [3], in the pigment network, the brown rings represent melanin in the rete ridges. The thinner suprapapillary epidermis, which overlies the tips of the dermal papillae, contains less melanin and appears relatively hypomelanotic (×70)

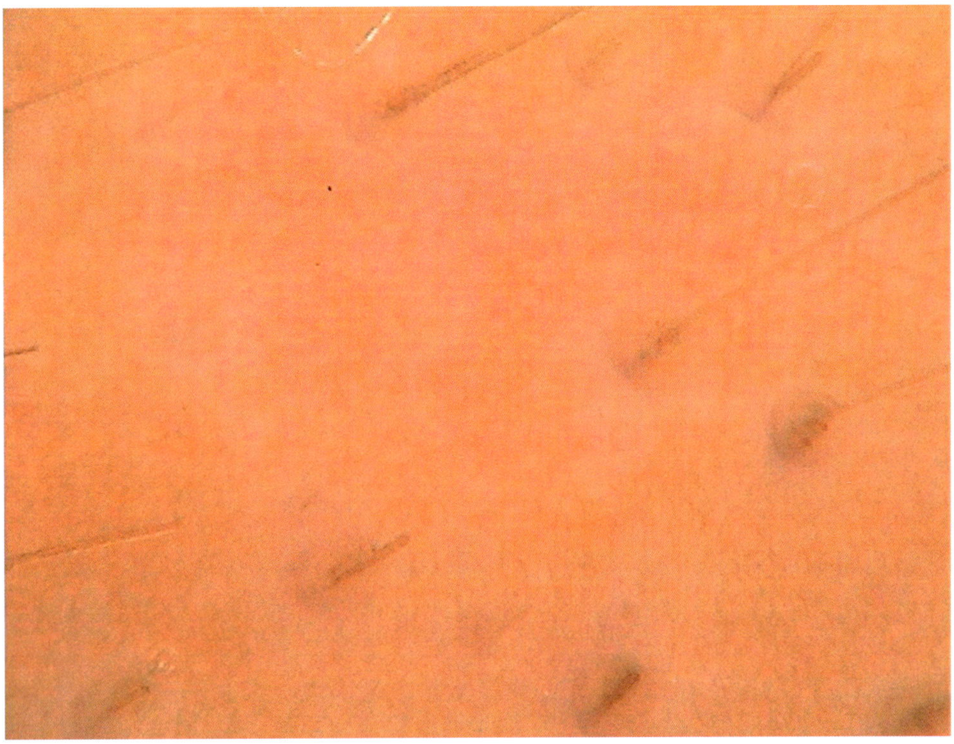

Fig. 4.14 Honeycomb pigmentation in a Caucasian patient with androgenetic alopecia. In this patient with phototype II and hair loss in the course of androgenetic alopecia, the honeycomb pattern pigmentation developed as a result of extensive sun exposure. In persons with light skin phototypes, the grid is light to medium brown. The extent of pigmentation correlates with the degree of hair loss; it is diffuse on bald scalps and less pronounced in patients with partial hair loss. This difference results from sun protection provided by the hair (×70)

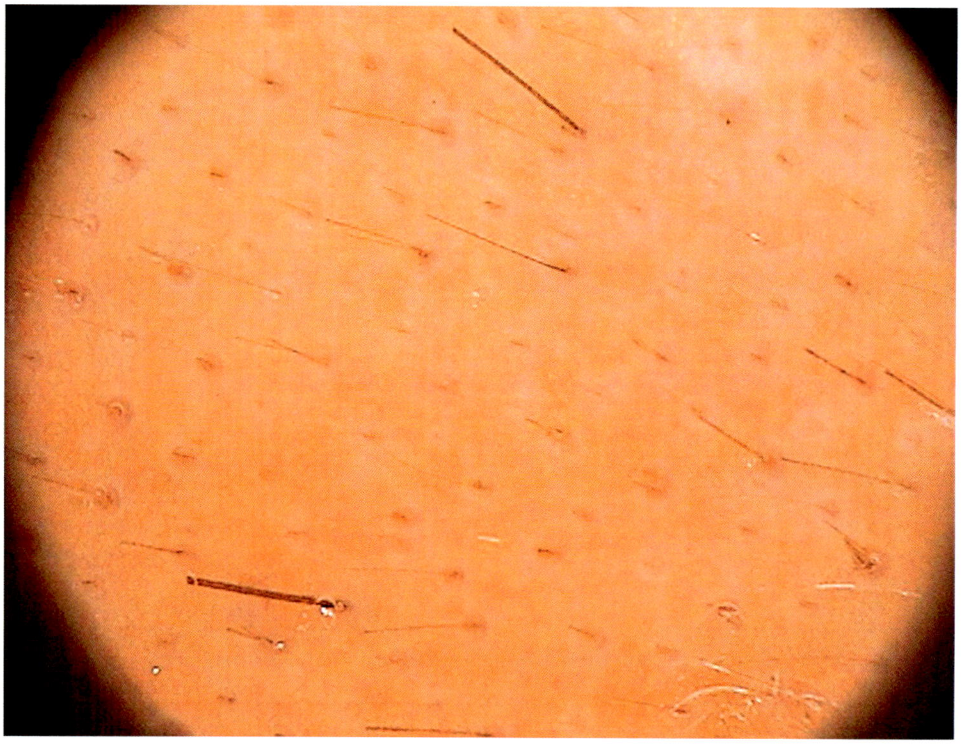

Fig. 4.15 Honeycomb hyperpigmentation. This image, taken at 20-fold magnification in the same patient as in Fig. 4.14, shows that the pattern becomes confluent and barely visible at lower magnifications (×20)

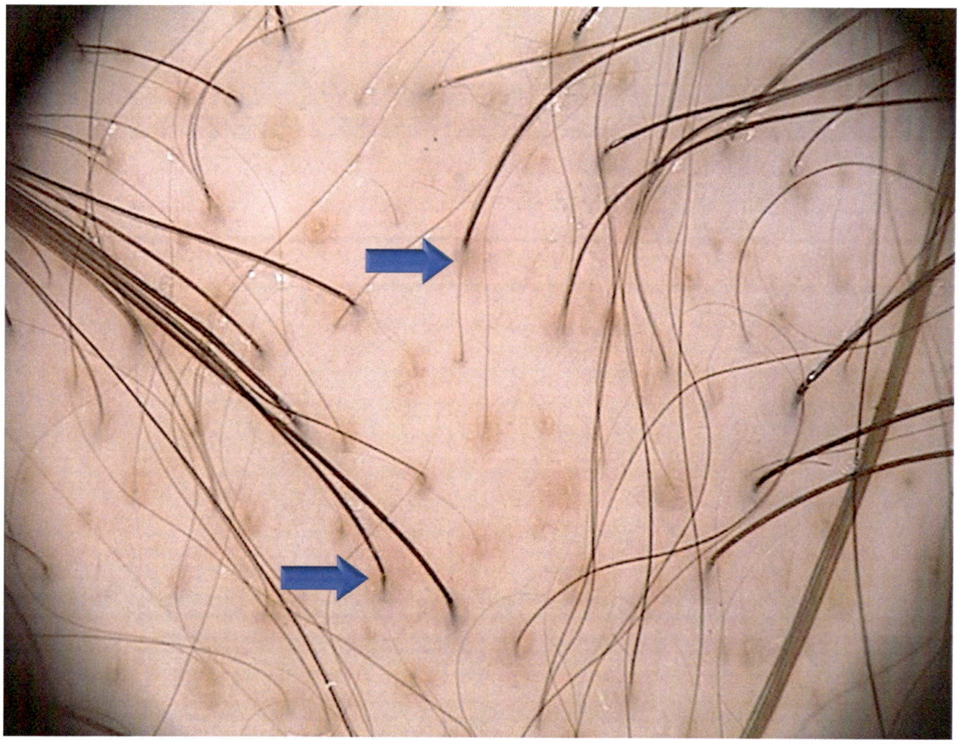

Fig. 4.16 Peripilar sign in androgenetic alopecia. The peripilar sign, first described by Deloche et al. [4], is a brown or brown-gray circular, perifollicular discoloration (*arrows*). The peripilar sign has been linked to superficial perifollicular lymphocytic infiltrates; however, the exact mechanism leading to the change in the color of the perifollicular skin surface is unknown. The peripilar sign is observed in 2–7 % of hair follicle openings in healthy individuals [10]. A higher percentage of hair follicle openings with perifollicular discoloration may be observed in persons with androgenetic alopecia (average, 41 %) and occasionally is observed in telogen effluvium [4, 5, 10, 11]. The peripilar sign may have a yellowish tint due to the sebum content (×20)

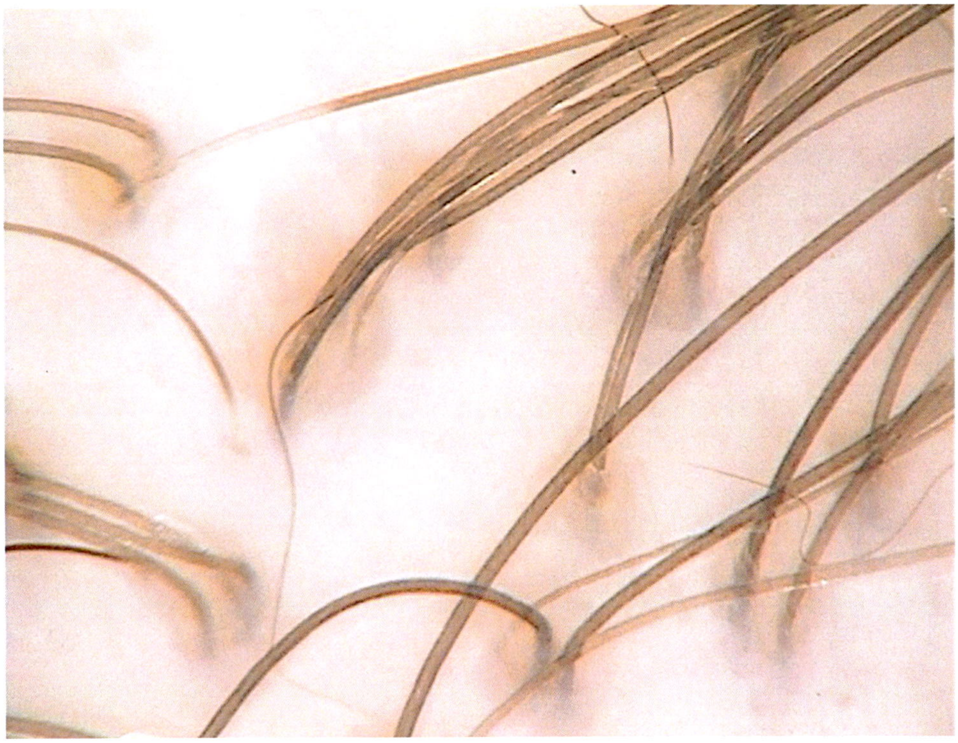

Fig. 4.17 Peripilar sign in acute telogen effluvium. High magnification shows a blurred margin of perifollicular discoloration. In follicular units with multiple hairs, the brown area surrounds all the hairs in the unit. In this image, almost 100 % of the hair follicle openings show the peripilar sign. In our experience, this is a negative prognostic factor for hair loss in the upcoming months (×70)

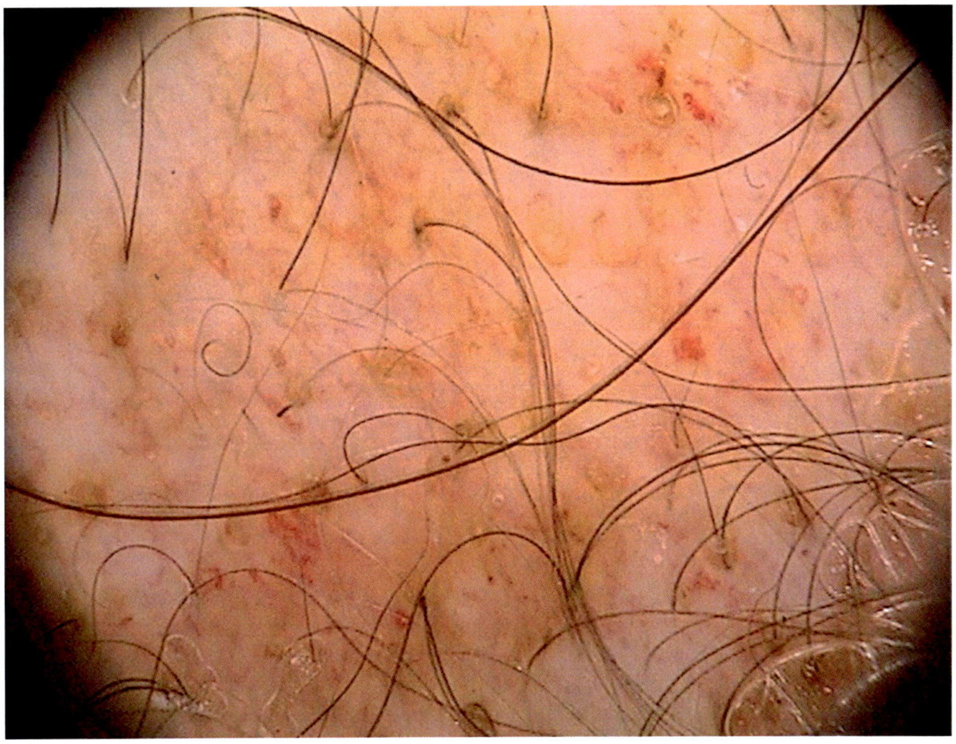

Fig. 4.18 Scattered brown skin pigmentation in discoid lupus erythematosus. The "dirty skin" appearance in discoid lupus erythematosus corresponds to pigment incontinence on histopathology [2, 8]. Pigment incontinence appears brown on trichoscopy of lesions with atrophic epidermis, such as discoid lupus erythematosus. In diseases with epidermal hyperplasia, such as lichen planopilaris, pigment incontinence appears bluish or violaceous. Scattered brown pigmentation in discoid lupus erythematosus must be differentiated from artificial pigmentation due to hair coloring (×20)

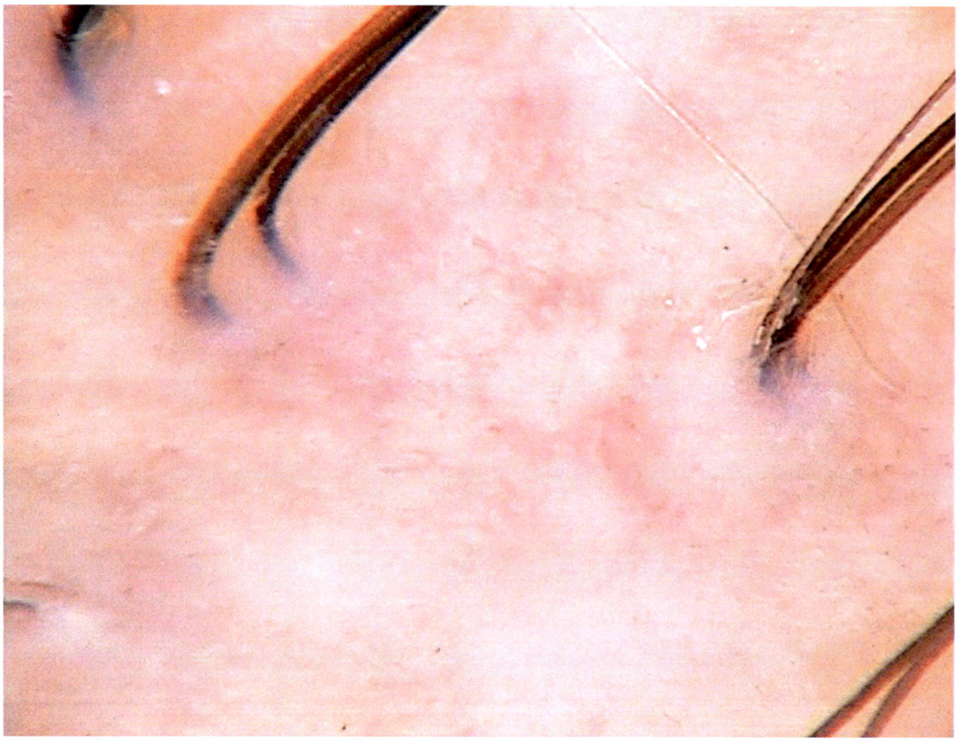

Fig. 4.19 White areas of fibrosis in lichen planopilaris. In lichen planopilaris, white dots become confluent and form white areas of fibrosis. This feature is seen best at the hair-bearing margin of cicatricial alopecia (×70)

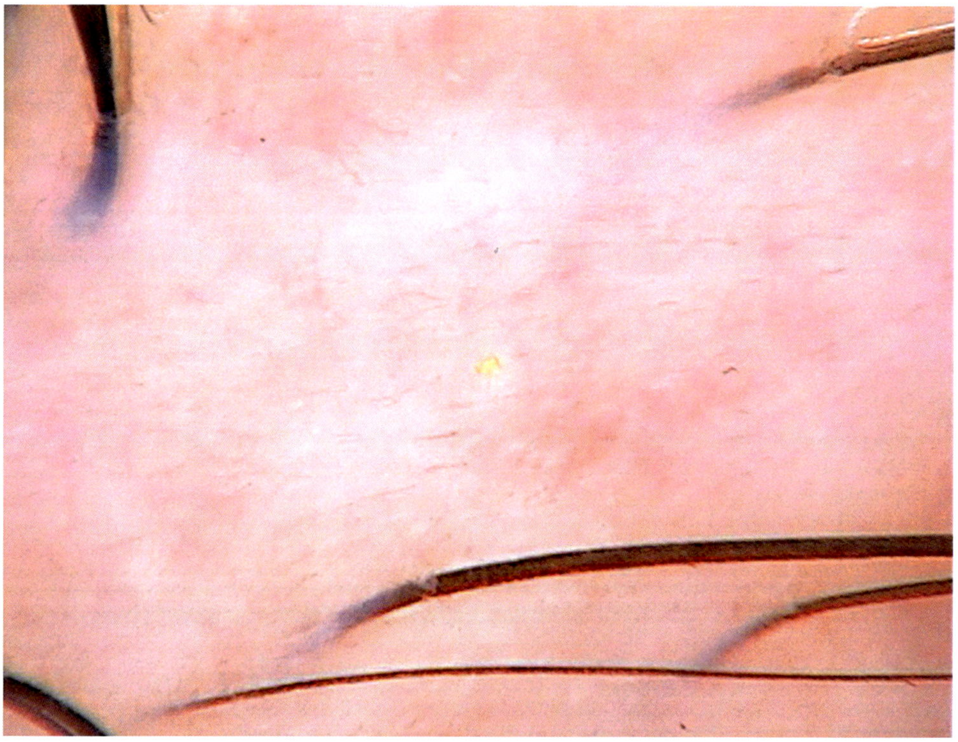

Fig. 4.20 White and pink areas of fibrosis in cicatricial alopecia. The coexistence of white dots, white areas of end-stage fibrosis, and pink areas, which correspond to fibrosis of recent onset, gives the skin a characteristic strawberry ice cream appearance. This finding is most common in lichen planopilaris but also may be observed in other types of cicatricial alopecia (×70)

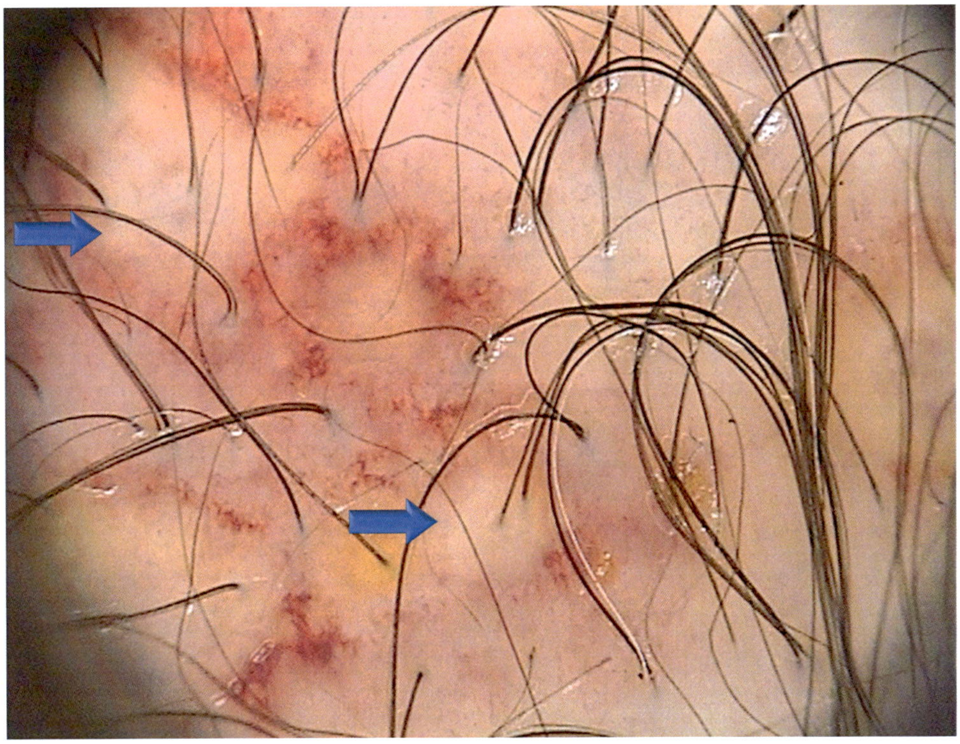

Fig. 4.21 White areas due to epidermal detachment in herpes zoster. White areas of fibrosis (*arrows*) must be differentiated from the white color corresponding to epidermal detachment observed in zoster, herpes simplex infections, erythema multiforme, pemphigoid, or pemphigus. In these diseases, the white areas have clear-cut borders and coexisting features of an active inflammatory process (×20)

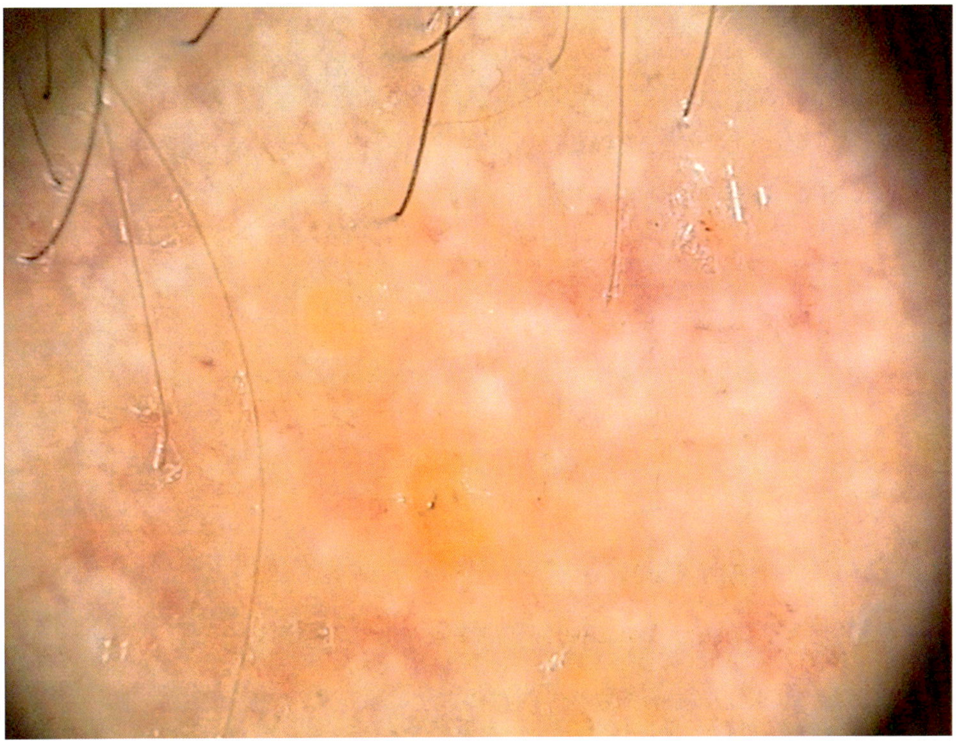

Fig. 4.22 White areas in Langerhans cell histiocytosis. Shown is a trichoscopic image from a patient with Langerhans cell histiocytosis.
On histopathology, rounded cotton wool–like, cloudy structures corresponded to a collection of Langerhans cells with accompanying interstitial edema in the upper dermis. How common this finding occurs in Langerhans cell histiocytosis remains to be evaluated (×20)

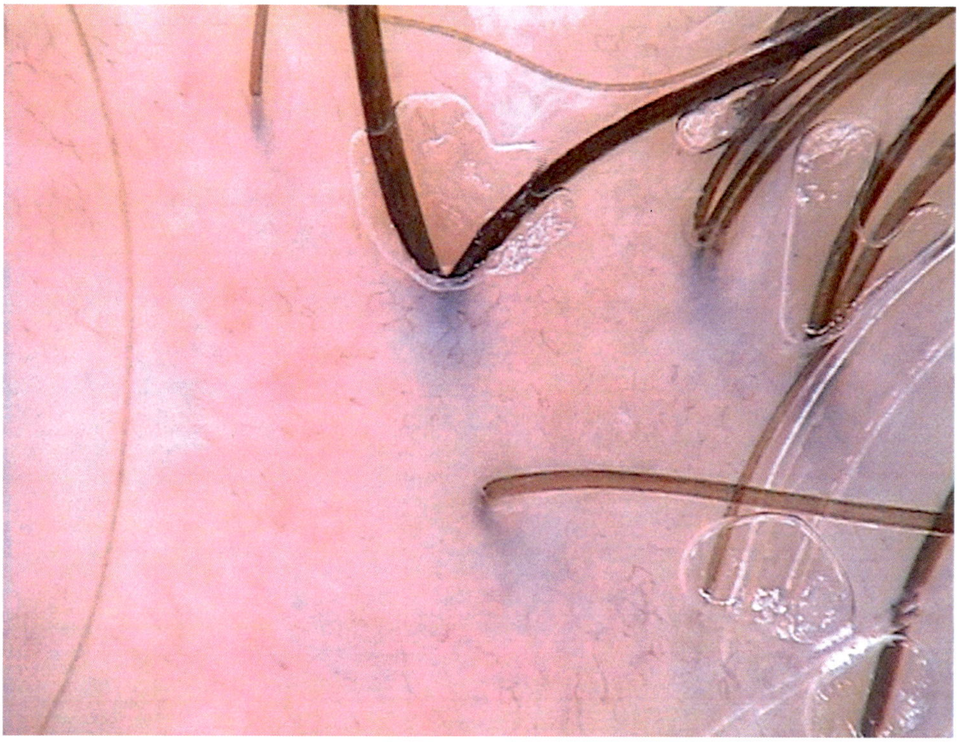

Fig. 4.23 Pink areas in cicatricial alopecia. Strawberry ice cream–colored areas devoid of hair follicle openings are characteristic of cicatricial alopecia with fibrosis of recent onset. Elongated blood vessels reflect the ongoing inflammatory process (×70)

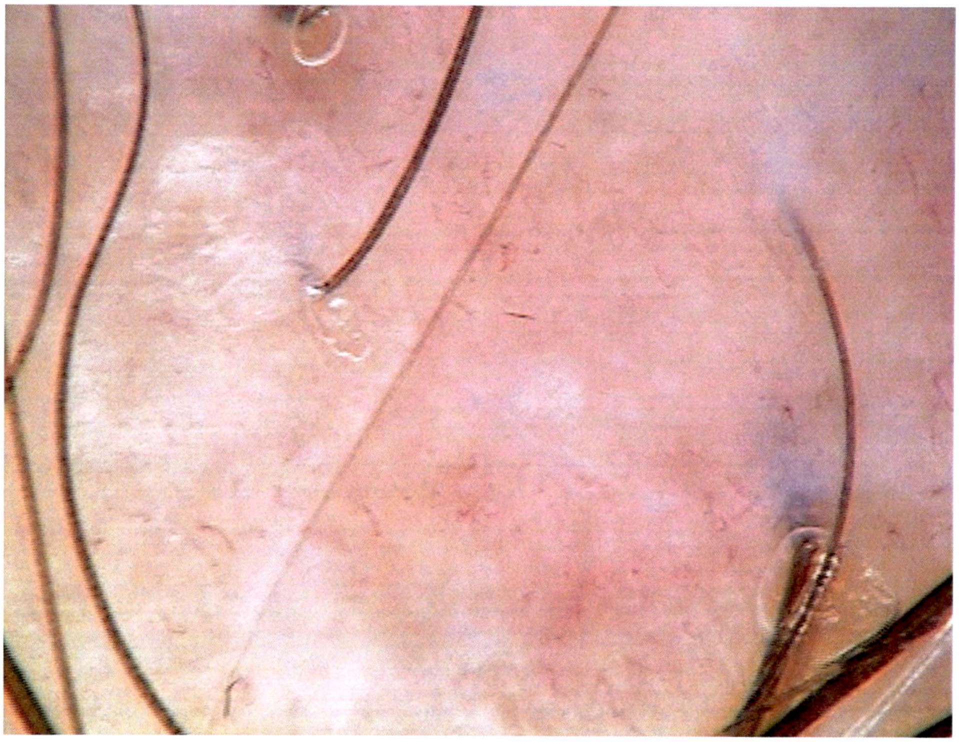

Fig. 4.24 Pink areas in lichen planopilaris. Pink, strawberry ice cream–colored areas devoid of hair follicle openings may be observed in every type of primary or secondary alopecia. The coexistence of pink areas with white dots and irregular white areas of end-stage fibrosis is characteristic of lichen planopilaris (×70)

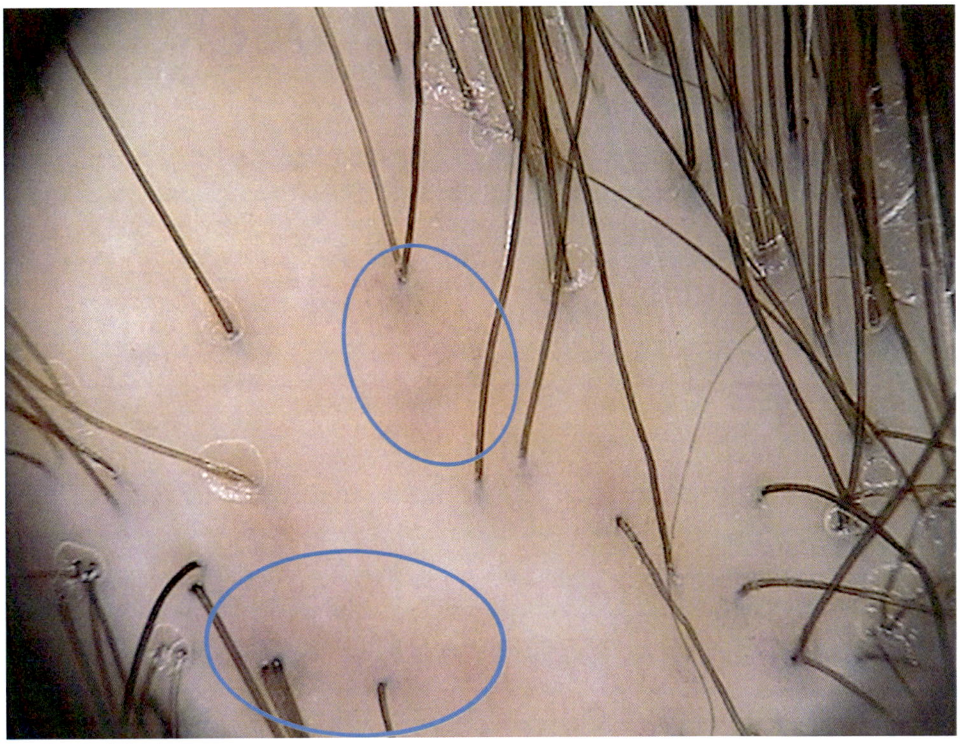

Fig. 4.25 Violaceous areas in lichen planopilaris. Violet-gray or violet-brown areas, commonly present in perifollicular localization, correspond to the pigment incontinence observed on histopathology. In lichen planopilaris, an inflammatory process in the epidermis stimulates melanin synthesis. Melanin then is transferred to the surrounding keratinocytes, released from the injured basal layer, and trapped by macrophages in the papillary dermis. Because of the Tyndall effect, melanin in the papillary dermis appears blue-gray on dermoscopy. In this trichoscopic image, the violaceous areas (*blue rings*) are altered further by the epidermal changes in lichen planopilaris (×20)

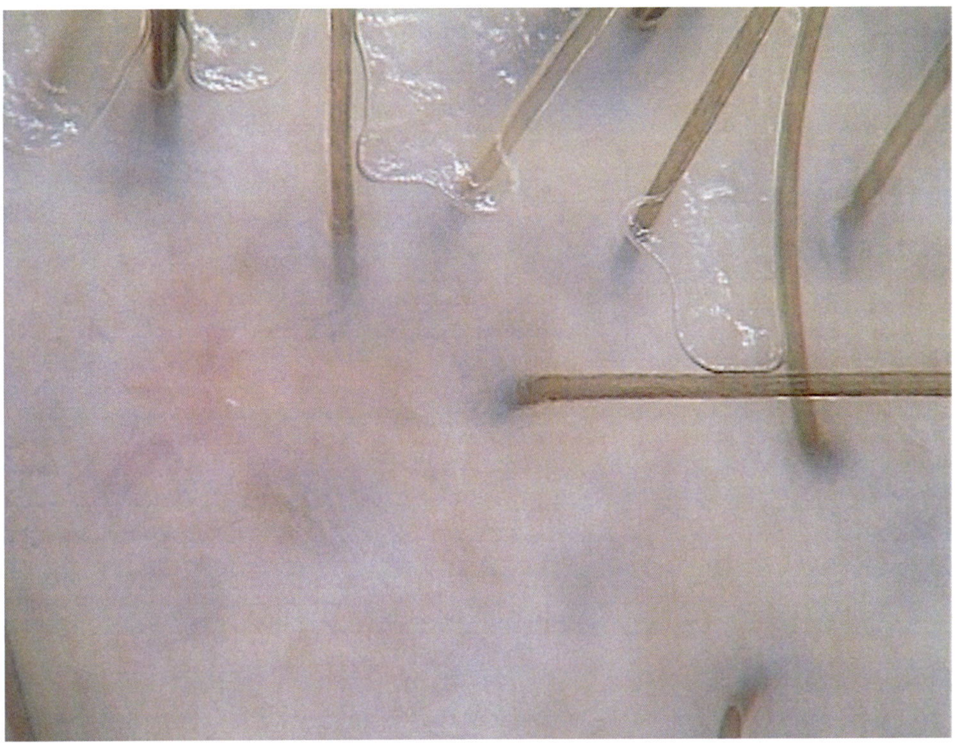

Fig. 4.26 Violaceous areas in lichen planopilaris. High magnification reveals the blurred structure and fading color intensity of the violaceous areas. Monitoring of these areas shows they may persist over months or years. The redness and elongated blood vessels reflect an ongoing inflammatory process in direct proximity to the violaceous area (×70)

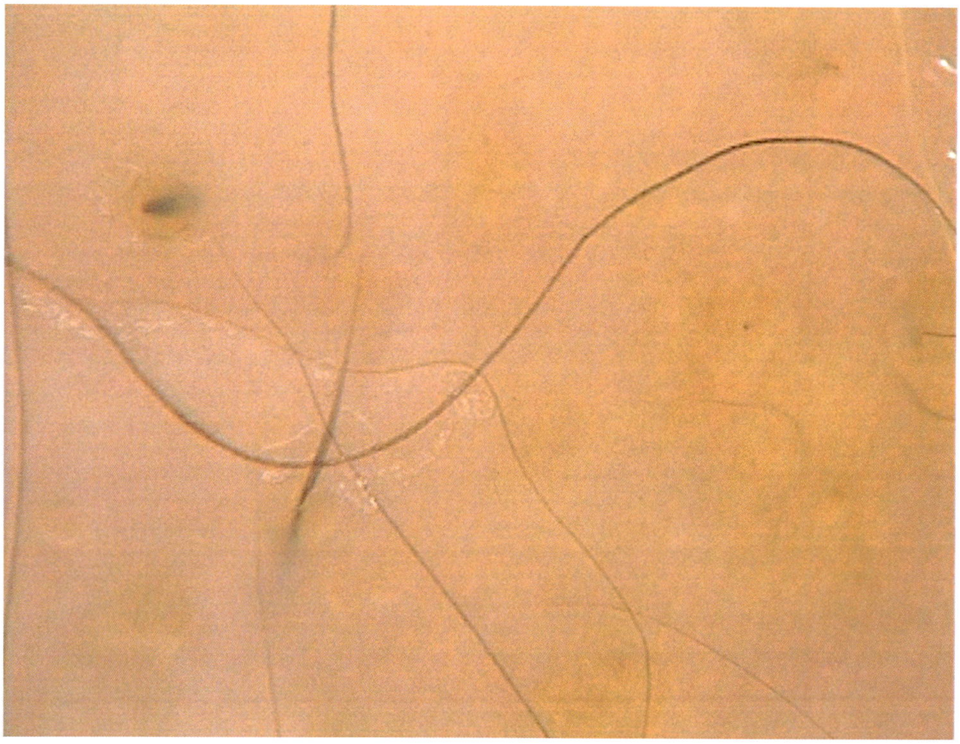

Fig. 4.27 Yellow amorphous areas in dissecting cellulitis. Amorphous yellow areas in dissecting cellulitis correspond to neutrophilic and lymphoplasmacytic infiltrates on histopathology. These structures tend to be oval to circular and multicentric. In the *upper left part* of the image, a characteristic three-dimensional yellow dot containing residual pigmented hair is visible (×70)

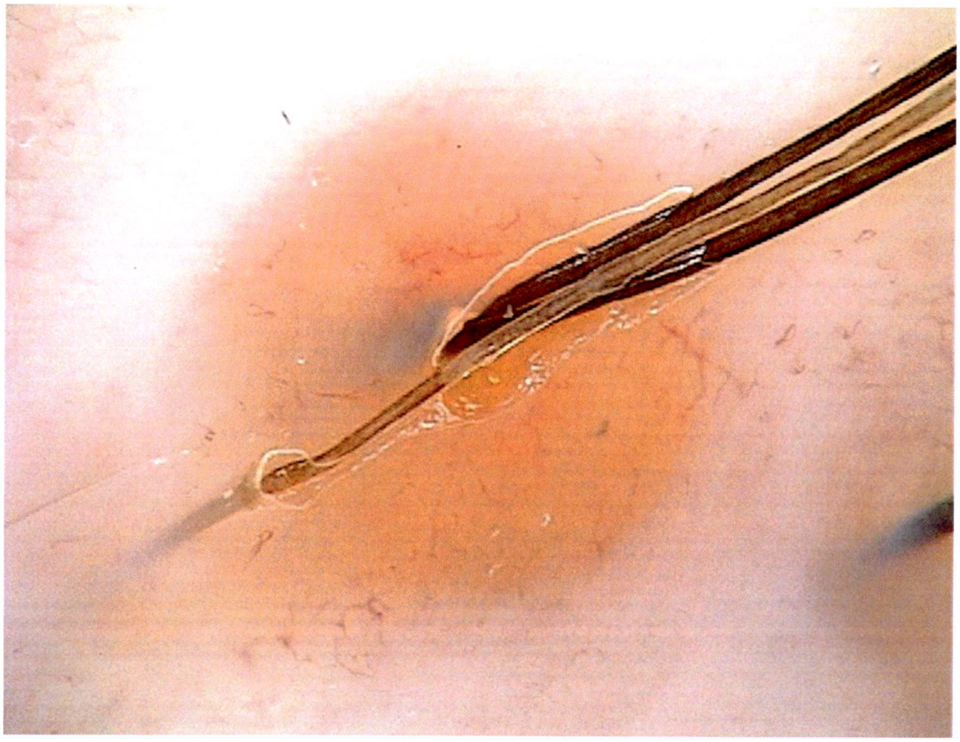

Fig. 4.28 Yellow follicular pustule in folliculitis decalvans. A large dark-yellow follicular pustule with an emerging hair shaft is a frequent finding in folliculitis decalvans. Differential diagnosis is bacterial folliculitis. Multiple, partly concentrically aligned vessels overlying the pustule favor the suspicion of folliculitis decalvans (×70)

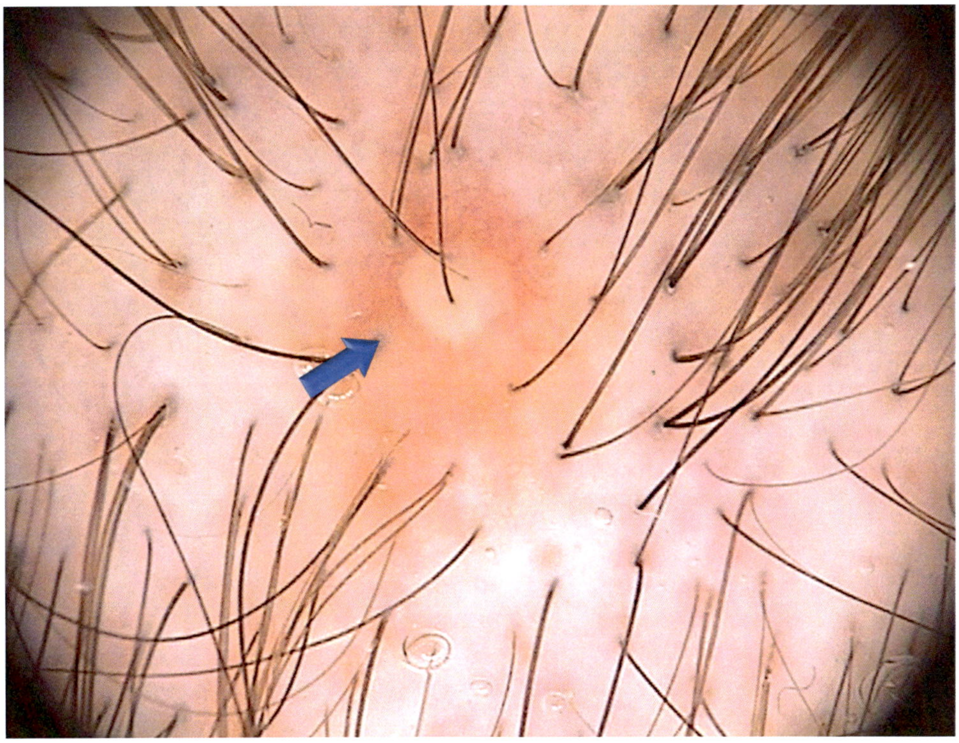

Fig. 4.29 Yellow pustule in bacterial folliculitis. Pustules in bacterial folliculitis (*arrow*) show a more pronounced inflammatory reaction at the periphery of the lesion compared with pustules in folliculitis decalvans. There is no vascular network overlying the pustule (×20)

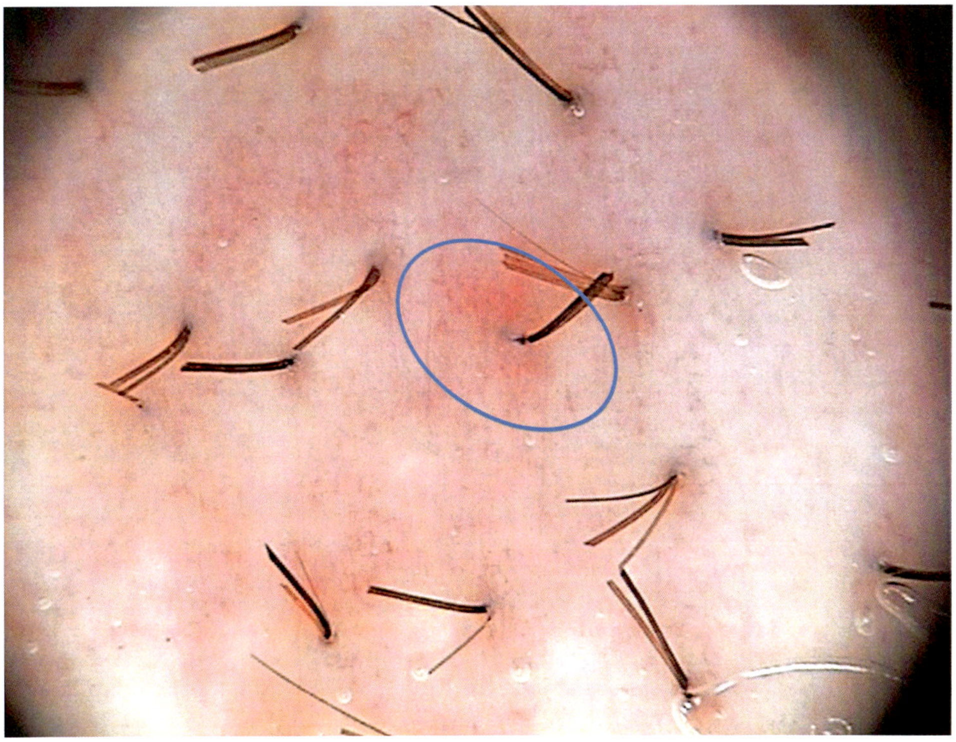

Fig. 4.30 Red areas: a manifestation of perifollicular inflammation. Red areas on trichoscopy represent inflammation, extravasation, or blood vessels, which are clearly distinguishable by their structure. This image shows perifollicular inflammation (*blue ring*), visible as red areas around pilosebaceous units in a patient with folliculitis decalvans. Pink areas correspond to a sequela of inflammation and fibrosis of recent onset. Diffuse white areas and white dots correspond with fibrosis (×20)

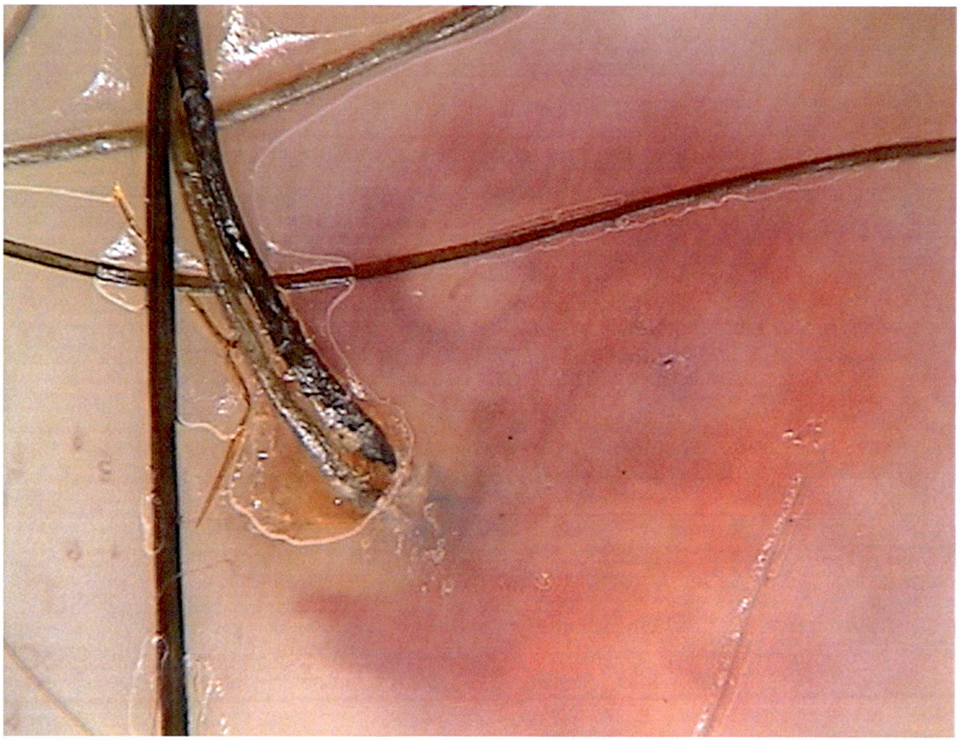

Fig. 4.31 Red areas: a manifestation of perifollicular inflammation. Deep red areas surrounding follicular openings correspond to perifollicular inflammation. This image shows perifollicular inflammation in a patient with a chronic inflammatory reaction to hair transplantation (×70)

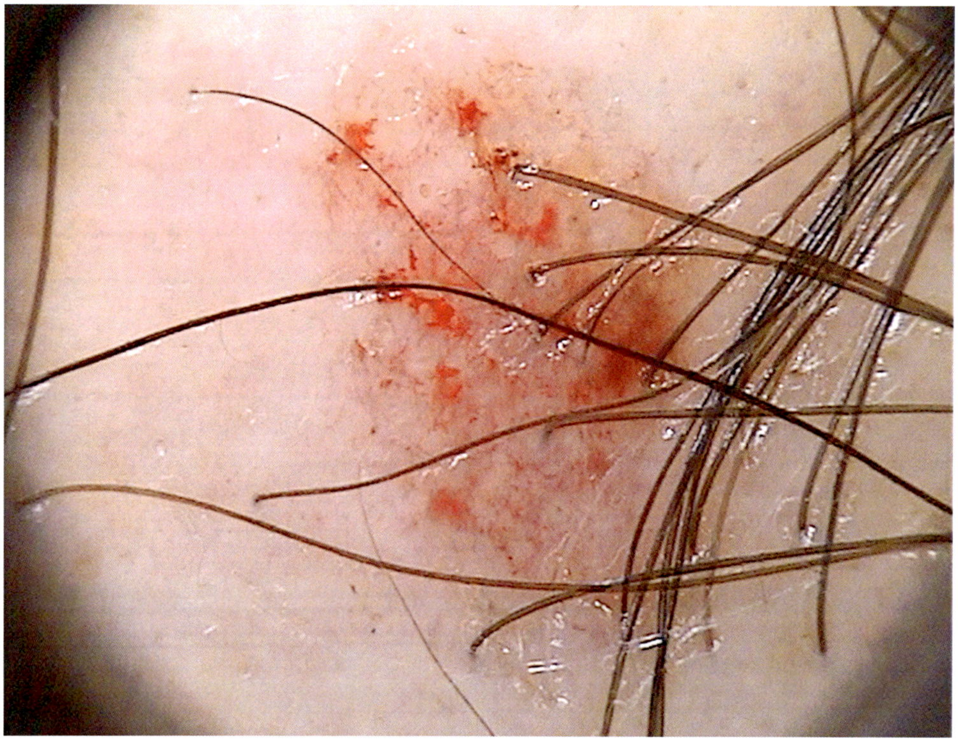

Fig. 4.32 Red areas: a manifestation of extravasation. This image shows intra- and subepidermal extravasations within a sharply demarcated blister in pemphigus vulgaris. Every type of recent-onset extravasation will appear similarly on trichoscopy (×20)

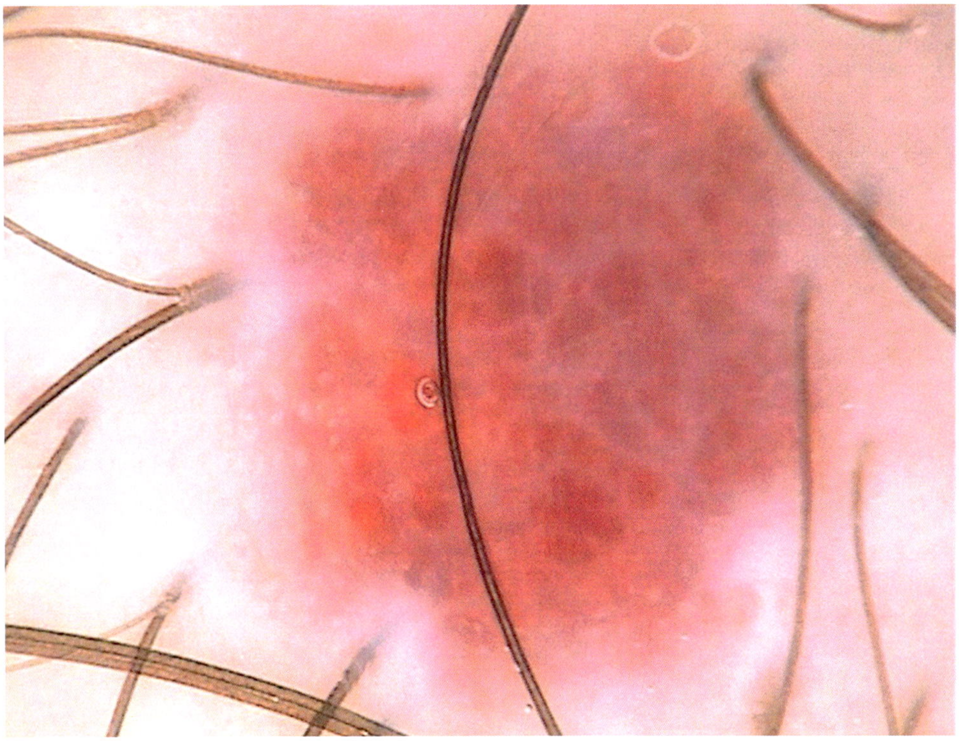

Fig. 4.33 Red areas: a manifestation of blood vessels and vascular tumors. Blood vessels and hemangiomas (seen here) usually are easy to identify by their characteristic structure (×70)

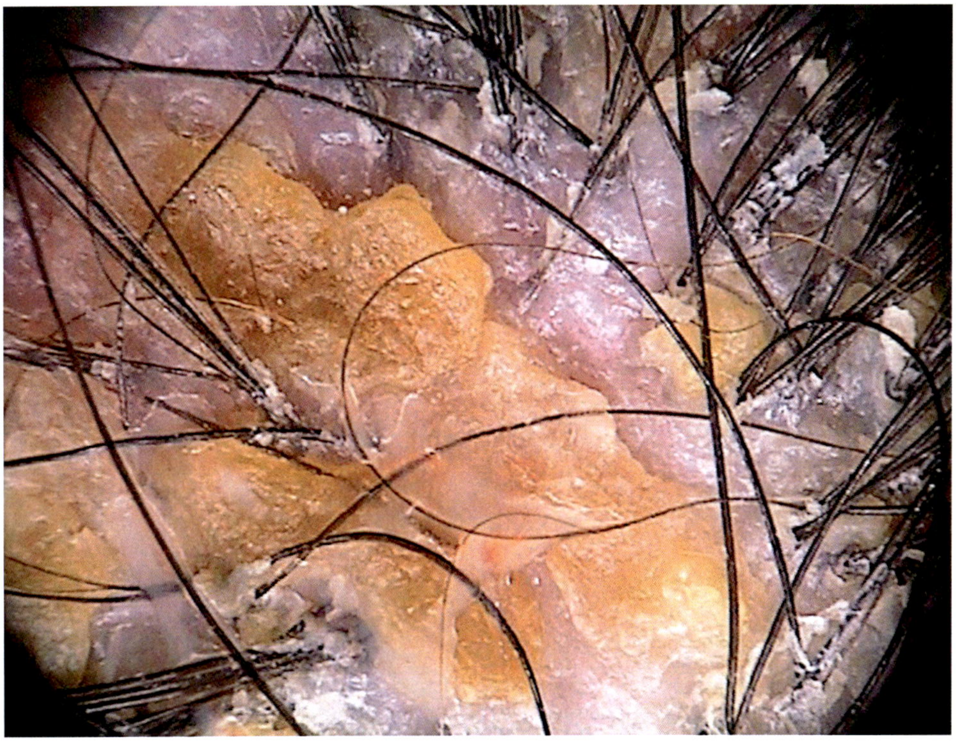

Fig. 4.34 Yellow exudate in folliculitis decalvans. A yellow purulent exudate may be associated with an infectious disease, dissecting cellulitis, or folliculitis decalvans. This image shows a dried exudate in a patient with folliculitis decalvans (×20)

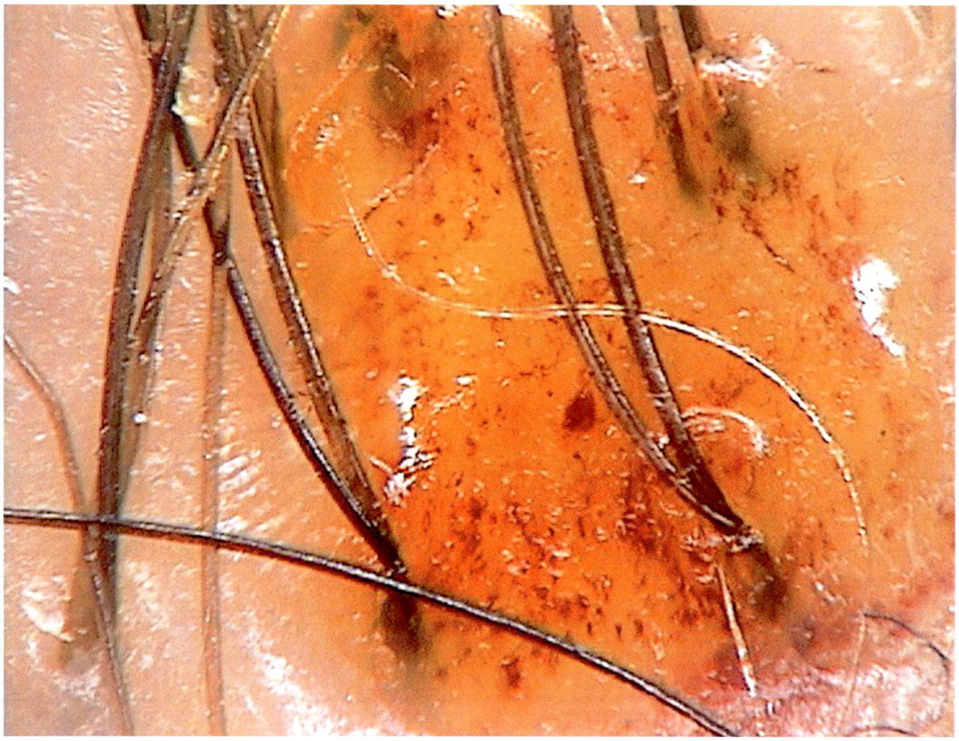

Fig. 4.35 Yellow exudate/amicrobial pustule in discoid lupus erythematosus. Amicrobial pustular dermatosis involving the scalp is rare in discoid lupus erythematosus [12]. Histologic examination shows acanthosis, neutrophilic exocytosis to the epidermis, and neutrophilic and lymphocytic infiltration with nuclear dust in the dermis. Direct immunofluorescence may be negative. Trichoscopy shows a large bulging, yellow, glossy pustule. Several short linear blood vessels and small extravasations may be seen through the translucent roof of the pustule. A purulent yellow-red exudate may be observed, depending on the evolutionary stage of the pustule (×70)

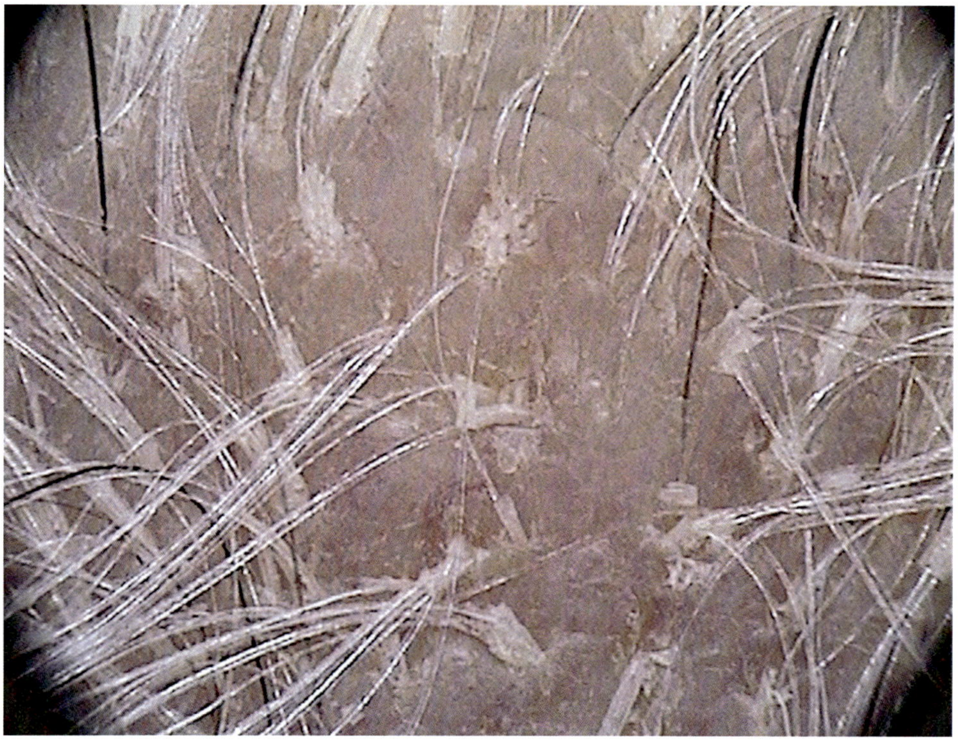

Fig. 4.36 Follicular spicules and hair casts in monoclonal gammopathy. Pseudo-hyperkeratotic follicular spicules are a rare but highly characteristic paraneoplastic feature associated with multiple myeloma. The spicules usually occur on the scalp, nose, and neck, and occasionally on the extremities. They consist of multiple myeloma paraprotein [13, 14]. This image shows follicular spicules in a patient with multiple myeloma (dry trichoscopy; ×20)

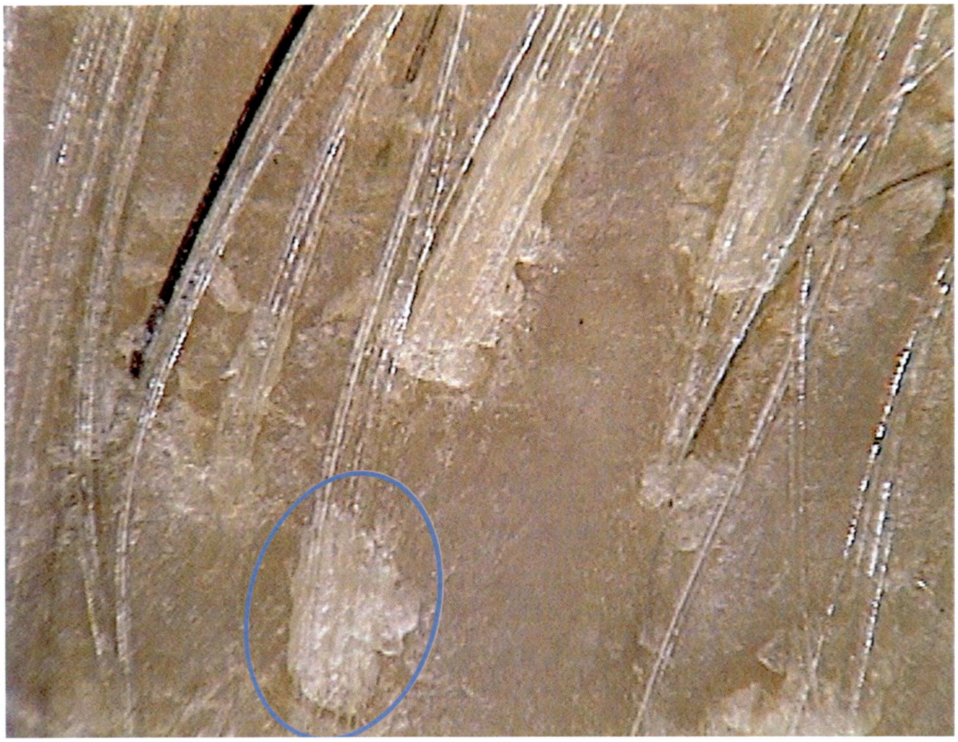

Fig. 4.37 Follicular spicules and hair casts in monoclonal gammopathy. High magnification of follicular spicules from the previous image shows white rectangular structures (*blue ring*) associated almost exclusively with hair follicle openings and hair shafts. They have a "soft" or "wet" homogenous structure and are freely movable along the hair shafts. There is no perifollicular scaling, which is a hallmark of lichen planopilaris. Also, no significant interfollicular scaling is visible. Differential diagnosis of paraneoplastic pseudo-hyperkeratotic follicular spicules with psoriasis, seborrheic dermatitis, lichen planopilaris, or folliculitis decalvans may be extremely difficult. Diagnosis should not rely on trichoscopy (dry trichoscopy; ×70)

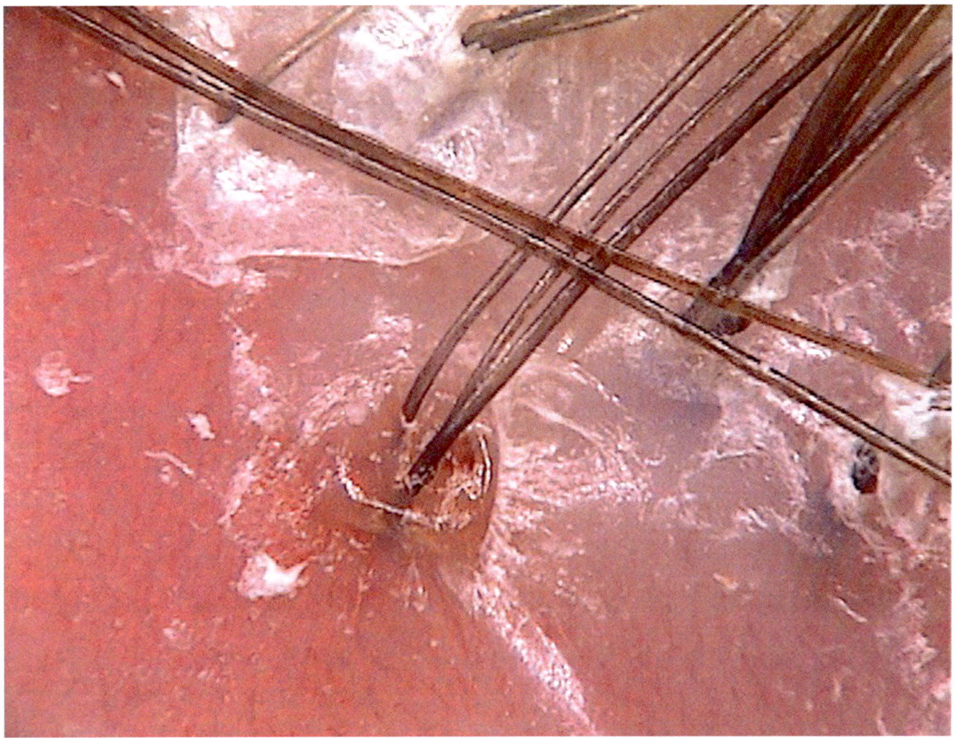

Fig. 4.38 Starburst pattern hyperplasia in folliculitis decalvans. Epidermal hyperplasia and fibrosis in folliculitis decalvans form areas of thickened skin, which are arranged concentrically around the hair follicles. This feature is called *starburst pattern hyperplasia*. The image shows an initial stage of starburst pattern hyperplasia formation (×70)

References

1. Rudnicka L, Olszewska M, Rakowska A, Kowalska-Oledzka E, Slowinska M. Trichoscopy: a new method for diagnosing hair loss. J Drugs Dermatol. 2008;7(7):651–4.
2. Rudnicka L, Olszewska M, Rakowska A, Slowinska M. Trichoscopy update 2011. J Dermatol Case Rep. 2011;5(4):82–8.
3. Ross EK, Vincenzi C, Tosti A. Videodermoscopy in the evaluation of hair and scalp disorders. J Am Acad Dermatol. 2006;55(5):799–806.
4. Deloche C, de Lacharriere O, Misciali C, Piraccini BM, Vincenzi C, Bastien P, et al. Histological features of peripilar signs associated with androgenetic alopecia. Arch Dermatol Res. 2004;295(10):422–8.
5. Wallace MP, de Berker DA. Hair diagnoses and signs: the use of dermatoscopy. Clin Exp Dermatol. 2010;35(1):41–6.
6. Inui S. Trichoscopy for common hair loss diseases: algorithmic method for diagnosis. J Dermatol. 2011;38(1):71–5.
7. Rakowska A. Trichoscopy (hair and scalp videodermoscopy) in the healthy female. Method standardization and norms for measurable parameters. J Dermatol Case Rep. 2009;3(1):14–9.
8. Rakowska A, Slowinska M, Kowalska-Oledzka E, Olszewska M, Rudnicka L. Trichoscopy in cicatricial alopecia. J Drugs Dermatol. 2012;11(6):753–8.
9. Inui S, Nakajima T, Itami S. Coudability hairs: a revisited sign of alopecia areata assessed by trichoscopy. Clin Exp Dermatol. 2010;35(4):361–5.
10. Rakowska A, Slowinska M, Kowalska-Oledzka E, Olszewska M, Rudnicka L. Dermoscopy in female androgenic alopecia: method standardization and diagnostic criteria. Int J Trichol. 2009;1(2):123–30.
11. Inui S, Nakajima T, Itami S. Scalp dermoscopy of androgenetic alopecia in Asian people. J Dermatol. 2009;36(2):82–5.
12. Kuyama M, Fujimoto W, Kambara H, Egusa M, Saitoh M, Yamasaki O, et al. Amicrobial pustular dermatosis in two patients with immunological abnormalities. Clin Exp Dermatol. 2002;27(4):286–9.
13. Tay LK, Lim FL, Ng HJ, Lee HY, Pang SM, Thirumoorthy T. Cutaneous follicular hyperkeratotic spicules—the first clinical sign of multiple myeloma progression or relapse. Int J Dermatol. 2010;49(8):934–6.
14. Weibel L, Berger M, Regenass S, Kamarashev J, Hafner J, French LE. Follicular spicules of the nose and ears—quiz case. Arch Dermatol. 2009;145(4):479–84.

Blood Vessels

5

Adriana Rakowska, Lidia Rudnicka,
Malgorzata Olszewska, and Marta Kurzeja

Abstract

Trichoscopy allows the detection of diverse vascular structures that may be present in healthy individuals or in patients with inflammatory scalp diseases. These vascular structures include (1) comma vessels, (2) dotted vessels, (3) vessels with a whitish halo, (4) hairpin vessels, (5) elongated hairpin vessels, (6) linear vessels, (7) thin arborizing vessels, (8) thick arborizing vessels, (9) capillary blood extravasations, (10) perifollicular-concentric vessels, (11) milky red globules, (12) linear helical vessels, (13) lace-like vessels, (14) glomerular (coiled) vessels, (15) serpentine vessels, (16) vessels in a crown arrangement, (17) thick root-like vessels, and (18) vessel nets. In a significant majority of cases, these are the same types of blood vessels identified previously on dermoscopy in skin tumors.

Keywords

Blood vessels • Healthy scalp • Vascular structures • Vessels

The spectrum of blood vessel arrangements in the normal scalp is very wide, and blood vessels do not seem to play as vital a role in diagnosing most scalp diseases as they do in skin tumors. An abundance of vessels with distinct morphologic structures, rather than a specific type of vessel, may be an indicator for diverse inflammatory scalp diseases.

The visualization of vascular structures depends partly on the optical device and the technique of dermoscopic examination [1]. When a contact dermoscope is used, the lens must be set carefully on the skin surface with the roll-on technique [2] and minimal downward pressure [1]. The use of alcohol or oil as an immersion fluid usually requires the application of considerable pressure against the skin, which reduces blood flow in the cutaneous capillaries and decreases their visibility. Translucent ultrasound gel allows one to apply the lens against the skin gently and to visualize the blood vessels better [1]. Green ultrasound gel or a green filter may even enhance the visibility of vessels, because green filters allow green light to pass through while blocking red light, making red objects (vessels) appear slightly darker [3]. It has been shown that 390–410 nm light also may improve the visibility of blood vessels on dermoscopy [4].

Noncontact dermoscopy does not require a liquid interphase between the lens and the skin; however, scaly scalp skin may cause reflections, which may limit the visualization of underlying vascular structures. In such cases, the application of immersion fluid to the skin may help diminish this surface reflection and improve the visualization of vessels [1].

We identified 18 types of blood vessel arrangements on the scalp [5]:

1. Comma vessels
2. Dotted vessels
3. Vessels with a whitish halo

A. Rakowska • M. Kurzeja
Department of Dermatology, CSK MSW, Warsaw, Poland

L. Rudnicka (✉)
Faculty of Health Sciences, Medical University of Warsaw, Poland

Department of Dermatology, CSK MSW,
Woloska 137, Warsaw 02-502, Poland
e-mail: lidia.rudnicka@euderm.eu

M. Olszewska
Department of Dermatology, Medical University of Warsaw,
Warsaw, Poland

L. Rudnicka et al. (eds.), *Atlas of Trichoscopy*,
DOI 10.1007/978-1-4471-4486-1_5, © Springer-Verlag London 2012

4. Hairpin vessels
5. Elongated hairpin vessels
6. Linear vessels
7. Thin arborizing vessels
8. Thick arborizing vessels
9. Capillary blood extravasations
10. Concentric perifollicular vessels
11. Milky red globules
12. Linear helical vessels
13. Lace-like vessels
14. Glomerular (coiled) vessels
15. Serpentine vessels
16. Vessels in a crown arrangement
17. Thick root-like vessels
18. Vessel nets

In a significant number of cases, these are the same types of blood vessels identified previously in skin tumors [1, 6, 7].

The specific arrangement of blood vessels may be a clue to the diagnosis of some scalp diseases, such as psoriasis, discoid lupus erythematous, or lichen planopilaris. Details are discussed in the chapters devoted to those diseases. This chapter focuses on the specific types of blood vessel shapes and arrangements observed on trichoscopy.

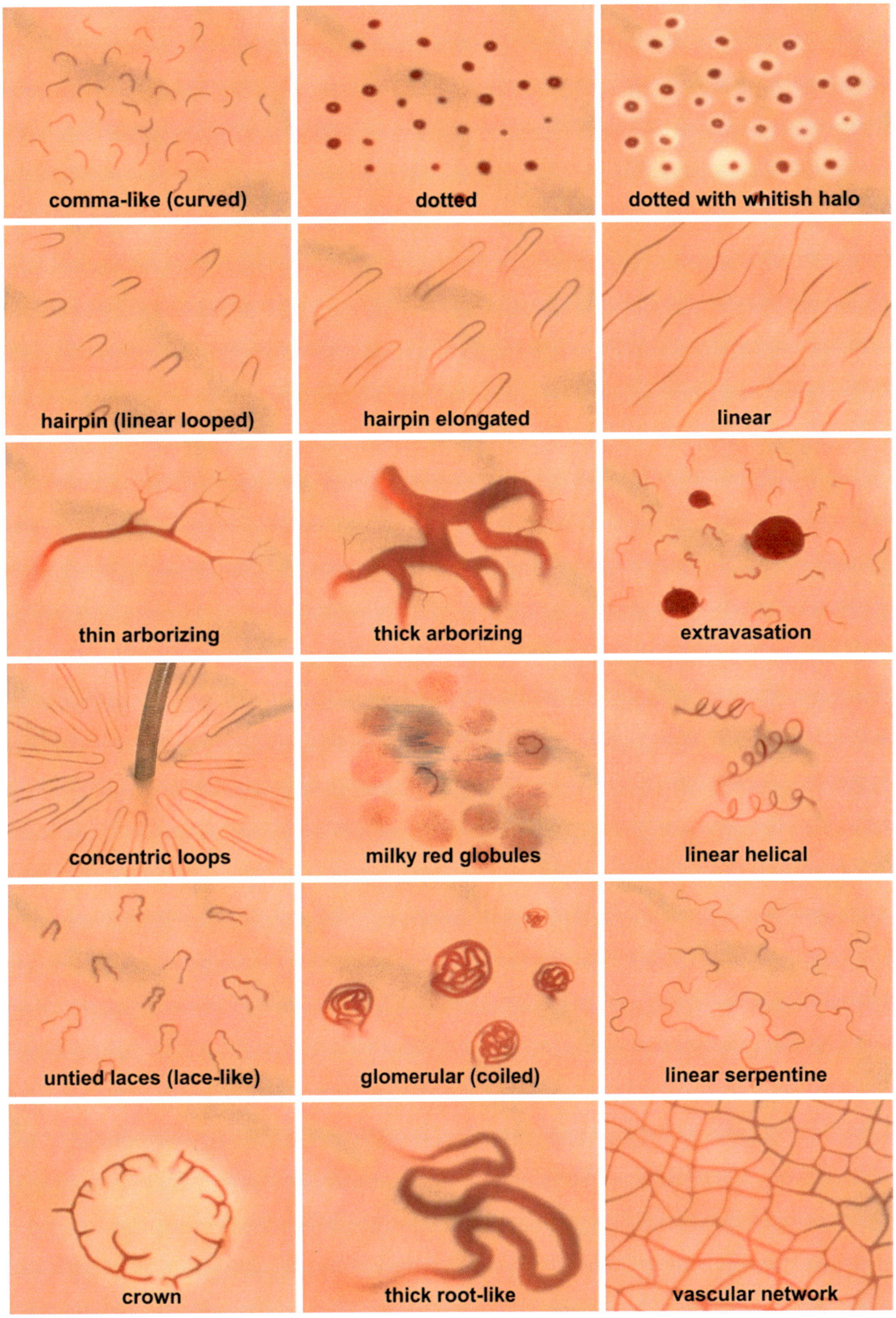

Fig. 5.1 Blood vessels observed on trichoscopy (*Graphics by* Dr. Wawrzyniec Podrzucki, *courtesy of* Journal of Dermatological Case Reports)

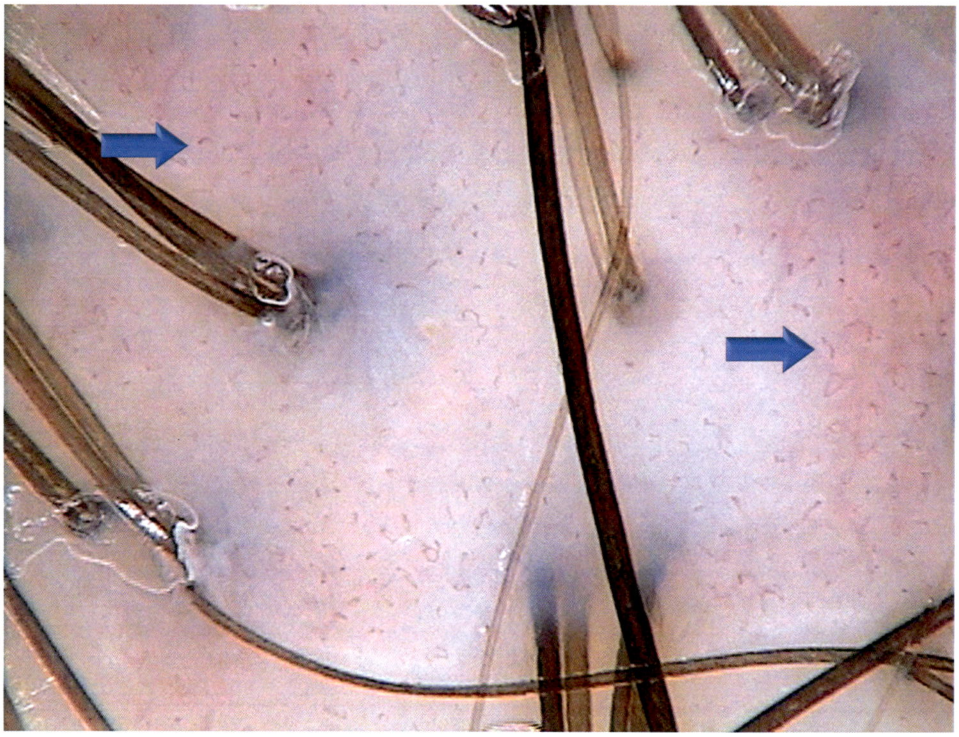

Fig. 5.2 **Comma vessels**. Comma (linear curved) vessels (*arrows*) are C-shaped or slightly curved vessels with no branching. They are common in inflammatory scalp diseases, such as seborrheic dermatitis and psoriasis, but also may be observed in healthy individuals (×70)

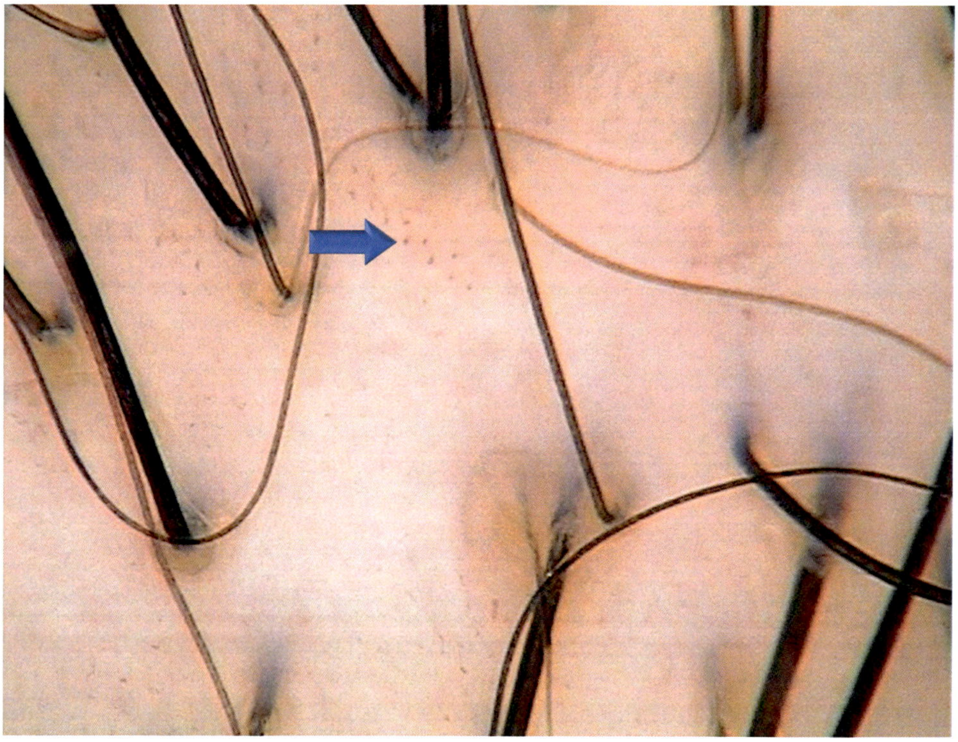

Fig. 5.3 **Dotted vessels**. By definition, dotted vessels (*arrow*) are tiny red dots densely aligned next to each other. They are a normal finding in healthy individuals and are present predominantly in the frontal scalp area [8]. The number of these vessels is increased in some inflammatory scalp diseases, such as eczema (×70)

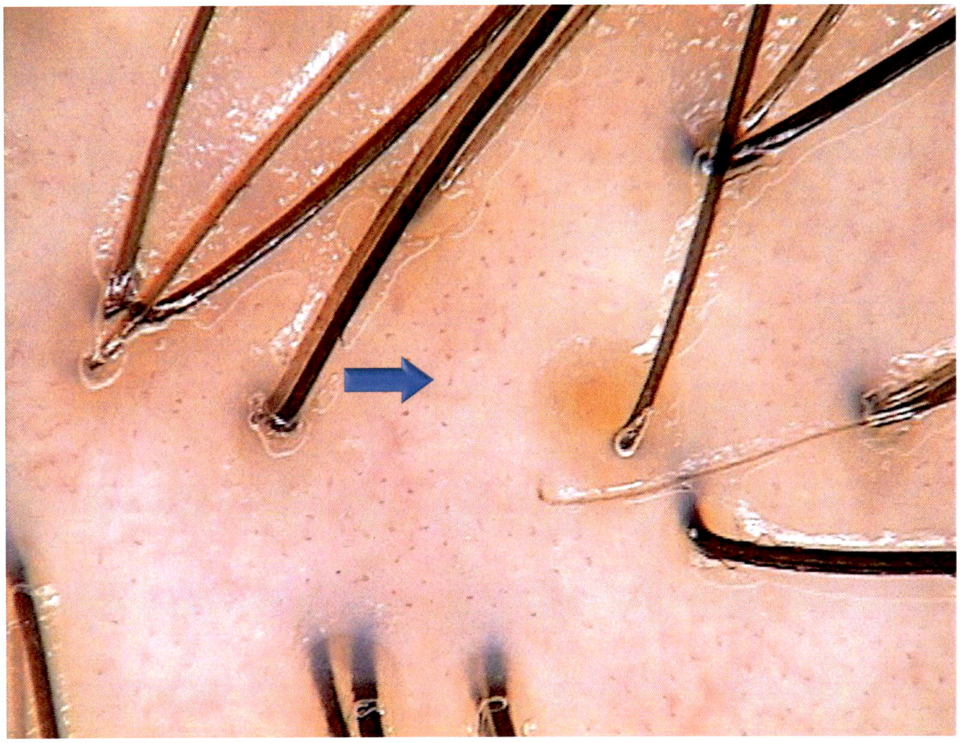

Fig. 5.4 Dotted vessels with a whitish halo. Dotted vessels with a whitish halo (*arrow*) are a characteristic trichoscopic feature of dissecting cellulitis [9], but occasionally may be present in patients with no hair or scalp disorders. They are observed with increased frequency in patients with thyroid disorders, most probably because of mucin deposits in the skin [5] (×70)

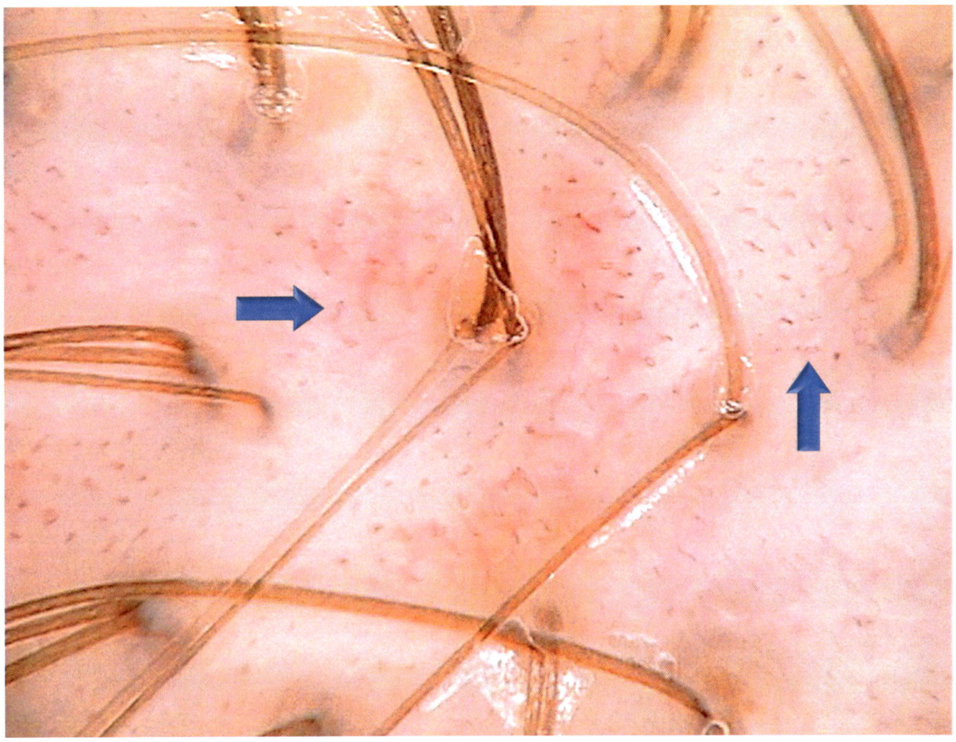

Fig. 5.5 Hairpin (linear looped) vessels. Small linear looped vessels (*arrows*) usually are seen in normal scalp skin in the frontal area. In the occipital and temporal areas, thin arborizing vessels are the predominant vessel type (×70)

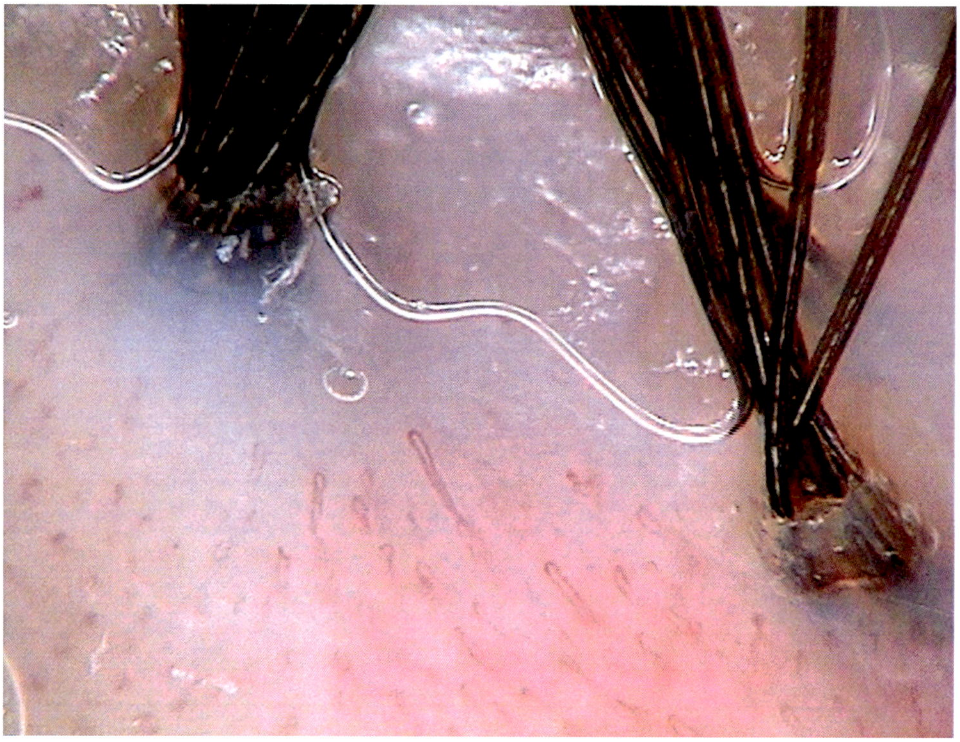

Fig. 5.6 Hairpin (linear looped) elongated vessels. Hairpin elongated vessels are characteristic of cicatricial alopecia and are observed most frequently in classic lichen planopilaris and folliculitis decalvans. This vessel type typically is found in the perifollicular area, especially adjacent to tufted hairs. Their closed end is oriented toward the follicular unit, which differentiates these vessels from the hairpin elongated vessels occasionally observed in cutaneous T-cell lymphoma (×70)

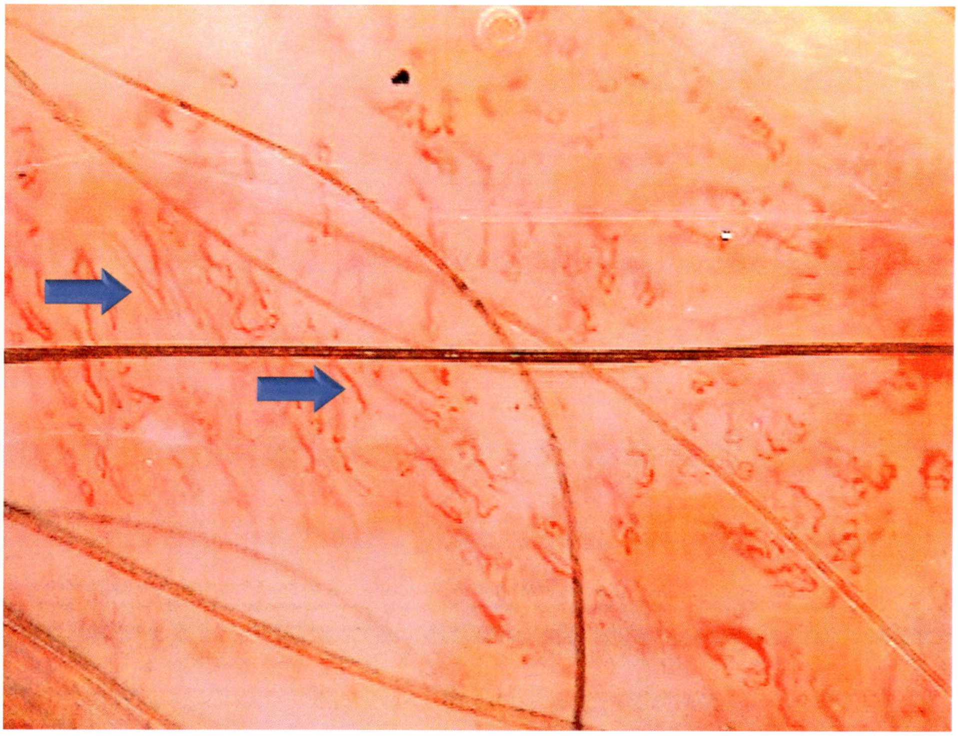

Fig. 5.7 Straight linear vessels. Linear vessels may be straight (*arrows*), serpentine, or helical. All these types are very rare in scalp skin. This image shows prominent linear vessels in a patient with active pemphigus vulgaris (×70)

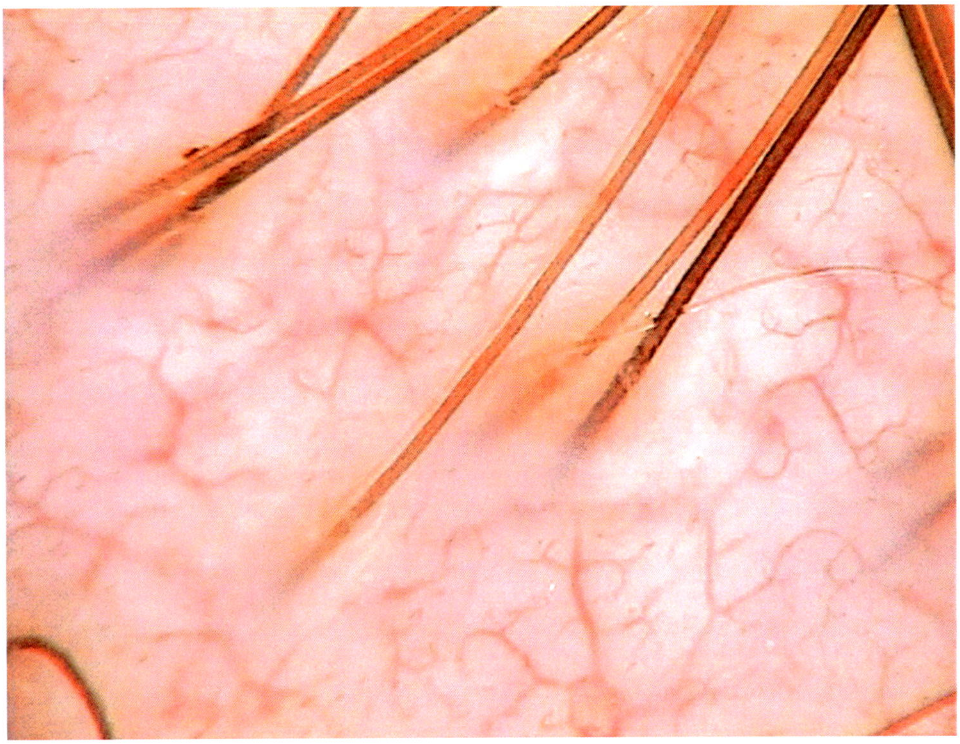

Fig. 5.8 Thin arborizing vessels. Thin arborizing vessels usually are thinner than the average hair on the trichoscopic image. They are a normal finding in the scalp, especially in the occipital and temporal areas [8]. They are distributed regularly between follicular units. Some authors suggest that thin arborizing vessels are characteristic of seborrheic dermatitis; however, thus far, studies have not compared patients with seborrheic dermatitis with healthy controls (×70)

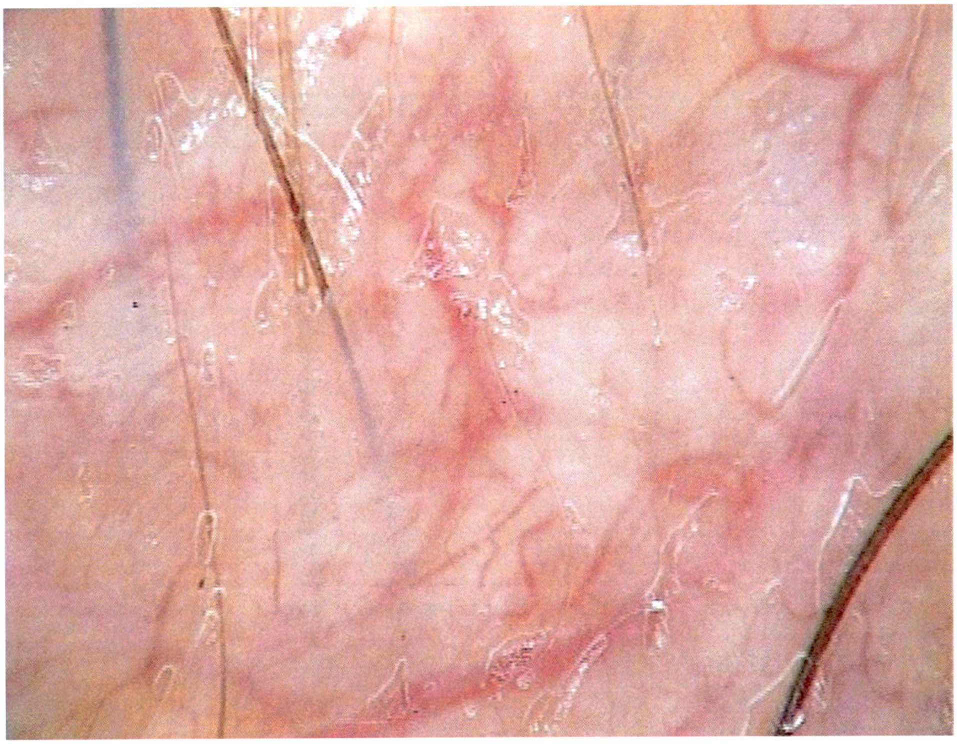

Fig. 5.9 Thick arborizing vessels. Thick arborizing vessels are thicker than the average terminal hair in the field of view (*see* Fig. 23.4 for details regarding the "vessel-hair test"). This type of vascular structure is most characteristic of discoid lupus erythematosus. The main differential diagnosis is basal cell carcinoma. In basal cell carcinoma, however, the vessels tend to be more sharply focused and deep amaranth in color (Iris Zalaudek, personal communication) (×70)

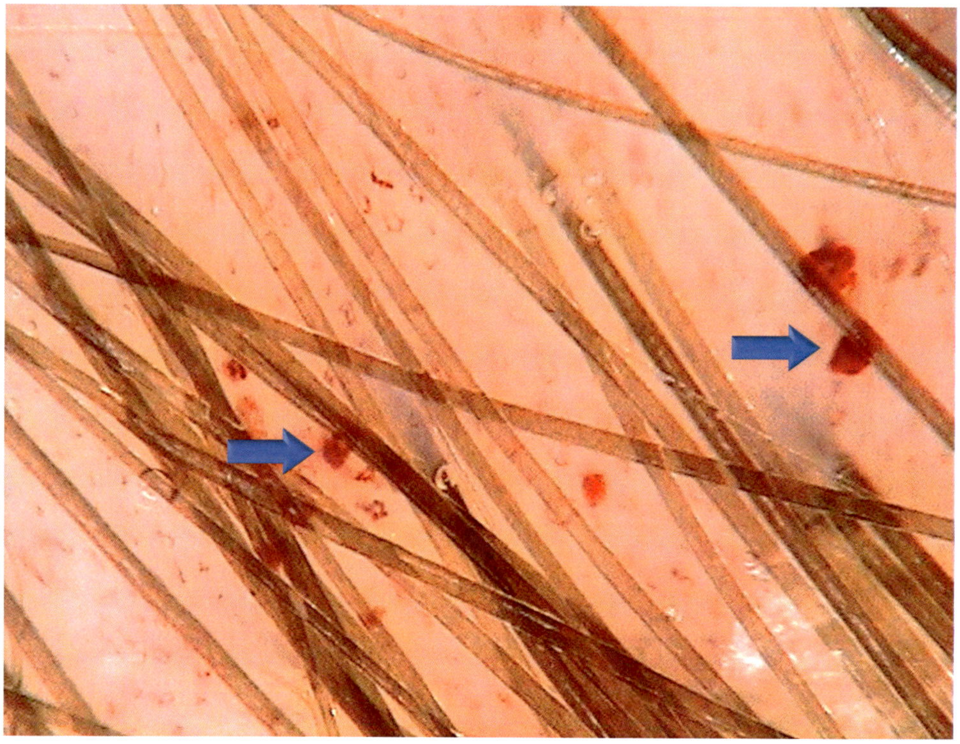

Fig. 5.10 Blood extravasations from capillaries (splinter hemorrhages). Blood extravasations from capillaries (*arrows*) are visible on trichoscopy as round or oval, sharply demarcated, intensely red areas. They are 100–300 μm in diameter. Frequently, the associated capillary is visible. Blood extravasations from capillaries are characteristic of active psoriasis. They correspond most probably to splinter hemorrhages in the nails. These blood extravasations usually develop in areas covered by glomerular (coiled) vessels (×70)

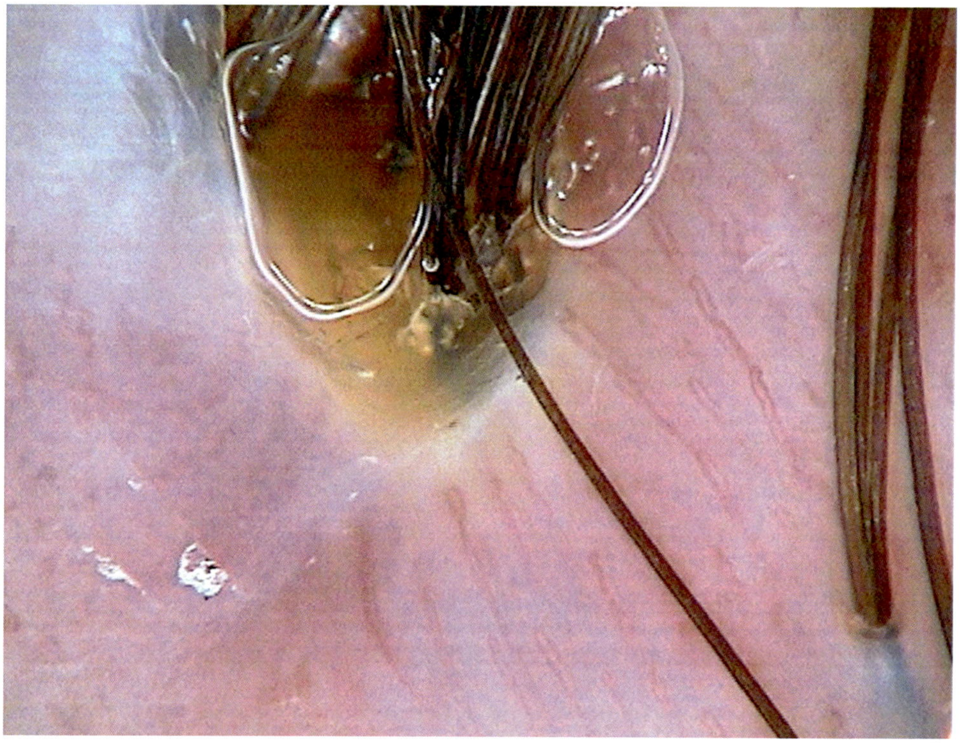

Fig. 5.11 Concentric perifollicular vessels. Concentric perifollicular vessels are vessels arranged concentrically around a follicular unit. Usually, elongated loops are observed in this arrangement, but linear and other types of vessels also may be arranged concentrically. This type of vessel arrangement is most characteristic of a folliculocentric cicatricial alopecia, such as lichen planopilaris or folliculitis decalvans (×70)

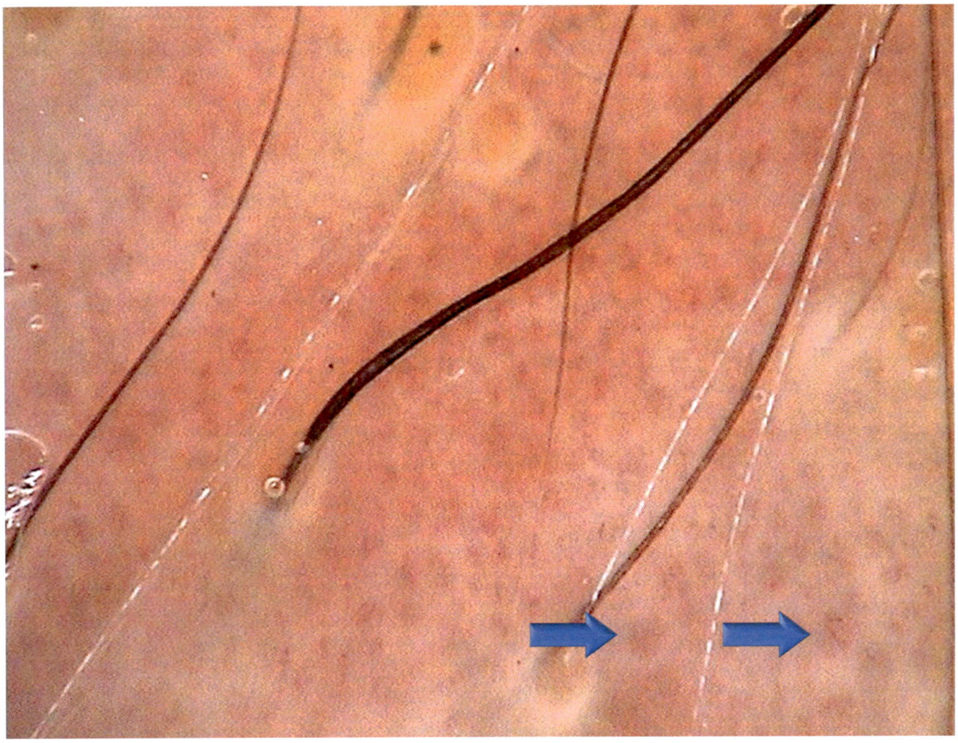

Fig. 5.12 Milky red globules. Milky red globules (*arrows*) are globules or larger areas of a fuzzy or unfocused milky red color. Thin capillaries may be visible within these areas. Shown is an example of milky red globules widely distributed throughout the scalp in a patient with cutaneous T-cell lymphoma (mycosis fungoides). Occasionally, milky red globules also may be observed in scalp psoriasis with scaling (×70)

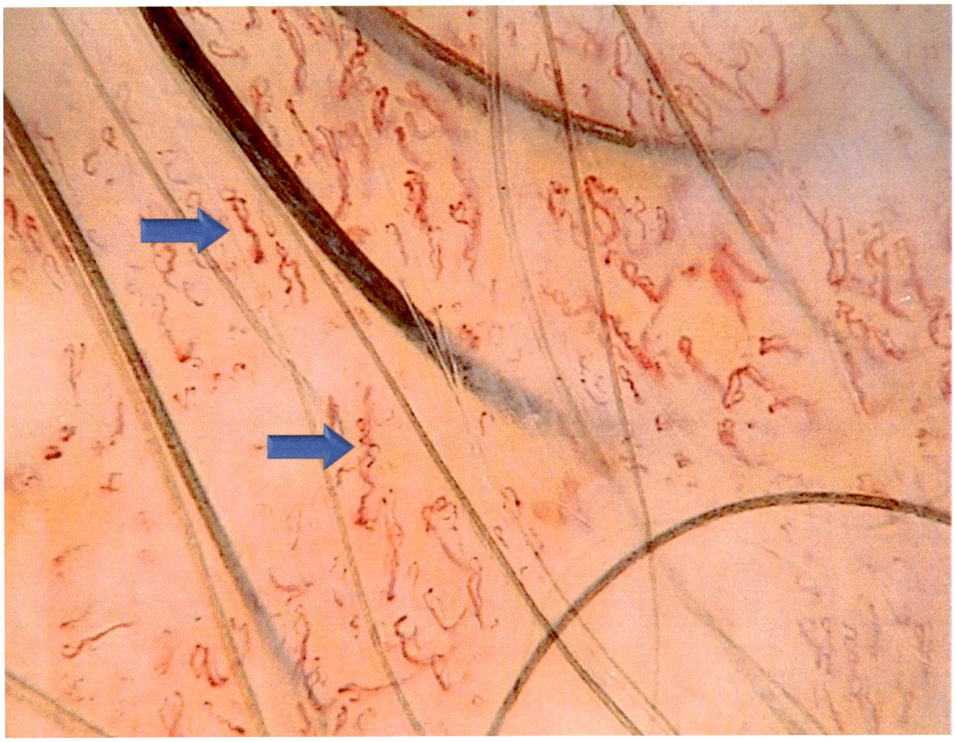

Fig. 5.13 Helical vessels. Helical (corkscrew) vessels (*arrows*) are linear vessels twisted along a central axis. They are observed rarely in scalp skin and never in healthy individuals. In noncancerous lesions, linear helical vessels are a marker of severe inflammation and are observed in severe scalp psoriasis, pemphigus, and cutaneous T-cell lymphoma. Shown is a trichoscopic image from a patient with pemphigus vulgaris (×70)

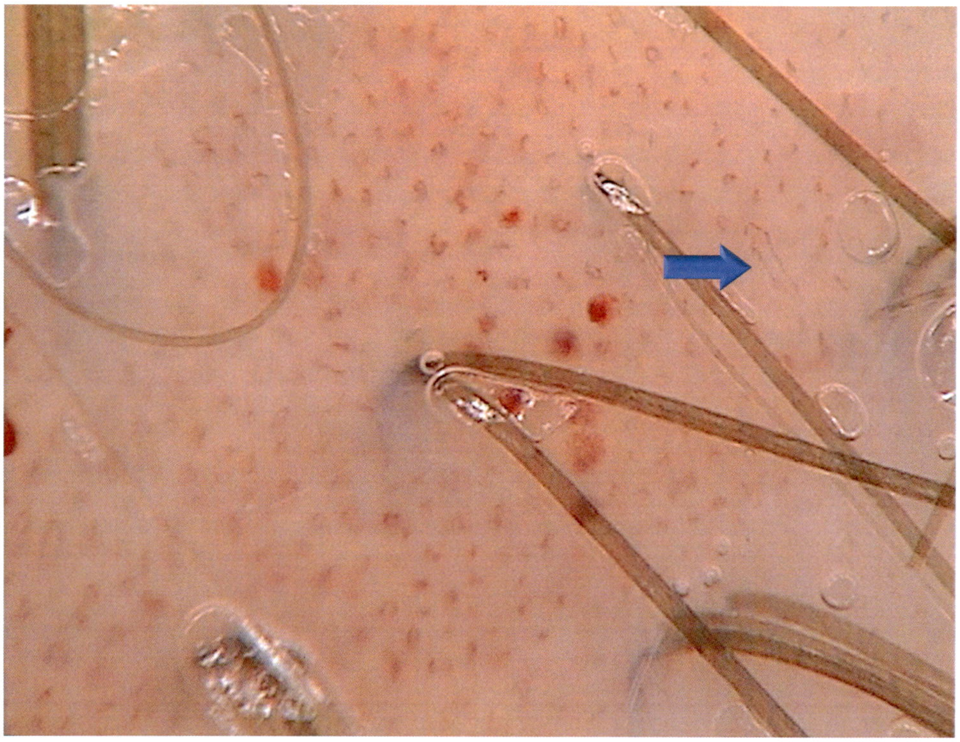

Fig. 5.14 **Lace-like vessels**. Lace-like vessels (*arrow*) are a combination of serpentine and looped vessels. These capillaries have a serpentine shape and open ends that usually are spaced widely. These vessels are most characteristic of psoriasis and correspond to the tortuous and dilated blood vessels within the elongated dermal papillae seen on histopathology (×70)

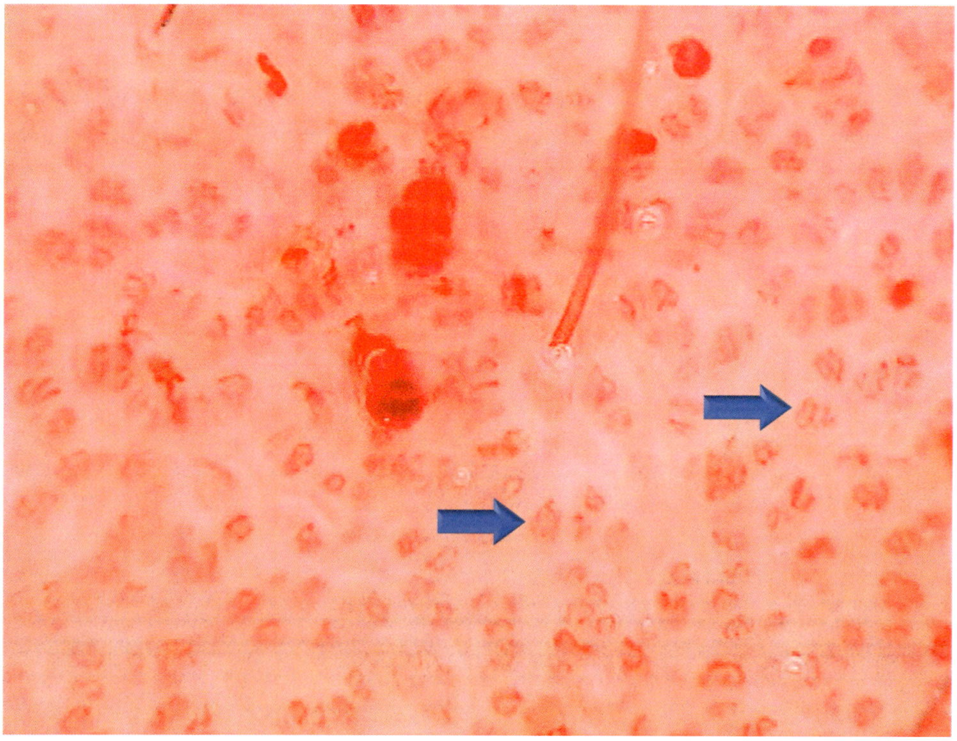

Fig. 5.15 **Glomerular (coiled) vessels**. Glomerular (i.e., coiled or twisted) vessels (*arrows*), are most characteristic of psoriasis [10, 11]. They usually are regularly arranged in lines or circles (*rings*). At lower magnification, these circles appear as "red globular rings" [12] (×70)

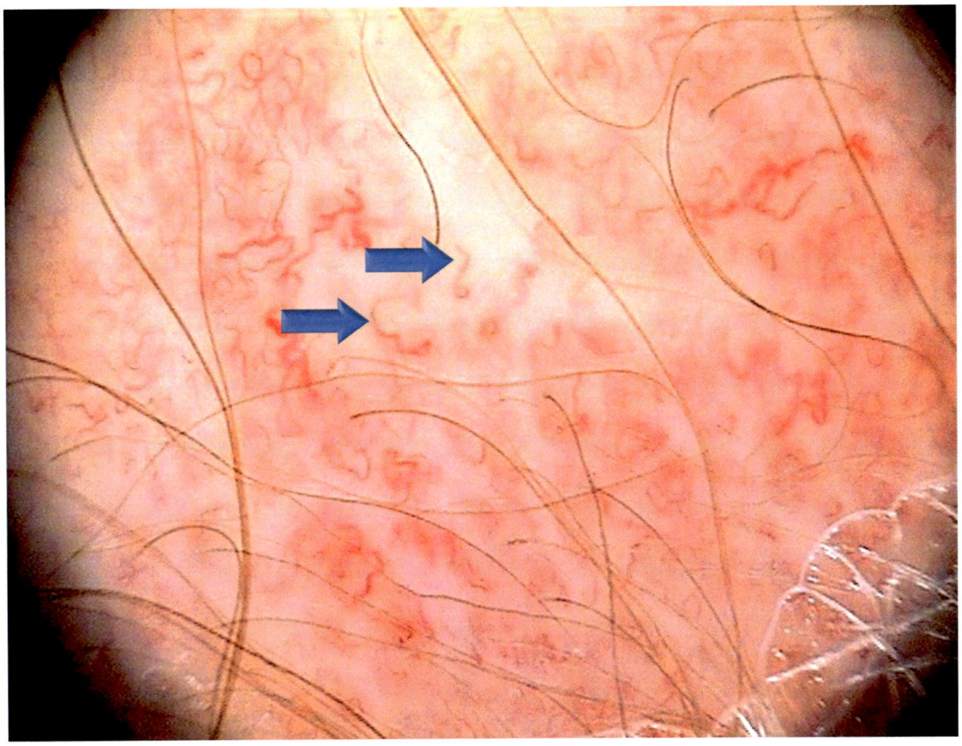

Fig. 5.16 Serpentine vessels. Linear serpentine vessels (*arrows*) are orderly bending, scarcely branching vessels. They rarely are observed in scalp lesions. Shown is a trichoscopic image from a patient with cicatricial alopecia in the course of discoid (cutaneous) lupus erythematosus (×20)

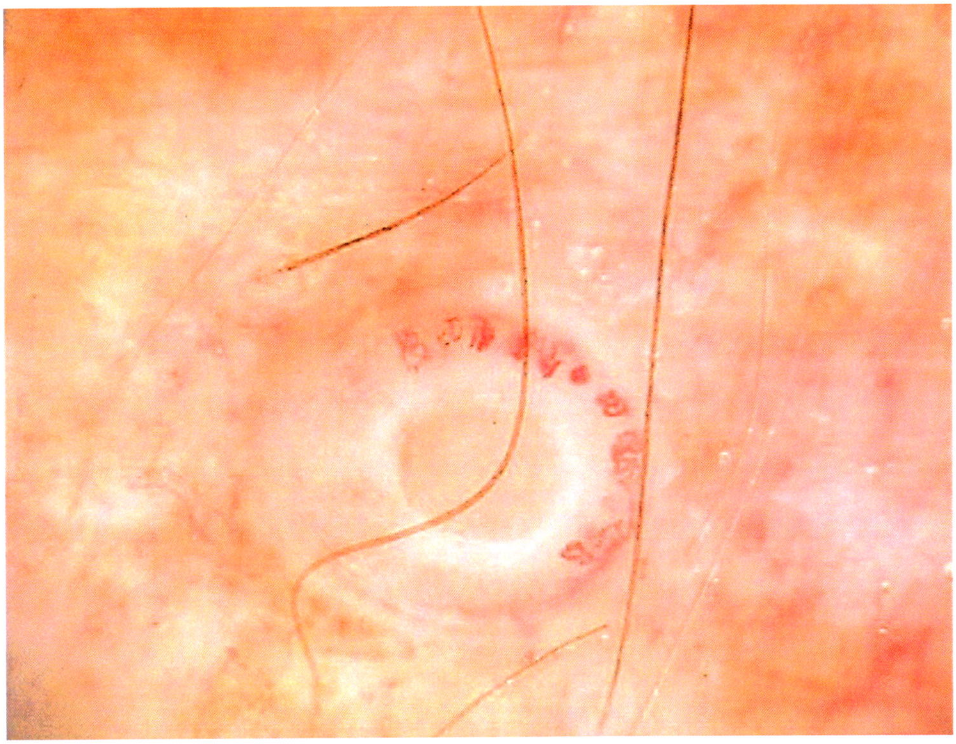

Fig. 5.17 Crown-like arrangement of vessels. Rarely, a crown-like arrangement of blood vessels is observed in the scalp. This image shows a small keratoacanthoma on the bald scalp of a patient with xeroderma pigmentosum (×70)

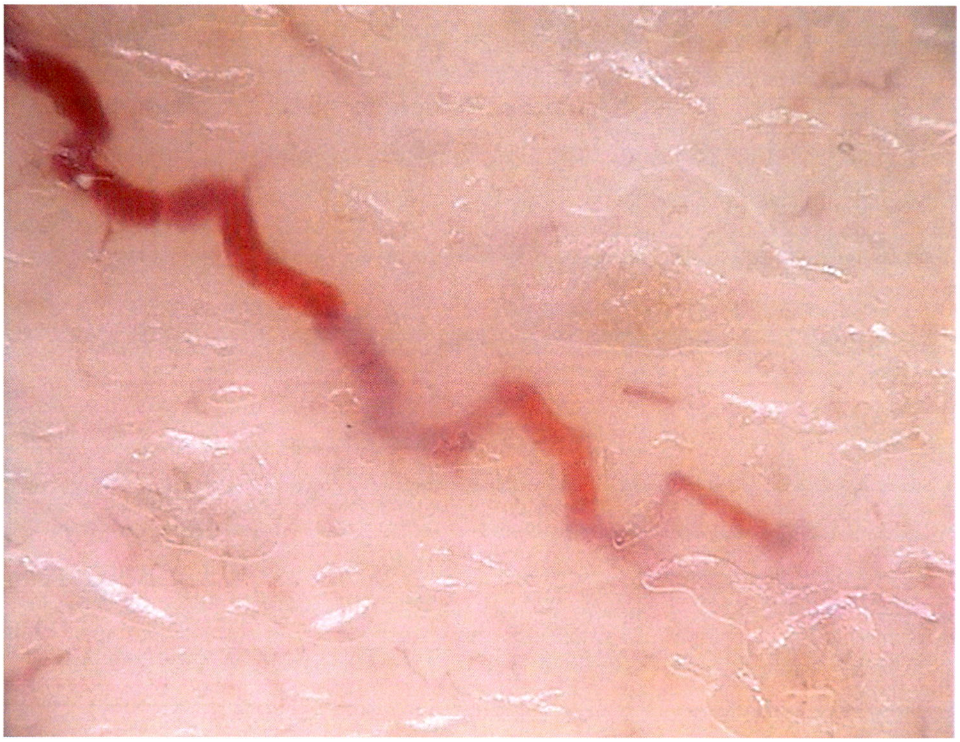

Fig. 5.18 Thick root-like vessels. Thick root-like vessels are thick, irregularly banded, linear vessels. They differ from arborizing vessels in that they do not have a tendency to branch. This type of vessel is observed most commonly in discoid lupus erythematosus and congenital capillary malformations (×70)

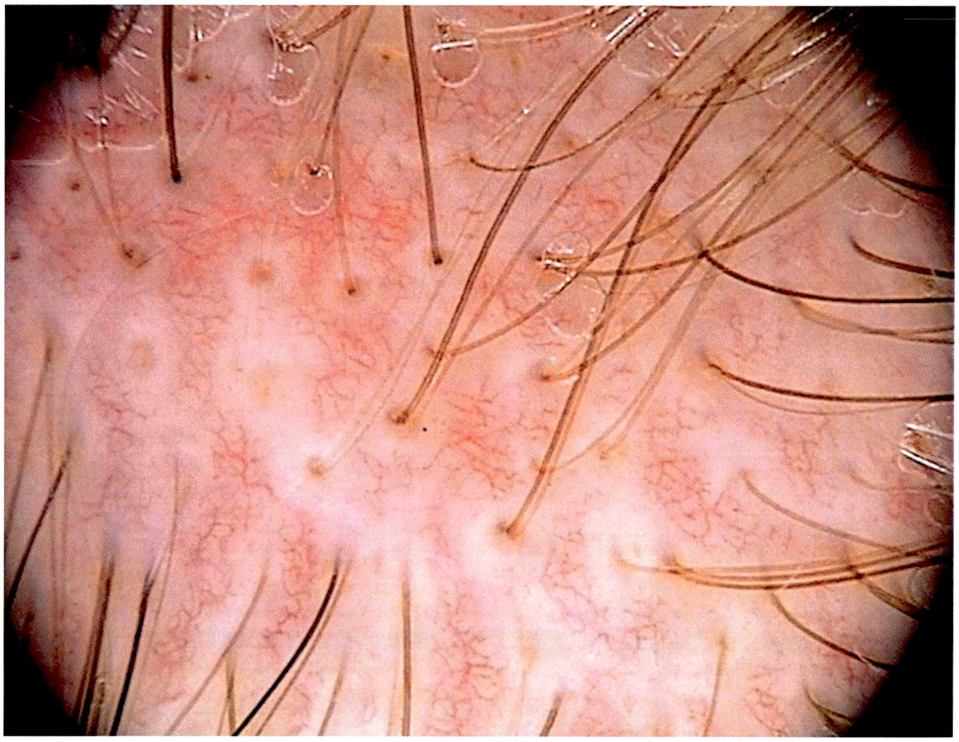

Fig. 5.19 Vessel net. In healthy individuals, trichoscopy often reveals a fine interfollicular network of blood vessels. This type of network is most common in the occipital area. The visibility of these vessels may be enhanced by skin atrophy in patients with a history of chronic use of potent topical corticosteroids. Note that in direct proximity to the follicular openings, the vessel net is not visible (×20)

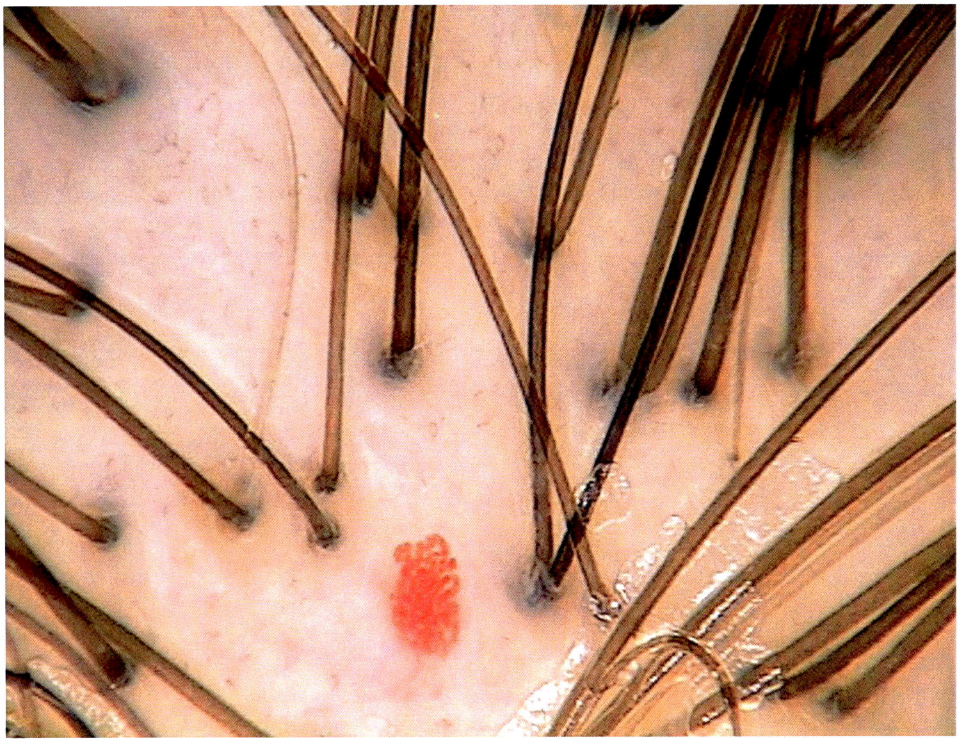

Fig. 5.20 Hemangioma. Small hemangiomas may be found incidentally during routine trichoscopy. Although they have no medical significance, they may be used as markers for a scalp area chosen for monitoring (×70)

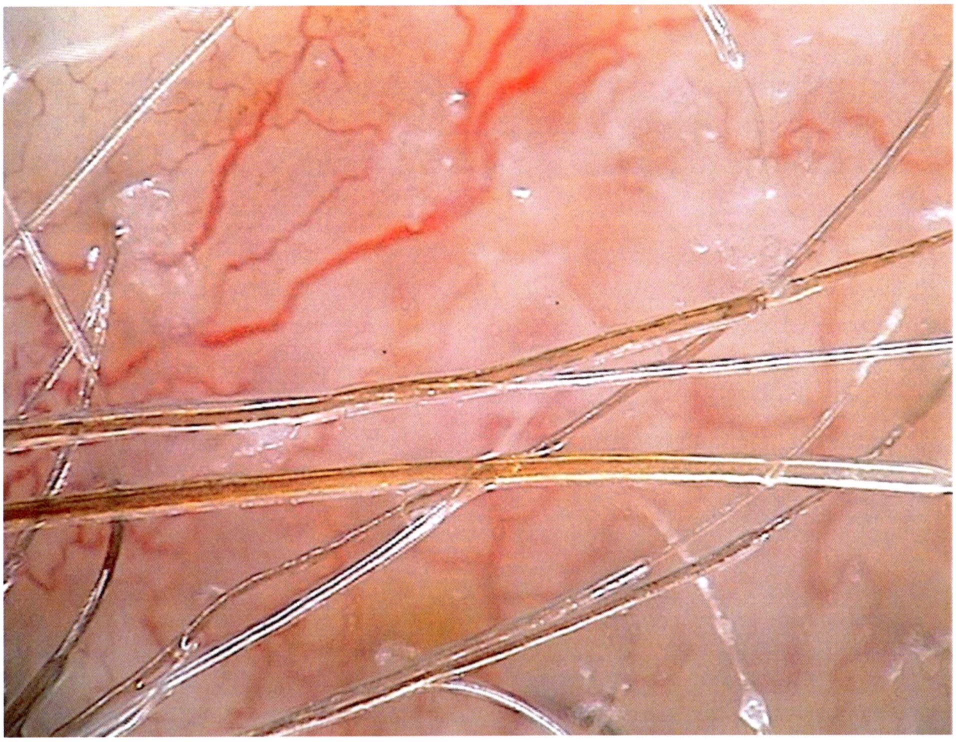

Fig. 5.21 Vessels in scalp tumors. As mentioned in this chapter, vascular structures previously thought to be associated with melanoma and nonmelanoma skin cancer may be present on the scalp of healthy individuals and in inflammatory scalp diseases. An example is thick arborizing vessels, which are a well-known hallmark of basal cell carcinoma [13, 14]. New data show that similar vessels are observed in discoid lupus erythematosus, a disease that requires a therapeutic approach entirely different from that of cancer [5, 9]. However, we should never lower our index of suspicion when evaluating scalp lesions. This image shows arborizing vessels in a patient with discoid lupus erythematosus who developed basal cell carcinoma of the scalp (×70)

References

1. Zalaudek I, Kreusch J, Giacomel J, Ferrara G, Catricala C, Argenziano G. How to diagnose nonpigmented skin tumors: a review of vascular structures seen with dermoscopy: part I. Melanocytic skin tumors. J Am Acad Dermatol. 2010;63(3):361–74; quiz 75–6.
2. Gewirtzman AJ, Saurat JH, Braun RP. An evaluation of dermoscopy fluids and application techniques. Br J Dermatol. 2003;149(1):59–63.
3. Rudnicka L, Olszewska M, Rakowska A, Slowinska M. Trichoscopy update 2011. J Dermatol Case Rep. 2011;5(4):82–8.
4. Lacarrubba F, Potenza MC, Micali G. Enhanced videodermoscopic visualization of superficial vascular patterns on skin using a 390- to 410-nm light. Arch Dermatol. 2012;148(2):276.
5. Rakowska A, Olszewska M, Rudnicka L. Vacular structures in scalp dermoscopy. J Dermatol Case Rep. 2013 (in press).
6. Zalaudek I, Kreusch J, Giacomel J, Ferrara G, Catricala C, Argenziano G. How to diagnose nonpigmented skin tumors: a review of vascular structures seen with dermoscopy: part II. Nonmelanocytic skin tumors. J Am Acad Dermatol. 2010;63(3):377–86; quiz 87–8.
7. Kittler H, Riedl E, Rosendahl C, Cameron A. Dermatoscopy of unpigmented lesions of the skin: a new classification of vessel morphology based on pattern analysis. Dermatopathol Pract Conceptual. 2008;14(4):3.
8. Rakowska A. Trichoscopy (hair and scalp videodermoscopy) in the healthy female. Method standardization and norms for measurable parameters. J Dermatol Case Rep. 2009;3(1):14–9.
9. Rakowska A, Slowinska M, Kowalska-Oledzka E, Olszewska M, Rudnicka L. Trichoscopy in cicatricial alopecia. J Drugs Dermatol. 2012;11:753–8.
10. Micali G, Lacarrubba F, Massimino D, Schwartz RA. Dermatoscopy: alternative uses in daily clinical practice. J Am Acad Dermatol. 2011;64(6):1135–46.
11. Kim GW, Jung HJ, Ko HC, Kim MB, Lee WJ, Lee SJ, et al. Dermoscopy can be useful in differentiating scalp psoriasis from seborrhoeic dermatitis. Br J Dermatol. 2011;164(3):652–6.
12. Vazquez-Lopez F, Zaballos P, Fueyo-Casado A, Sanchez-Martin J. A dermoscopy subpattern of plaque-type psoriasis: red globular rings. Arch Dermatol. 2007;143(12):1612.
13. Puig S, Cecilia N, Malvehy J. Dermoscopic criteria and basal cell carcinoma. G Ital Dermatol Venereol. 2012;147(2):135–40.
14. Liebman TN, Jaimes-Lopez N, Balagula Y, Rabinovitz HS, Wang SQ, Dusza SW, et al. Dermoscopic features of basal cell carcinomas: differences in appearance under non-polarized and polarized light. Dermatol Surg. 2012;38(3):392–9.

Part III

Normal Values in Trichoscopy

6 Normal Values in Trichoscopy

Adriana Rakowska and Lidia Rudnicka

Abstract
Diagnosis of scalp and hair abnormalities by trichoscopy requires knowledge of the normal range of trichoscopic results in healthy individuals. This chapter focuses on trichoscopic features and normal values for measurable parameters in healthy individuals.

Keywords
Children • Follicular openings • Follicular units • Hair shaft • Healthy individual • Normal values • Vellus hairs • Vessels

Trichoscopy in healthy individuals has not been studied extensively; results of only a few studies have been published [1, 2]. These studies focused on the appearance of the hair shafts, follicular openings, and blood vessels.

On trichoscopy, normal terminal hair shafts are uniform in thickness and color [1, 3]. Hair shaft thickness may be estimated roughly (i.e., as thin, normal, or thick) with a handheld dermoscope or may be calculated precisely with adequate software in a digital dermoscope. Thin hairs may account for up to 20 % of the total number of hairs. A higher percentage of thin hairs is considered a marker of hair follicle miniaturization [4, 5].

On the scalp, hair follicles and shafts are grouped into follicular units consisting of one to three hairs [6]. Follicular units with four or more hairs are rare and account for less than 5 % of all follicular units in healthy individuals [1]. Based on trichoscopic calculations, the average number of hairs in one follicular unit in healthy Caucasian females is 2.6 [1, 7]. The percentage of follicular units with only one hair should be less than 35 % in the frontal, 30 % in the occipital, and 40 % in the temporal areas [1].

Interestingly, in the temporal areas of healthy women, the percentage of follicular units with only one hair is high and the distance between follicular units is above average. This observation indicates that, physiologically, the temporal areas have lower hair density than other scalp areas [1, 7, 8].

The number of hairs per follicular unit is decreased in hair loss, especially in androgenetic alopecia and telogen effluvium [5, 7, 9]. In children, this is a common finding in ectodermal dysplasias.

Empty follicular openings and yellow dots are seen occasionally in healthy individuals [1, 7]. Small, sharply demarcated pinpoint white dots correspond to follicular and eccrine sweat gland openings. They are a normal finding in patients with dark skin phototypes and may be visible on sun-exposed scalp skin in Caucasians [10].

Brownish perifollicular discoloration, also known as the peripilar sign of androgenetic alopecia [11], also may be present in some healthy individuals [1]. In healthy persons, up to about 15 % of follicular units may be surrounded by a brownish halo [1, 7].

Two types of blood vessels are most common in healthy individuals. Dotted vessels are observed mainly in the frontal scalp, and thin arborizing vessels predominate in the occipital and temporal areas [1, 7].

Some trichoscopic features of disease, such as solitary black dots, broken hairs, or comma hairs, occasionally may be seen in healthy individuals [1, 7]. Usually, no more than one or two such hairs are present in a healthy individual, and they have no diagnostic significance.

A. Rakowska
Department of Dermatology, CSK MSW, Warsaw, Poland

L. Rudnicka (✉)
Faculty of Health Sciences, Medical University of Warsaw, Poland

Department of Dermatology, CSK MSW, Woloska 137, Warsaw 02-502, Poland
e-mail: lidia.rudnicka@euderm.eu

L. Rudnicka et al. (eds.), *Atlas of Trichoscopy*,
DOI 10.1007/978-1-4471-4486-1_6, © Springer-Verlag London 2012

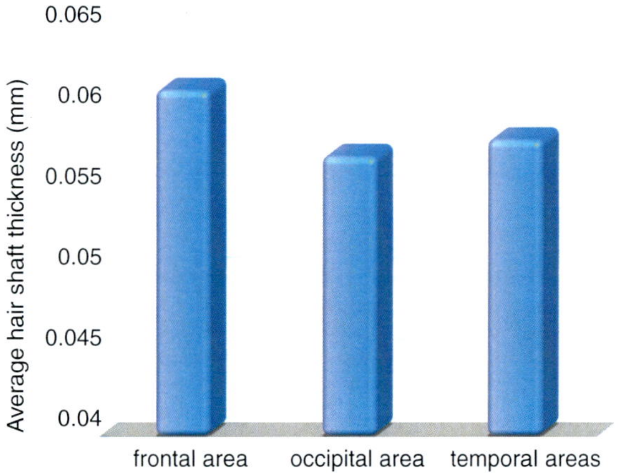

Fig. 6.1 Average hair thickness in the frontal, occipital, and temporal areas in healthy females. Hair thickness may differ between scalp areas in the same person. The greatest hair shaft thickness is observed in the frontal area, whereas in the occipital area, the hair shafts are significantly thinner. The proportion of thin hairs (<0.03 mm) is highest in the temporal areas (*Graph adapted from* Rakowska [1])

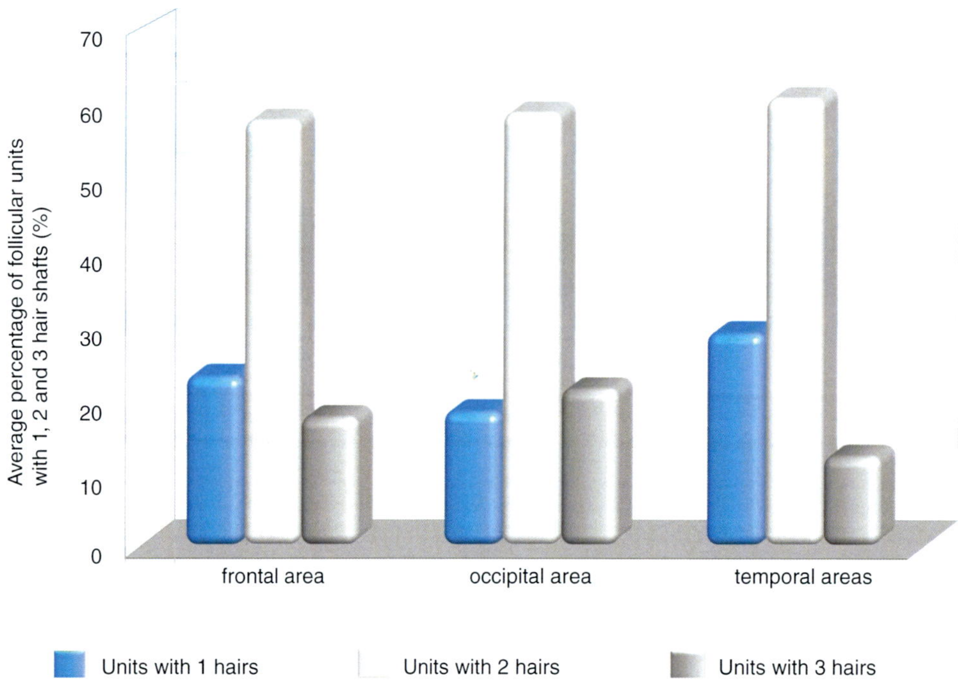

Fig. 6.2 Average percentage of follicular units with one, two, or three hairs in the frontal, occipital, and temporal areas in healthy females. Most follicular units consist of two hairs. Follicular units with three hairs are less common. The number of hairs per follicular unit provides important information about the hair's condition. Usually, a decreased proportion of follicular units with three hairs is the first sign of hair loss. The proportion of follicular units with only one hair is greatest in the temporal area. The distance between follicular units is above average in this area. Thus, diffuse hair loss, which affects the whole scalp proportionally will be most visible clinically in the temporal areas. This phenomenon is observed in telogen effluvium. It is important to emphasize that in diffuse hair loss, trichoscopy should be performed in at least three areas: the occipital, the frontal, and one of the temporal areas. Research data indicate there is no difference in trichoscopic results between the left and right temporal areas [12] (*Graph adapted from* Rakowska [1])

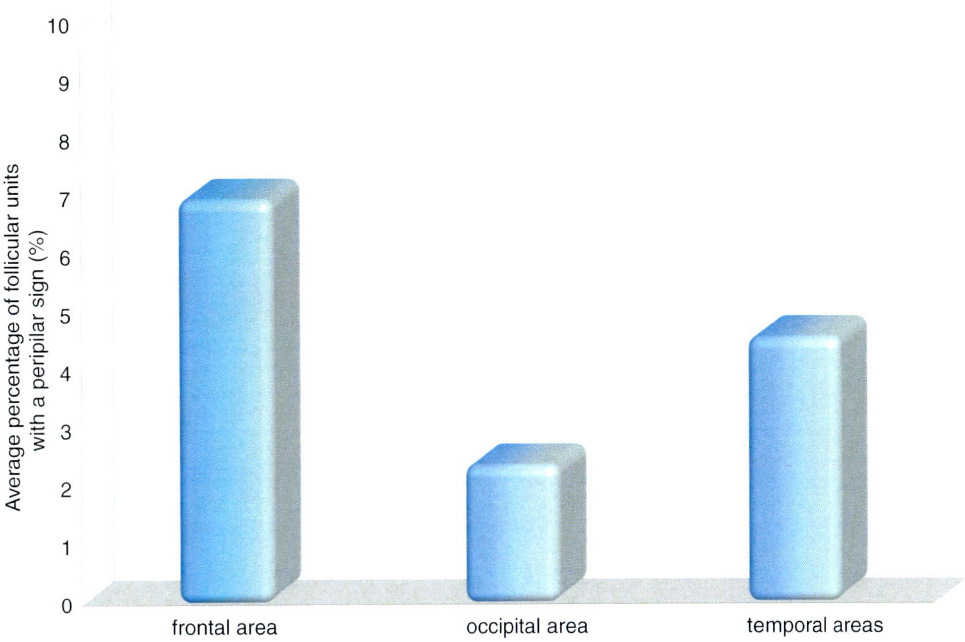

Fig. 6.3 Average percentage of follicular units with brownish perifollicular discoloration in healthy females. Perifollicular discoloration (peripilar sign) is observed in the area surrounding 7 ± 20.2 % of follicular units in the frontal area, 2.4 ± 13.4 % in the occipital area, and 4.6 ± 15.7 % in the temporal area in females with no features of hair loss. A large proportion of follicular units with the peripilar sign is typical of androgenetic alopecia [11] but also may be observed in telogen effluvium. When performing trichoscopy, one should keep in mind that androgenetic alopecia and telogen effluvium both are very common. Accordingly, the coexistence of both diseases also is frequent in clinical practice. Other combinations of two or more diseases are less frequent, but this possibility also must be considered. A single trichoscopic examination allows differentiation of most of these diseases (*Graph adapted from* Rakowska [1])

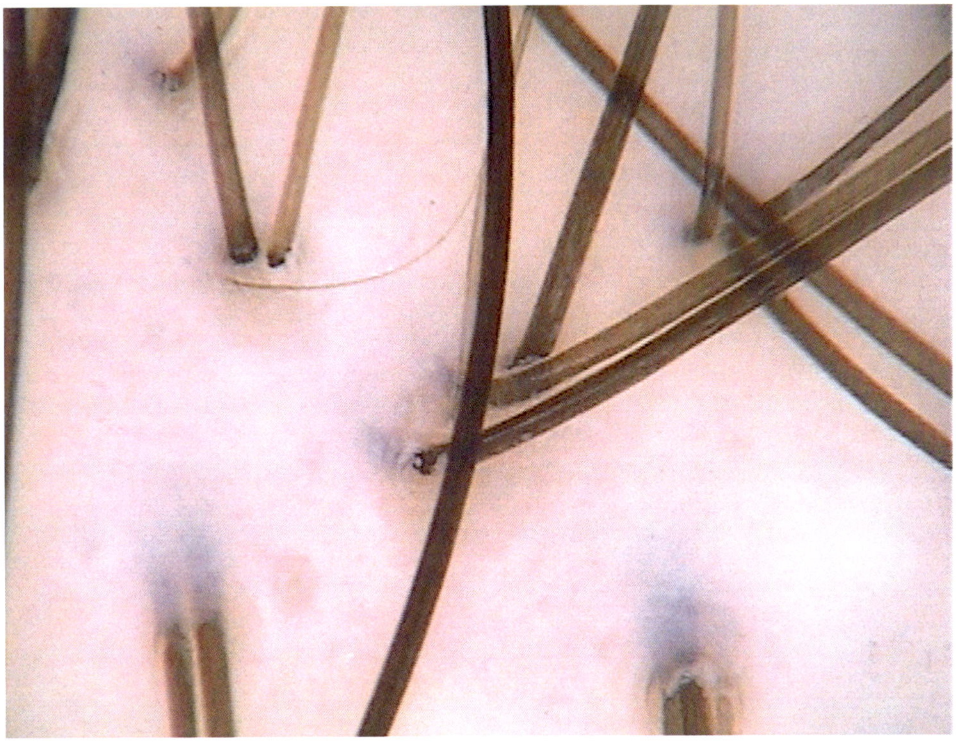

Fig. 6.4 Trichoscopy in a healthy individual. The hair shafts are homogenous and uniform in thickness and color. Thin hairs may account for up to 20 % of the total number of hairs. In this image, 22 hair shafts are visible, two of which are thin hairs. Thus, 2 of 22 hairs (9 %) are thin, which is in the normal range. Hairs usually grow in groups of one to three. These small groups are called "follicular units"(*see* Chap. 2 for details). In this image, most follicular units consist of two or three hairs. Hair shafts in one follicular unit may, but most do not, emerge from the same follicular opening (×70)

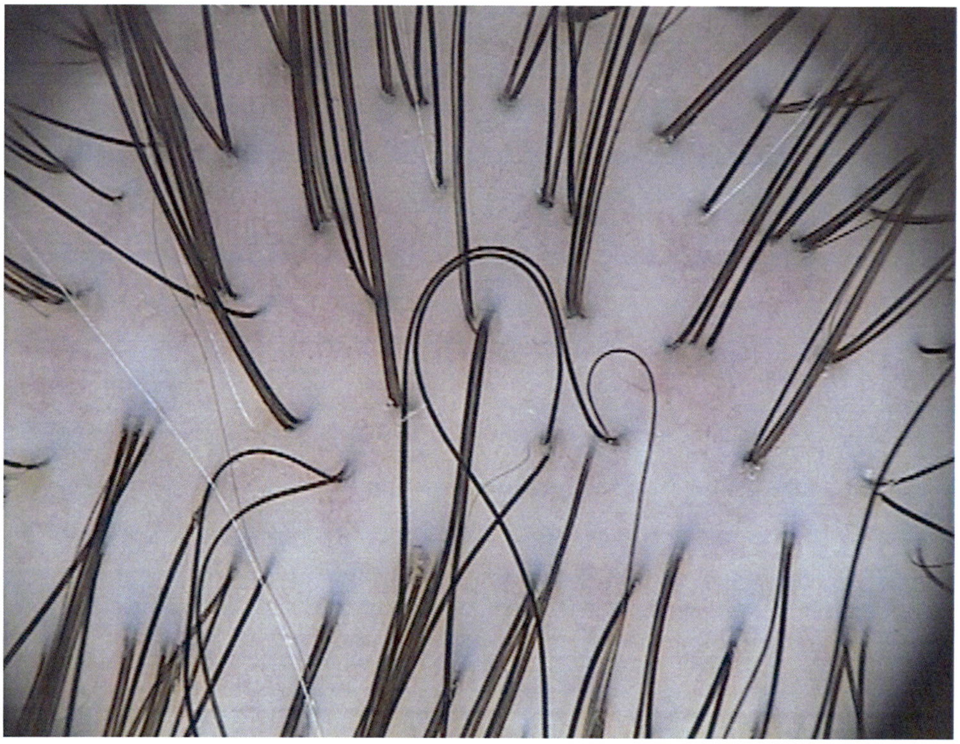

Fig. 6.5 Trichoscopy in a healthy individual (frontal area). The hairs are uniform in thickness and color. Thin hairs account for less than 20 %. Most follicular units consist of two to four hairs. Note that for easy trichoscopic evaluation, it is beneficial to distribute the hairs in a 2:1 ratio (*top to bottom* of the image). In the *upper part* of the image, more follicular units may be evaluated, whereas in the *bottom part*, the perifollicular area may be visualized better because it is not covered by hair (×20)

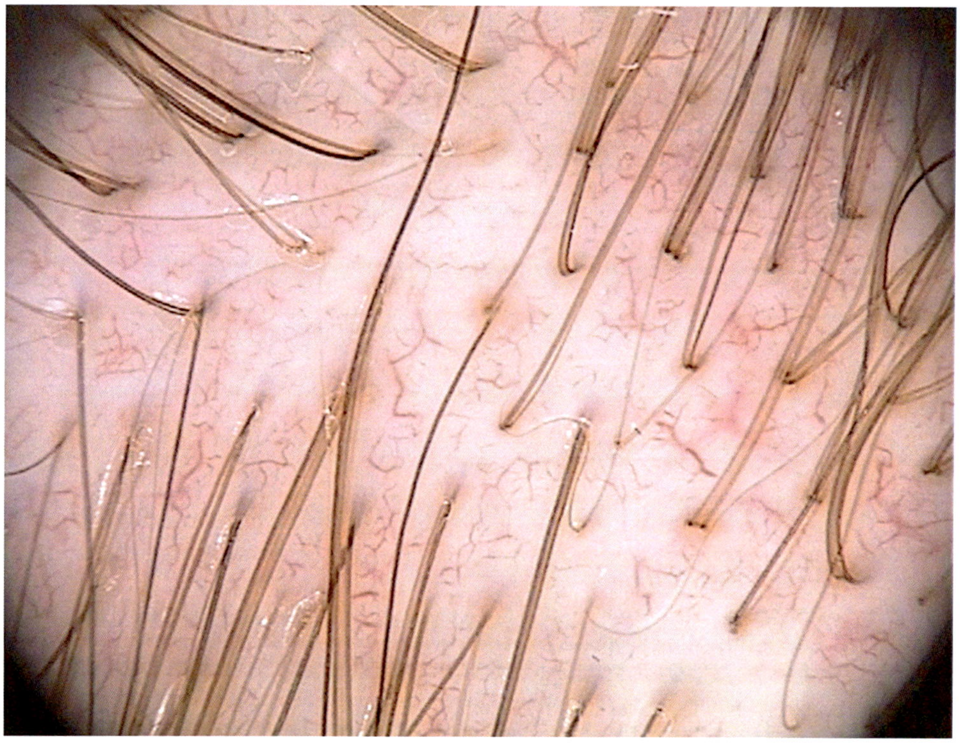

Fig. 6.6 Blood vessels in a healthy individual (temporal area). The presence of thin arborizing vessels between follicular units is a normal finding. Most of these vessels appear in the occipital and temporal areas, whereas in the frontal area, dotted vessels predominate (×20)

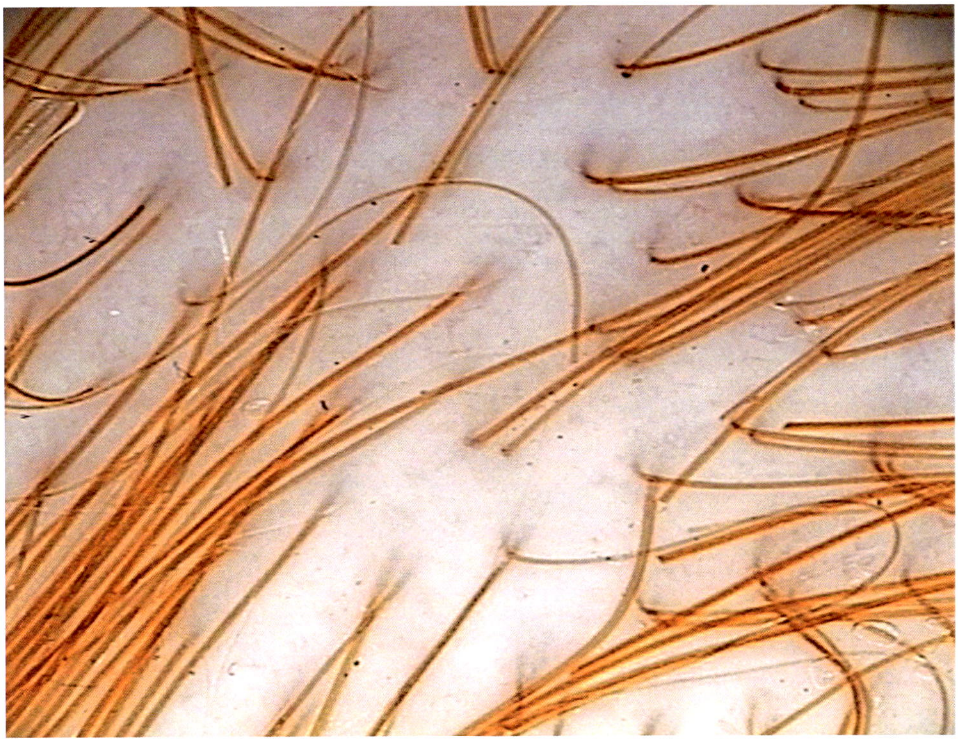

Fig. 6.7 Hair color in healthy individuals. Patients with any hair color may be evaluated by trichoscopy. In patients with light blond or gray hair, contact dermoscopy with immersion fluid should not be used. To maintain good visibility in patients with light-colored hair, contact dermoscopes should be used without immersion fluid (dry trichoscopy). This image shows red hair in a healthy child. Dirty dots (small brown environmental particles) [13] are visible. Trichoscopy of light-colored hairs and dirty dots is described in detail in Chap. 7 (×20)

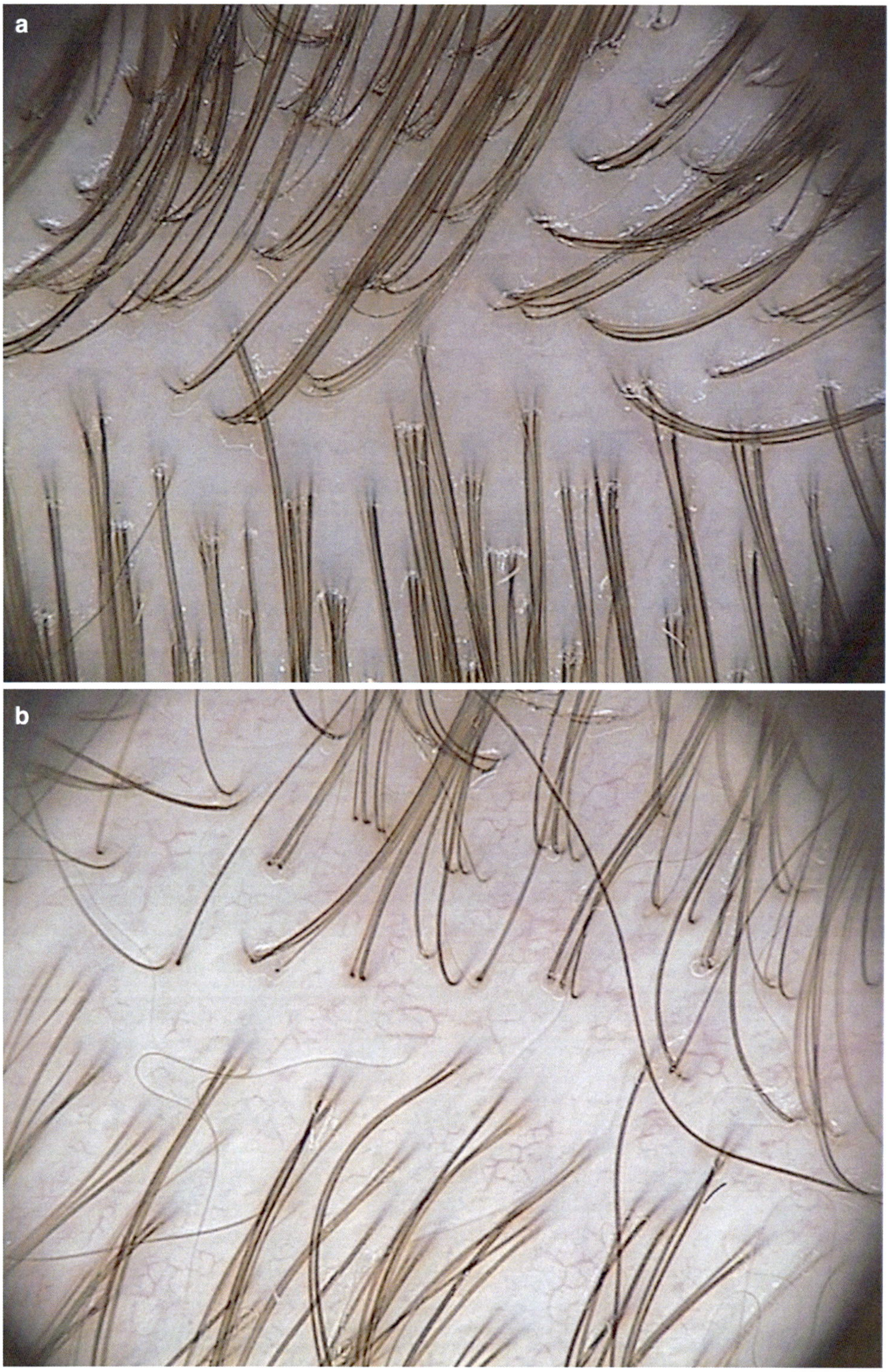

Fig. 6.8 Occipital versus temporal areas in a healthy individual. The images show trichoscopy of (**a**) the occipital area and (**b**) the temporal area performed in a female patient on the same day. These two areas differ with respect to the average number of hairs per follicular unit (more in the occipital area) and the distance between follicular units (greater in the temporal area). Thus, when evaluating trichoscopic images, it often is vital to know from which scalp area they were taken (×20)

References

1. Rakowska A. Trichoscopy (hair and scalp videodermoscopy) in the healthy female. Method standardization and norms for measurable parameters. J Dermatol Case Rep. 2009;3(1):14–9.
2. Ross EK, Vincenzi C, Tosti A. Videodermoscopy in the evaluation of hair and scalp disorders. J Am Acad Dermatol. 2006;55(5):799–806.
3. Vogt A, McElwee KJ, Blume-Peytavi U. Biology of the hair follicle. In: Blume-Peytavi U, Tosti A, Whiting D, Trüeb R, editors. Hair growth and disorders. Berlin: Springer; 2008. p. 1–22.
4. de Lacharriere O, Deloche C, Misciali C, Piraccini BM, Vincenzi C, Bastien P, et al. Hair diameter diversity: a clinical sign reflecting the follicle miniaturization. Arch Dermatol. 2001;137(5):641–6.
5. Miteva M, Tosti A. Hair and scalp dermatoscopy. J Am Acad Dermatol. doi: 10.1016/J.jaad.2012.05.041. Accessed on Sep 03, 2012.
6. Jimenez-Acosta F, Ponce I. Follicular unit hair transplantation: current technique [in Spanish]. Actas Dermosifiliogr. 2010;101(4):291–306.
7. Rakowska A, Slowinska M, Kowalska-Oledzka E, Olszewska M, Rudnicka L. Dermoscopy in female androgenic alopecia: method standardization and diagnostic criteria. Int J Trichol. 2009;1(2): 123–30.
8. Yazdabadi A, Magee J, Harrison S, Sinclair R. The Ludwig pattern of androgenetic alopecia is due to a hierarchy of androgen sensitivity within follicular units that leads to selective miniaturization and a reduction in the number of terminal hairs per follicular unit. Br J Dermatol. 2008;159(6):1300–2.
9. Rudnicka L, Olszewska M, Rakowska A, Slowinska M. Trichoscopy update 2011. J Dermatol Case Rep. 2011;5(4):82–8.
10. Abraham LS, Pineiro-Maceira J, Duque-Estrada B, Barcaui CB, Sodre CT. Pinpoint white dots in the scalp: dermoscopic and histopathologic correlation. J Am Acad Dermatol. 2010;63(4):721–2.
11. Deloche C, de Lacharriere O, Misciali C, Piraccini BM, Vincenzi C, Bastien P, et al. Histological features of peripilar signs associated with androgenetic alopecia. Arch Dermatol Res. 2004;295(10): 422–8.
12. Rakowska A. Trichoscopy: a new imaging technique in differential diagnosis of hair and scalp diseases [PhD thesis]. Warsaw Medical University, Warsaw; 2010.
13. Fu JM, Starace M, Tosti A. A new dermoscopic finding in healthy children. Arch Dermatol. 2009;145(5):596–7.

Part IV

Tips, Tricks, and Artifacts

Tips, Tricks, and Artifacts in Trichoscopy

7

Lidia Rudnicka and Adriana Rakowska

Abstract

In this chapter, we share some practical ideas on how to get better results from trichoscopic examinations and how to avoid the most common technical problems. Issues related to dermoscope use, immersion fluids, artifacts, and optical illusions in trichoscopy are discussed.

Keywords

Artifacts • Black dots • Dermoscope • Dirty dots • Eyelash • Eyebrow • Hair colorization • Hair dye dots • Light reflection • Immersion fluid • Optical illusion • Pili annulati • Tips • Tricks UV-enhanced trichoscopy (UVET)

In this chapter, we share some practical ideas on how to get better results from trichoscopic examinations and how to avoid the most common technical problems. Issues related to dermoscope use, immersion fluids, artifacts, and optical illusions in trichoscopy are discussed. Some tips, tricks, and artifacts are as follows:

1. Any contact or noncontact dermoscope may be used to perform trichoscopy.
2. When using a contact dermoscope, start with dry trichoscopy to look for scaling and features of blond or gray hairs; then, add immersion fluid.
3. Any immersion fluid may be used. We prefer alcohol solutions because they ensure clear visibility, evaporate immediately, have antibacterial properties, and have a relatively low potential to generate air bubbles.
4. Avoid air bubbles if possible, especially when taking photographs for later evaluation. Air bubbles decrease the image quality and reduce the visibility of trichoscopic structures.
5. Use the roll-on technique to place a contact dermoscope on the scalp. Place the dermoscope's edge on the skin first, then "roll" until the glass plate is located flat against the skin. This technique allows one to increase the pressure slowly while observing the field of view.
6. Blood vessels are best evaluated when the pressure exerted on the dermoscope is low. High outside pressure reduces blood flow and decreases the visibility of blood vessels.
7. Eyebrows and eyelashes are best inspected with a noncontact dermoscope. If using a contact dermoscope, take special caution to avoid irritating the conjunctiva. Never use alcoholic immersion fluids for eyebrows and eyelashes.
8. Hair washing may destroy the most important findings. Ask patients not to wash their hair for at least 2–3 days before a trichoscopic examination, if possible. This is important in doubtful cases.
9. In patients who dye their hair from blond or gray to a darker color, trichoscopy should be performed after hair dyeing, because visibility of dark hair is better than that of light-colored hair. Ideally, in these patients, trichoscopy should be performed after hair dyeing and after washing the hair once or twice to remove any leftover dye.

L. Rudnicka (✉)
Faculty of Health Sciences,
Medical University of Warsaw, Poland

Department of Dermatology, CSK MSW,
Woloska 137, Warsaw 02-502, Poland
e-mail: lidia.rudnicka@euderm.eu

A. Rakowska
Department of Dermatology, CSK MSW, Warsaw, Poland

L. Rudnicka et al. (eds.), *Atlas of Trichoscopy*,
DOI 10.1007/978-1-4471-4486-1_7, © Springer-Verlag London 2012

10. Patients with intense scaling may be asked to apply a keratolytic product to the scalp for 1–2 weeks, then trichoscopy may be performed again. Removing the scaly coating layer improves visibility of the blood vessels.
11. Objects on the scalp that may hinder diagnosis include dirty dots (in children), leftover hair dye, makeup foundation, textile fibers, or cosmetic hair fibers.
12. Ultraviolet-enhanced trichoscopy (UVET) may facilitate the diagnosis of diseases that exhibit fluorescence on Wood's light (e.g., tinea capitis caused by *Microsporum canis*).
13. Use trichoscopy in every patient with a hair or scalp problem. You may be surprised by the result, and your patients will feel they have received special care.

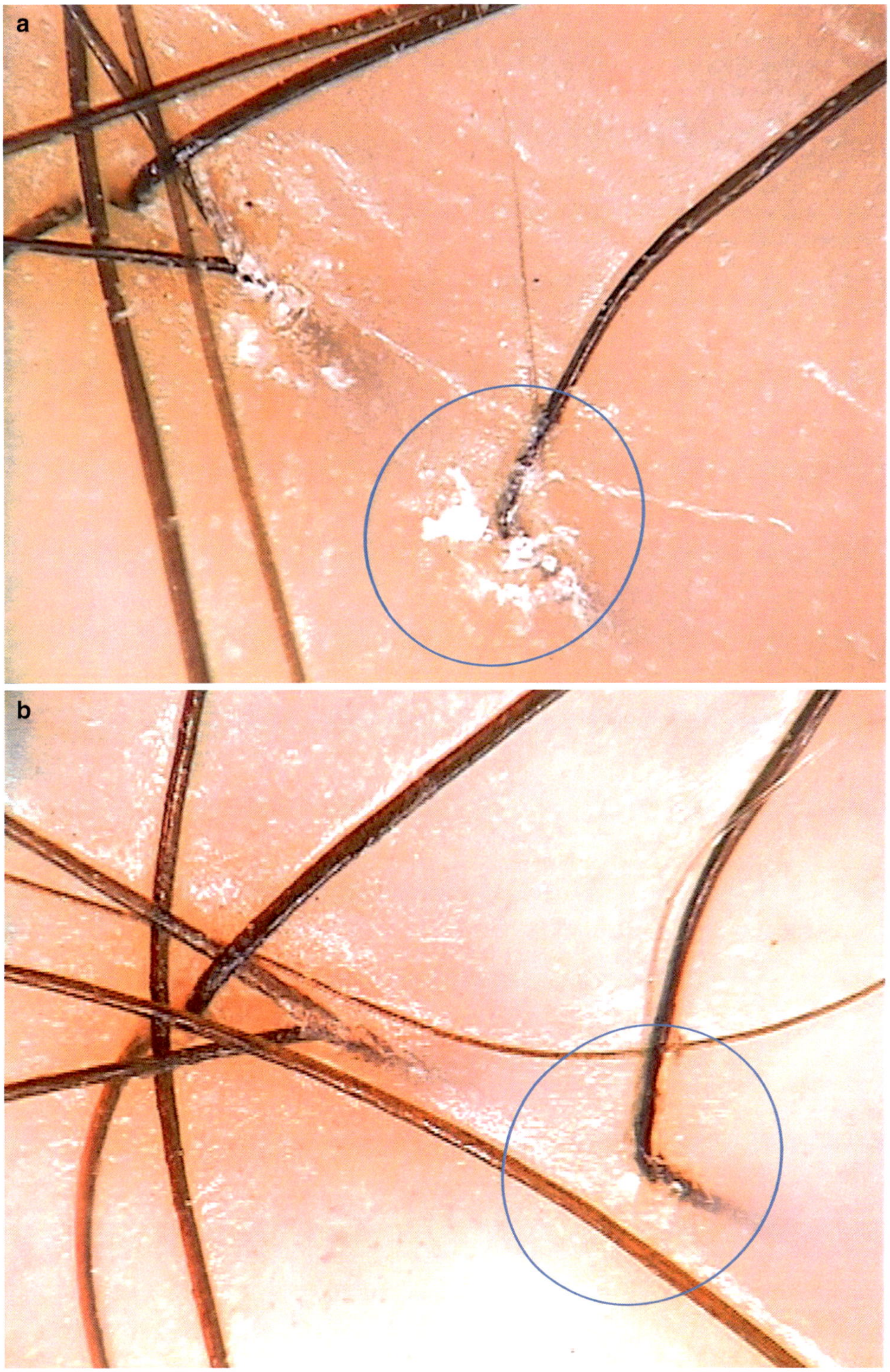

Fig. 7.1 Perifollicular scaling: dry trichoscopy versus immersion fluid. These two images show the same field of view in a patient with lichen planopilaris seen on dry trichoscopy (**a**) and with immersion fluid (**b**). Dry trichoscopy allows better visualization of perifollicular scaling (*blue rings*) [1, 2]. On trichoscopy with immersion fluid, these areas appear slightly erythematous. Severe scaling may appear as irregular white areas. These images show that perifollicular scaling may be easily missed when trichoscopy is performed with immersion fluid only (×70)

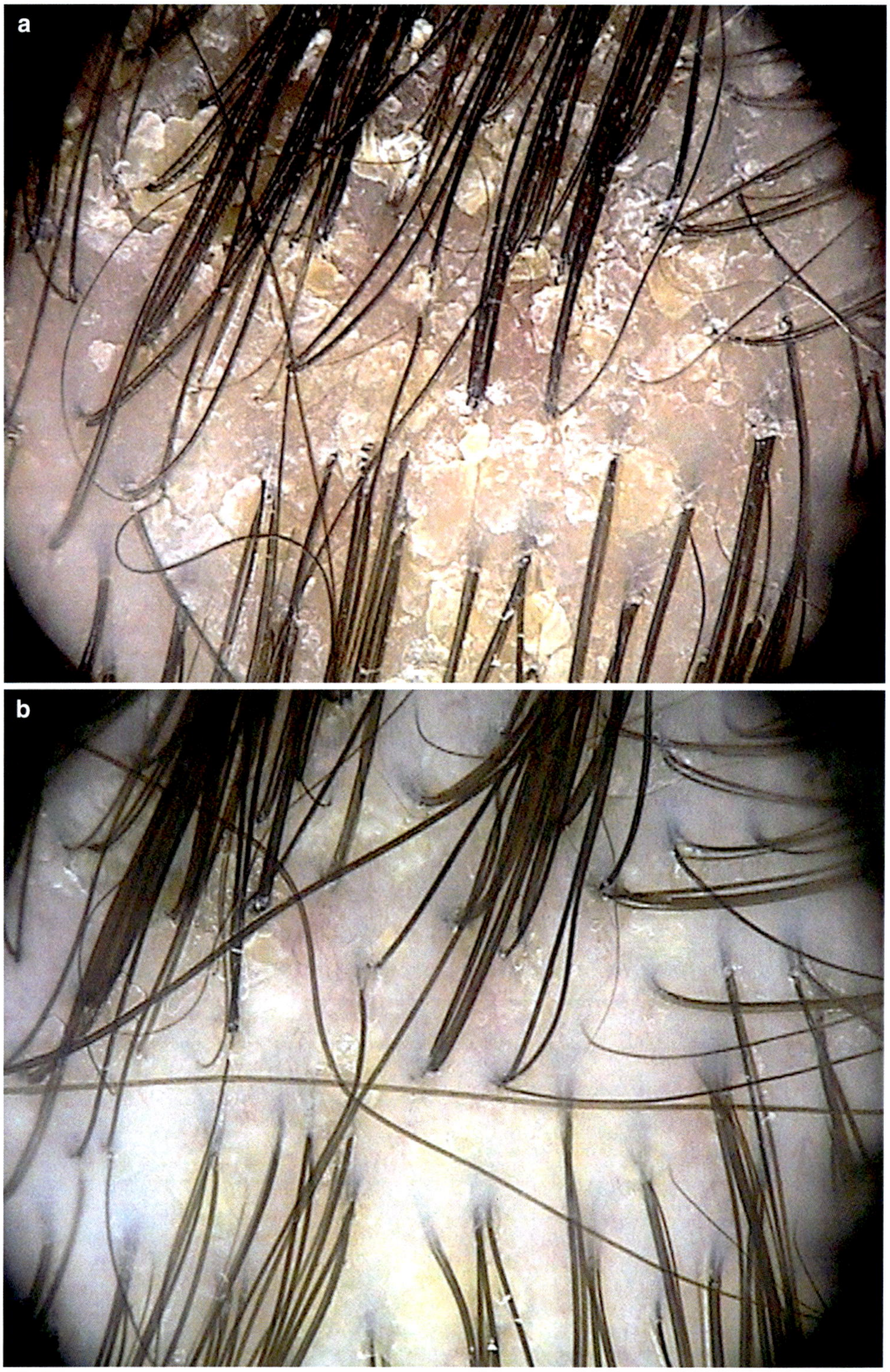

Fig. 7.2 Diffuse scaling: dry trichoscopy versus immersion fluid. These two images show the same scalp area in a patient with seborrheic dermatitis seen on dry trichoscopy (**a**) and with immersion fluid (**b**). Dry trichoscopy reveals diffuse yellow scaling, which is characteristic of seborrheic dermatitis. When immersion fluid is added, only a yellowish hue can be observed (×20)

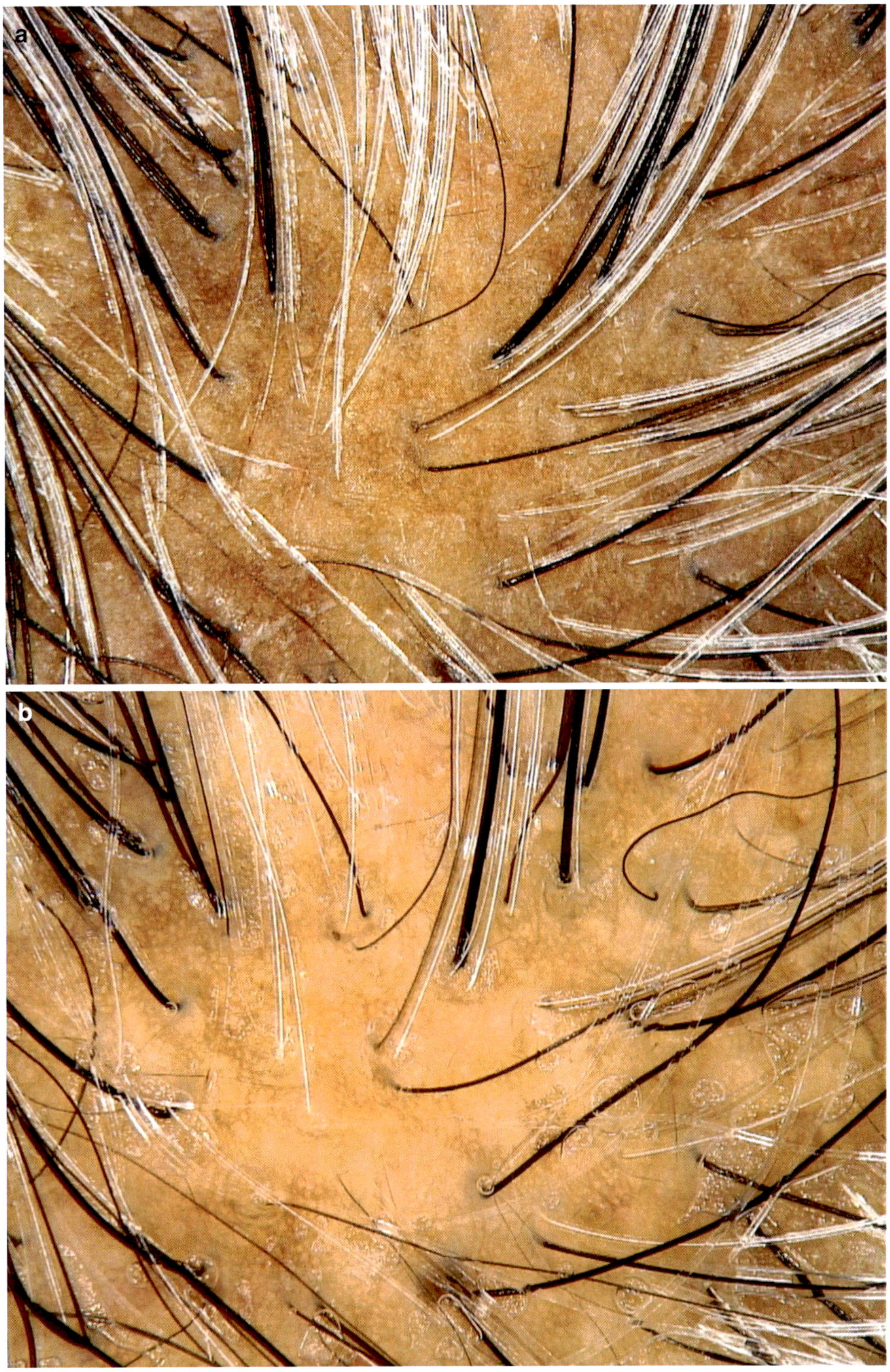

Fig. 7.3 **Gray hair: dry trichoscopy versus immersion fluid**. These two images show the same field of view in a patient with gray hair seen on dry trichoscopy (**a**) and with immersion fluid (**b**). The number of hair shafts seems to differ between the images, because hypopigmented hair shafts are visualized better on dry trichoscopy. When immersion fluid is used, light reflection from these hairs is suppressed (i.e., the hairs become "translucent") and these hair shafts may easily be missed. Thus, trichoscopy in patients with gray or light blond hair is easier with dry (or noncontact) trichoscopy. For patients who dye their hair, we recommend performing trichoscopy within 7–14 days after hair dyeing so that hair shaft visibility is increased (×20)

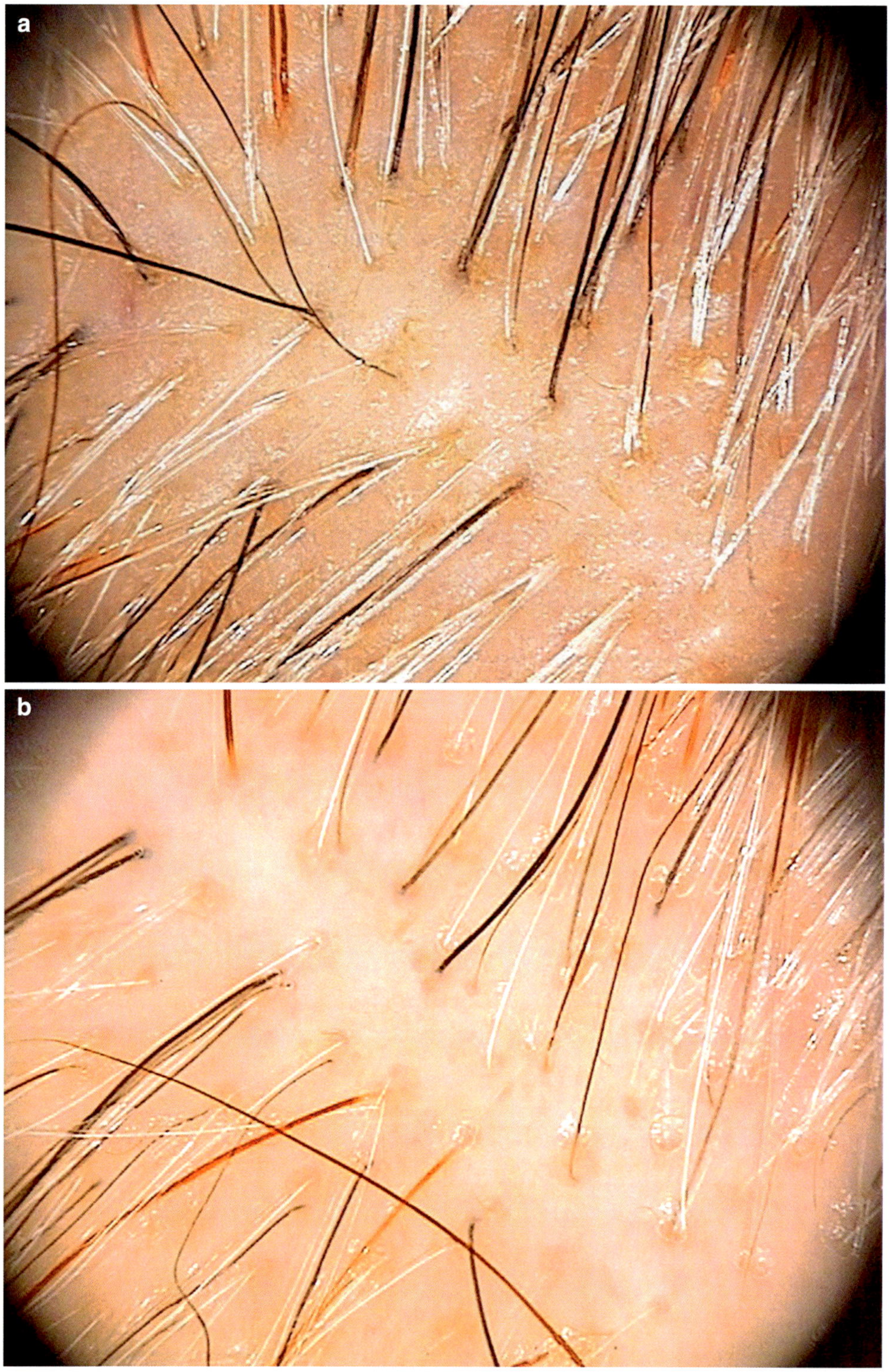

Fig. 7.4 Gray hairs: dry trichoscopy versus immersion fluid. These two images show the scalp area of a patient with gray hair seen on dry trichoscopy (**a**) and with immersion fluid (**b**). The hair appears denser on dry trichoscopy than on trichoscopy with immersion fluid. The detail in *panel b* shows hypopigmented hairs, which become "translucent" with the addition of immersion fluid (×20)

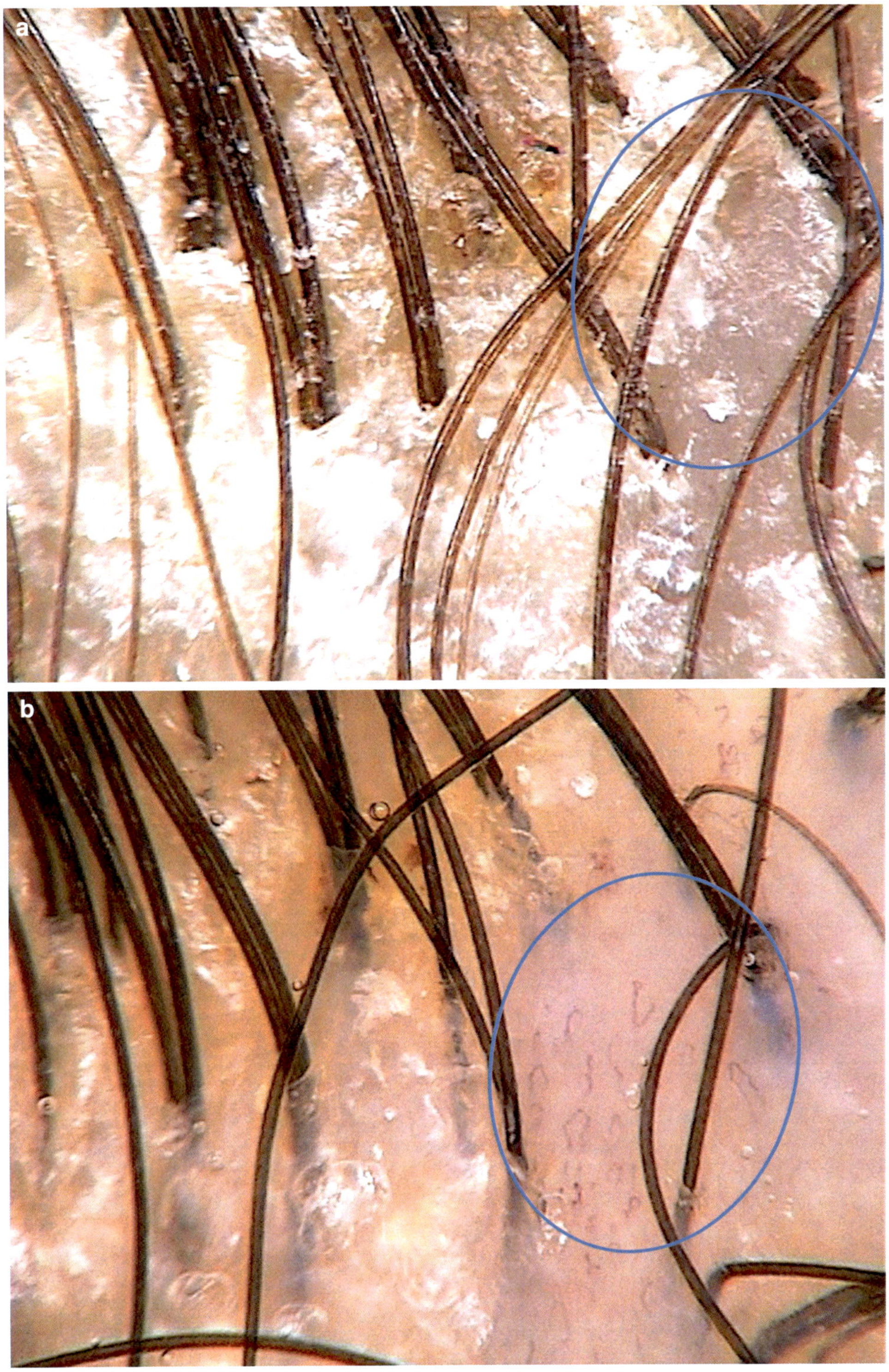

Fig. 7.5 Blood vessels: dry trichoscopy versus immersion fluid. These two images show the same field of view in a patient with psoriasis seen on dry trichoscopy (**a**) and with immersion fluid (**b**). The *blue rings* indicate the exact same area in both images, showing only diffuse white scaling in *panel a* (dry trichoscopy). When immersion fluid is added (**b**), the reflection from the scales is suppressed and multiple lace-like vessels in regular distribution and linear alignment are visible. This trichoscopic feature, which is highly characteristic for psoriasis, might be missed on dry trichoscopy (×70)

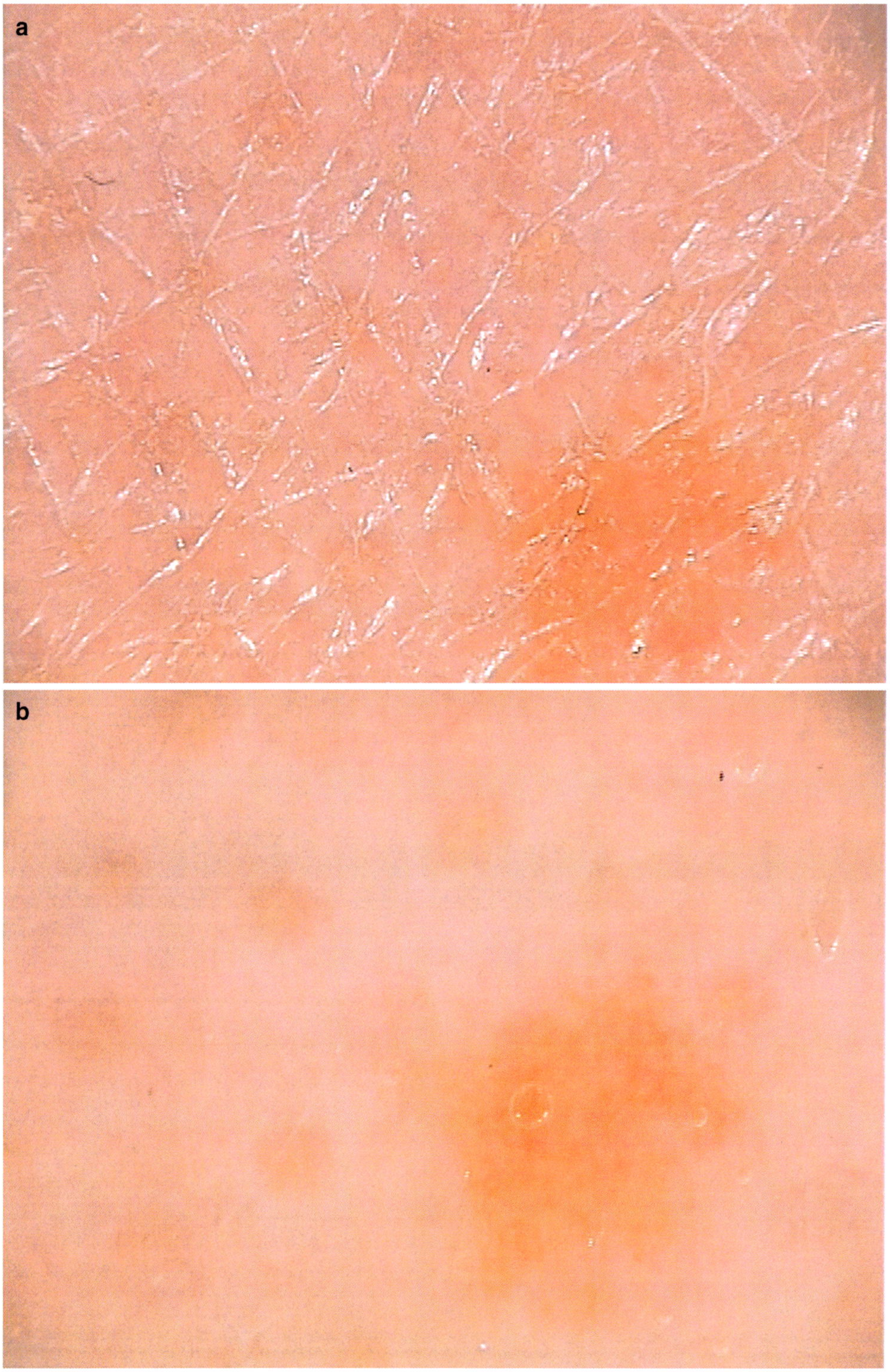

Fig. 7.6 Yellow dots: dry trichoscopy versus immersion fluid. These two images show the same field of view in a patient with alopecia areata seen on dry trichoscopy (**a**) and with immersion fluid (**b**). The nevus (*bottom right*) may serve as an orientation point. A comparison of these images shows that yellow dots are visualized better when contact dermoscopy with immersion fluid is used. Considering that the visibility of some trichoscopic structures is better with immersion fluid and that others are more visible with dry trichoscopy, we perform both examinations in our patients. First, we perform dry trichoscopy; then, we add immersion fluid. Dermatologists who use noncontact dermoscopes should be aware of the slight differences in visibility of the structures (×70)

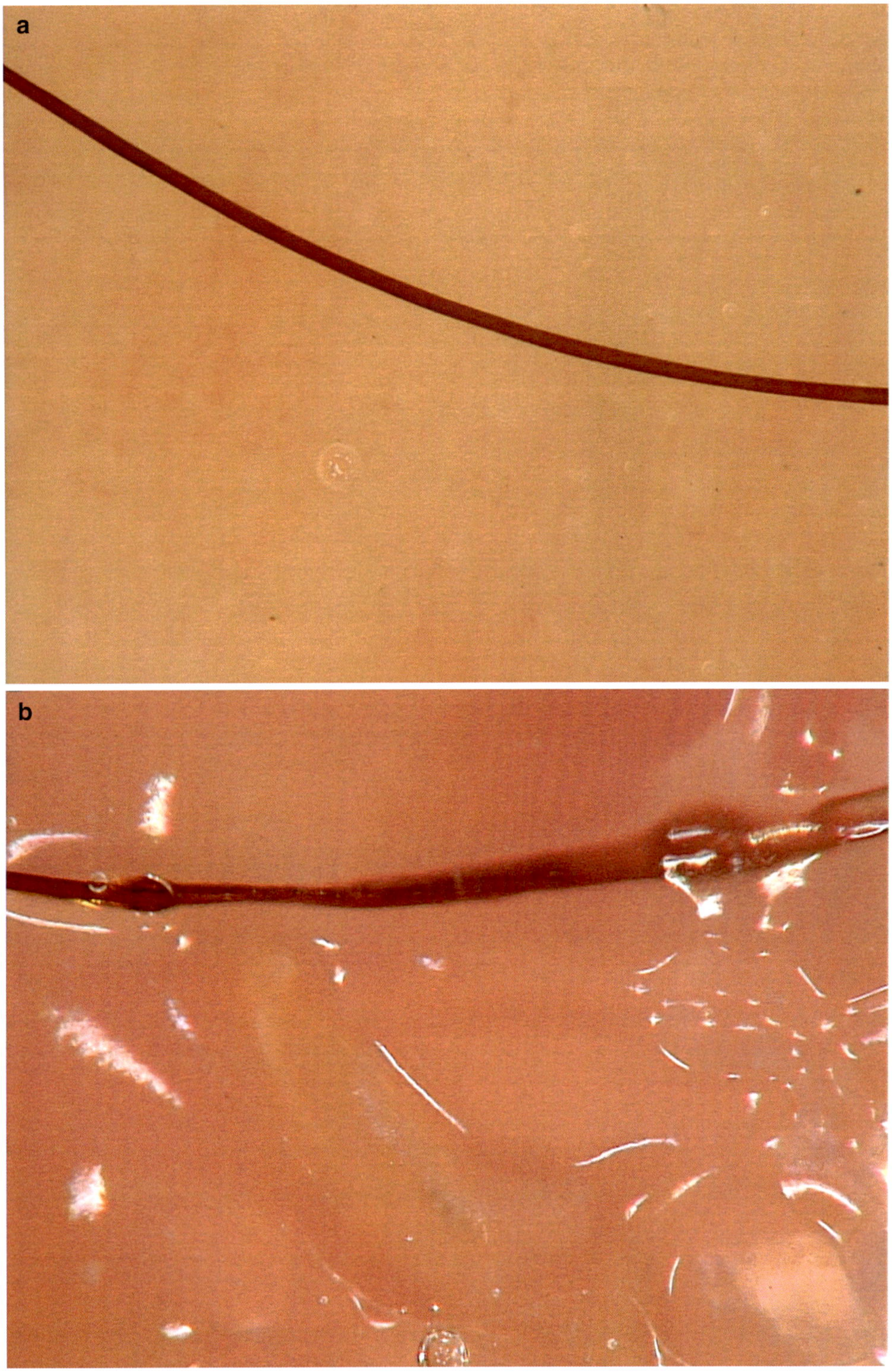

Fig. 7.7 Hair shaft artifact caused by immersion gel and low dermoscope pressure. These two images show the same normal hair shaft observed with immersion (ultrasound) gel in both images. (**a**) Sufficient pressure was applied to the dermoscope to minimize the gap between the dermoscope lens and the skin. The hair is uniform in thickness and color. (**b**) Light pressure was applied to the dermoscope, and a gel-filled gap was created between the lens and the skin. Irregular distribution of the gel and air inclusions (air bubbles) cause an optical illusion, which changes the appearance of the hair shaft. Air bubbles in immersion fluid should be avoided, if possible, to increase the quality of the image. In some cases of protruding, irregularly shaped structures, avoidance of air bubbles may be especially difficult. Air bubbles are easier to avoid with alcoholic immersion fluids than with other solutions [3] (×70)

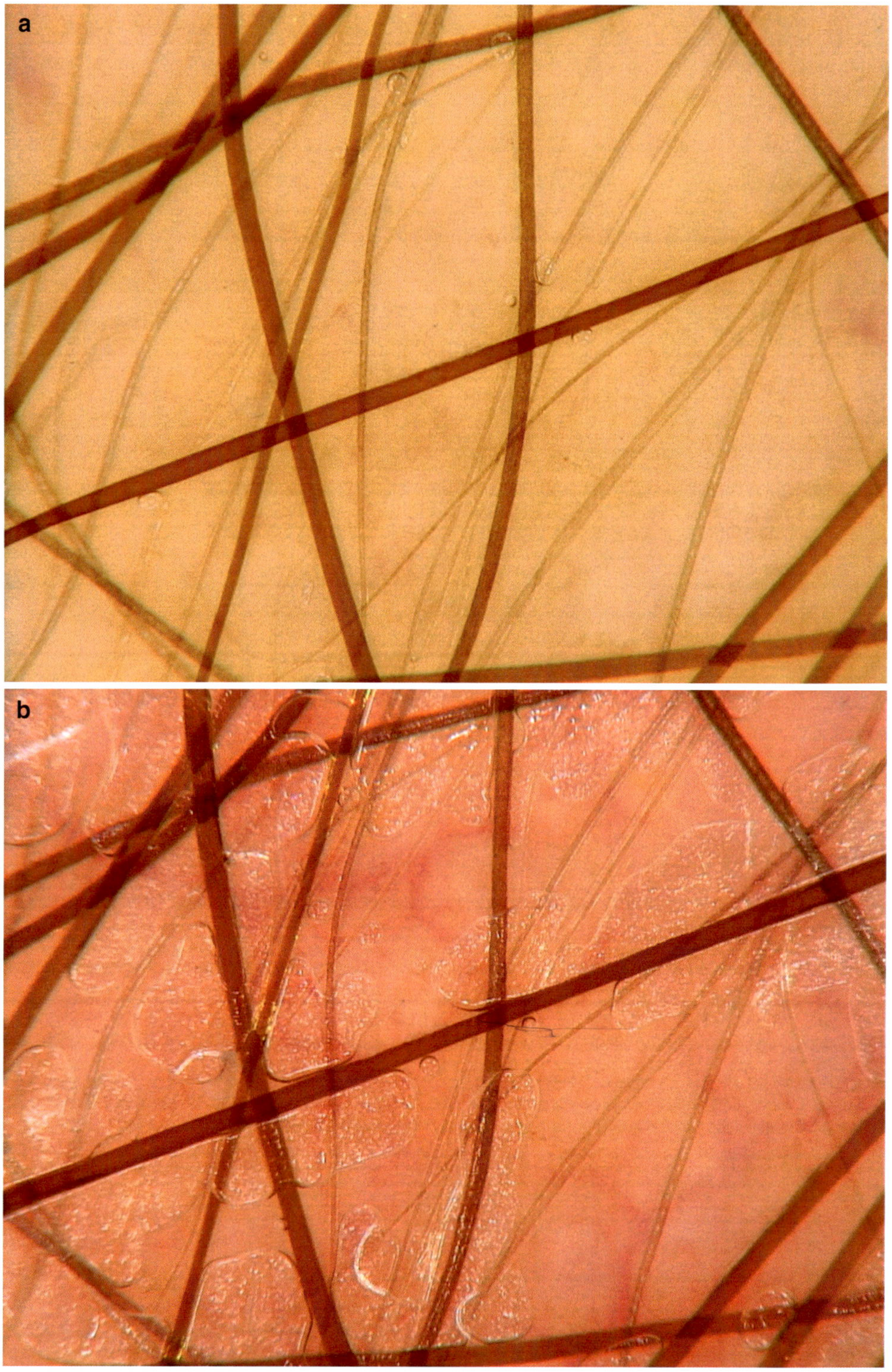

Fig. 7.8 Air bubbles: heavy versus light pressure on the dermoscope. These two images show the same field of view on trichoscopy with heavy (**a**) and light (**b**) pressure applied to the dermoscope. If the pressure of the dermoscope against the skin is too great, blood vessels may be missed; however, if it is too light, air bubbles will be seen in the immersion fluid. One way to avoid this problem is the roll-on technique for using a contact dermoscope [3]. The dermoscope's edge is placed on the skin first and then "rolled" until the glass plate lies flat against the skin. This technique allows one to increase the pressure slowly while observing the field of view (×70)

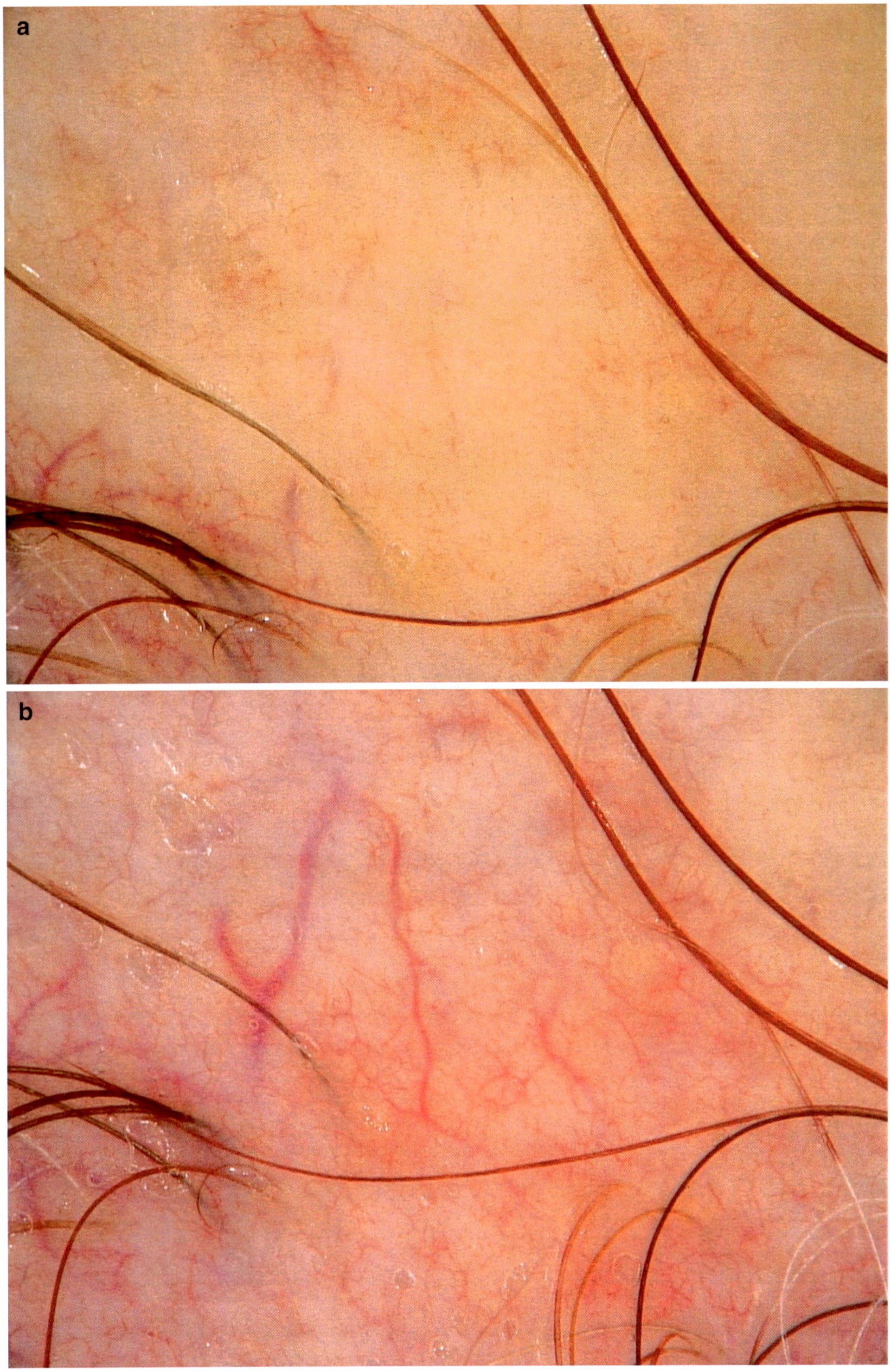

Fig. 7.9 Blood vessels: applying heavy versus light pressure to the dermoscope. These two images show the same field of view on trichoscopy with less (**a**) and more (**b**) pressure applied to the dermoscope. When the pressure of the dermoscope against the skin is too great, blood vessels may be suppressed, reducing blood flow and worsening visibility (×70)

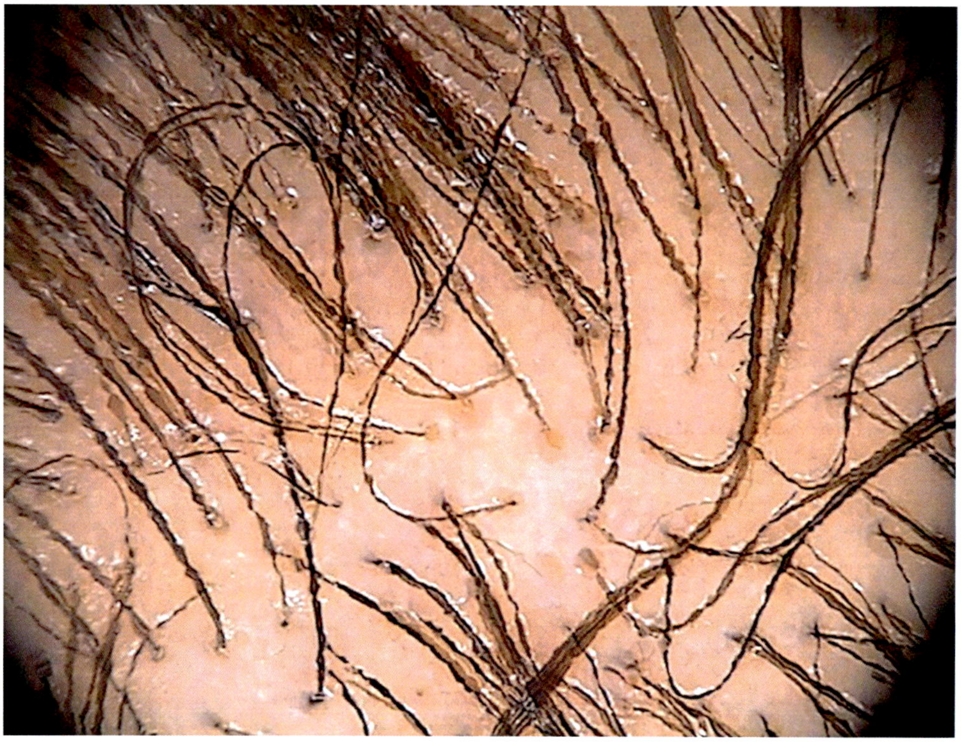

Fig. 7.10 Hair shafts: artifacts caused by immersion gel. Immersion (ultrasound) gel adhering to hair shafts creates an optical illusion of nodosities and constrictions in these hairs. This phenomenon may be mistaken for true monilethrix or monilethrix-like hairs. To verify the diagnosis, more gel should be added or trichoscopy should be performed with an aqueous or alcoholic immersion fluid (×20)

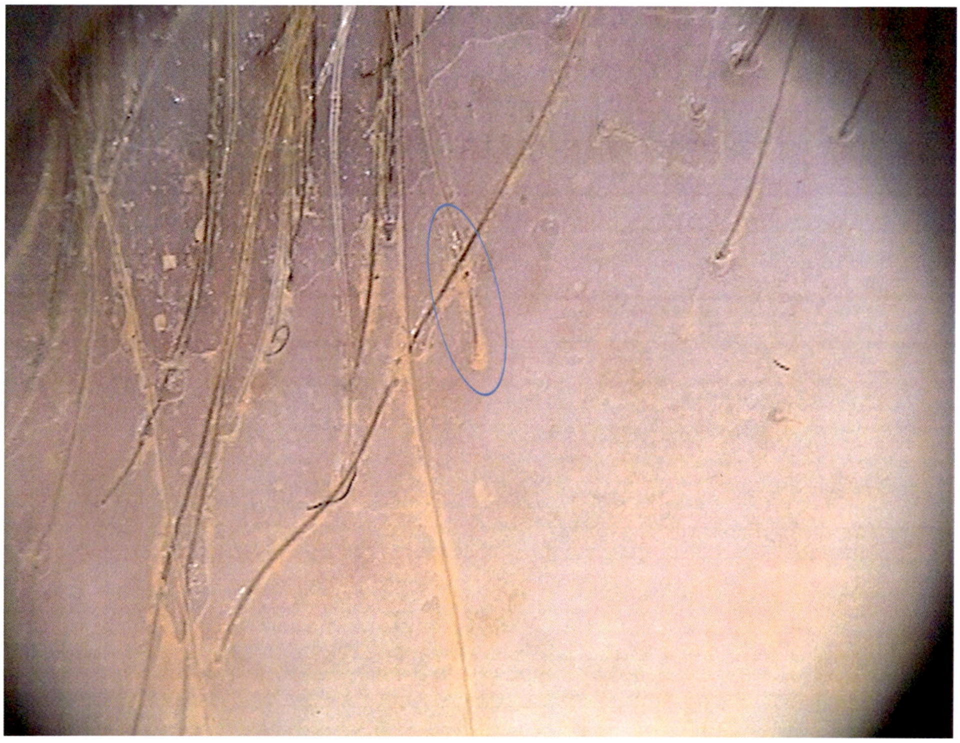

Fig. 7.11 Hair shafts: artifacts caused by makeup foundation. Makeup foundation commonly adheres to hairs at the frontal hair-bearing margin (*blue ring*), but this manifestation may occasionally be observed in other locations. It should not be mistaken for trichomycosis axillaris caused by *Corynebacterium tenuis* or for white piedra caused by *Trichosporon* spp. (×20)

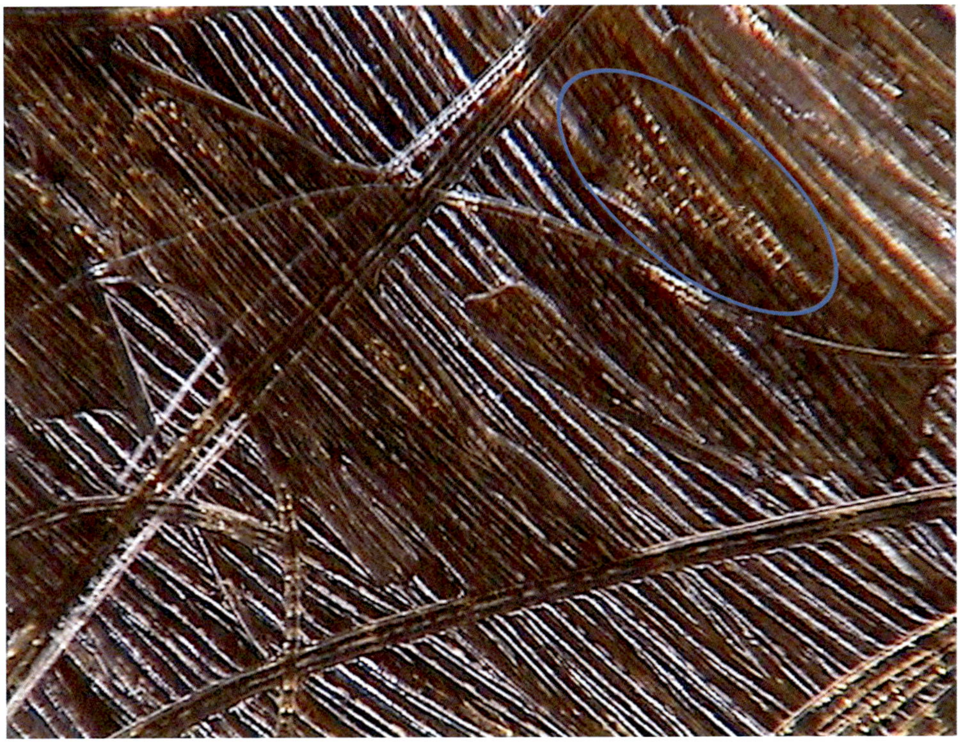

Fig. 7.12 Tiger tail: optical illusion. This optical manifestation of transverse bands in the hair shafts (hairs in the *blue ring*) may be observed when a small amount of alcoholic immersion fluid is used and light pressure is applied. The true "tiger tail" bands observed under polarizing light microscopy in patients with trichothiodystrophy are not visible on trichoscopy [4] (×50)

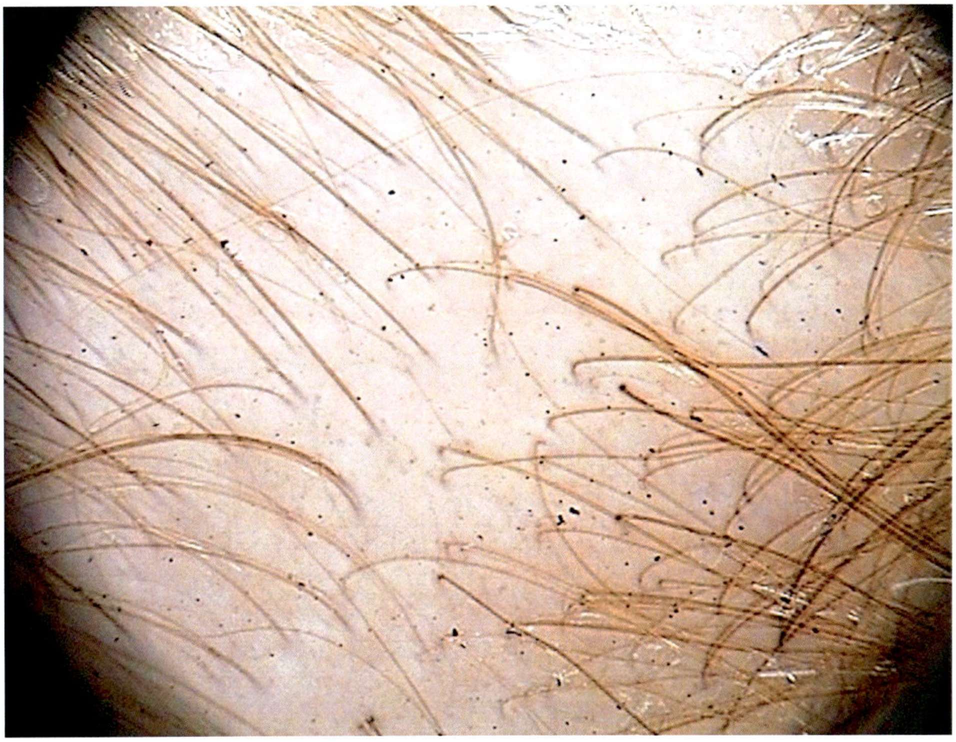

Fig. 7.13 Dirty dots. Dirty dots appear as brown particles irregularly distributed on the scalp. They are environmental particles observed in children after playing in the backyard or garden [5]. Dirty dots should not be mistaken for black dots, which are present in alopecia areata, tinea capitis, and other diseases (×20)

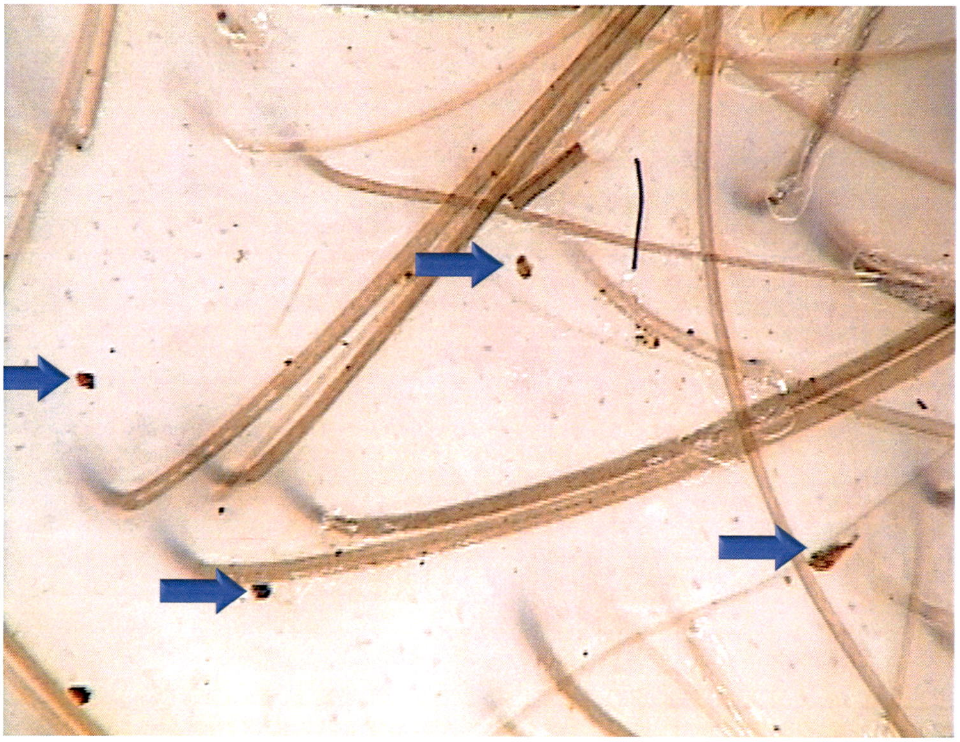

Fig. 7.14 Dirty dots and hat fibers. Higher magnifications show that dirty dots (*arrows*) have different shapes, sizes, and shades of brown. They are not associated with follicular openings. Dirty dots are particles of dirt collected by children from the environment while playing outdoors. They are removed with hair washing [5]. Dirty dots are not present in adults. In both children and adults, fibers from a hat or cap may be seen during trichoscopy. In most cases, they are easy to distinguish from other trichoscopic structures by their color and shape (×70)

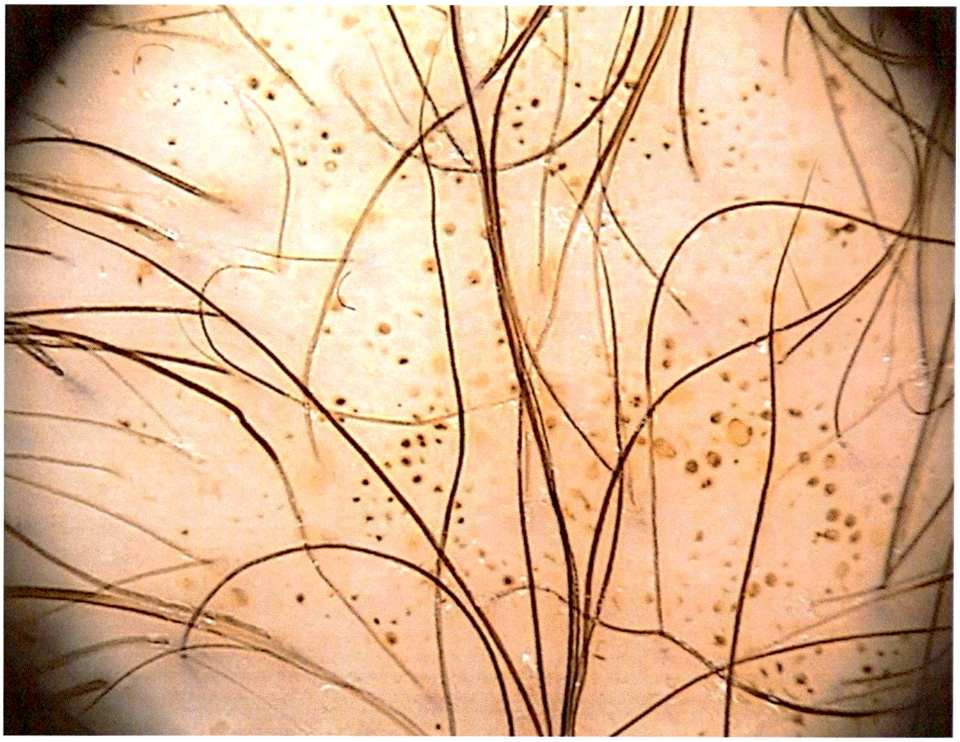

Fig. 7.15 Hair dye dots. These numerous dark dots are the remains of hair dye. Their unusual distribution results from the preferential adherence of hair dye to openings of empty follicles and apocrine gland ducts. We observe this type of hair dye distribution most frequently in patients with alopecia areata (×20)

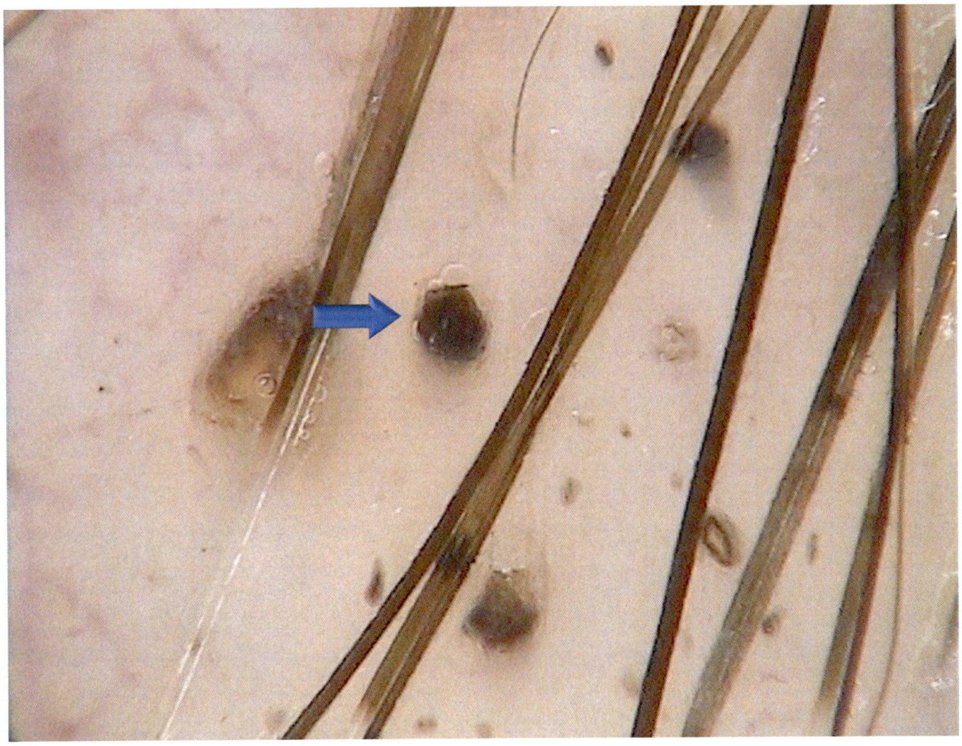

Fig. 7.16 Hair dye dots. These black areas (*arrow*) are the remains of hair dye, which strongly adhere to keratotic material in empty follicular openings. They should not be mistaken for true black dots, which represent residues of pigmented hairs destroyed or broken at scalp level (×70)

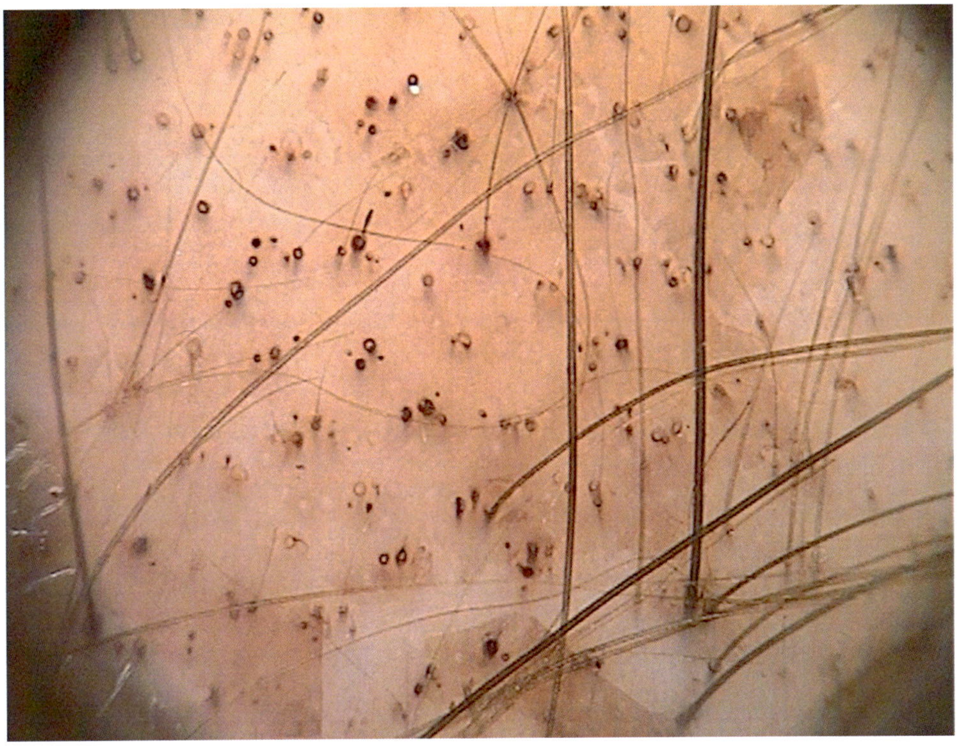

Fig. 7.17 Hair dye in follicular and interfollicular distribution. Brownish rhomboidal structures between follicular units are characteristic of hair dye staining. Within these structures, hair dye dots are visible. They are grouped by two or three, which reflects the hair follicle openings in follicular units. The spared central part of these dots may be a hint to distinguish hair dye dots from true black dots. In doubtful cases, hair dye may be removed from the investigated area with an alcohol swab (×20)

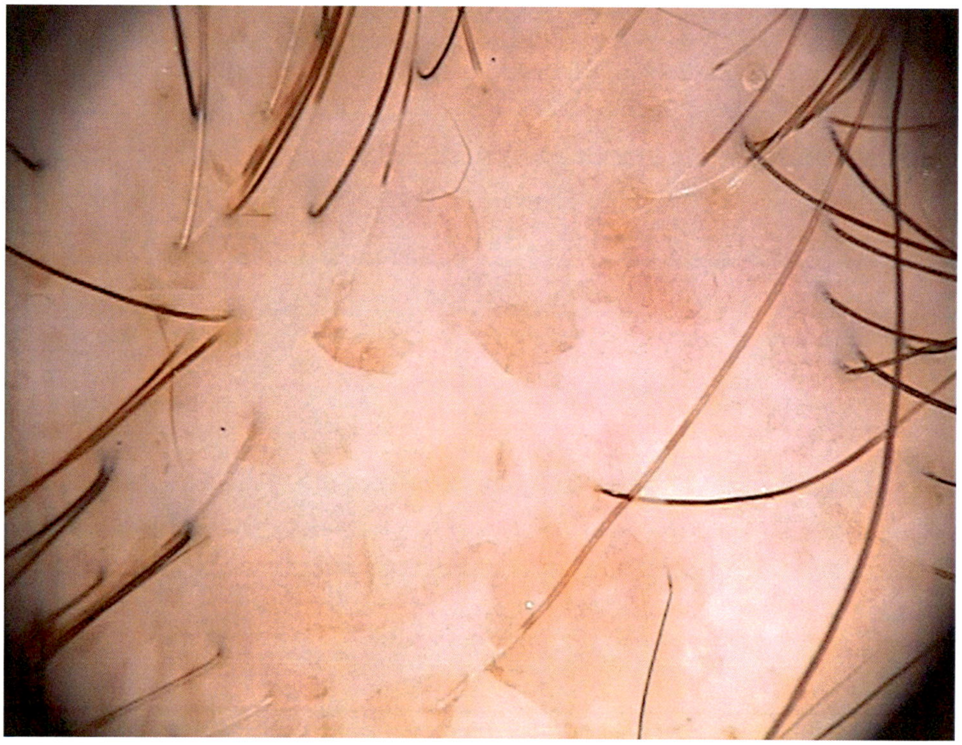

Fig. 7.18 Hair dye in interfollicular distribution. Multiple brownish rhomboidal structures between follicular units are residues of hair dye. They should not be mistaken for hyperpigmentation. Irregularly colored bands on hair shafts show features of recent incomplete hair dyeing (×20)

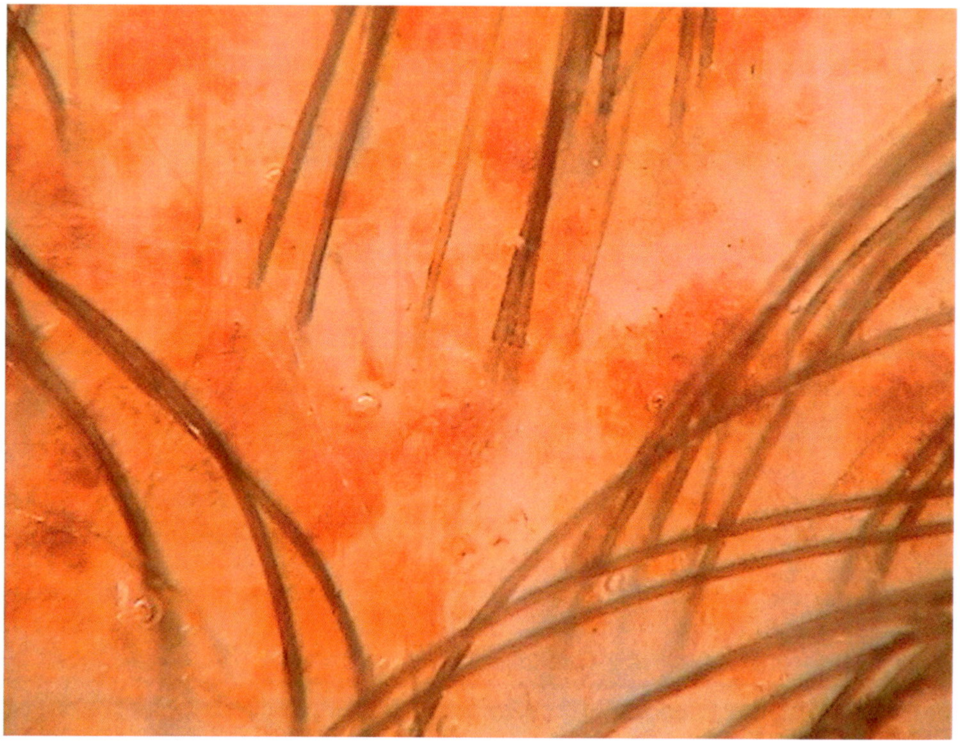

Fig. 7.19 Henna hair dye in interfollicular distribution. Irregular copper-brown rhomboidal structures between follicular units are residues of henna hair dye. They should not be mistaken for hyperpigmentation or blood extravasation. We recommend that patients wash their hair once or twice after colorization to remove leftover hair dye (×70)

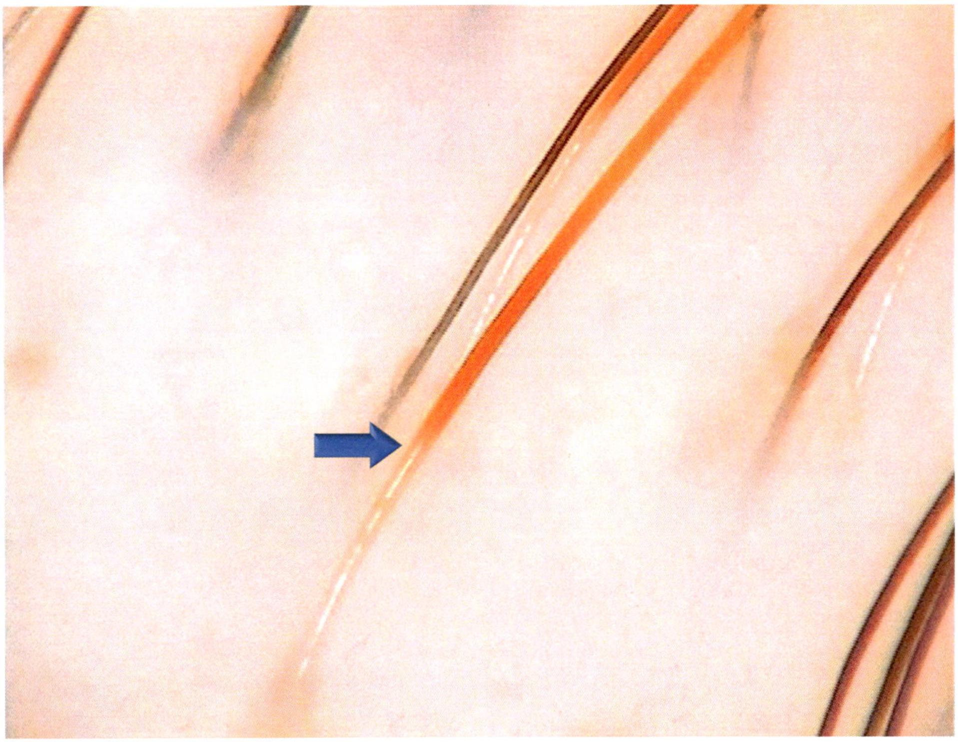

Fig. 7.20 Medulla covered by hair dye. The medulla of the hair shaft may appear on trichoscopy as continuous, interrupted, fragmented, or absent. This image shows a fragment of undyed hair shaft with a visible continuous medulla (*arrow*). The medulla becomes invisible in the dyed portion of the hair. In most well-dyed hairs, the medulla is not visible (×20)

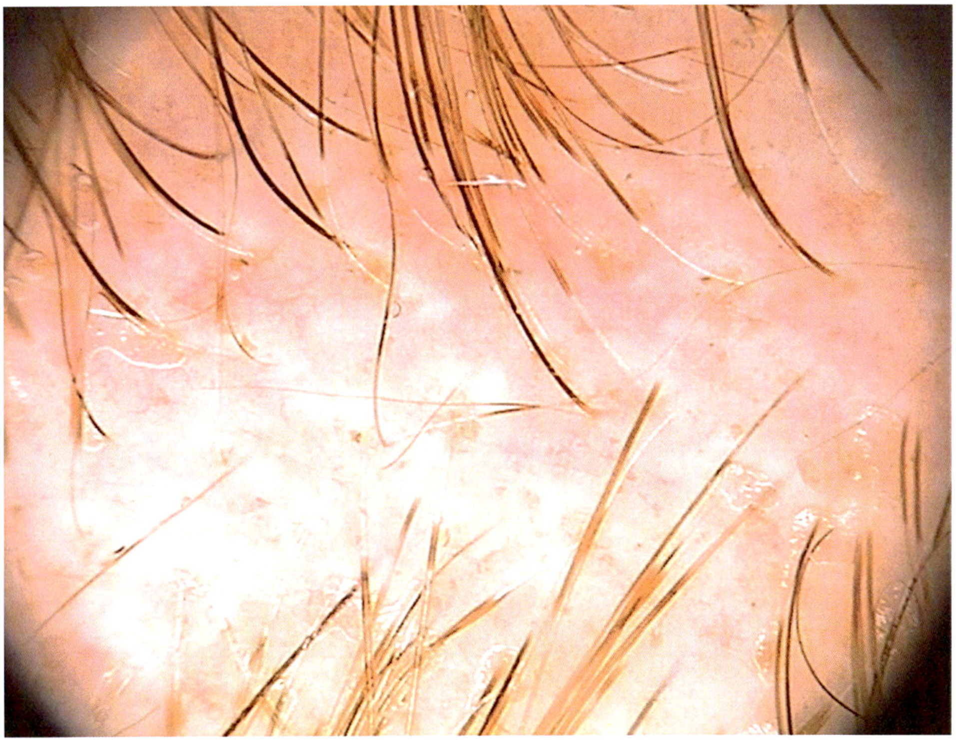

Fig. 7.21 Pili annulati–like effect of irregular hair dyeing. This image shows hairs resembling pili annulati (dark and white bands). Closer examination reveals that the transverse banding is caused by irregular hair dyeing. Unlike true pili annulati, white bands are irregular in size and distribution. In some hair shafts, hair dyeing is indicated by the clear-cut loss of a visible medulla (×20)

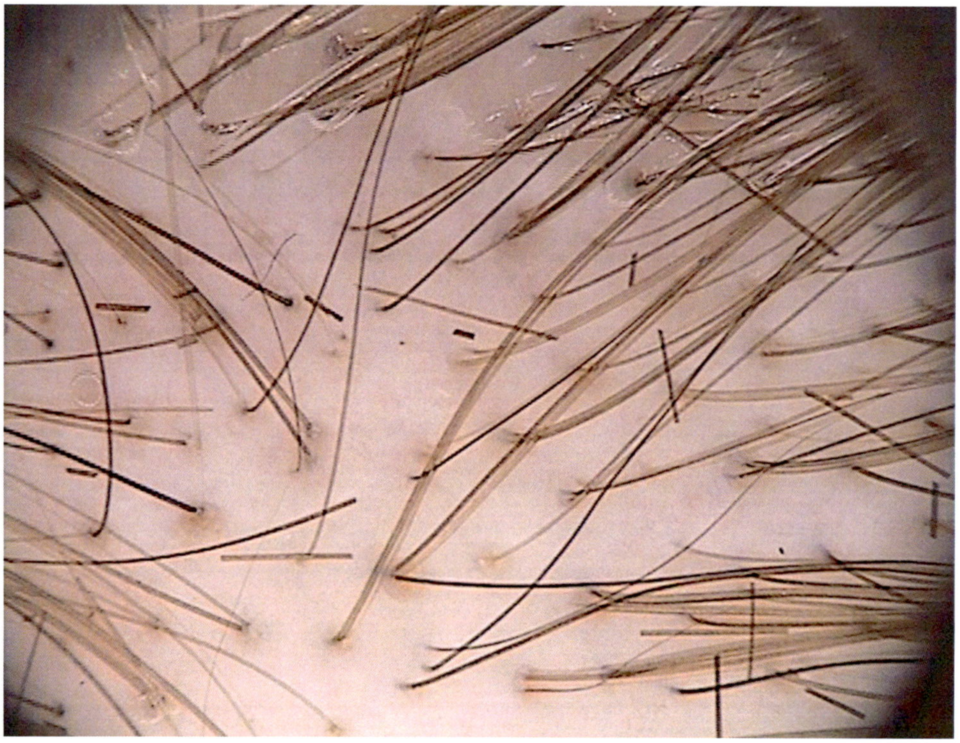

Fig. 7.22 Hair shaft fragments cut by a hairdresser. The short hairs visible in this picture are hair shaft fragments cut during a hairdressing procedure. They are not attached to the skin surface. They differ in length and are irregularly distributed. In this patient, trichoscopy was performed a few hours after her hair was cut (×20)

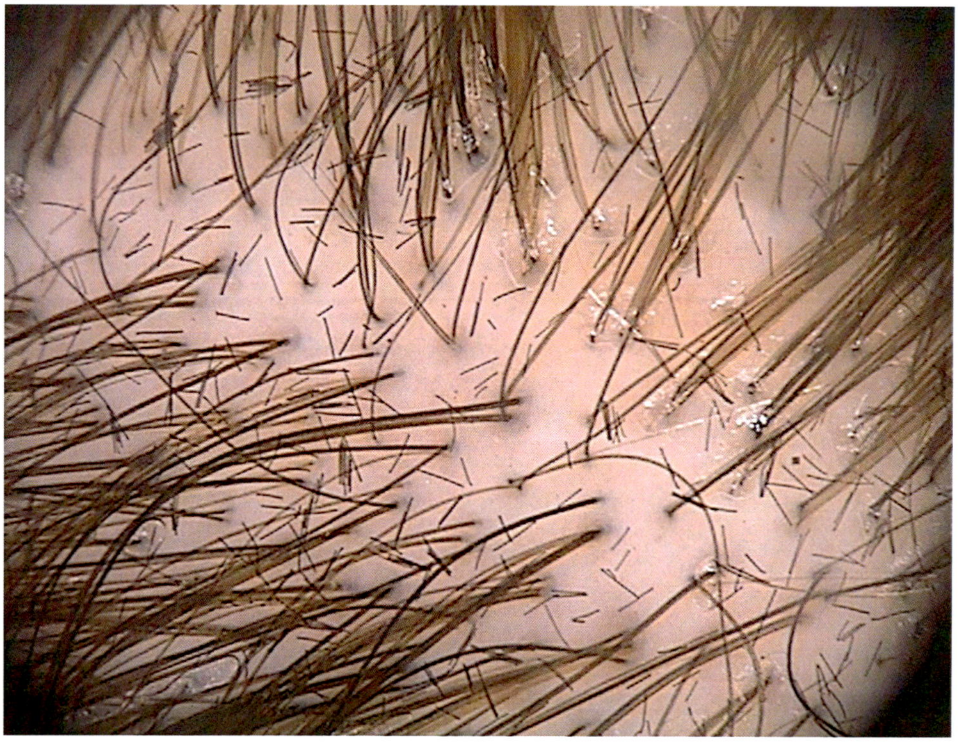

Fig. 7.23 Cosmetic hair fibers. These short lines are dark brown cosmetic hair fibers, which match the color of naturally growing hairs. Cosmetic hair fibers most commonly consist of keratin proteins and/or synthetic ingredients. They are used to mask decreased hair density or hair thinning (×20)

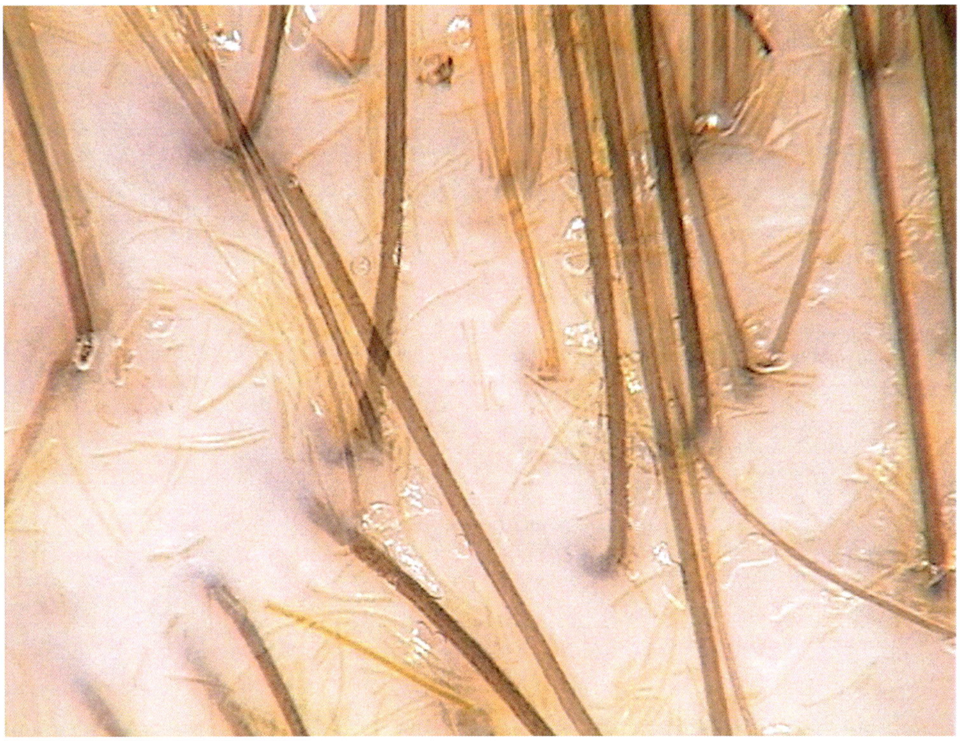

Fig. 7.24 **Cosmetic hair fibers**. The patient shown here has used cosmetic hair fibers matching the color of her dark blond hair. High magnification reveals that they are significantly thinner than the natural hair shafts. Cosmetic hair fibers usually vary somewhat in thickness and length (×70)

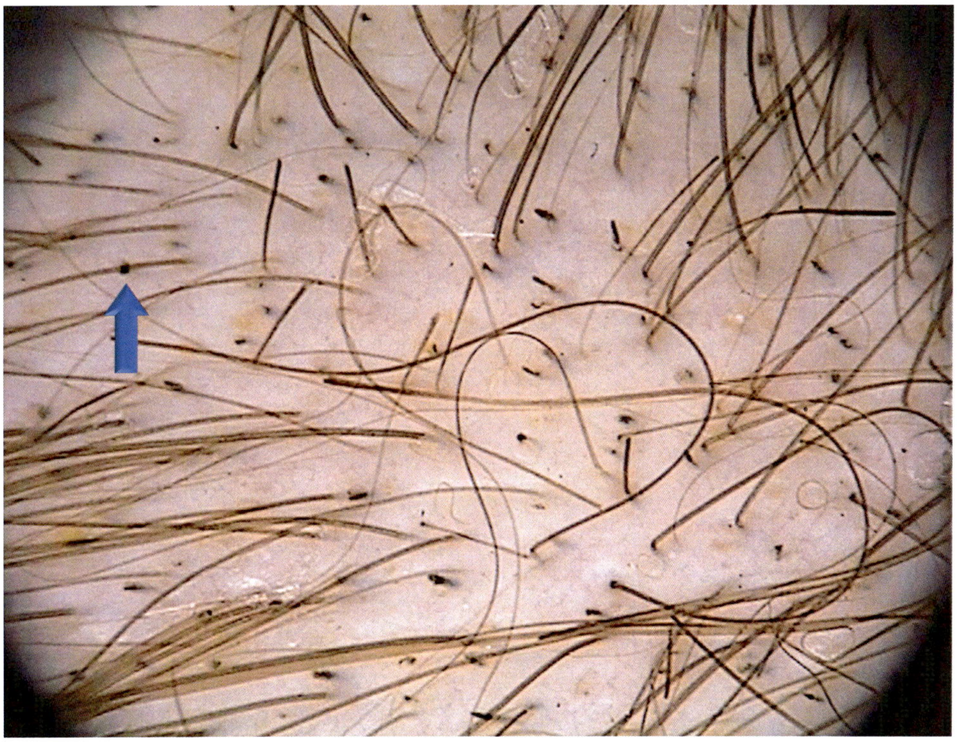

Fig. 7.25 **Trichorrhexis invaginata–like optical illusion**. In this image, a hair shaft overlaps a black dot (*arrow*). This may give the impression of a nodule in the hair shaft and lead to a misdiagnosis of Netherton's syndrome. A similar illusion of hair shaft nodules may be created by clusters of hair dye (*see* Chap. 9 for details). In such cases, Netherton's syndrome may be excluded based on other trichoscopic features and the clinical appearance (×20)

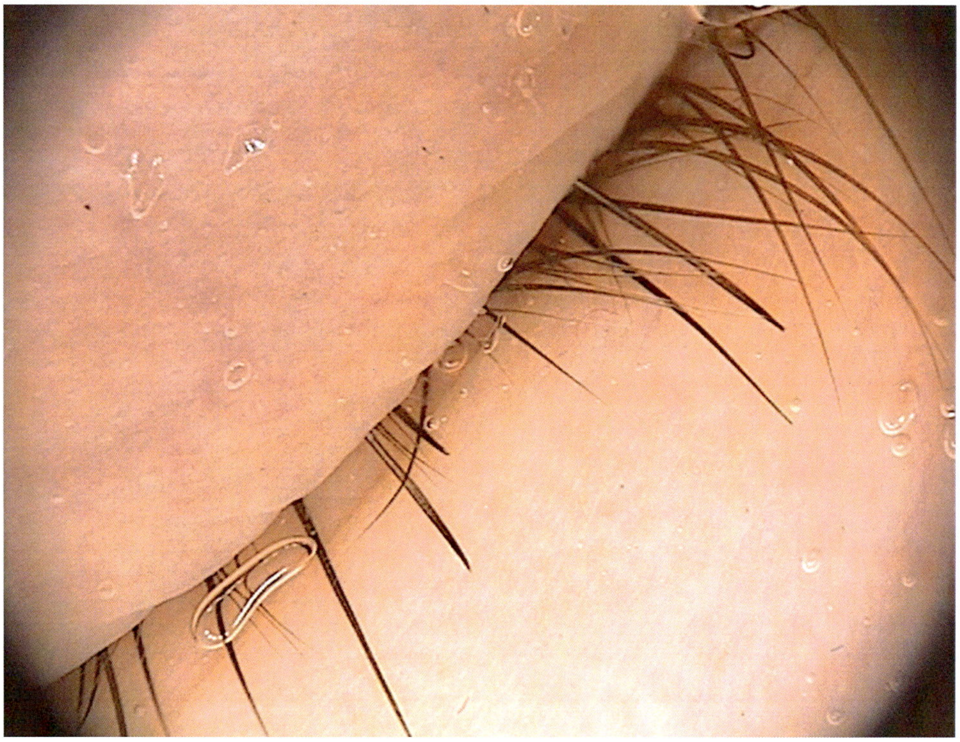

Fig. 7.26 Eyelash and eyebrow trichoscopy. Eyelash and eyebrow trichoscopy may give significant insight into diagnosing isolated madarosis and may be valuable in diagnosing diseases with scalp hair loss, such as trichorrhexis invaginata or frontal fibrosing alopecia. Noncontact dermoscopes are best for evaluating the eye area. If using a contact dermoscope, it is vital to avoid conjunctival irritation by not using alcoholic immersion fluids. We use ultrasound gel for the eyebrows and normal saline (0.9 % NaCl) for the eyelashes. Special caution is needed, when examining the eye area in children (×20)

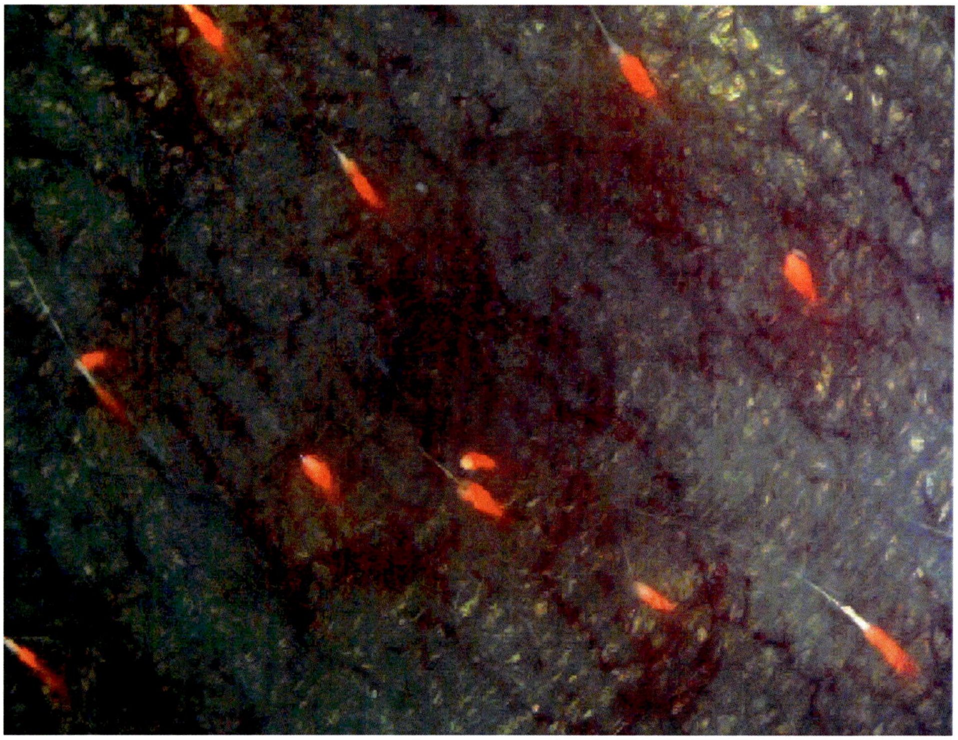

Fig. 7.27 Ultraviolet-enhanced trichoscopy. With some digital videodermoscopes, the user has the option to switch from visible to UV light. This option is used in UVET [2], a technique combining the capabilities of trichoscopy with those of a Wood's lamp. Fluorescence may be observed in greater detail and the examination may be performed in an office with normal lighting. The following fluorescence may be expected: blue green (*Microsporum audouinii*, *M. canis*), yellow (*Microsporum gypseum*), blue (*Trichophyton schoenleinii*, *Pseudomonas* spp.), or orange (*Malassezia furfur*) [2, 3]. This image shows orange fluorescence associated with hair follicle openings and vellus hairs in a patient with *Pityrosporum* folliculitis (Bomtech Kong UV Camera, Republic of Korea)

References

1. Rakowska A, Slowinska M, Kowalska-Oledzka E, Olszewska M, Rudnicka L. Trichoscopy in cicatricial alopecia. J Drugs Dermatol. 2012;11:753–8.
2. Inui S, Nakajima T, Itami S. Dry dermoscopy in clinical treatment of alopecia areata. J Dermatol. 2007;34(9):635–9.
3. Gewirtzman AJ, Saurat JH, Braun RP. An evaluation of dermoscopy fluids and application techniques. Br J Dermatol. 2003;149(1): 59–63.
4. Rakowska A, Slowinska M, Kowalska-Oledzka E, Rudnicka L. Trichoscopy in genetic hair shaft abnormalities. J Dermatol Case Rep. 2008;2(2):14–20.
5. Fu JM, Starace M, Tosti A. A new dermoscopic finding in healthy children. Arch Dermatol. 2009;145(5):596–7.

Part V

Genetic Hair Shaft Disorders

8 Monilethrix, Pseudomonilethrix, and Monilethrix-Like Hairs

Adriana Rakowska and Lidia Rudnicka

Abstract

In monilethrix, trichoscopy shows abnormalities in terminal and vellus hairs of the scalp. Hair shafts show uniform elliptical nodosities and intermittent constrictions causing regular variation in hair shaft thickness. Hairs bend and break at constriction sites. Horny follicular papules appear as big yellow dots when evaluated on trichoscopy with immersion fluid. Perifollicular scaling and keratotic follicular plugs are be best visible on dry trichoscopy. Differential diagnosis includes monilethrix-like congenital hypotrichosis, pseudomonilethrix, and acquired monilethrix-like hair shaft appearance.

Keywords

Alopecia areata • Chemotherapy-induced alopecia • Monilethrix • Monilethrix-like congenital hypotrichosis • Monilethrix-like hair • Nails • Lichen planopilaris • Pseudomonilethrix

Monilethrix is an autosomal dominant hair disorder characterized by regular, periodic thinning of hair shafts and a tendency for the hair to fracture at constricted points. Nodosities correspond to the normal hair caliber, whereas the defect is in the constricted sections [1]. The term *monilethrix*—derived from the Latin *monile*, meaning necklace, and Greek *trichos*, meaning hair—refers to the necklace-like appearance of hair shafts with intermittent constrictions and nodosities.

Most commonly, the disease results from a mutation in the human hair keratin *hHb6* gene [2]. However, cases of monilethrix caused by mutations in genes encoding *hHb1* or *hHb3* have been reported. Mutations in the desmoglein 4 gene (*DSG4*) have been associated with autosomal recessive monilethrix and monilethrix-like congenital hypotrichosis, which differs from classic monilethrix by barely visible internodes, which do not show constant periodicity [3–5].

The phenotype of monilethrix is variable, even within families, and may range from macroscopically normal hair or mild occipital hair loss to near total alopecia.

From early childhood, patients with monilethrix present with short and fragile hairs that never grow long enough to require a haircut. Noninvolved hairs seldom are longer than 5–8 cm [6, 7]. Other hairy areas, such as eyebrows or eyelashes, or axillary, pubic, and body hair also may be involved [6].

Follicular abnormalities observed in monilethrix range from subtle perifollicular erythema to large hyperkeratotic follicular papules. Other, rare ectodermal symptoms in these patients may include koilonychia, brittle nails, syndactyly, juvenile cataract, decreased visual field, and dental abnormalities [6].

Trichoscopy shows abnormalities in terminal and vellus hairs of the scalp. Usually, not all scalp hairs are affected. Hair shafts show uniform elliptical nodosities and intermittent constrictions causing variation in hair shaft thickness. Hairs are bent regularly at multiple locations and have a tendency to fracture at constriction sites [7–10]. The term "regularly bent ribbon sign" was suggested to differentiate

A. Rakowska
Department of Dermatology, CSK MSW,
Warsaw, Poland

L. Rudnicka (✉)
Faculty of Health Sciences, Medical University of Warsaw,
Erazma Ciolka 27, Warsaw 01-445, Poland

Department of Dermatology, CSK MSW,
Warsaw, Woloska 137 02-507, Poland
e-mail: lidia.rudnicka@euderm.eu

L. Rudnicka et al. (eds.), *Atlas of Trichoscopy*,
DOI 10.1007/978-1-4471-4486-1_8, © Springer-Verlag London 2012

the trichoscopic features of monilethrix from pseudomonilethrix and other causes of hair loss. Horny follicular papules appear as big yellow dots when evaluated on trichoscopy with immersion fluid. Perifollicular scaling and keratotic follicular plugs are be best visible on dry trichoscopy.

Pseudomonilethrix is characterized by irregular square-shaped flattening of hair shafts. It remains controversial whether pseudomonilethrix is a true disease or an artifact produced either by the preparation of hairs for microscopic examination or by excessive use of cosmetic hair care products [11, 12].

Pseudomonilethrix must be distinguished from "monilethrix-like" hairs, which show the same type of ovoid constrictions as in monilethrix, but without the regularity characteristic of true monilethrix (Table 8.1).

Monilethrix-like hair shafts may be observed in diseases with a variable course, such as alopecia areata and lichen planopilaris, or in patients undergoing chemotherapy. A similar monilethrix-like effect may be observed in patients who use hairstyling gels [8]. Thus, patients should be advised not to use these products between hair washing and trichoscopy. Also, ultrasound gel used as an immersion fluid can make hair shafts appear irregularly constricted [8].

Table 8.1 Monilethrix-like hair shafts on trichoscopy

Monilethrix
Monilethrix-like congenital hypotrichosis
Alopecia areata with variable activity in the course of disease
Primary cicatricial alopecia (border of fibrotic area)
Chemotherapy-induced alopecia
Monilethrix-like effect from hair styling gel
Monilethrix-like effect from immersion gel
Pseudomonilethrix

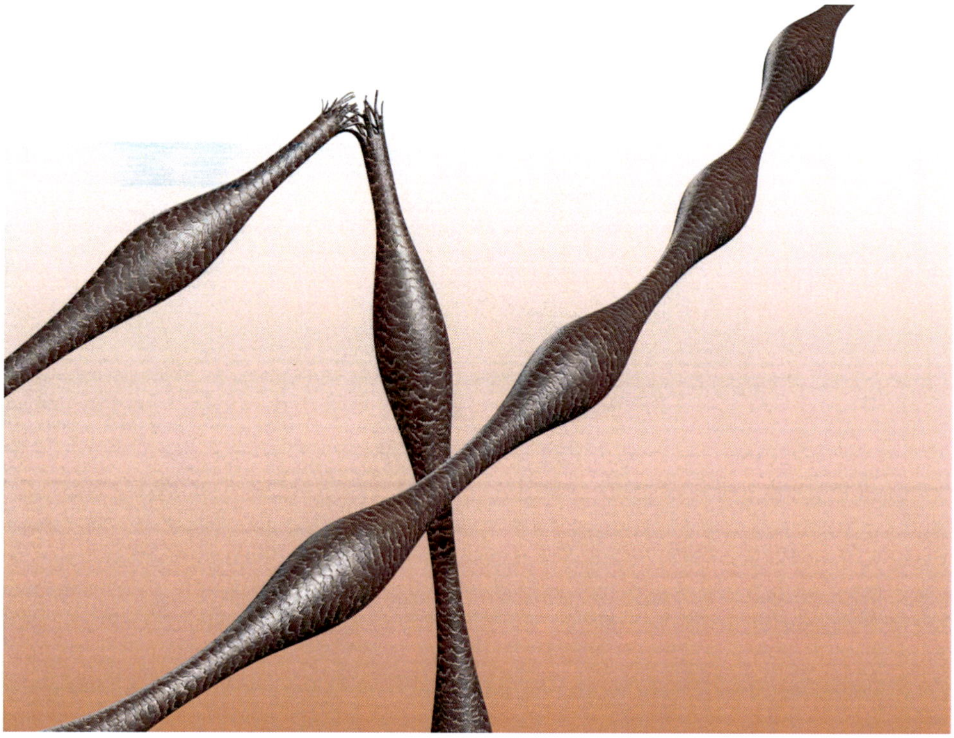

Fig. 8.1 **Monilethrix**. Monilethrix is characterized by regular, periodic thinning of the hair shafts. Nodosities correspond to the normal hair caliber, whereas the defect is in the constricted sections. Hair shafts have a tendency to fracture at constricted sites. The interval length is constant in an individual patient but may differ between patients. (*Graphic by* Dr. Wawrzyniec Podrzucki)

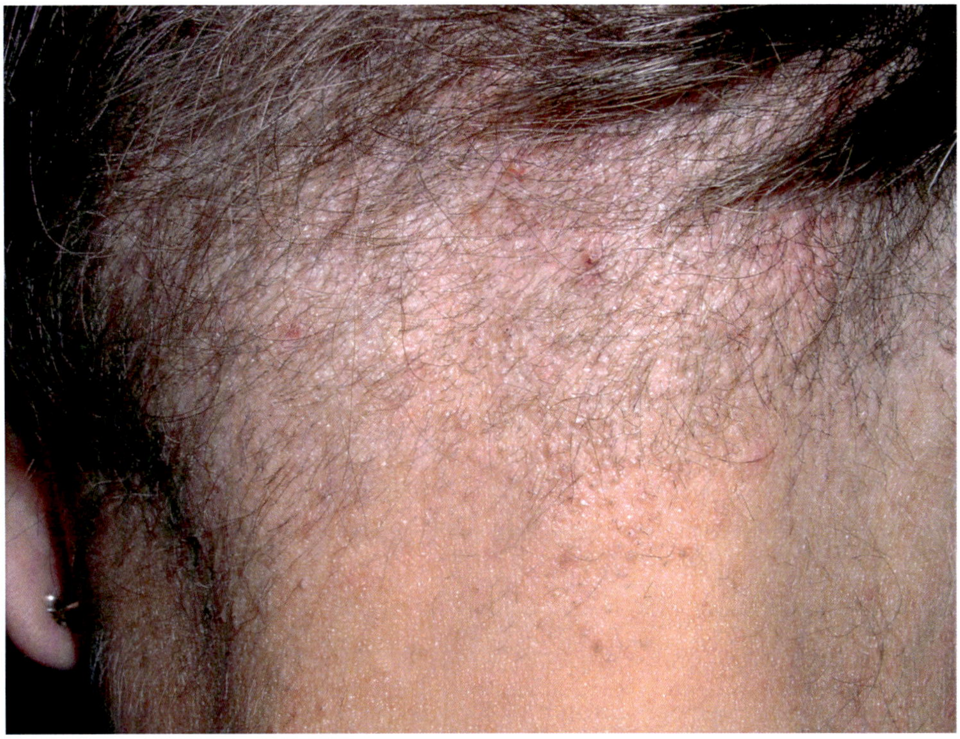

Fig. 8.2 Female patient with monilethrix. The hairs are short and fragile, never requiring cutting. Most commonly, the occipital and temporal regions are affected, but any scalp or body area may be involved. In rare cases, monilethrix distribution may mimic androgenic alopecia [10]. Hair loss is associated with follicular hyperkeratosis, which makes the skin feel rough, especially in the occipital region and back of the neck [2]

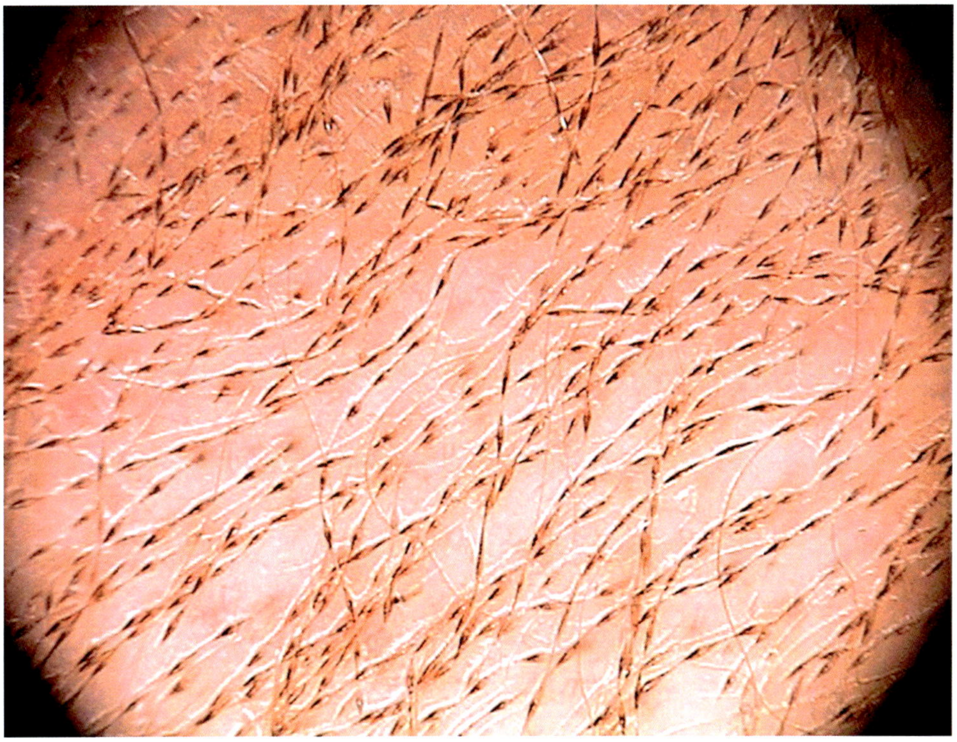

Fig. 8.3 Monilethrix. Multiple regular elliptical nodes (0.7–1 mm long) and constricted regions along the hair shaft produce the appearance of a necklace [10]. This image was taken with dry trichoscopy (no immersion fluid), which sometimes allows better visualization of the nodosities in thin light-colored hair shafts (×20)

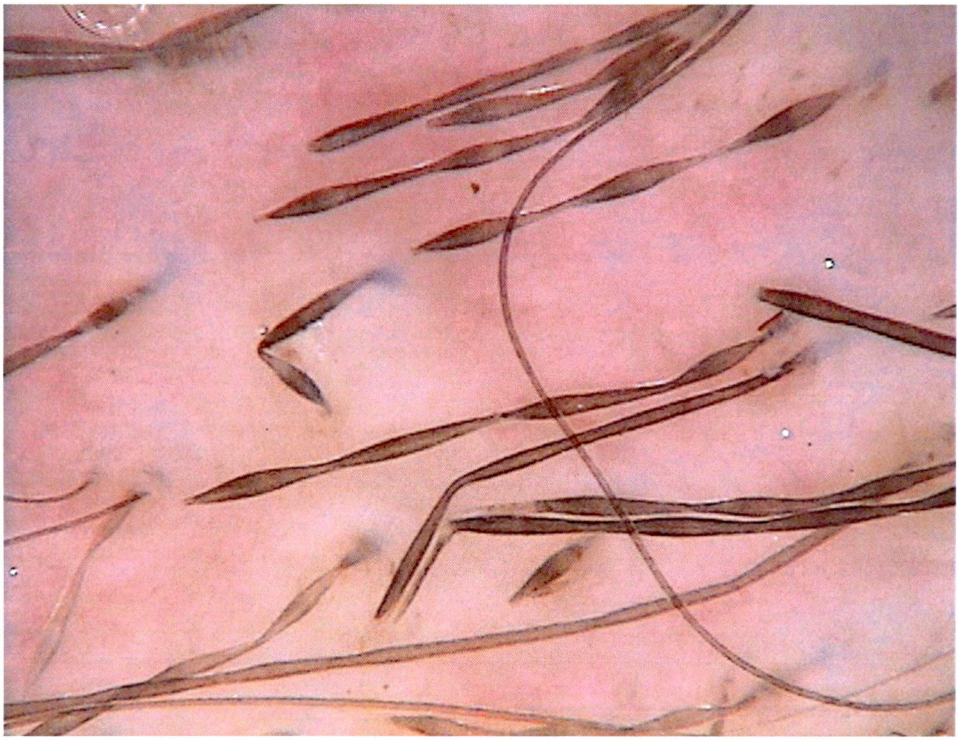

Fig. 8.4 **Monilethrix**. Trichoscopic image of a "regularly bent ribbon sign." Regular, uniform elliptical nodes and intermittent constrictions (internodes). This feature is characteristic of monilethrix [8]. Hairs have tendency to bend in different directions and fracture at constriction sites (×70)

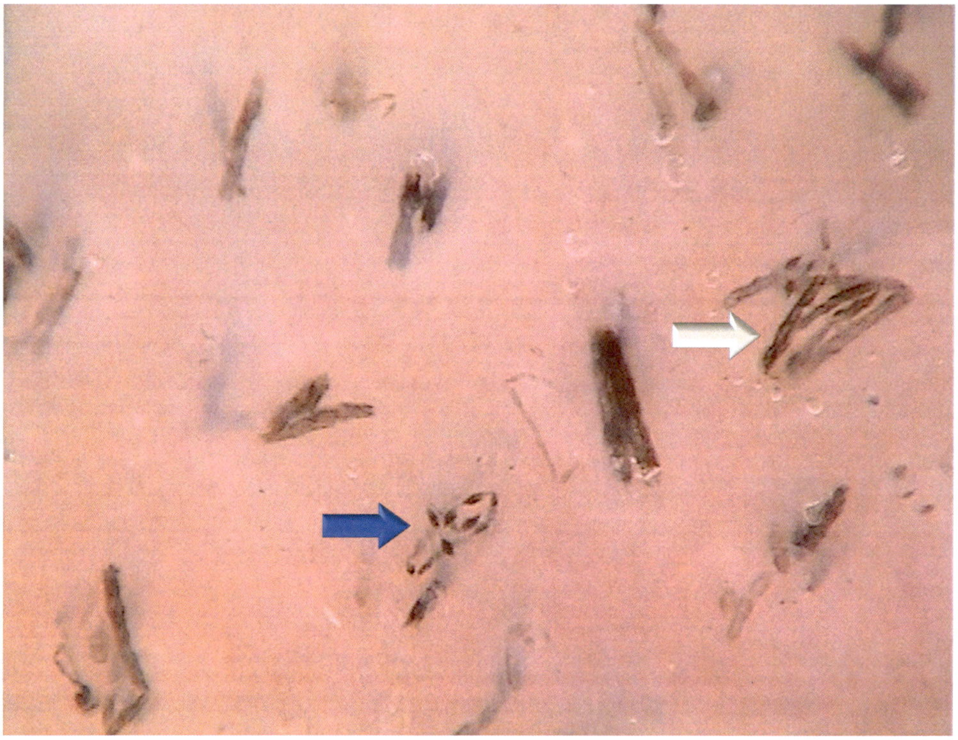

Fig. 8.5 **Monilethrix-like congenital hypotrichosis**. This term corresponds to the rare cases of monilethrix with nonvertical transmission and mutation in the desmoglein 4 gene [3]. Trichoscopy shows internodes very close to each other, as well as very short nodosities (*blue arrow*). In thick hairs, the internodes are hardly visible (*white arrow*). The hairs break in the internodes, which is visualized more easily in thinner hairs (×70)

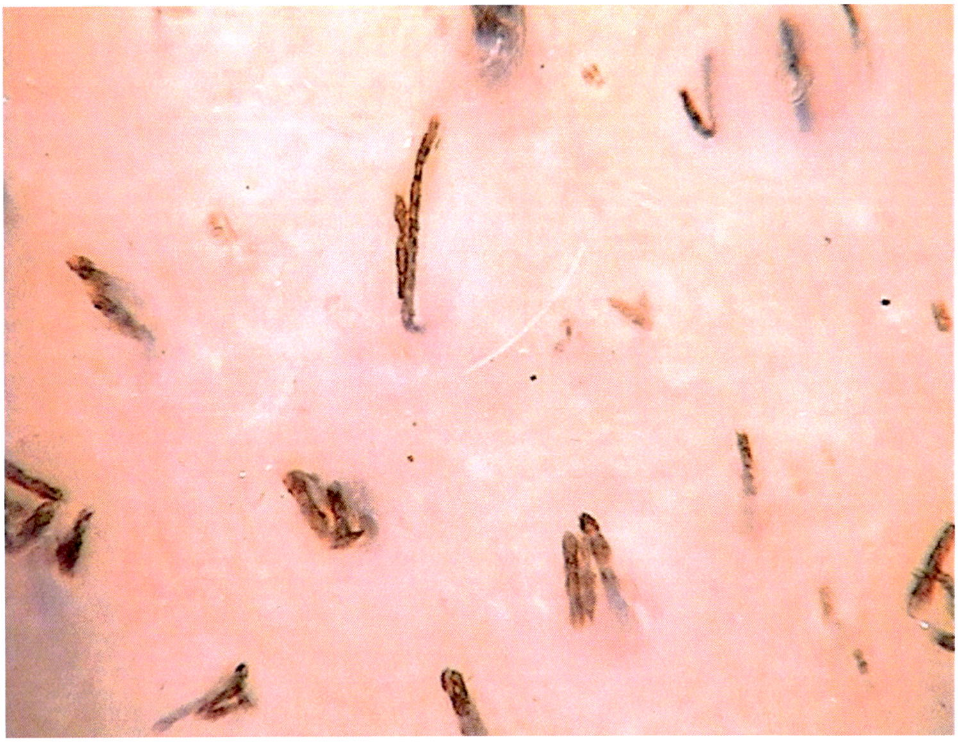

Fig. 8.6 Monilethrix-like congenital hypotrichosis caused by a mutation in the desmoglein 4 gene. Constrictions are regularly distributed but are shallow and very close to each other, barely visible in thick hair shafts. Hairs are very short and fracture easily, which causes clinically more severe hair loss compared with monilethrix caused by mutations in hair keratin genes (×70)

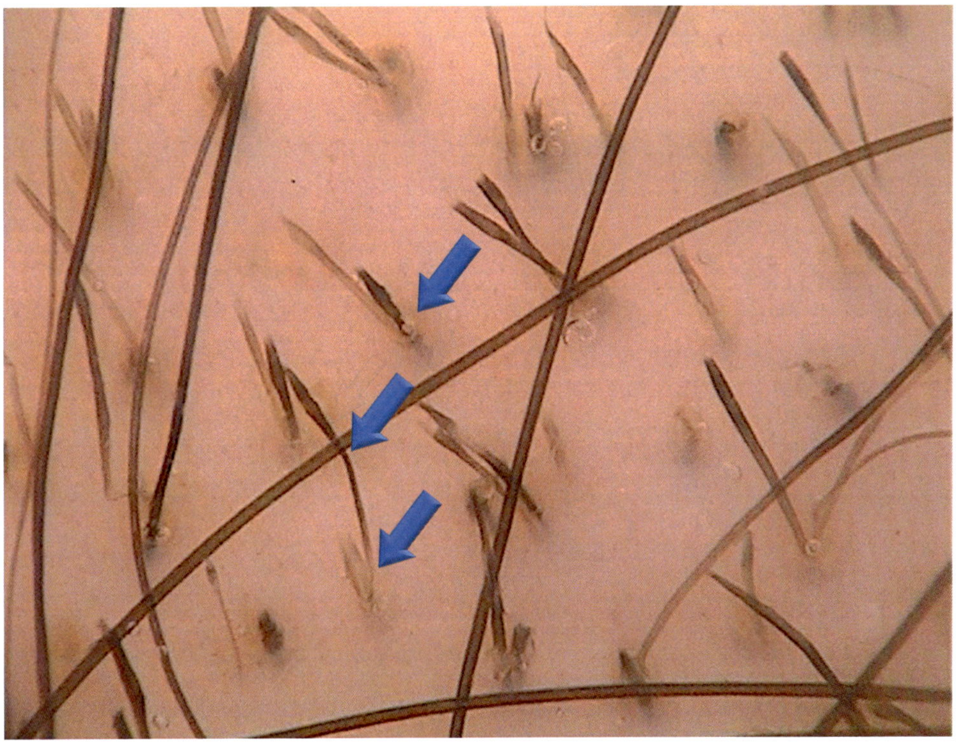

Fig. 8.7 Monilethrix-like phenomenon in alopecia areata. Monilethrix-like hairs may be observed in diseases with a variable course, such as alopecia areata. The growing hair shaft becomes thinner (*arrows*) during high disease activity and thicker during remission. This effect creates hair shafts with variable thickness resembling monilethrix, but with an uneven length of nodosities and irregular intervals between constrictions. In this patient alopecia areata coexisted with trichotillomania (×70)

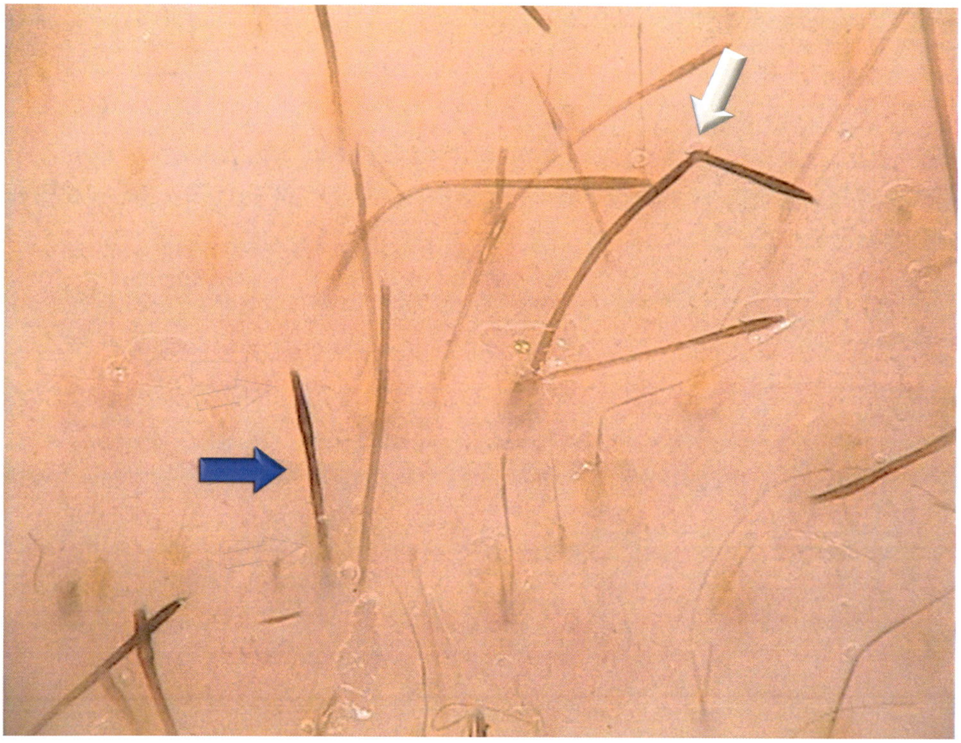

Fig. 8.8 **Monilethrix-like phenomenon in alopecia areata**. Trichoscopy shows an uneven length of intervals between constrictions (*blue arrow*). Hairs bend (*white arrow*) and break at constriction sites. Additional features of alopecia areata are visible: yellow dots, black dots, and exclamation mark hairs (×70)

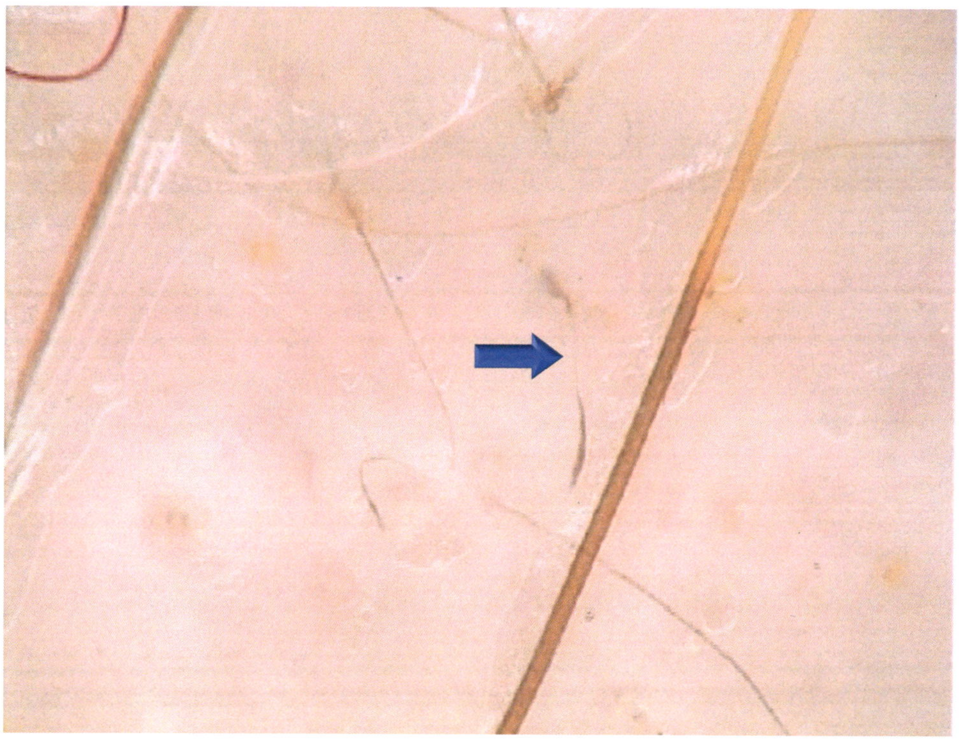

Fig. 8.9 **Monilethrix-like phenomenon in chemotherapy-induced alopecia**. High doses of chemotherapy cause an arrest in mitotic activity of hair follicle cells and a sharp hair shaft constriction (Pohl-Pinkus constriction), at which point the hair fractures. With lower doses, there may be only a segmental thinning or narrowing of the shaft (*arrow*) without fracture and a temporary arrest in growth. Another course of the drug reproduces these changes, creating a monilethrix-like appearance of the hair shaft. Similar monilethrix-like constrictions in the hair shaft may be induced by exposure to toxins (e.g., heavy metals, plant toxins) or x-rays [13, 14] (×70)

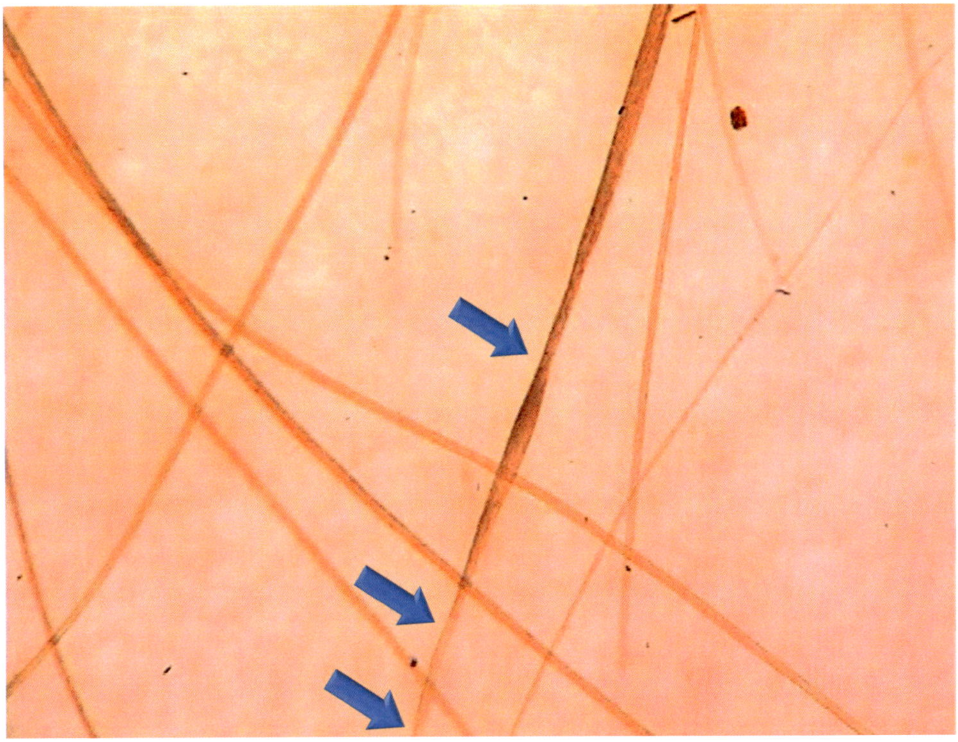

Fig. 8.10 Monilethrix-like hair shaft in lichen planopilaris. A hair shaft with irregular thinning or flattening may only theoretically fulfill the definition of pseudomonilethrix. Pseudomonilethrix was first described in 1973–1975 as a hair shaft abnormality affecting 1.9 % of the population in the Durban, South Africa area, including multiple members of five families. In these patients, scanning electron microscopy showed that "pseudomonilethrix nodes" were an optical illusion and that they were actually short square-shaped or rectangular indentations in the hair shaft (see Fig. 2.18 for details). Since then, no other familial case of true pseudomonilethrix has been reported, which makes us think pseudomonilethrix is a hair shaft abnormality confined to the South Africa area and that further investigation is worthwhile. Some authors from other regions indicated that pseudomonilethrix may be an optical artifact [11, 12]; others extended the definition of pseudomonilethrix to any type of irregular hair shaft constrictions [15]. Pseudomonilethrix (with rectangular indentations) must be distinguished from "monilethrix-like" hairs, which show the same type of ovoid constrictions (*arrows*) as in monilethrix, but with no regularity characteristic for true monilethrix. Monilethrix-like hair shafts may be observed in diseases with a variable course, such as alopecia areata and lichen planopilaris, or in patients undergoing chemotherapy. A monilethrix-like effect may be created in patients who use hair styling gels [8] or when ultrasound gel is used as an immersion fluid (see Fig. 7.7 for details) (×70)

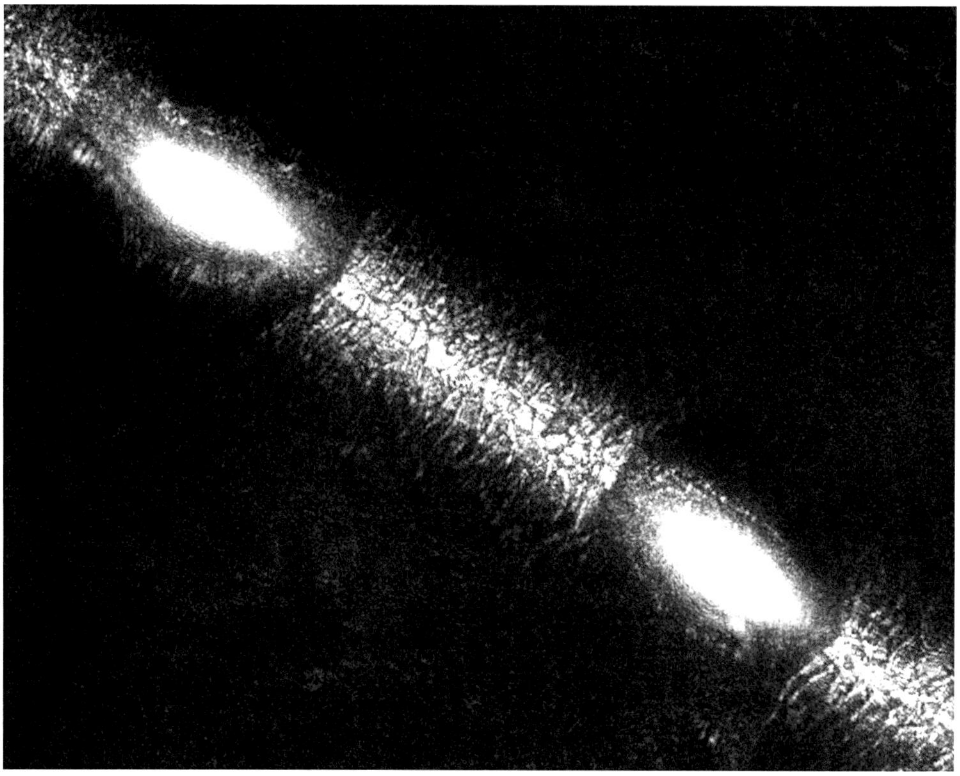

Fig. 8.11 Reflectance microscopic image of monilethrix. Reflectance confocal microscopy shows regular, uniform elliptical nodes and intermittent constrictions. In patients in whom monilethrix is suspected, reflectance confocal microscopy is easiest to perform on hairs preselected by trichoscopy

References

1. Neila Iglesias J, Rodriguez Pichardo A, Garcia Bravo B, Camacho Martinez F. Masquerading of trichotillomania in a family with monilethrix. Eur J Dermatol. 2011;21(1):133.
2. Djabali K, Panteleyev AA, Lalin T, Garzon MC, Longley BJ, Bickers DR, et al. Recurrent missense mutations in the hair keratin gene hHb6 in monilethrix. Clin Exp Dermatol. 2003;28(2):206–10.
3. Shimomura Y, Sakamoto F, Kariya N, Matsunaga K, Ito M. Mutations in the desmoglein 4 gene are associated with monilethrix-like congenital hypotrichosis. J Invest Dermatol. 2006;126(6):1281–5.
4. Farooq M, Ito M, Naito M, Shimomura Y. A case of monilethrix caused by novel compound heterozygous mutations in the desmoglein 4 (DSG4) gene. Br J Dermatol. 2011;165(2):425–31.
5. Zlotogorski A, Marek D, Horev L, Abu A, Ben-Amitai D, Gerad L, et al. An autosomal recessive form of monilethrix is caused by mutations in DSG4: clinical overlap with localized autosomal recessive hypotrichosis. J Invest Dermatol. 2006;126(6):1292–6.
6. Mirmirani P, Huang KP, Price VH. A practical, algorithmic approach to diagnosing hair shaft disorders. Int J Dermatol. 2011; 50(1):1–12.
7. Rakowska A, Slowinska M, Kowalska-Oledzka E, Rudnicka L. Trichoscopy in genetic hair shaft abnormalities. J Dermatol Case Rep. 2008;2(2):14–20.
8. Rakowska A, Slowinska M, Czuwara J, Olszewska M, Rudnicka L. Dermoscopy as a tool for rapid diagnosis of monilethrix. J Drugs Dermatol. 2007;6(2):222–4.
9. Wallace MP, de Berker DA. Hair diagnoses and signs: the use of dermatoscopy. Clin Exp Dermatol. 2010;35(1):41–6.
10. Jain N, Khopkar U. Monilethrix in pattern distribution in siblings: diagnosis by trichoscopy. Int J Trichol. 2010;2(1):56–9.
11. Zitelli JA. Pseudomonilethrix. An artifact. Arch Dermatol. 1986; 122(6):688–90.
12. Itin PH, Schiller P, Mathys D, Guggenheim R. Cosmetically induced hair beads. J Am Acad Dermatol. 1997;36(2 Pt 1):260–1.
13. Trueb RM. Chemotherapy-induced alopecia. Curr Opin Support Palliat Care. 2010;4(4):281–4.
14. Yeager CE, Olsen EA. Treatment of chemotherapy-induced alopecia. Dermatol Ther. 2011;24(4):432–42.
15. Blume-Peytavi U, Fohles J, Schulz R, Wortmann G, Gollnick H, Orfanos CE. Hypotrichosis, hair structure defects, hypercysteine hair and glucosuria: a new genetic syndrome? Br J Dermatol. 1996;134(2):319–24.

Trichorrhexis Invaginata and Netherton's Syndrome

9

Adriana Rakowska, Malgorzata Olszewska, and Lidia Rudnicka

Abstract

Trichorrhexis invaginata (bamboo hair) is an abnormality of the hair in which the hair shaft telescopes into itself (invaginates) at several points along the shaft. On a handheld dermoscope, trichorrhexis invaginata appears as multiple small nodules spaced along the shaft. High magnifications produced by a videodermoscope show invagination of the distal portion of the hair shaft into its proximal portion, forming a "ball-in-cup" appearance. When the hair shaft ruptures at the site of this abnormality, the distal end of the remaining hair shaft shows a "golf tee-like" invagination. Trichorrhexis invaginata is pathognomonic of Netherton's syndrome.

Keywords

Ball-in-cup hairs • Bamboo hairs • Eyebrows • Golf tee hairs • Matchstick hairs • Netherton's syndrome • Nodules • Short hairs • Trichorrhexis invaginata • Trichorrhexis nodosa

Netherton's syndrome is a rare autosomal recessive disorder of cornification characterized clinically by the triad of ichthyosis (most commonly, ichthyosis linearis circumflexa), atopic diathesis, and trichorrhexis invaginata. The neonatal period is commonly complicated by congenital ichthyosiform erythroderma of variable expression [1, 2]. Ichthyosis linearis circumflexa, which consists of erythematous migratory polycyclic patches surrounded by serpiginous double-edged scales, is variable and episodic, evolving with recurrent acute attacks lasting a few weeks [3]. Other associated manifestations of Netherton's syndrome may include aminoaciduria, failure to thrive, mental and neurologic retardation, and immune abnormalities.

The disease is caused by loss-of-function mutations in the *SPINK5* gene, which encodes LEKTI (lymphoepithelial Kazal-type inhibitor), a serine protease inhibitor with antitrypsin activity. LEKTI is normally expressed in epithelial and lymphoid tissues and may play an important role in anti-inflammatory and antimicrobial effects [4, 5].

Patients with Netherton's syndrome have sparse hair, which is dry, short, spiky, and brittle. The diagnosis of Netherton's syndrome may be definitely established by identifying at least one hair shaft with trichorrhexis invaginata [3]. The term *trichorrhexis invaginata* is derived from the Greek *trichos*, meaning hair, and *rhexis*, meaning rupture and "invagination" of hair shafts within themselves at the keratinization zone [6].

Trichorrhexis invaginata, also called bamboo hair, is an abnormality of the hair in which the hair shaft telescopes in on itself (invaginates) at several points along the shaft. On low-magnification trichoscopy, this appears as multiple small nodules spaced along the shaft at irregular intervals. High-magnification trichoscopy shows an invagination of

A. Rakowska
Department of Dermatology, CSK MSW,
Warsaw, Poland

M. Olszewska
Department of Dermatology, Medical University of Warsaw,
Warsaw, Poland

L. Rudnicka (✉)
Faculty of Health Sciences, Medical University of Warsaw,
Poland

Department of Dermatology, CSK MSW,
Woloska 137, Warsaw 02-502, Poland
e-mail: lidia.rudnicka@euderm.eu

L. Rudnicka et al. (eds.), *Atlas of Trichoscopy*,
DOI 10.1007/978-1-4471-4486-1_9, © Springer-Verlag London 2012

the distal portion of the hair shaft into its proximal portion, forming a "ball-in-cup" appearance, which is considered pathognomonic of Netherton's syndrome. Occasionally, one may see ragged, cupped proximal hair ends in which the distal end has fractured. This abnormality is often referred to as "golf tee hairs" [7–9]. Recently, "matchstick" hairs were described in a patient with Netherton's syndrome [10]. These hairs are visible on a handheld dermoscope as short hair shafts with a bulging tip and are equivalent to golf tee hairs visible at higher magnifications.

Several authors have indicated that trichorrhexis invaginata (bamboo hairs) and golf tee hairs are easiest to find on trichoscopy of the eyebrow area [8, 10, 11], because the number of lesions per millimeter of hair shaft is 10 times higher in the eyebrow area than the scalp in patients with Netherton's syndrome [12]. Eyelashes also may exhibit trichoscopic features of trichorrhexis invaginata [13].

Other hair anomalies, such as pili torti, trichorrhexis nodosa, and helical hairs, may be found in patients with Netherton's syndrome but are not specific to the disease [2].

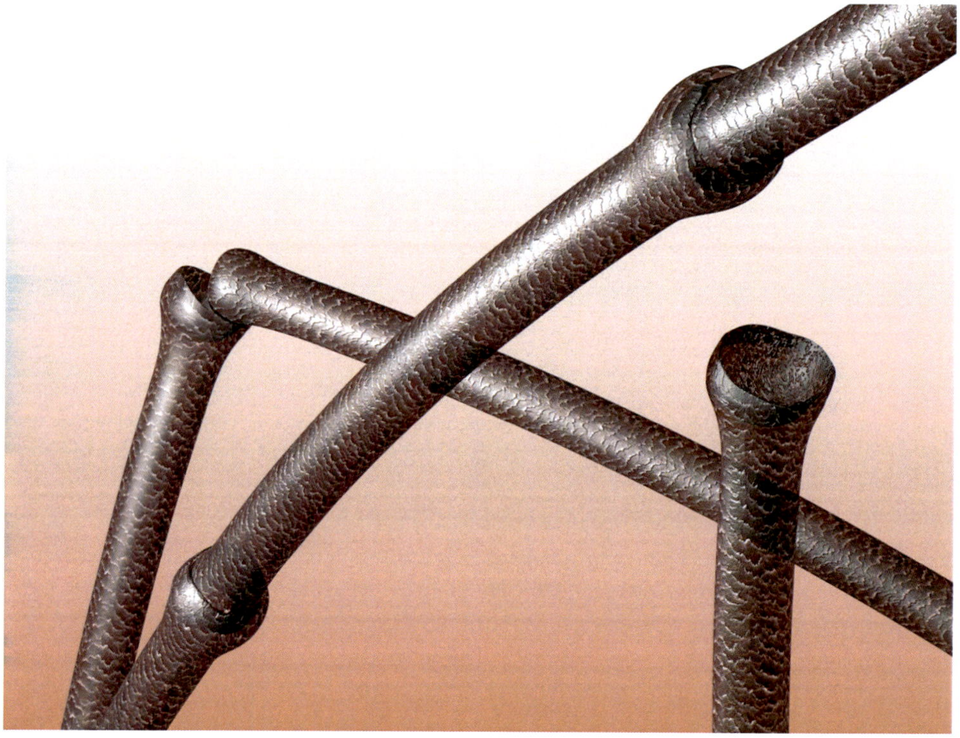

Fig. 9.1 Trichorrhexis invaginata. Trichorrhexis invaginata (bamboo hair) is an abnormality of the hair in which the hair shaft telescopes into itself (invaginates) at several points along the shaft. This is a pathognomonic sign of Netherton's syndrome. When the hair fractures, the proximal end of the hair shaft will appear cupped (invaginated). These hair fractures are also called golf tee hairs [7–9] because they resemble cupped tees, stands used to support golf balls

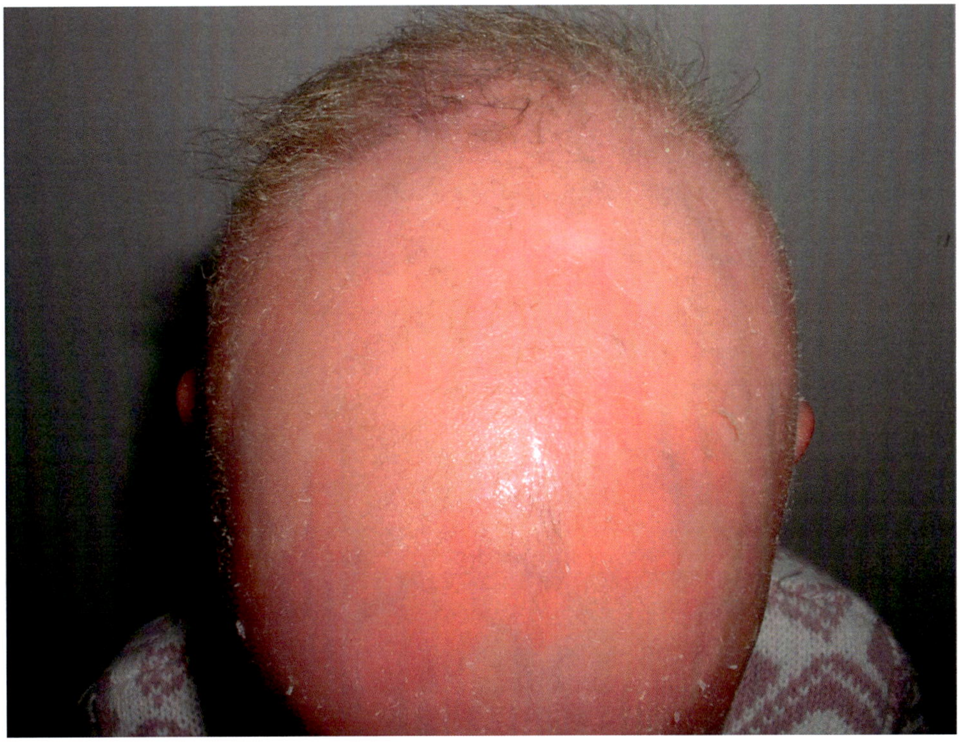

Fig. 9.2 Hair loss in a patient with Netherton's syndrome. Netherton's syndrome is characterized clinically by the triad of ichthyosis (most commonly, ichthyosis linearis circumflexa), atopic diathesis, and trichorrhexis invaginata [1, 2]. Clinically, in trichorrhexis invaginata, hair is sparse, dull, and brittle and has a tendency to fracture easily

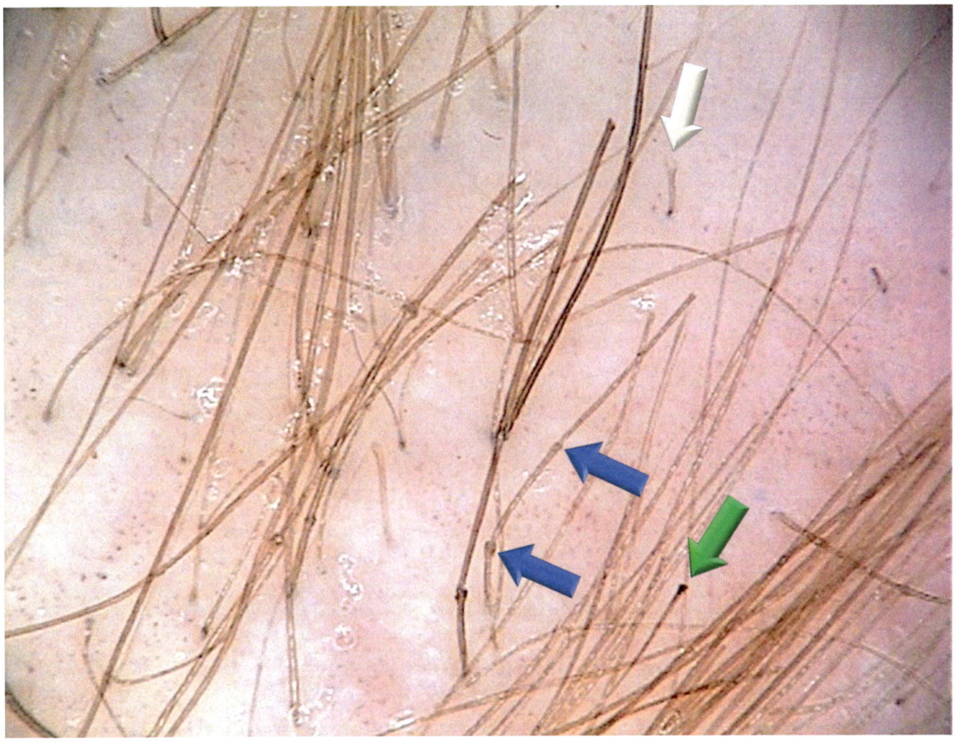

Fig. 9.3 Trichorrhexis invaginata. Invagination of the distal portion of the hair shaft into its proximal portion at several points along the shaft creates a bamboo-like hair appearance (*blue arrows*). Detection of only one bamboo hair is sufficient to establish the diagnosis of trichorrhexis invaginata. In this patient, about 20 % of the hairs are affected. Fractured bamboo hairs have an invaginated appearance at the distal end (*white arrow*). This type of hair is called golf tee hair. At low magnification, golf tee hairs may appear as light-colored hairs with a dark distal end (*green arrow*). These matchstick-like hairs appear very similar to the broken hairs in trichorrhexis nodosa and tulip hairs in alopecia areata (×20)

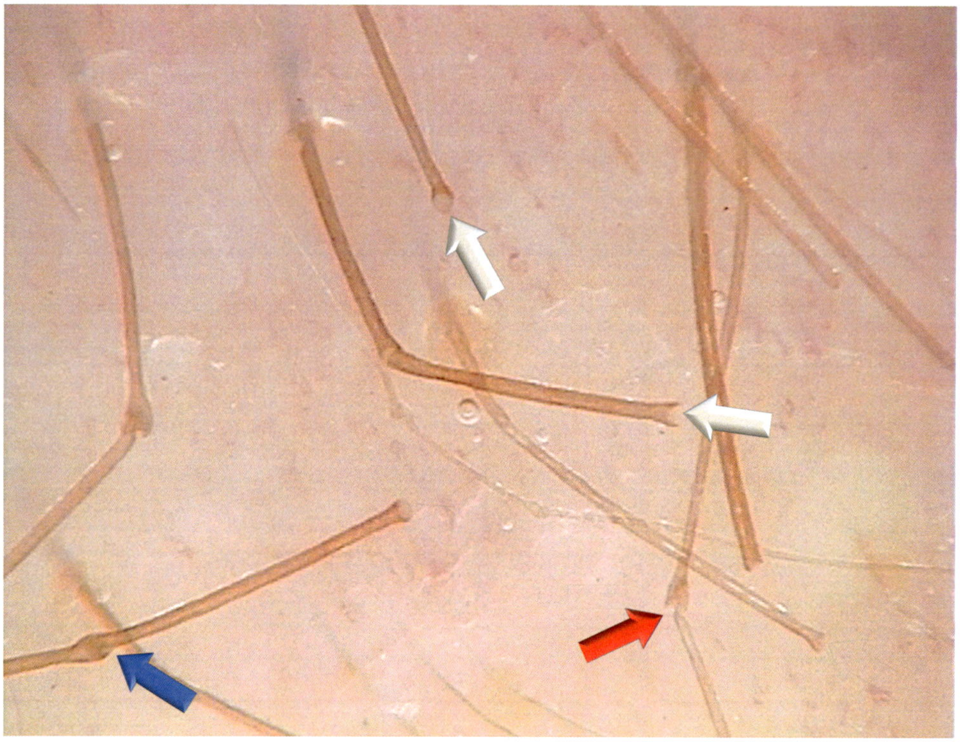

Fig. 9.4 Trichorrhexis invaginata. Multiple bamboo hairs with characteristic telescopic invaginations (*blue arrow*). At these sites, hair shafts fracture easily (*red arrow*), leaving cupped (invaginated) distal ends (*white arrows*). Note that hairs are very sparse, with only one hair emerging from one follicular unit (×70)

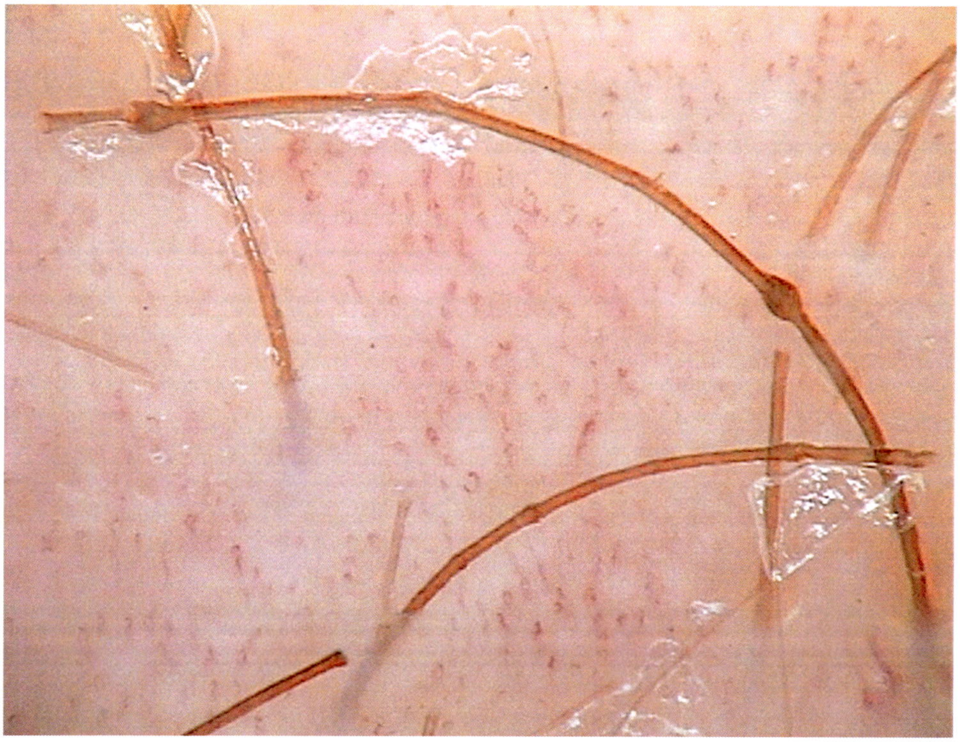

Fig. 9.5 Trichorrhexis invaginata. This image shows that the length and thickness of the abnormal parts of the hair shaft may differ significantly from one hair to another in the same patient. In the thicker hair in this image, the nodules is about 240 μm long and 160 μm wide. In the thinner hair, it is hardly visible at about 90 μm long and about 50 μm wide. The inner structure of the "nodules" shows characteristic telescopic invagination of the hair shaft. This feature is most visible in the thick hair shafts (×70)

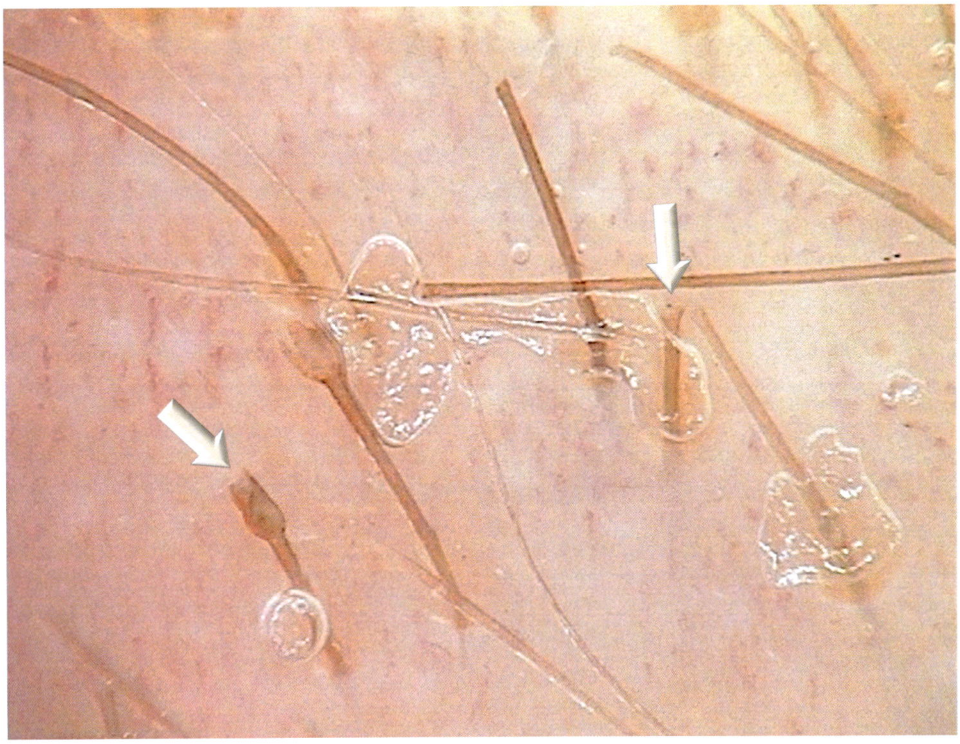

Fig. 9.6 Golf tee hairs in trichorrhexis invaginata. In this patient with trichorrhexis invaginata, only golf tee hairs are visible (*arrows*). They range from very deep to very shallow. The deep cupping in two hairs may indicate that the distal ends of the hairs were recently shed. Additionally, pressure from the dermoscope lens may flatten and optically increase the size of the hair shaft end. In other hair shafts, the distal, fractured end is ragged, creating a more characteristic shallow golf tee appearance. Multiple dilated blood vessels correspond to the inflammatory changes in the scalp skin (×70)

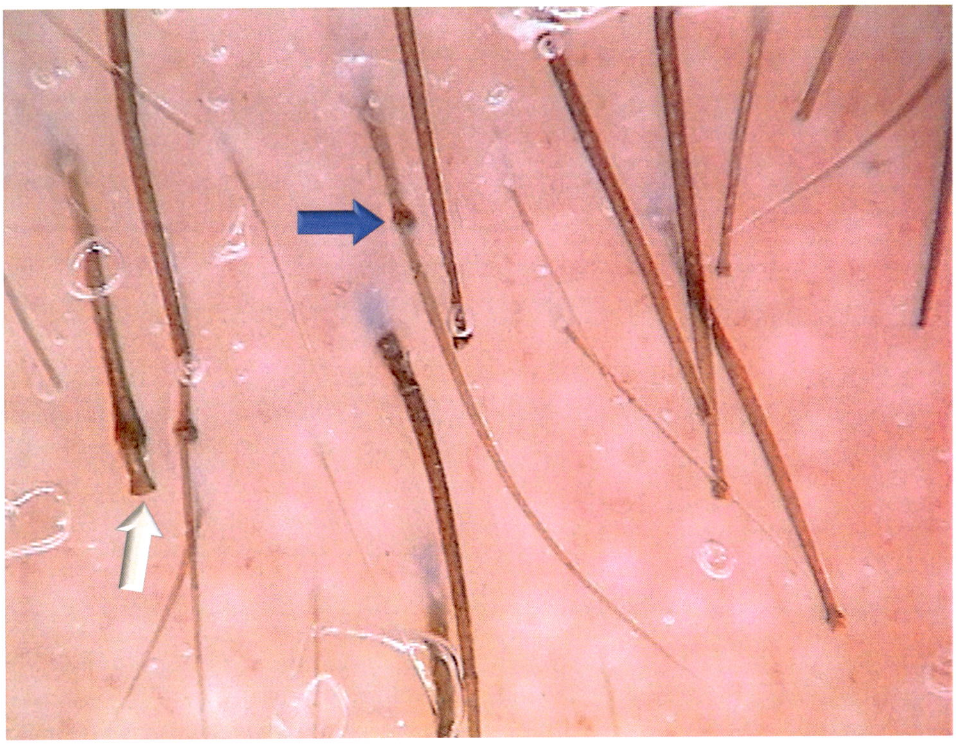

Fig. 9.7 Trichoscopy of eyebrows in trichorrhexis invaginata. Identification of at least one trichorrhexis invaginata hair is necessary to make the diagnosis of Netherton's syndrome. However, finding the abnormality may be difficult because the defect varies in time and location. Examination of the eyebrows may facilitate the diagnosis, because eyebrows are less commonly exposed to mechanical injury than is the scalp and there is a good chance of finding an intact invaginated trichorrhexis nodosa hair in this location. Eyebrow examination is especially important in patients with a total loss of scalp hairs in the course of trichorrhexis invaginata. Note several eyebrows with trichorrhexis invaginata (*blue arrow*) and fractured hairs (*white arrow*) with a cupped distal end (×70)

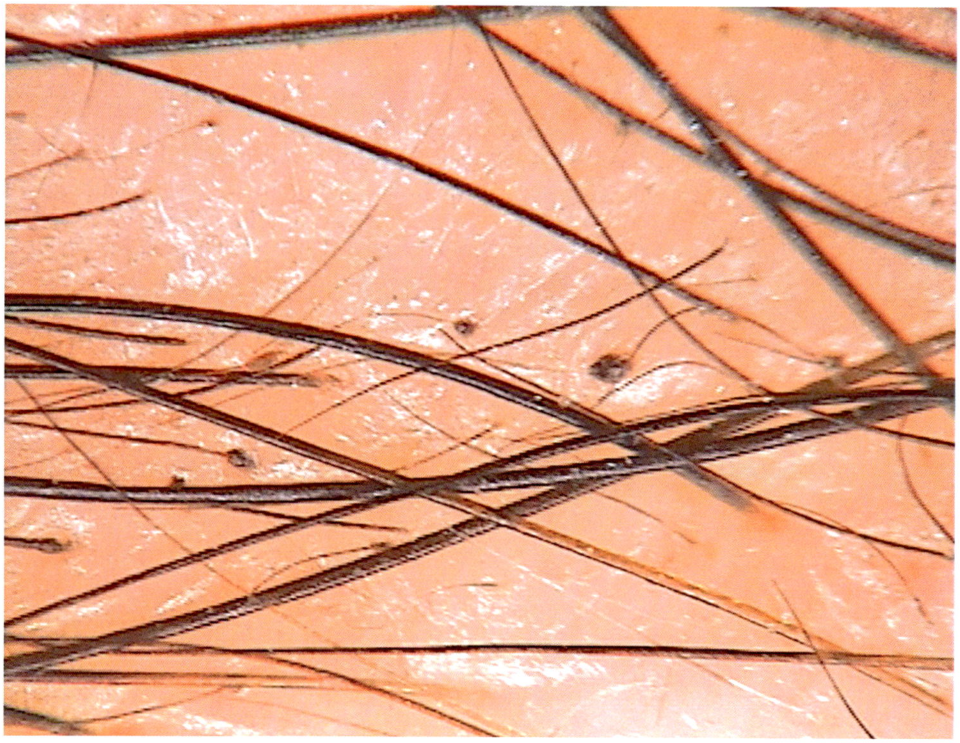

Fig. 9.8 Artifacts producing a trichorrhexis nodosa–like effect. In this patient, colorization of the eyebrows with henna produced an image of nodules along the hair shafts. These nodules differ from those of trichorrhexis invaginata by their location, predominantly at the base of the emerging hair, and by the lack of inner structure resulting from the telescopic invagination of the hair shaft. No broken eyebrows with cupped ends are visible (×70)

References

1. Mirmirani P, Huang KP, Price VH. A practical, algorithmic approach to diagnosing hair shaft disorders. Int J Dermatol. 2011;50(1):1–12.
2. Whiting DA, Dy LC. Office diagnosis of hair shaft defects. Semin Cutan Med Surg. 2006;25(1):24–34.
3. Boussofara L, Ghannouchi N, Ghariani N, Denguezli M, Belajouza C, Nouira R. Netherton's syndrome: the importance of eyebrow hair. Dermatol Online J. 2007;13(3):21.
4. Alpigiani MG, Salvati P, Schiaffino MC, Occella C, Castiglia D, Covaciu C, et al. A new SPINK5 mutation in a patient with Netherton syndrome: a case report. Pediatr Dermatol. 2012;29(4):521–2.
5. Fong K, Akdeniz S, Isi H, Taskesen M, McGrath JA, Lai-Cheong JE. New homozygous SPINK5 mutation, p.Gln333X, in a Turkish pedigree with Netherton syndrome. Clin Exp Dermatol. 2011;36(4):412–5.
6. Wilkinson RD, Curtis GH, Hawk WA. Netherton's disease; trichorrhexis invaginata (bamboo hair), congenital ichthyosiform erythroderma and the atopic diathesis. A histopathologic study. Arch Dermatol. 1964;89:46–54.
7. de Berker DA, Paige DG, Ferguson DJ, Dawber RP. Golf tee hairs in Netherton disease. Pediatr Dermatol. 1995;12(1):7–11.
8. Rakowska A, Kowalska-Oledzka E, Slowinska M, Rosinska D, Rudnicka L. Hair shaft videodermoscopy in Netherton syndrome. Pediatr Dermatol. 2009;26(3):320–2.
9. Burk C, Hu S, Lee C, Connelly EA. Netherton syndrome and trichorrhexis invaginata—a novel diagnostic approach. Pediatr Dermatol. 2008;25(2):287–8.
10. Goujon E, Beer F, Fraitag S, Hovnanian A, Vabres P. 'Matchstick' eyebrow hairs: a dermoscopic clue to the diagnosis of Netherton syndrome. J Eur Acad Dermatol Venereol. 2010;24(6):740–1.
11. Rakowska A, Slowinska M, Kowalska-Oledzka E, Rudnicka L. Trichoscopy in genetic hair shaft abnormalities. J Dermatol Case Rep. 2008;2(2):14–20.
12. Powell J. Increasing the likelihood of early diagnosis of Netherton syndrome by simple examination of eyebrow hairs. Arch Dermatol. 2000;136(3):423–4.
13. Neri I, Balestri R, Starace M, Bardazzi F, Patrizi A. Videodermoscopy of eyelashes in Netherton syndrome. J Eur Acad Dermatol Venereol. 2011;25(11):1360–1.

Trichorrhexis Nodosa

10

Lidia Rudnicka, Malgorzata Olszewska,
Adriana Rakowska, and Ana Maria Costa Pinheiro

Abstract

The trichoscopic appearance of trichorrhexis nodosa depends on the magnification and the presence of immersion fluid. At low magnifications, trichoscopy reveals nodular thickenings along hair shafts, and these thickenings appear lighter in the dark hair shafts. At these sites, the hairs bend with a rounded edge and eventually break, leaving a slightly thickened, rounded hair shaft end. At higher magnifications, trichoscopy reveals numerous small fibers, producing a picture that resembles two brooms or brushes aligned in opposition. To better visualize trichorrhexis nodosa, the hairs should be evaluated with dry trichoscopy.

Keywords

Dry trichoscopy • Ectodermal dysplasia • Hypothyroidism • Monilethrix • Physical trauma • Pruritus • Mental retardation • Trichoclasia • Trichoptilosis • Trichorrhexis nodosa • Zinc deficiency

Trichorrhexis nodosa is a condition in which a hair shaft splits longitudinally into many small fibers. This abnormality is restricted to a short area along the hair shaft. The outer fibers bulge outward, causing a segmental increase in hair diameter. Macroscopically, this may resemble nodules located along the hair shaft. Hairs eventually break at these points, leaving brush-like ends [1].

L. Rudnicka (✉)
Faculty of Health Sciences,
Medical University of Warsaw, Poland

Department of Dermatology, CSK MSW,
Woloska 137, Warsaw 02-502, Poland
e-mail: lidia.rudnicka@euderm.eu

M. Olszewska
Department of Dermatology,
Medical University of Warsaw, Warsaw, Poland

A. Rakowska
Department of Dermatology, CSK MSW, Warsaw, Poland

A.M.C. Pinheiro
Department of Internal Medicine,
Hospital Universitario de Brasilia, Brasilia, Brazil

The term *trichorrhexis nodosa* is derived from the Greek word *trichos*, meaning *hair*; the Latin *rhexis*, meaning *rupture*; and *nodosa* as *nodule*, and refers to easily breaking hair with nodular structures along the hairs. Trichorrhexis nodosa is observed most commonly in scalp hair but may affect hairs of the genitoinguinal area and other body hairs [2].

The condition rarely presents as an isolated, inherited abnormality. Trichorrhexis nodosa as a sole finding, not associated with other clinical symptoms, is observed in only 5.6 % of children with this condition [3].

Several inherited and acquired conditions are associated with an increased tendency to develop trichorrhexis nodosa (Table 10.1). This abnormality also may be induced by physical or chemical trauma and may be reproduced in vitro [2]. Trichorrhexis nodosa may be associated with severe pruritus in the affected areas and may resolve with control of the pruritus [2].

In patients with trichorrhexis nodosa, the hair appears clinically dry and brittle with a tendency to break at different lengths.

Trichoscopy may give slightly different images depending on magnification. At low magnifications, trichoscopy reveals nodular thickenings along the hair shafts, and these

L. Rudnicka et al. (eds.), *Atlas of Trichoscopy*,
DOI 10.1007/978-1-4471-4486-1_10, © Springer-Verlag London 2012

Table 10.1 Conditions associated with an increased tendency to develop trichorrhexis nodosa

Physical trauma [4, 5]
Chemical trauma [6]
Thermal trauma [7]
Scalp pruritus [2]
Mental retardation (e.g., Pollitt syndrome) [8]
Diarrhea (e.g., tricho-hepato-enteric syndrome) [9]
Argininosuccinic aciduria [10]
Kabuki syndrome [11]
Menkes disease [12]
Ectodermal dysplasias [13, 14]
Biotin deficiency [1]
Monilethrix-like congenital hypotrichosis [15]
Hypovitaminosis A[a] [16]
Seborrheic dermatitis [2]
Netherton's syndrome (as an additional, nonspecific finding) [1]
Mutation in the *XPD* gene [17]
Laron syndrome [18]
Congenital disorder of glycosylation[b] [19]
Zinc deficiency[b] [20, 21]
Hypotrichosis, hair structure defects, hypercysteine hair, and glucosuria (HHHG) syndrome[b] [22]
Bazex-Dupré-Christol syndrome[b] [23]
Hypothyroidism[a] [24]
Congenital trichorrhexis nodosa without coexisting defects [1]

[a]One case published, according to our literature search
[b]Three cases published, according to our literature search

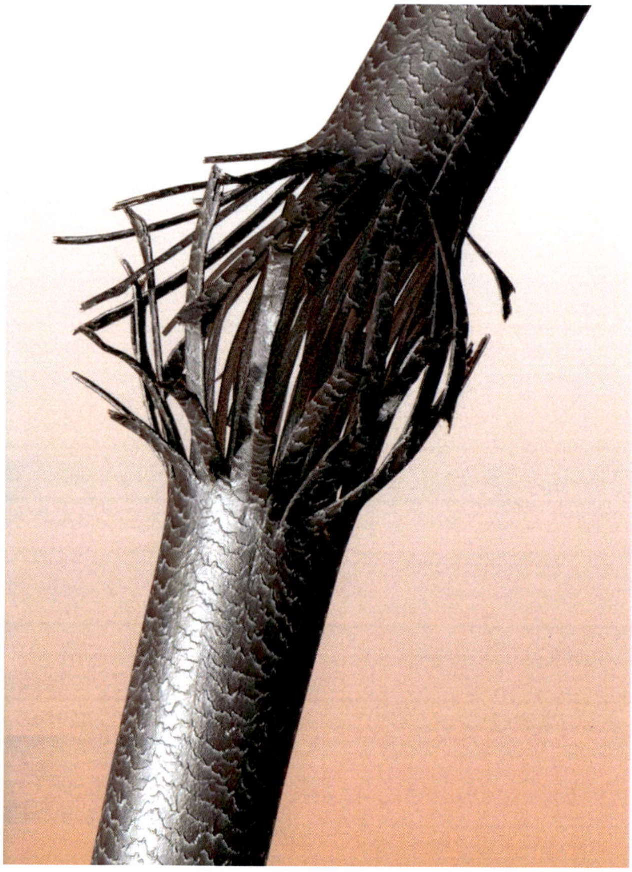

Fig. 10.1 **Trichorrhexis nodosa**. At random areas, the shaft splits longitudinally into numerous small fibers. The outer fibers bulge outward, resulting in a segmental increase in hair diameter. Macroscopically, this may resemble nodules located along the hair shaft. The fibers have a high tendency to break, producing an appearance suggesting two brushes aligned in opposition. Eventually, the hair shafts break at these sites, leaving shafts with brush-like ends (*Illustration by* Dr. Wawrzyniec Podrzucki.)

thickenings appear light in the darker hair shafts. The hair shaft is about 25 % thicker at the site of the "nodule" than at the adjacent part of the shaft. Trichoscopic results correspond to earlier light microscopy data, which show that the "nodes" differ in length—from 0.06 to 0.30 mm—and in width—from 0.04 to 0.13 mm [2]. At the level of these nodular thickenings, the hairs bend with a rounded edge. When a hair shaft breaks at the level of the nodule, it leaves a slightly thickened, rounded hair shaft end, which may appear darker than the light-colored hair shaft. On dry trichoscopy of dark hairs, these ends tend to appear lighter than the remaining hair shafts. At higher magnifications, trichoscopy reveals numerous small fibers, which produce a picture resembling two brooms or brushes aligned in opposition. Broken hairs leave brush-like ends with numerous small fibers at the distal end of the hair shaft.

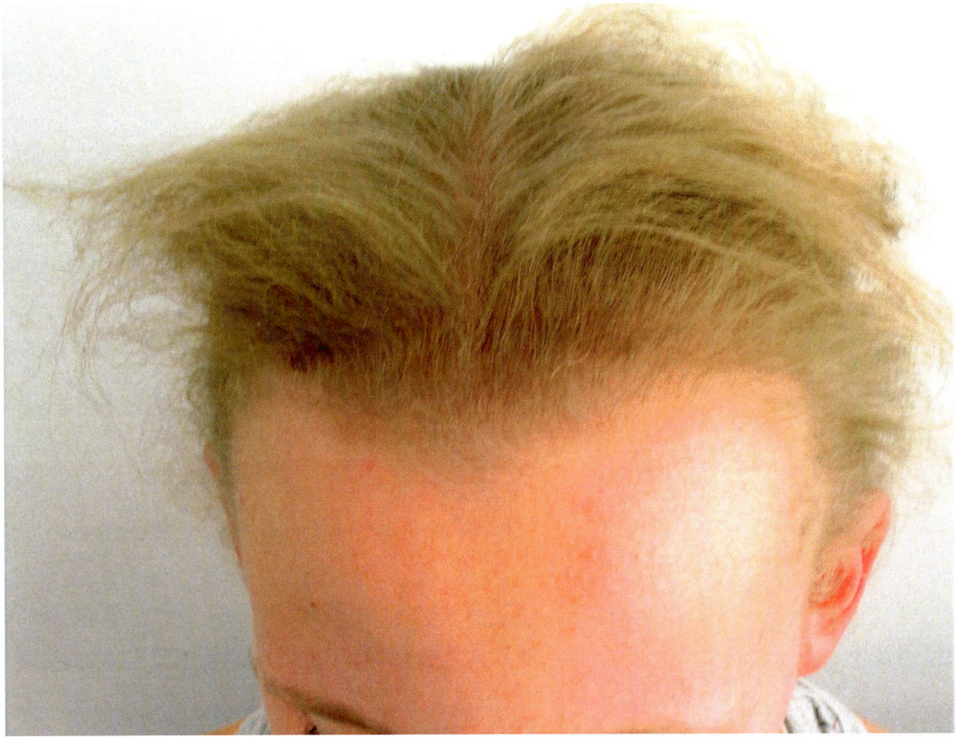

Fig. 10.2 Congenital trichorrhexis nodosa. Hairs are dry and brittle and break at different lengths. The clinical appearance depends on the number of hairs involved and the level of the fracture (distal or proximal). Occasionally the "nodes" may be visible macroscopically

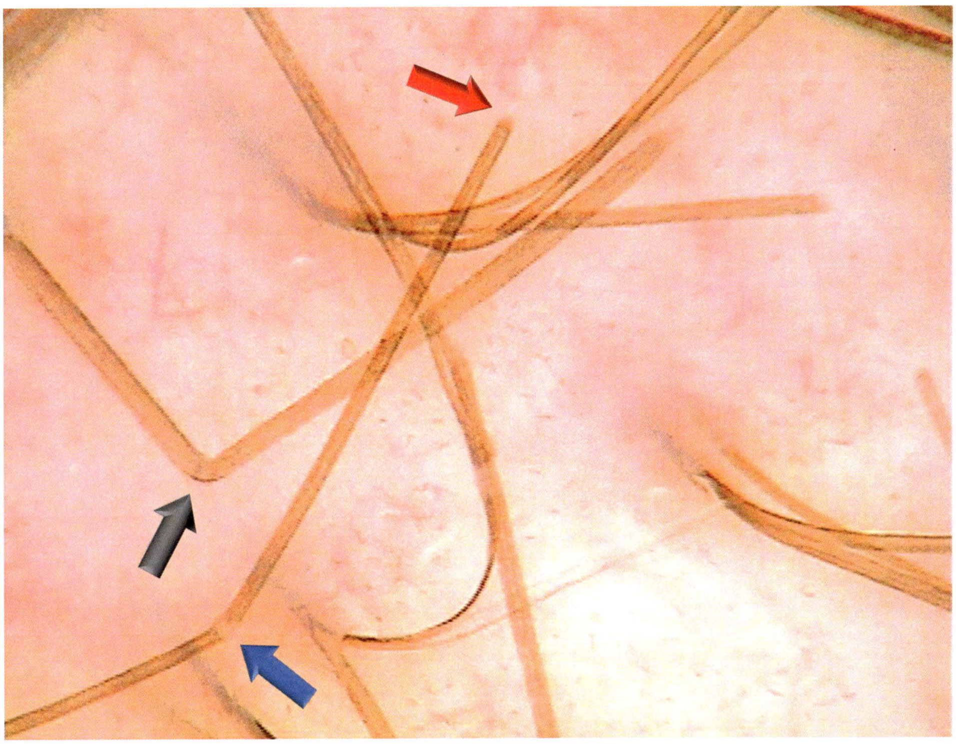

Fig. 10.3 Trichorrhexis nodosa. Trichoscopy shows nodular thickenings along the hair shafts, which appear lighter in the dark hair shafts. The hair shaft is about 25 % thicker at the site of the "nodule" (*blue arrow*) than at the adjacent part of the shaft. At the site of these nodular thickenings, the hairs bend with a rounded edge (*black arrow*) and eventually break, leaving distal hair shaft ends that appear rounded on trichoscopy (*red arrow*; ×70)

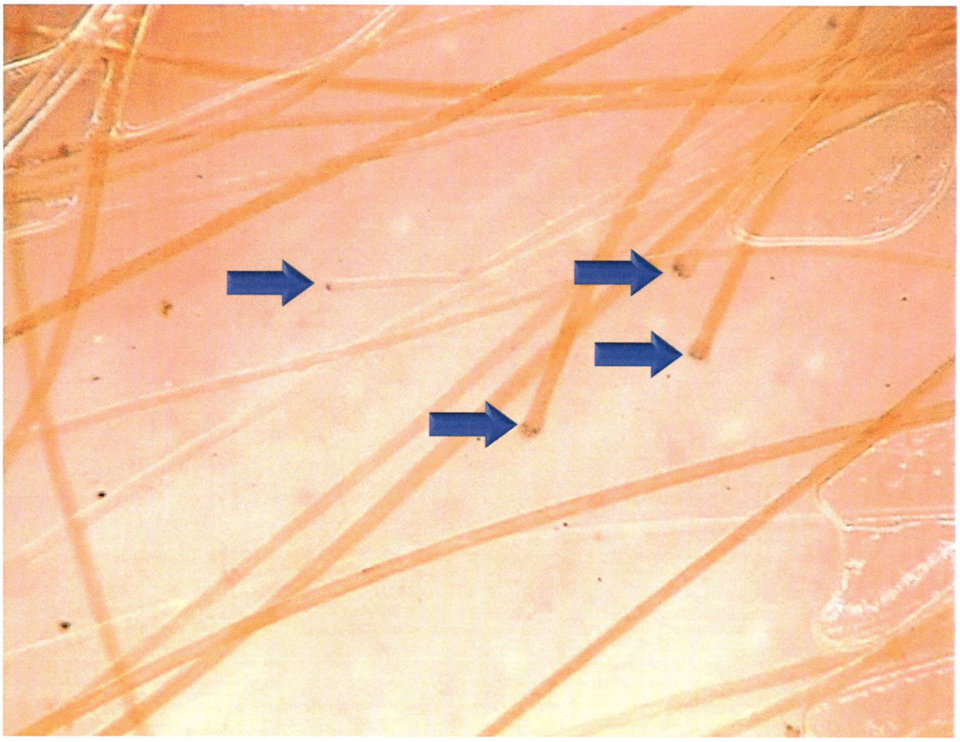

Fig. 10.4 Broken hair shafts in congenital trichorrhexis nodosa. The hair shafts have a tendency to break at the points of trichorrhexis nodosa, leaving rounded or brush-like ends (*arrows*). The color of the distal end of the broken hair is usually darker than the remaining portion of the hair shaft when evaluated on trichoscopy with immersion fluid (×70)

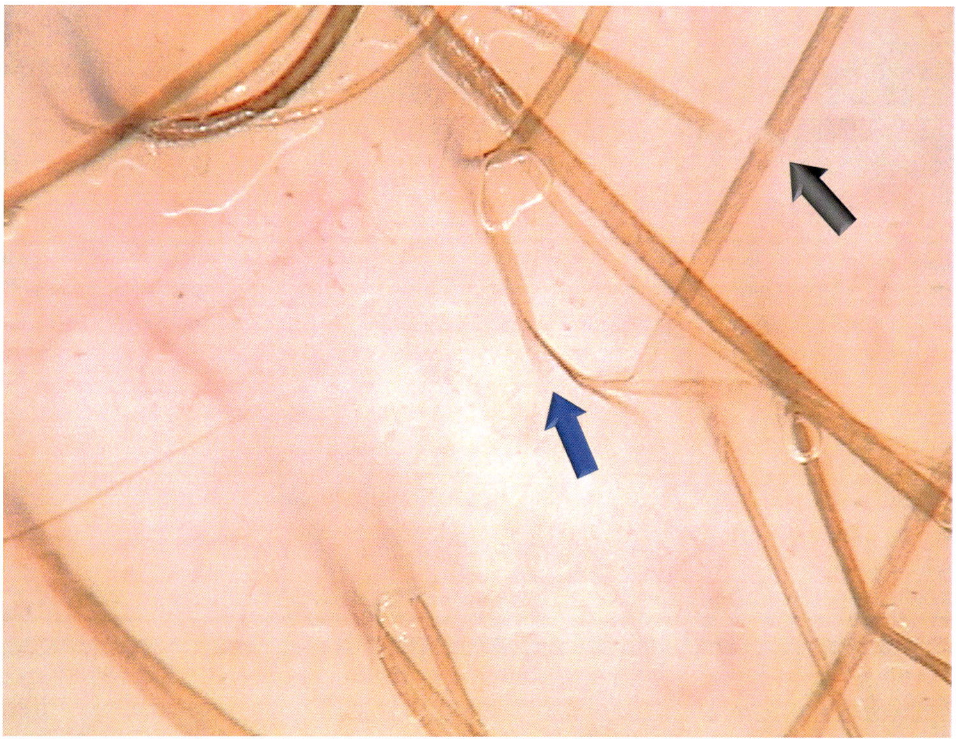

Fig. 10.5 Congenital trichorrhexis nodosa and trichoptilosis. Trichoptilosis is the longitudinal splitting of the hair shaft into two or more fibrils (*blue arrow*). This phenomenon differs from trichoclasia, which is a transverse fracture of the hair shaft at the midpart of the node from traction or bending. This trichoscopic image shows trichoptilosis in a patient with congenital trichorrhexis nodosa. A hair in the *upper right* part of the image (*black arrow*) shows a very light-colored trichorrhexis nodosa "nodule," which appears almost as a transverse gap in the shaft (×70)

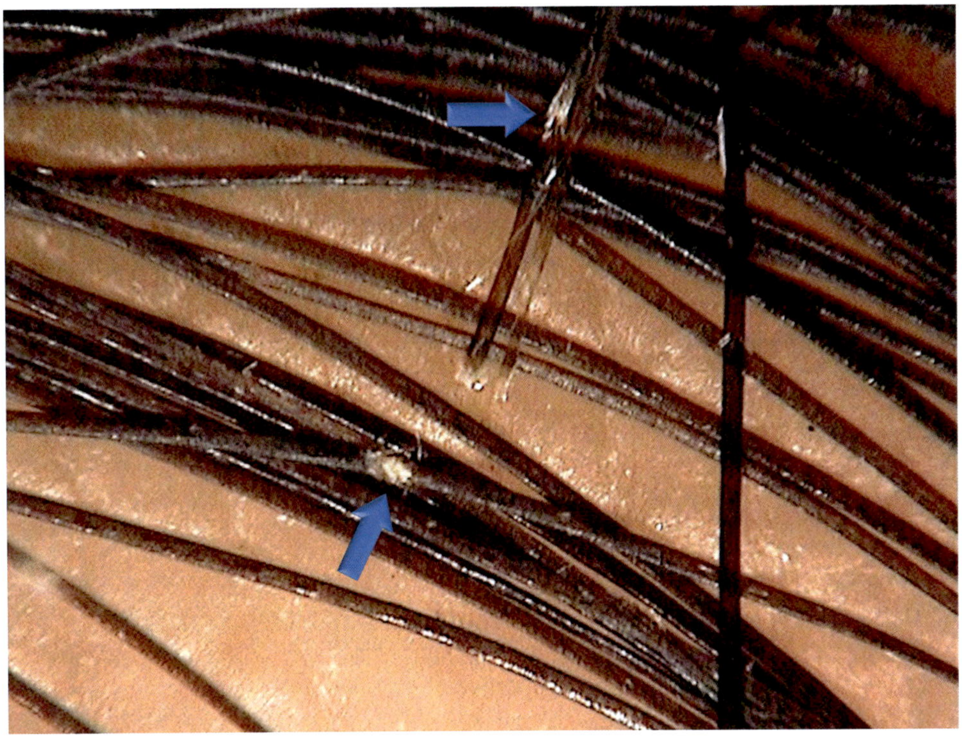

Fig. 10.6 Acquired trichorrhexis nodosa. In this Brazilian patient, trichorrhexis nodosa developed after a hairstyling procedure. The hair shaft abnormality appears on trichoscopy as whitish inclusions in dark brown hairs. The "nodes" in acquired trichorrhexis nodosa caused by physical trauma are significantly longer and more irregular compared with those in congenital trichorrhexis nodosa (×70)

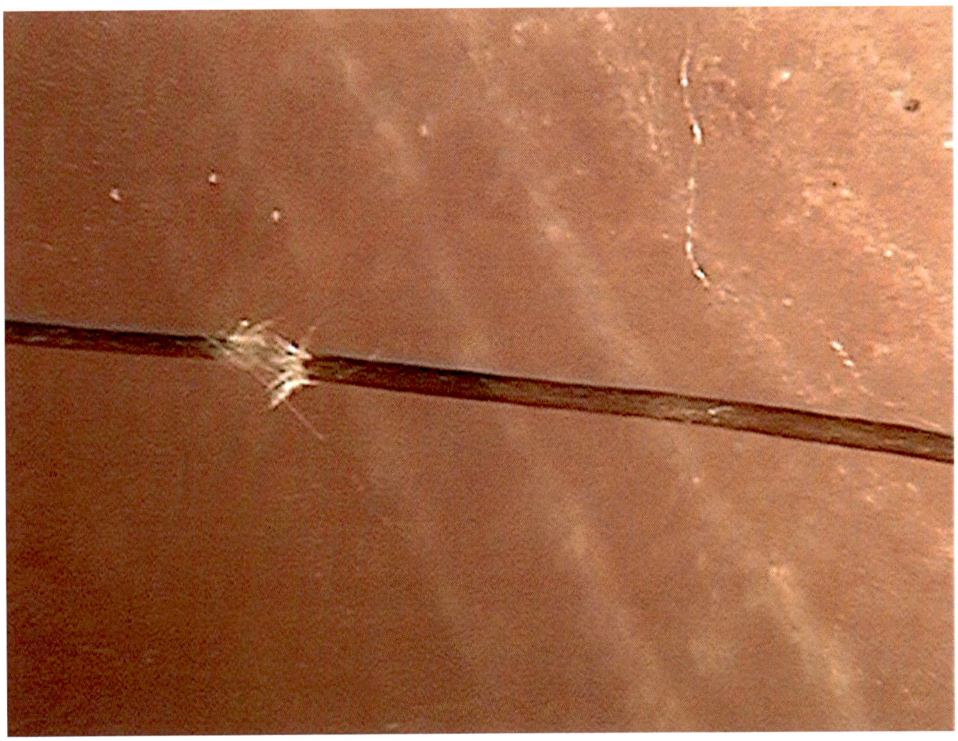

Fig. 10.7 Trichorrhexis nodosa. Trichoscopy shows a hair shaft split longitudinally into numerous small fibers, producing an appearance suggesting the ends of two brushes aligned in opposition. At this site, the hair shaft breaks transversely. Trichoscopy rarely shows this pathognomonic feature of trichorrhexis nodosa in such detail as seen in this 70-fold magnification. Under a handheld dermoscope, trichorrhexis nodosa appears as a white "nodule" or white irregular segment in the hair shaft. (×70)

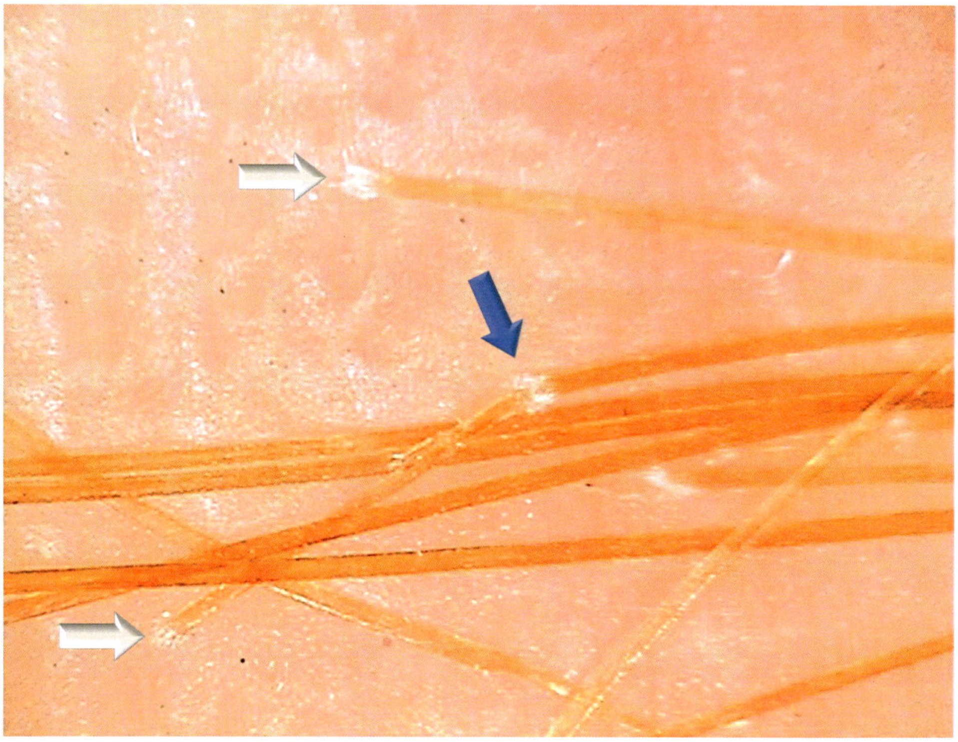

Fig. 10.8 Trichorrhexis nodosa in a child with ectodermal dysplasia. In this patient, hair shaft abnormalities coexisted with dental abnormalities, onychodysplasia, and dyshydrosis. The image shows a "nodule" (*blue arrow*) and the distal ends of broken hairs (*white arrows*). The image was obtained with dry trichoscopy to better visualize the fibers. Use of immersion fluid sometimes hinders the detection of trichorrhexis nodosa (×70)

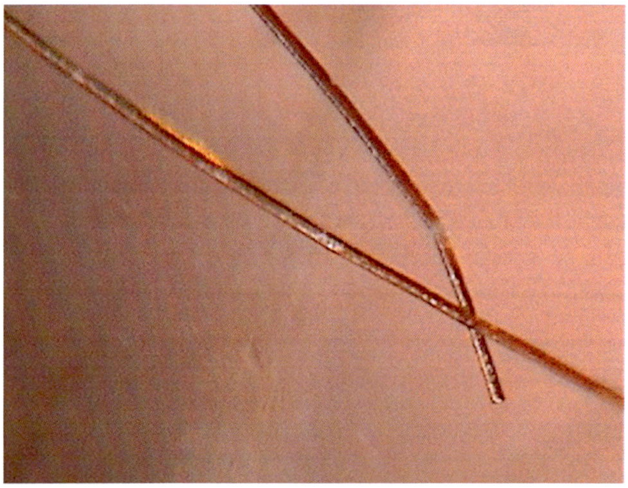

Fig. 10.9 Trichorrhexis nodosa "nodule" at the distal end of a hair shaft. Typically, in acquired trichorrhexis nodosa, the nodules are localized at the distal ends of the hair shafts. The best way for the examiner to find this abnormality is to hold a few or more hairs against his or her finger and to browse along the hair shafts. Acquired trichorrhexis nodosa is rare at the proximal end of the hair shafts and usually is not observed during regular inspection of the scalp with a dermoscope. Nodules at the proximal hair end are observed most commonly in congenital trichorrhexis nodosa (×70)

References

1. Bartels NG, Blume-Peytavi U. Hair loss in children. In: Blume-Peytavi U, Tosti A, Whiting D, Trüeb R, editors. Hair growth and disorders. Leipzig: Springer; 2008. p. 293–4.
2. Chernosky ME, Owens DW. Trichorrhexis nodosa. Clinical and investigative studies. Arch Dermatol. 1966;94(5):577–85.
3. Smith VV, Anderson G, Malone M, Sebire NJ. Light microscopic examination of scalp hair samples as an aid in the diagnosis of paediatric disorders: retrospective review of more than 300 cases from a single centre. J Clin Pathol. 2005;58(12):1294–8.
4. Martin AM, Sugathan P. Localised acquired trichorrhexis nodosa of the scalp hair induced by a specific comb and combing habit—a report of three cases. Int J Trichol. 2011;3(1):34–7.
5. Mirmirani P. Ceramic flat irons: improper use leading to acquired trichorrhexis nodosa. J Am Acad Dermatol. 2010;62(1):145–7.
6. Burkhart CG, Burkhart CN. Trichorrhexis nodosa revisited. Skinmed. 2007;6(2):57–8.
7. Callender VD, McMichael AJ, Cohen GF. Medical and surgical therapies for alopecias in black women. Dermatol Ther. 2004;17(2): 164–76.
8. Pollitt RJ, Jenner FA, Davies M. Sibs with mental and physical retardation and trichorrhexis nodosa with abnormal amino acid composition of the hair. Arch Dis Child. 1968;43(228):211–6.
9. Fabre A, Andre N, Breton A, Broue P, Badens C, Roquelaure B. Intractable diarrhea with "phenotypic anomalies" and tricho-hepato-enteric syndrome: two names for the same disorder. Am J Med Genet A. 2007;143(6):584–8.
10. Erez A, Nagamani SC, Lee B. Argininosuccinate lyase deficiency-argininosuccinic aciduria and beyond. Am J Med Genet C Semin Med Genet. 2011;157(1):45–53.
11. Abdel-Salam GM, Afifi HH, Eid MM, El-Badry TH, Kholoussi N. Ectodermal abnormalities in patients with Kabuki syndrome. Pediatr Dermatol. 2011;28(5):507–11.
12. Wang XH, Lu JL, Zhang LP, Zou LP, Wu HS, Wang X, et al. Clinical and laboratory features of the Menkes disease [in Chinese]. Zhonghua Er Ke Za Zhi. 2009;47(8):604–7.
13. Kelly SC, Ratajczak P, Keller M, Purcell SM, Griffin T, Richard G. A novel GJA 1 mutation in oculo-dento-digital dysplasia with curly hair and hyperkeratosis. Eur J Dermatol. 2006;16(3):241–5.
14. Rouse C, Siegfried E, Breer W, Nahass G. Hair and sweat glands in families with hypohidrotic ectodermal dysplasia: further characterization. Arch Dermatol. 2004;140(7):850–5.
15. Zlotogorski A, Marek D, Horev L, Abu A, Ben-Amitai D, Gerad L, et al. An autosomal recessive form of monilethrix is caused by mutations in DSG4: clinical overlap with localized autosomal recessive hypotrichosis. J Invest Dermatol. 2006;126(6):1292–6.
16. Colomb D, Cretin J, Vibert J, Steiner HG. Trichorrhexis nodosa in a hypothrepsic child with hypovitaminosis A [in French]. Lyon Med. 1970;223(5):337–8.
17. Botta E, Nardo T, Broughton BC, Marinoni S, Lehmann AR, Stefanini M. Analysis of mutations in the XPD gene in Italian patients with trichothiodystrophy: site of mutation correlates with repair deficiency, but gene dosage appears to determine clinical severity. Am J Hum Genet. 1998;63(4):1036–48.
18. Lurie R, Ben-Amitai D, Laron Z. Laron syndrome (primary growth hormone insensitivity): a unique model to explore the effect of insulin-like growth factor 1 deficiency on human hair. Dermatology. 2004;208(4):314–8.
19. Silengo M, Valenzise M, Pagliardini S, Spada M. Hair changes in congenital disorders of glycosylation (CDG type 1). Eur J Pediatr. 2003;162(2):114–5.
20. Traupe H, Happle R, Grobe H, Bertram HP. Polarization microscopy of hair in acrodermatitis enteropathica. Pediatr Dermatol. 1986;3(4):300–3.
21. Slonim AE, Sadick N, Pugliese M, Meyers-Seifer CH. Clinical response of alopecia, trichorrhexis nodosa, and dry, scaly skin to zinc supplementation. J Pediatr. 1992;121(6):890–5.
22. Blume-Peytavi U, Fohles J, Schulz R, Wortmann G, Gollnick H, Orfanos CE. Hypotrichosis, hair structure defects, hypercysteine hair and glucosuria: a new genetic syndrome? Br J Dermatol. 1996;134(2):319–24.
23. Colomb D, Ducros B, Boussuge N. Bazex, Dupre and Christol syndrome. Apropos of a case with prolymphocytic leukemia [in French]. Ann Dermatol Venereol. 1989;116(5):381–7.
24. Lurie R, Hodak E, Ginzburg A, David M. Trichorrhexis nodosa: a manifestation of hypothyroidism. Cutis. 1996;57(5):358–9.

Pili Torti

11

Malgorzata Olszewska and Adriana Rakowska

Abstract

In pili torti, sections of hair are flattened at irregular intervals and rotated 180° around their own axis. The condition may be either inherited or acquired. Trichoscopy of pili torti shows twists of hair shafts along their long axis. The abnormality is best evaluated with dry trichoscopy and at high magnification.

Keywords

Alopecia areata • Björnstad syndrome • Cicatricial alopecia • Ectodermal dysplasia • Hair transplantation • Lichen planopilaris • Menkes syndrome • Pili torti • Retinoids • Schöpf-Schulz-Passarge syndrome • Scleroderma • Trichothiodystrophy

Pili torti means "twisted hair" (Latin: *pili=hair, torti=twisted*) [1]. In pili torti, sections of a hair shaft are flattened at irregular intervals and then rotated 180° around its long axis [2]. Pili torti may be either inherited or acquired.

The condition affects mainly scalp hair, but eyebrows, eyelashes, and axillary hair may show features of pili torti. Hairs are brittle and dry, and break before they grow long [1]. The abnormality is probably caused by alterations in the inner root sheath. The genetic background of most inherited diseases associated with pili torti is unknown.

Pili torti was first described and named by Galewsky in 1932 and independently, by Ronchese, also in 1932 [1, 3]. Currently, two types of the inherited variant of the disease are distinguished: (1) the early-onset, classic type (Ronchese), and (2) the late-onset type (Beare).

In the classic (Ronchese) form, the abnormality is observed beginning in early childhood. The disease onset is between the third month and third year of life. It typically occurs in girls with blond hair. The foci of alopecia are located predominantly in the temporal and occipital areas, and are associated with increased friction in these areas. This type of pili torti may coexist with leukonychia, keratosis pilaris, dystrophic nails, ichthyosis, and dental abnormalities (in ectodermal syndromes). Inheritance is autosomal dominant or recessive.

The second, late-onset (Beare) type occurs after puberty and is more frequently associated with dark hair. Inheritance is autosomal dominant [1].

In 1965, Björnstad presented a group of patients with deafness and pili torti; since then, the term *Björnstad syndrome* has been used to describe the coexistence of pili torti and sensorineural hearing loss with autosomal recessive inheritance. The disease is associated with mutations in gene *BCS1L* [3–5].

Pili torti also may be associated with several other, rare inherited diseases and syndromes.

M. Olszewska (✉)
Department of Dermatology, Medical University of Warsaw, Koszykowa 82A, Warsaw 02-008, Poland
e-mail: malgorzata.olszewska@wum.edu.pl

A. Rakowska
Department of Dermatology, CSK MSW, Woloska 137, Warsaw 02-507, Poland

L. Rudnicka et al. (eds.), *Atlas of Trichoscopy*,
DOI 10.1007/978-1-4471-4486-1_11, © Springer-Verlag London 2012

Acquired forms of pili torti may result from repetitive trauma, oral retinoid treatment [6], hair follicle changes in cicatricial alopecia [7], and scleroderma. We observed one case of pili torti associated with alopecia areata in a child.

Light microscopy shows twists at irregular intervals along the shaft. Only some of the hairs in a sample and only part of the hair length are affected.

Table 11.1 Conditions associated with pili torti

Congenital
Pili torti
Ronchese type
Beare type
Autosomal recessive ichthyosis with hypotrichosis (ARIH)
Basex syndrome
Beare syndrome
Björnstad syndrome
Congenital disorder of glycosylation, type Ia
Crandall syndrome
Hypohidrotic ectodermal dysplasia
HOPP (hypotrichosis–osteolysis–periodontitis–palmoplantar keratoderma) syndrome
Menkes syndrome
Pseudomonilethrix
Rapp-Hodgkin syndrome
Trichodysplasia xeroderma
Trichothiodystrophy (photosensitive)
Schöpf-Schulz-Passarge syndrome
Acquired
Alopecia areata
Cicatricial alopecia
Hair transplantation
Repetitive trauma
Retinoid treatment
Scleroderma (systemic sclerosis)

Trichoscopy of pili torti shows twists of hair shafts along the long axis. Images taken at low magnifications may demonstrate hair shafts bending at different angles at irregular intervals. The abnormality is best observed on dry trichoscopy at high magnification [8].

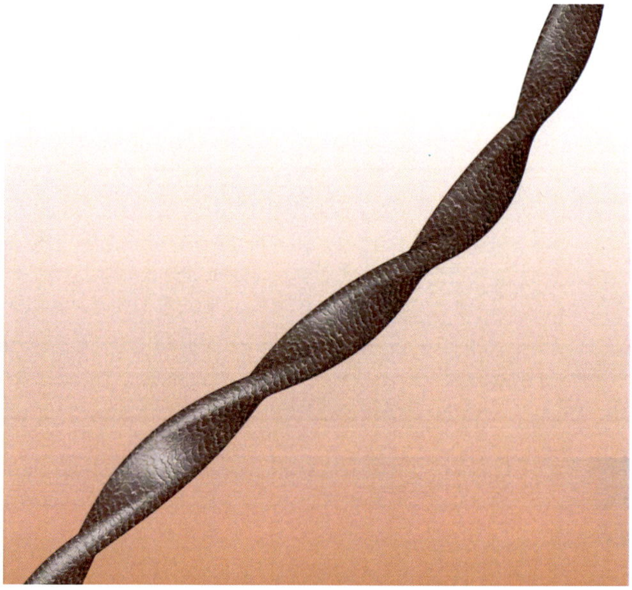

Fig. 11.1 **Pili torti**. In pili torti, sections of a hair shaft are flattened at irregular intervals and rotated 180° around its long axis [2]. This condition affects mainly the scalp hair, but eyebrows, eyelashes, and axillary hair also may show features of pili torti. Inherited and acquired forms exist

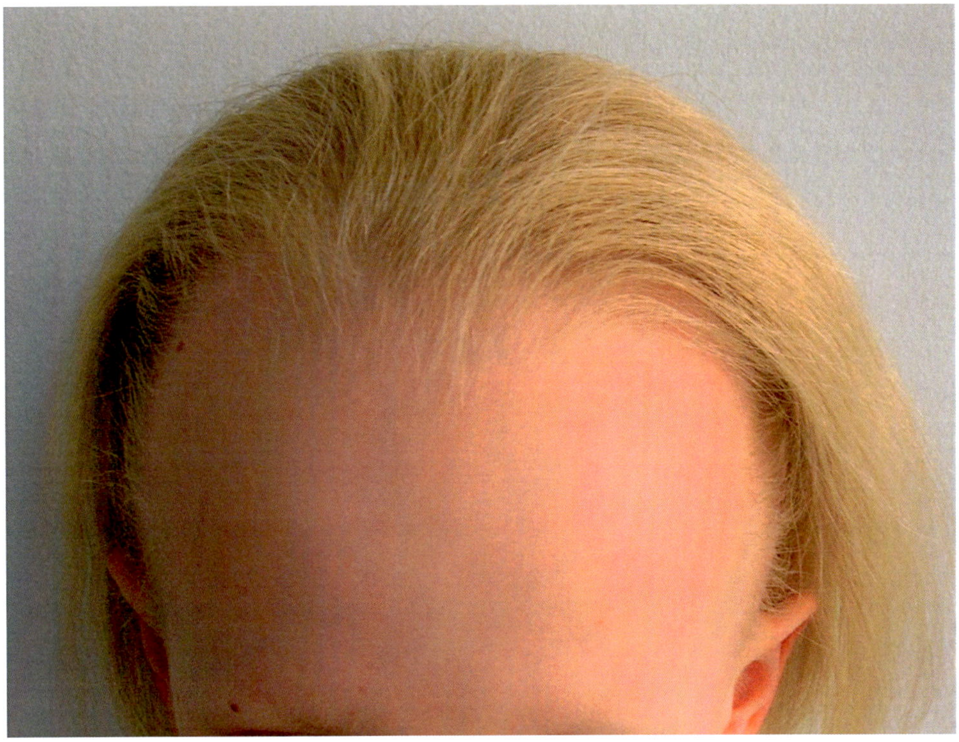

Fig. 11.2 Ronchese type of pili torti. The early-onset, Ronchese type of pili torti typically occurs in girls with blond hair. Hairs are sparse, coarse, dry, and fragile; break at different lengths; and never require cutting. In most cases, not all hairs are affected. Hairs with the abnormality are easiest to find in the temporal and occipital areas

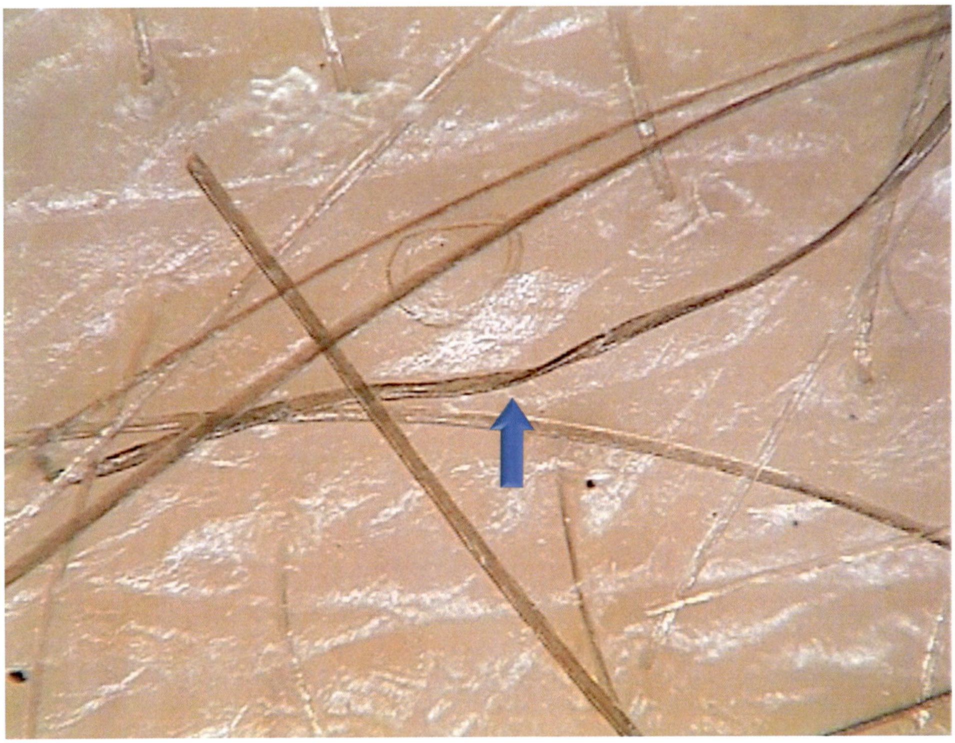

Fig. 11.3 Pili torti. Sections of the hair shaft are flattened at irregular intervals and rotated 180° (*arrow*). Usually, not all the hairs in a field of view are affected and only part of an affected hair shaft shows the abnormality [9, 10]. The twists are most visible on dry trichoscopy at high magnification (dry trichoscopy; ×70)

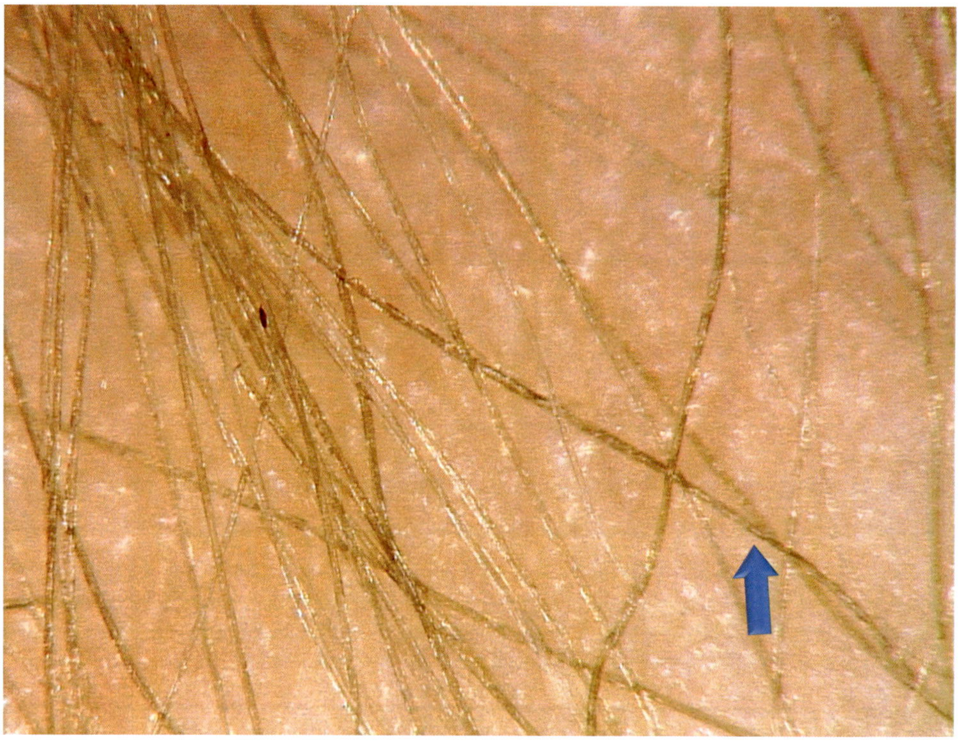

Fig. 11.4 Pili torti in a child with ectodermal dysplasia. In this child with thin, sparse hairs, pili torti (*arrow*) may be easy to miss. Other features of ectodermal dysplasia, such as the presence of hypopigmented hairs, may be observed in this image. The characteristic twists of pili torti also affect the hypopigmented hairs (×60)

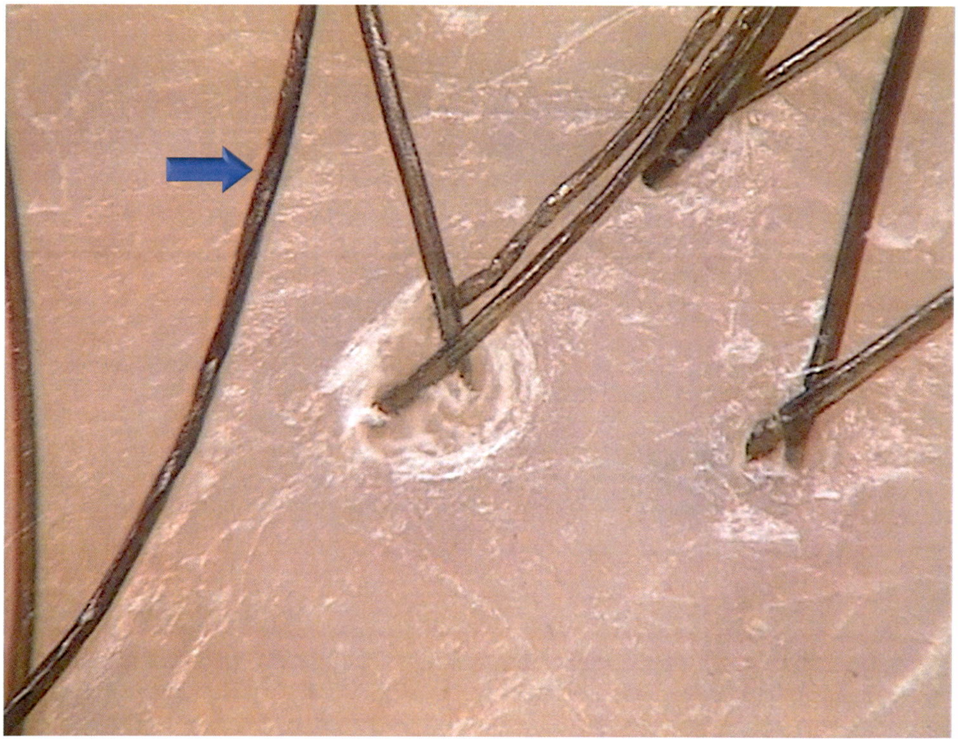

Fig. 11.5 Pili torti in cicatricial alopecia. In cicatricial alopecia, pili torti most probably results from hair follicle deformation during the process of perifollicular fibrosis. This image shows pili torti (*arrow*) in a patient with lichen planopilaris. Characteristic perifollicular scaling is visible (×70)

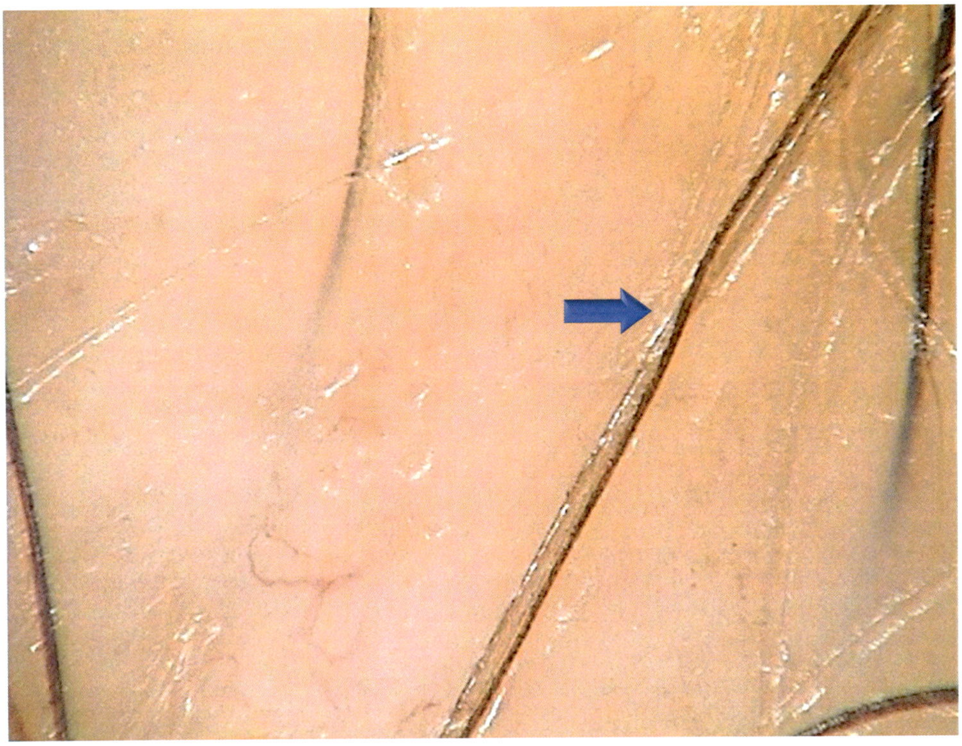

Fig. 11.6 Pili torti in scleroderma (systemic sclerosis). In systemic sclerosis, the mechanism leading to pili torti is most probably similar to cicatricial alopecia. The image shows pili torti (*arrow*) in a patient with longstanding systemic sclerosis. Typical elongated vessels are visible. In patients with systemic sclerosis of recent onset, trichoscopy does not reveal any abnormalities

References

1. Mirmirani P, Samimi SS, Mostow E. Pili torti: clinical findings, associated disorders, and new insights into mechanisms of hair twisting. Cutis. 2009;84(3):143–7.
2. Whiting DA, Dy LC. Office diagnosis of hair shaft defects. Semin Cutan Med Surg. 2006;25(1):24–34.
3. Selvaag E. Pili torti and sensorineural hearing loss. A follow-up of Bjornstad's original patients and a review of the literature. Eur J Dermatol. 2000;10(2):91–7.
4. Richards KA4, Mancini AJ. Three members of a family with pili torti and sensorineural hearing loss: the Bjornstad syndrome. J Am Acad Dermatol. 2002;46(2):301–3.
5. Hinson JT, Fantin VR, Schonberger J, Breivik N, Siem G, McDonough B, et al. Missense mutations in the BCS1L gene as a cause of the Bjornstad syndrome. N Engl J Med. 2007;356(8):809–19.
6. Hays SB, Camisa C. Acquired pili torti in two patients treated with synthetic retinoids. Cutis. 1985;35(5):466–8.
7. Sakamoto F, Ito M, Saito R. Ultrastructural study of acquired pili torti-like hair defects accompanying pseudopelade. J Dermatol. 2002;29(4):197–201.
8. Rakowska A, Slowinska M, Kowalska-Oledzka E, Rudnicka L. Trichoscopy in genetic hair shaft abnormalities. J Dermatol Case Rep. 2008;2(2):14–20.
9. de Berker D. Clinical relevance of hair microscopy in alopecia. Clin Exp Dermatol. 2002;27(5):366–72.
10. Rogers M. Hair shaft abnormalities: part I. Australas J Dermatol. 1995;36(4):179–84; quiz 85–6.

Pili Annulati

12

Adriana Rakowska and Malgorzata Olszewska

Abstract
Trichoscopy of pili annulati demonstrates hair shafts with alternating white and dark bands. The white bands are subtle, cloudy, and shorter than the remaining, dark portion of the hair shaft. About 20–80 % of hairs are affected, and the bands tend to disappear distally. Trichoscopic differential diagnosis includes fragmented medulla, inaccurate hair colorization, and pseudopili annulati.

Keywords
Bands • Hair colorization • Medulla • Pili annulati • Pseudopili annulati

Pili annulati is the Latin expression for *ring hair*. The term refers to an autosomal dominant disorder characterized by hair shafts with alternating white and dark bands [1]. A locus for pili annulati was mapped to chromosome 12q24.32–24.33 [2], but it remains unknown which gene is responsible for the disease. There is no consensus on the origin of the white bands. Most authors indicate that the bands are the result of air-filled gaps in the cortex [3, 4].

Pili annulati appears at birth or during infancy. The characteristic bands may be seen on clinical examination. The hair often appears shiny but is otherwise normal. The hairs are not excessively fragile; however, in some patients, increased sensitivity to weathering may occur in the light bands [5]. The abnormality usually is limited to scalp hair, but axillary, beard, and pubic hair also may be affected [1]. Pili annulati is more easily detected in blond hair, because the banding pattern tends to be masked by the additional pigment in dark hair [1]. Pili annulati is not associated with other hair or systemic abnormalities. Although cases of pili annulati associated with alopecia areata have been reported, they likely have been a coincidental concomitant manifestation rather than a true pathogenetic association [6].

Scanning and transmission electron microscopy may give the most accurate diagnosis of pili annulati; however, these methods rarely are used for diagnosing hair shaft abnormalities in clinical practice.

On light microscopy, hair shafts show alternating light and dark bands. Bands that appear white macroscopically and trichoscopically look dark on light microscopy, because light does not pass through the air-filled gaps in the cortex.

Trichoscopy demonstrates hair shafts with alternating white and dark bands in both dark and blond hairs [7]. About 20–80 % of hairs are affected in individuals with pili annulati, and the number of white bands is reduced distally [6, 8]. It is unclear why the bands tend to disappear as the hair grows. It may be because of a weathering process resulting in collapse of the cavities or because of damage to the cuticle, allowing immersion fluid to penetrate into the cavities.

On trichoscopy, pili annulati must be differentiated from a fragmented or intermittent medulla in healthy individuals.

A. Rakowska (✉)
Department of Dermatology, CSK MSW,
Woloska 137, Warsaw 02-507, Poland
e-mail: adrianarak@op.pl

M. Olszewska
Department of Dermatology, Medical University of Warsaw,
Koszykowa 82A, Warsaw 02-008, Poland

L. Rudnicka et al. (eds.), *Atlas of Trichoscopy*,
DOI 10.1007/978-1-4471-4486-1_12, © Springer-Verlag London 2012

An intermittent medulla is visible on trichoscopy as a longitudinal white structure covering less than 50 % of the hair shaft width. In pili annulati, which is an abnormality of the cortex, the light-colored bands cover 50–100 % of the hair shaft thickness.

Another differential diagnosis is pseudo–pili annulati [9], in which the banded clinical appearance of hairs is an optical effect resulting from the partial twisting of the hair shaft in an oscillating manner. In such cases, trichoscopy will show no white bands, only twisted hairs.

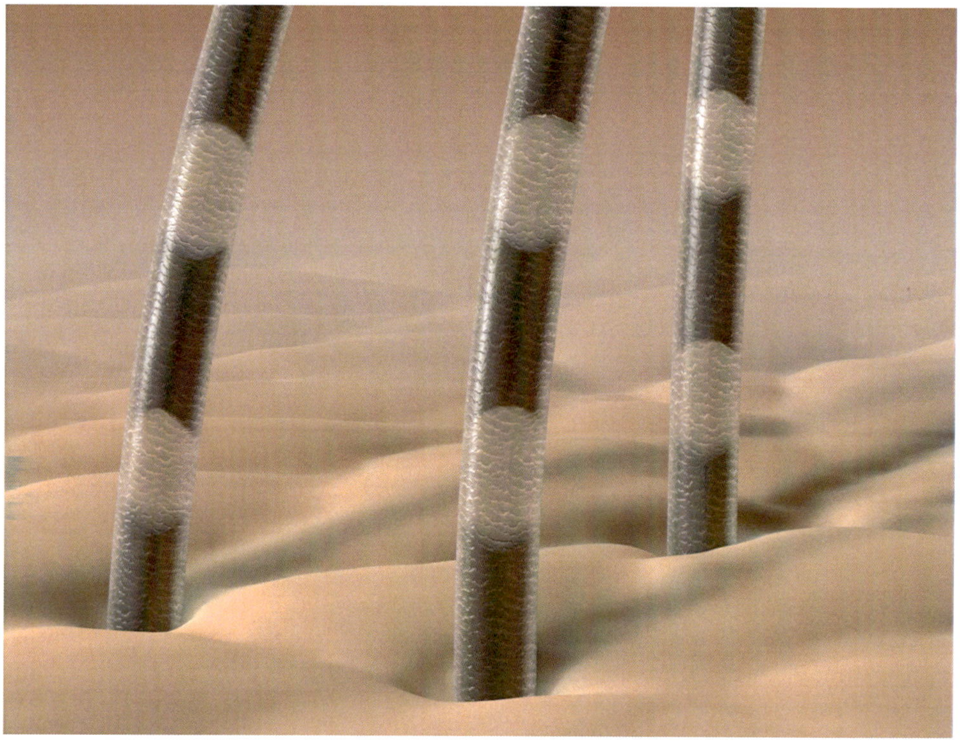

Fig. 12.1 Pili annulati. This disorder is characterized by alternating white and dark bands (rings) in the hair shafts that cover 50–100 % of the hair shaft thickness. Otherwise, the hair appears normal and may grow long. The hairs usually are not excessively fragile

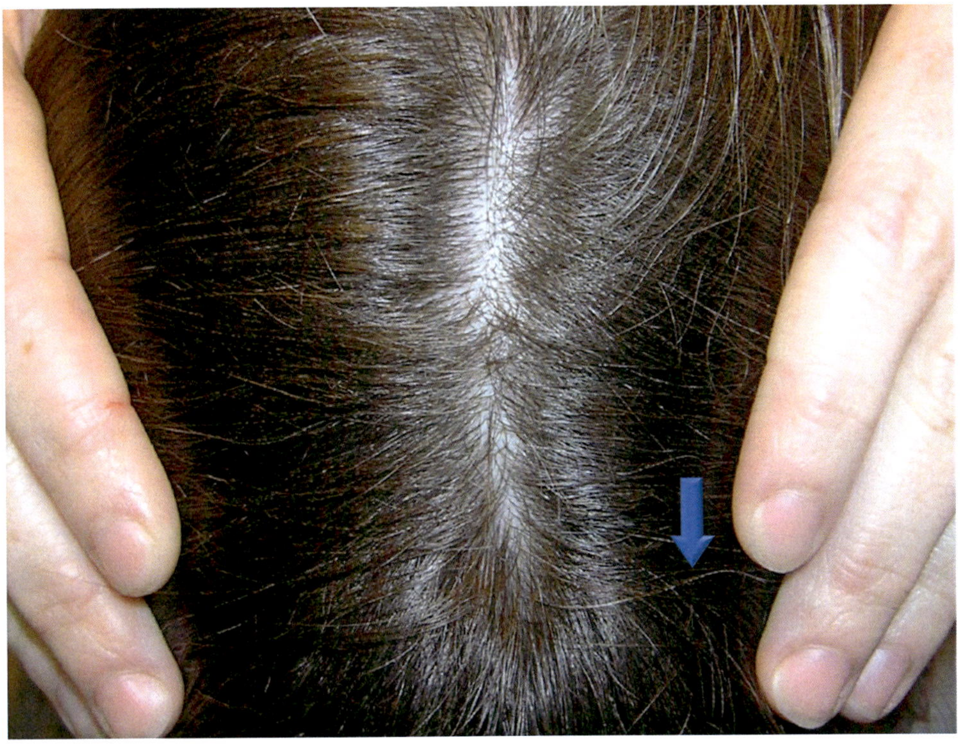

Fig. 12.2 Pili annulati. A clinical photograph of hair in an 18-year-old female patient with pili annulati. The characteristic alternating light and dark bands (*arrow*) are visible in most of the hair shafts. The hair is clinically normal otherwise

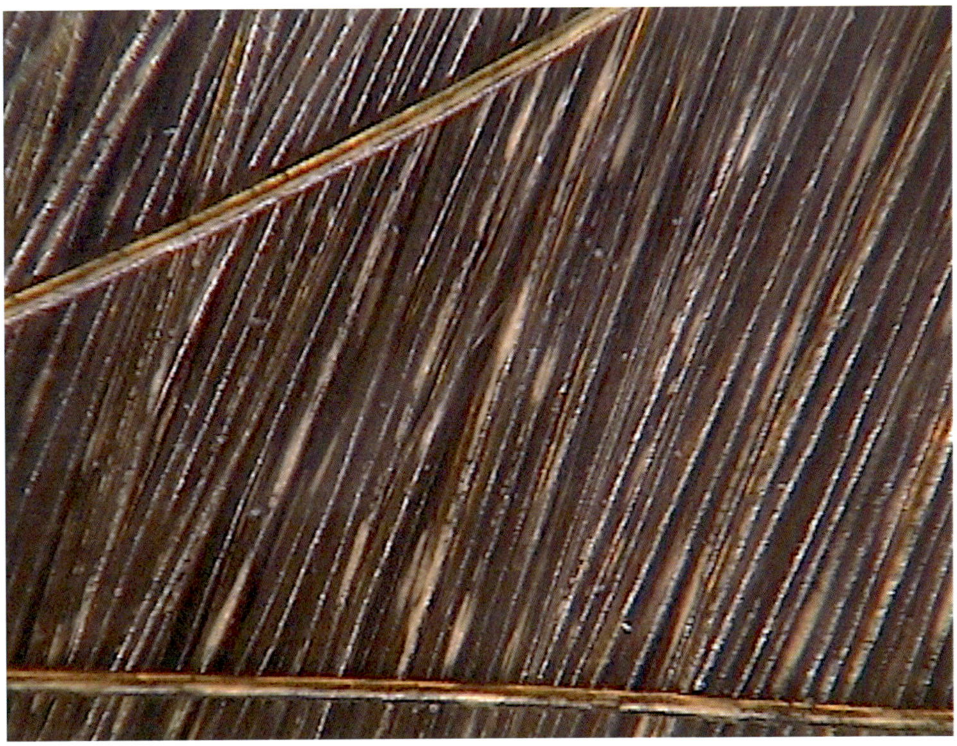

Fig. 12.3 Pili annulati. Trichoscopy demonstrates hair shafts with alternating white and dark bands. The borders of the light bands are not clear-cut, but rather subtle, cloudy, and misty. The bands are shorter than the remaining, dark portion of the hair shaft. The term *light cloudy bands* has been suggested for this finding [7]. Other authors describe the bands as subtle, spangled, and shimmering in appearance [10]. Usually, about 20–80 % of hairs are affected. The white bands tend to disappear distally (×70)

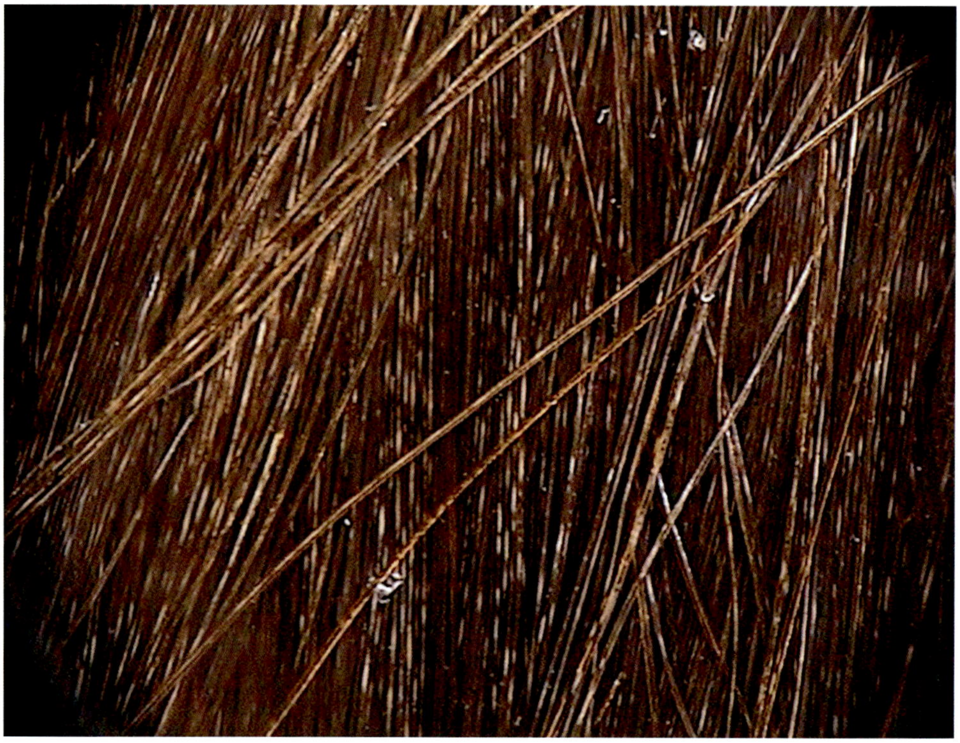

Fig. 12.4 Pili annulati. Low-magnification trichoscopy (i.e., performed with a handheld dermoscope) allows visualization of the characteristic white bands of pili annulati, with less detailed visualization of the cloudy, shimmering inner structure. The characteristic bands are seen better with immersion fluid (compared with dry trichoscopy) and when placing the dermoscope lens against a bundle of several hairs, or against a dark background (×20)

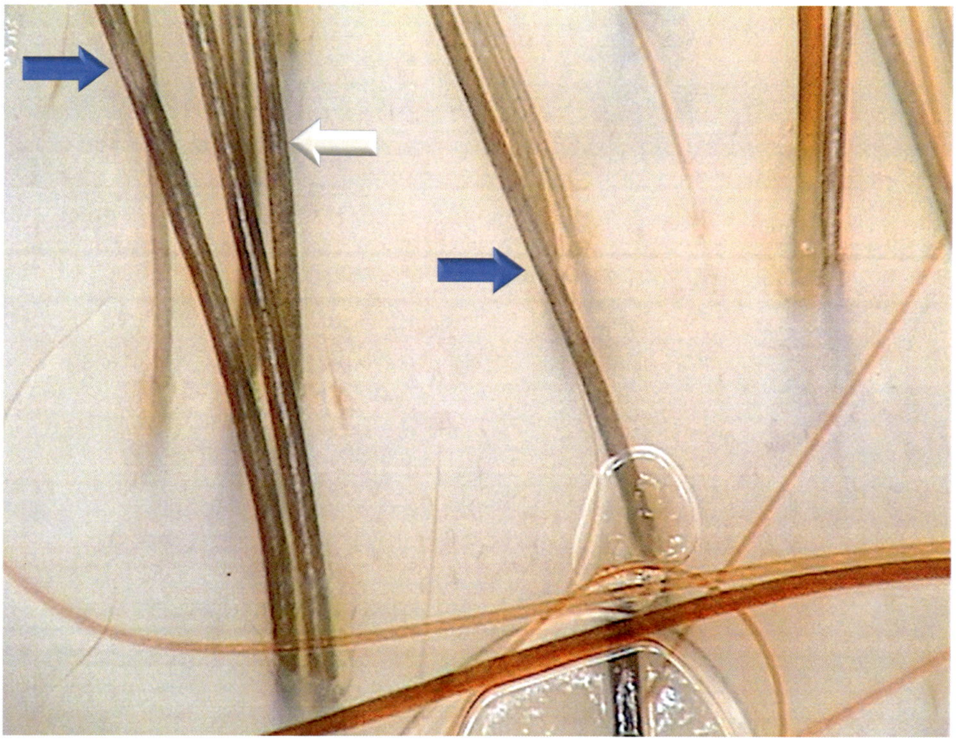

Fig. 12.5 Pili annulati and fragmented medulla. White pili annulati bands (*blue arrows*) may be differentiated clearly from a fragmented medulla (*white arrow*). The white bands in pili annulati are subtle and cloudy, do not have clear-cut borders, and cover 50–100 % of the hair shaft thickness. The white fragmented longitudinal medulla is centrally located in the hair shaft, covers less than 50 % (usually about 30 %) of the hair shaft thickness, and is characterized by clear borders separating the medulla from the remaining, darker part of the hair (×70)

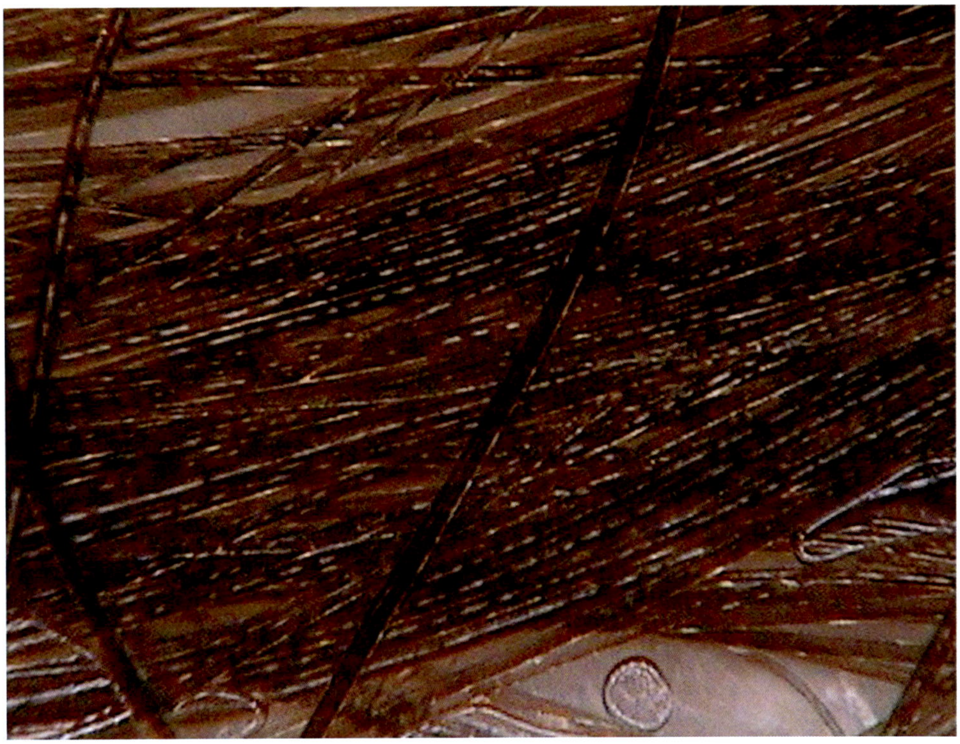

Fig. 12.6 Fragmented and intermittent medulla in a healthy individual. On trichoscopy, the white bands of pili annulati must be differentiated from bands generated by the white medulla. The medulla may be continuous, interrupted, fragmented, or absent in healthy individuals [11]. A continuous medulla is visible on trichoscopy as a light-colored longitudinal structure located centrally in the hair shaft. The trichoscopic impression of the "fragmented" medulla is in fact a thick medulla separated by fragments of thinner medulla, which is not visible on trichoscopy. This produces an image of white fragments within hair shafts. These thin white fragments, demonstrated in this image, should be differentiated from pili annulati (×20)

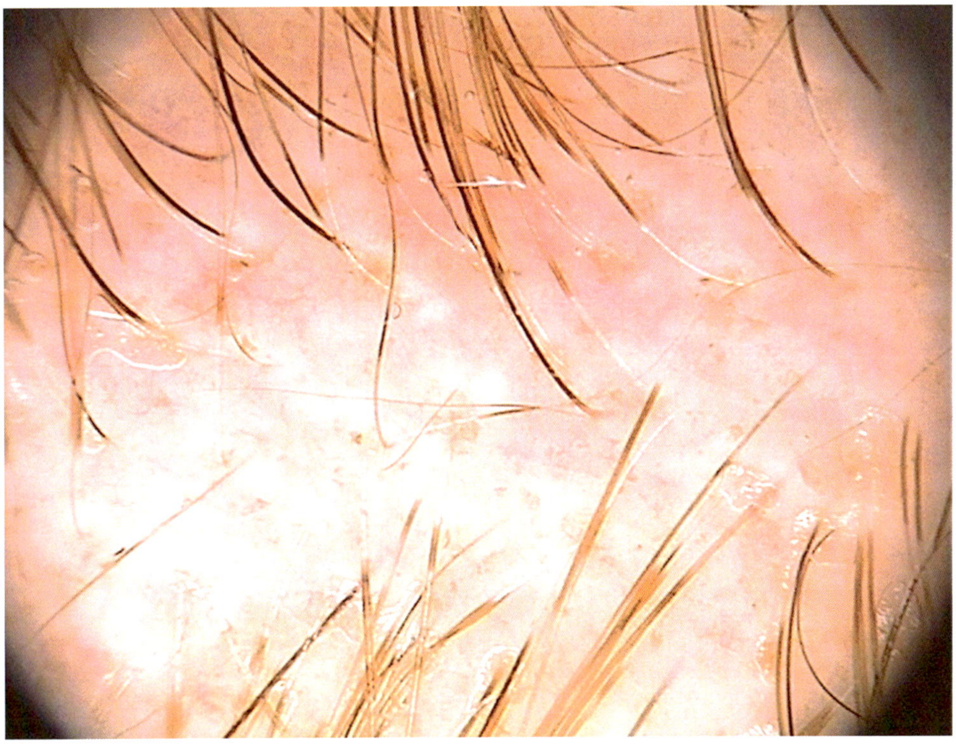

Fig. 12.7 Artificial white bands from inaccurate hair colorization. The differential diagnosis of pili annulati should include artificial bands produced by hair colorization. In this 61-year-old patient with female androgenetic alopecia, the white bands are the result of inaccurate dyeing with a home hair-coloring kit. These white bands do not have a subtle spangled and shimmering appearance, as in pili annulati (×20)

References

1. Cheng AS, Bayliss SJ. The genetics of hair shaft disorders. J Am Acad Dermatol. 2008;59(1):1–22; quiz 3–6.
2. Giehl KA, Rogers MA, Radivojkov M, Tosti A, de Berker DA, Weinlich G, et al. Pili annulati: refinement of the locus on chromosome 12q24.33 to a 2.9-Mb interval and candidate gene analysis. Br J Dermatol. 2009;160(3):527–33.
3. Streck AP, Moncores M, Sarmento DF, Barbosa HS, Weissmuller G, Baetas-Da-Cruz W. Study of nanomechanical properties of human hair shaft in a case of pili annulati by atomic force microscopy. J Eur Acad Dermatol Venereol. 2007;21(8):1109–10.
4. Giehl KA, Schmuth M, Tosti A, De Berker DA, Crispin A, Wolff H, et al. Concomitant manifestation of pili annulati and alopecia areata: coincidental rather than true association. Acta Derm Venereol. 2011;91(4):459–62.
5. Feldmann KA, Dawber RP, Pittelkow MR, Ferguson DJ. Newly described weathering pattern in pili annulati hair shafts: a scanning electron microscopic study. J Am Acad Dermatol. 2001;45(4):625–7.
6. Giehl KA, Ferguson DJ, Dawber RP, Pittelkow MR, Foehles J, de Berker DA. Update on detection, morphology and fragility in pili annulati in three kindreds. J Eur Acad Dermatol Venereol. 2004;18(6):654–8.
7. Rakowska A, Slowinska M, Kowalska-Oledzka E, Rudnicka L. Trichoscopy in genetic hair shaft abnormalities. J Dermatol Case Rep. 2008;2(2):14–20.
8. Rudnicka L, Olszewska M, Rakowska A, Slowinska M. Trichoscopy update 2011. J Dermatol Case Rep. 2011;5(4):82–8.
9. Lee SS, Lee YS, Giam YC. Pseudopili annulati in a dark-haired individual: a light and electron microscopic study. Pediatr Dermatol. 2001;18(1):27–30.
10. Wallace MP, de Berker DA. Hair diagnoses and signs: the use of dermatoscopy. Clin Exp Dermatol. 2010;35(1):41–6.
11. Wagner R, Joekes I. Hair medulla morphology and mechanical properties. J Cosmet Sci. 2007;58(4):359–68.

Woolly Hair

13

Adriana Rakowska and Malgorzata Olszewska

Abstract

In woolly hair, trichoscopy demonstrates hair shafts with waves at very short intervals, giving the hair a "crawling snake" appearance. Hair shaft thickness appears uneven because of the twists that are typical for this condition. Entangled and broken hairs may be present. Trichoscopy is not decisive for diagnosis.

Keywords

Black dots • Broken hairs • Cicatricial alopecia • Pili annulati • Trichorrhexis nodosa Woolly hair

The term *woolly hair* refers to an abnormal variant of fine, tightly curled hair with 180° longitudinal twisting and an increased tendency to fracture. Transverse sections of hair shafts show varying ovoid shapes of different morphology [1, 2]. Hair may be sparse and hypopigmented [1]. Trichorrhexis nodosa and pili annulati may coexist [1].

Hutchinson et al. [3] classified the condition into three variants: (1) woolly hair nevus, (2) autosomal dominant (hereditary) woolly hair, and (3) autosomal recessive (familial) woolly hair.

The nonsyndromic autosomal recessive inherited form is associated with mutations in genes *P2RY5*, *LIPH*, *LPA*, and *mPA-PLA1* [4–8]. In the autosomal dominant type, a mutation in the helix initiation motif of keratin 74 (*KRT74*) was described [9]. Depending on the type of genetic background, the clinical appearance of the disease varies from hair curling to hypotrichosis or total alopecia.

A. Rakowska (✉)
Department of Dermatology, CSK MSW,
Woloska 137, Warsaw 02-507, Poland
e-mail: adrianarak@op.pl

M. Olszewska
Department of Dermatology, Medical University of Warsaw,
Koszykowa 82A, Warsaw 02-008, Poland

Woolly hair may be a trichologic manifestation of various inherited syndromes. The Naxos and Carvajal syndromes consist of woolly hair, palmoplantar keratoderma, and right (Naxos) or left (Carvajal) ventricular cardiac disease [1, 10, 11]. Mutations in genes encoding plakoglobin in Naxos syndrome and desmoplakin in Carvajal syndrome were described. Defects in the desmoplakin gene also may cause the woolly hair–skin fragility syndrome with no cardiac abnormalities and cardiomyopathy with woolly hair, palmoplantar keratoderma, extensive skin blistering, and enamel abnormalities [12].

Woolly hair also is a symptom of cardiofaciocutaneous syndrome, Noonan syndrome, and Costello syndrome, characterized by growth failure, heart defects, mental retardation, and ectodermal abnormalities [13]. There is no consensus regarding the differences among these syndromes. There are reports of the occurrence of woolly hair in Olmsted syndrome (symmetric, mutilating palmoplantar keratoderma and periorificial hyperkeratosis), curly hair–ankyloblepharon–nail dysplasia (CHANDS) syndrome, and trichodento-osseous syndrome [14].

Woolly hair nevus is a non–genetically determined condition presenting clinically as a localized area with a well-circumscribed border. Hair in this area is tightly curled and sometimes hypopigmented. The first manifestation is at birth or during the first 2 years of life [15].

L. Rudnicka et al. (eds.), *Atlas of Trichoscopy*,
DOI 10.1007/978-1-4471-4486-1_13, © Springer-Verlag London 2012

In woolly hair, trichoscopy demonstrates intensely wavy hair with a "crawling snake" appearance and broken hair shafts. Trichoscopy is not decisive for diagnosis, but the typical wavy appearance of the hair may indicate the need for detailed clinical evaluation [16].

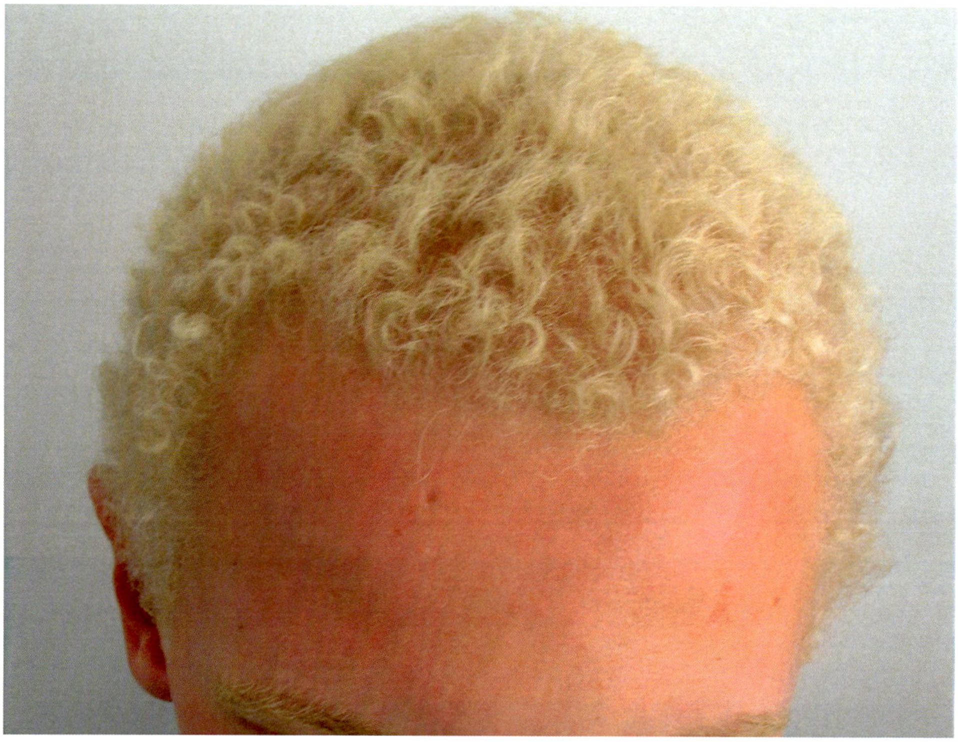

Fig. 13.1 **Woolly hair**. Shown is a patient with autosomal dominant woolly hair (hereditary woolly hair). The hairs are tightly curled, short, hypopigmented, and sparse. Woolly hair sometimes is wrongly compared with curly hair or with ethnic hair in African Americans. Woolly hair differs from healthy curly hair in its tendency to fracture. In patients with woolly hair, the hair grows no longer than about 5 cm (2 in). It also is very tightly curled, with 180° longitudinal twisting

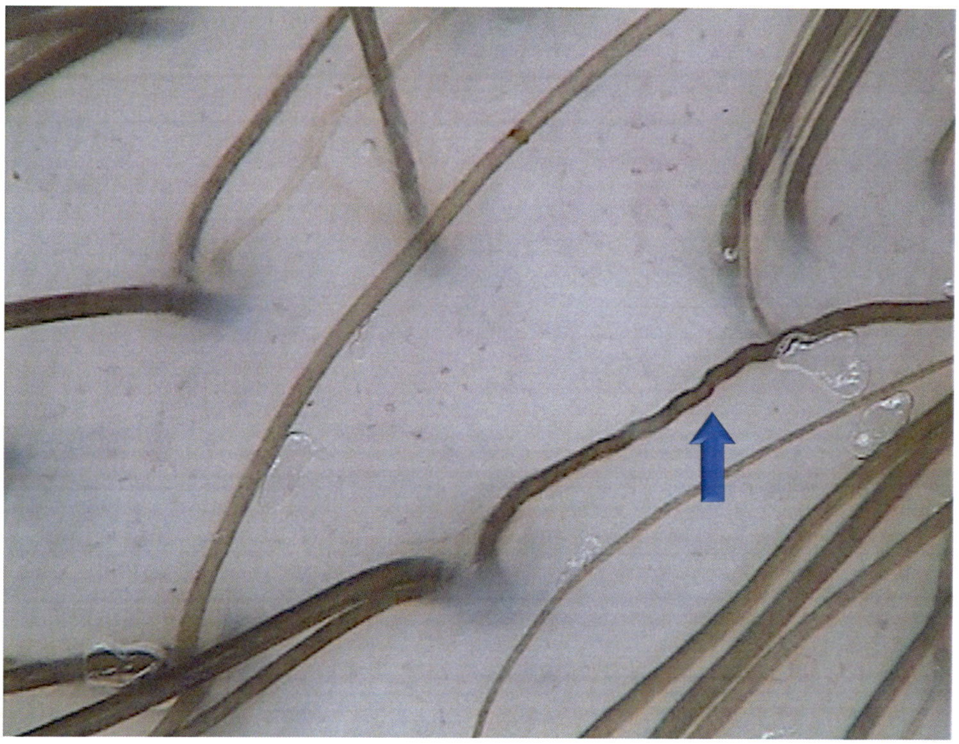

Fig. 13.2 **Woolly hair**. Trichoscopy demonstrates a hair shaft with waves at very short intervals, giving the hair a "crawling snake" look (*blue arrow*). The appearance of variable hair shaft thickness results from twists, which are typical for this condition. Entangled hairs are visible. Trichoscopy is not decisive for diagnosis, but the typical wavy hairs with waves at very short intervals and a twisted appearance may indicate the need for detailed clinical evaluation (×70)

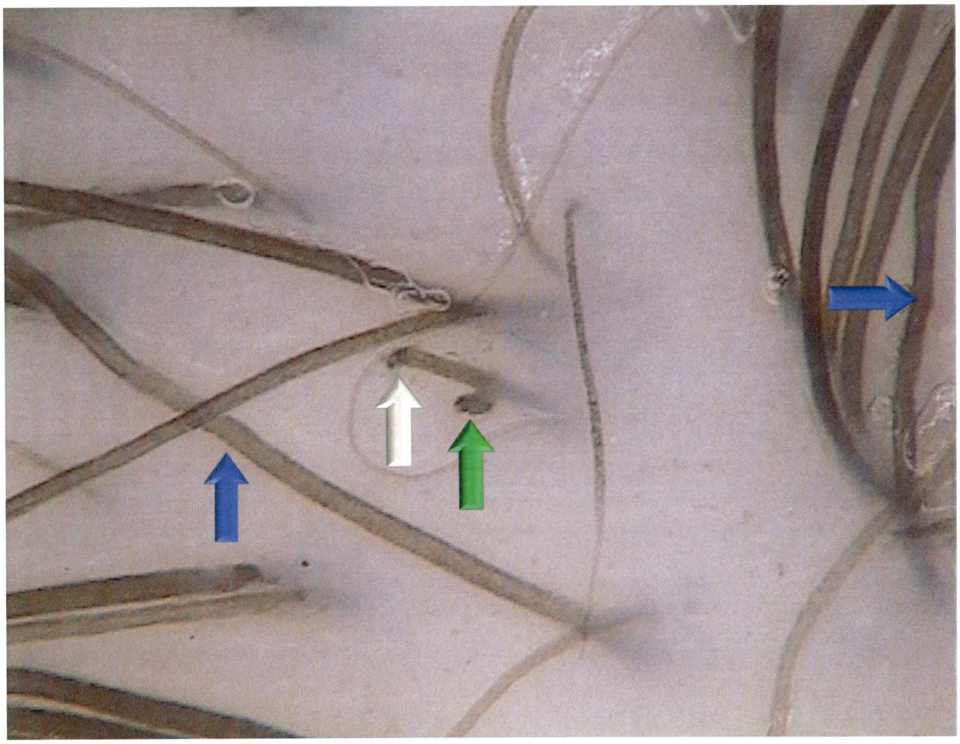

Fig. 13.3 Woolly hair. A few wavy hairs are visible (*blue arrows*). The presence of broken hairs (*white arrow*) is a trichoscopic finding that helps differentiate woolly hair from normal, intensely curled hair. A black dot results from hair fracture at the level of the scalp (*green arrow*; ×70)

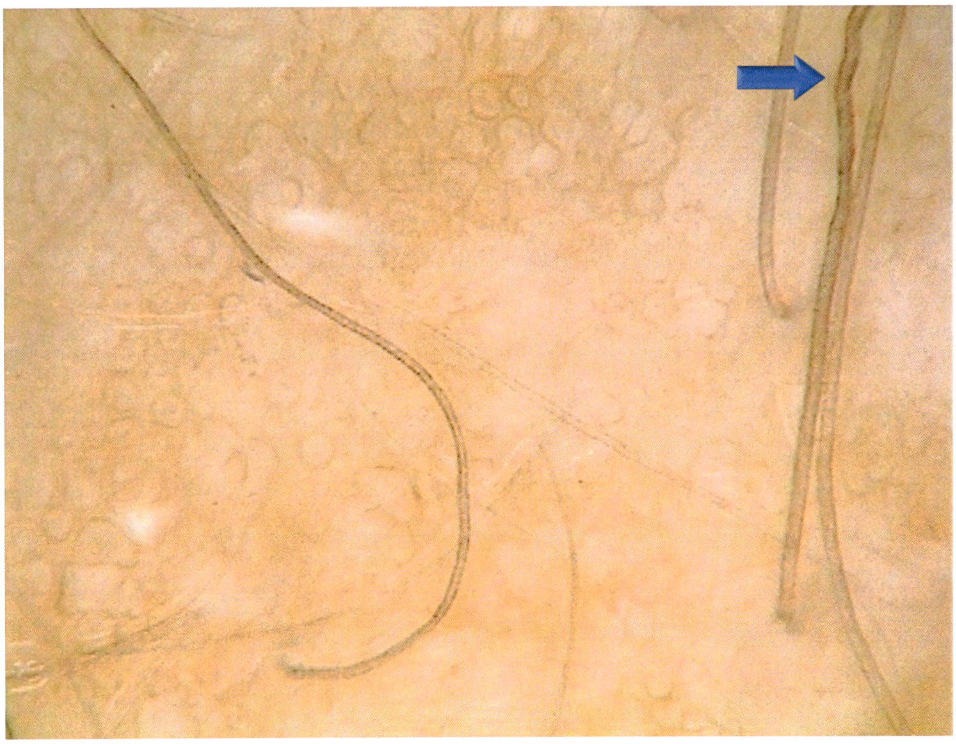

Fig. 13.4 A wavy, twisted hair in cicatricial alopecia. The image shows a wavy, twisted hair (*arrow*) in a 56-year-old patient with cicatricial alopecia and no clinical features of woolly hair. The hair shaft is practically indistinguishable from that seen in woolly hair, which indicates the need for wide differential diagnostics in the trichoscopy of woolly hair (×70)

References

1. Chien AJ, Valentine MC, Sybert VP. Hereditary woolly hair and keratosis pilaris. J Am Acad Dermatol. 2006;54(2 Suppl):S35–9.
2. Jimenez-Sanchez MD, Garcia-Hernandez MJ, Camacho FM. Woolly hair with alopecia areata in a Caucasian girl. Eur J Dermatol. 2010;20(2):245–6.
3. Hutchinson PE, Cairns RJ, Wells RS. Woolly hair. Clinical and general aspects. Trans St Johns Hosp Dermatol Soc. 1974;60(2):160–77.
4. Horev L, Tosti A, Rosen I, Hershko K, Vincenzi C, Nanova K, et al. Mutations in lipase H cause autosomal recessive hypotrichosis simplex with woolly hair. J Am Acad Dermatol. 2009;61(5):813–8.
5. Horev L, Babay S, Ramot Y, Saad-Edin B, Moorad S, Ingber A, et al. Mutations in two genes on chromosome 13 resulting in a complex hair and skin phenotype due to two rare genodermatoses: KLICK and autosomal recessive woolly hair/hypotrichosis simplex. Br J Dermatol. 2011;164(5):1113–6.
6. Horev L, Saad-Edin B, Ingber A, Zlotogorski A. A novel deletion mutation in P2RY5/LPA(6) gene cause autosomal recessive woolly hair with hypotrichosis. J Eur Acad Dermatol Venereol. 2010;24(7):858–9.
7. Shimomura Y, Wajid M, Ishii Y, Shapiro L, Petukhova L, Gordon D, et al. Disruption of P2RY5, an orphan G protein-coupled receptor, underlies autosomal recessive woolly hair. Nat Genet. 2008;40(3):335–9.
8. Shimomura Y, Ito M, Christiano AM. Mutations in the LIPH gene in three Japanese families with autosomal recessive woolly hair/hypotrichosis. J Dermatol Sci. 2009;56(3):205–7.
9. Shimomura Y, Wajid M, Petukhova L, Kurban M, Christiano AM. Autosomal-dominant woolly hair resulting from disruption of keratin 74 (KRT74), a potential determinant of human hair texture. Am J Hum Genet. 2010;86(4):632–8. PMCID: 2850421.
10. Bolling MC, Jonkman MF. Skin and heart: une liaison dangereuse. Exp Dermatol. 2009;18(8):658–68.
11. Koumantaki E, Gregoriou S, Kakrida M, Christofidou E, Katsambas A. What is your diagnosis? Diffuse nonepidermolytic palmoplantar keratoderma with woolly hair and cardiomyopathy (Naxos-Carvajal syndrome). Cutis. 2010;85(4):180, 9–90.
12. Al-Owain M, Wakil S, Shareef F, Al-Fatani A, Hamadah E, Haider M, et al. Novel homozygous mutation in DSP causing skin fragility-woolly hair syndrome: report of a large family and review of the desmoplakin-related phenotypes. Clin Genet. 2011;80(1):50–8.
13. Weiss G, Confino Y, Shemer A, Trau H. Cutaneous manifestations in the cardiofaciocutaneous syndrome, a variant of the classical Noonan syndrome. Report of a case and review of the literature. J Eur Acad Dermatol Venereol. 2004;18(3):324–7.
14. Tharini GK, Hema N, Jayakumar S, Parveen B. Olmsted syndrome: report of two cases. Indian J Dermatol. 2011;56(5):591–3.
15. Kumaran S, Dogra S, Handa S, Kanwar AJ. Woolly hair nevus. Pediatr Dermatol. 2004;21(5):609–10.
16. Rakowska A, Slowinska M, Kowalska-Oledzka E, Rudnicka L. Trichoscopy in genetic hair shaft abnormalities. J Dermatol Case Rep. 2008;2(2):14–20.

Trichothiodystrophy

14

Adriana Rakowska and Malgorzata Olszewska

Abstract
Trichoscopy does not allow visualization of the most specific feature of trichothiodystrophy: the "tiger tail" bands. Thus, trichothiodystrophy cannot be diagnosed based on trichoscopy. Nonspecific findings are a nonhomogenous structure of hair shafts, resembling grains of sand, and a very slightly wavy contour. Trichoschisis may be observed, but distinction between trichoschisis and trichoclasis is not possible by trichoscopy.

Keywords
Brittle hair • Eyelashes • Eyebrows • Grains of sand • Tiger tail • Trichoclasis • Trichoschisis
Trichothiodystrophy

Trichothiodystrophy (TTD), or sulfur-deficient brittle hair, identifies a group of neuroectodermal disorders with remarkable clinical heterogeneity [1]. The term *trichothiodystrophy* was introduced by Price et al. [2] in 1980. Several manifestations may be observed in TTD: mental and growth retardation, micrognathia, a small nose, large ears, microcephaly, nail dysplasia, teeth abnormalities, ichthyosis, reduced stature, osseous anomalies, and hypogonadism [3]. In the past, various acronyms were used to describe TTD subtypes, such as BIDS, IBIDS, and PIBIDS (from: brittle hair, ichthyosis, impaired intelligence, decreased fertility, short stature, and photosensitivity) [4]. The new clinicogenetic classification of TTD distinguishes three types of disease [3]: (1) the photosensitive type with mutations in genes encoding transcription/repair factor IIH (TFIIH) subunits (XPD, XPB, TTDA); (2) the non-photosensitive type with TTDN1 mutation; and (3) the non-photosensitive type with no mutation in the gene encoding TTDN1 and no identified genetic basis [3, 4].

Clinical symptoms of TTD vary widely in type and severity. The single common feature in all patients is fragile hair [5]. In addition, hair loss may occur with periodic cyclicity. Increased hair loss during infections has been observed [6]. Scalp hair, eyebrows, and eyelashes are brittle, unruly, and of variable lengths. Some authors indicate that eyelashes may be long in TTD [4].

Light microscopy shows hair shafts with an irregular, undulating contour and clean transverse fractures through the hair shaft (trichoschisis) [7].

The basis for diagnosis is examination of the hair shafts on polarized light microscopy. Under polarized light, the hair shafts show alternating bright and dark bands, often called "tiger tail" banding [1].

The structural abnormality that causes the transverse lines is not fully understood. An x-ray microanalysis revealed an alternating sulfur content along the long axis of the hair [8]. The x-ray results also showed that calcium was absent in the tracts corresponding to the dark bands, whereas it was normally present in the light bands [9]. Amino acid analysis of the hair in TTD reveals a notably low cysteine content (less than half the normal amount), which parallels the low total

A. Rakowska
Department of Dermatology, CSK MSW,
Woloska 137, Warsaw 02-507, Poland

M. Olszewska (✉)
Department of Dermatology, Medical University of Warsaw,
Koszykowa 82A, Warsaw 02-008, Poland
e-mail: malgorzata.olszewska@wum.edu.pl

L. Rudnicka et al. (eds.), *Atlas of Trichoscopy*,
DOI 10.1007/978-1-4471-4486-1_14, © Springer-Verlag London 2012

sulfur content [6]. Cross-sectional examination of the hair cuticle shows the lack of an exocuticle and A layer [7].

The diagnosis of TTD on polarized light microscopy should not be made based on a few hairs that appear to have alternating bright and dark bands. Rather, all hair should show the tiger tail pattern [1].

Trichoscopy has limited value in identifying TTD because it does not reveal the characteristic phenomena observed under polarized light microscopy. Trichoscopic examination can only suggest the need for further diagnosis of TTD when hair shafts assessed at high magnification have a nonhomogenous structure resembling grains of sand and their contour is very slightly wavy [10]. Trichoschisis may be observed on trichoscopy, but a distinction between trichoschisis and trichoclasis rarely can be made [10].

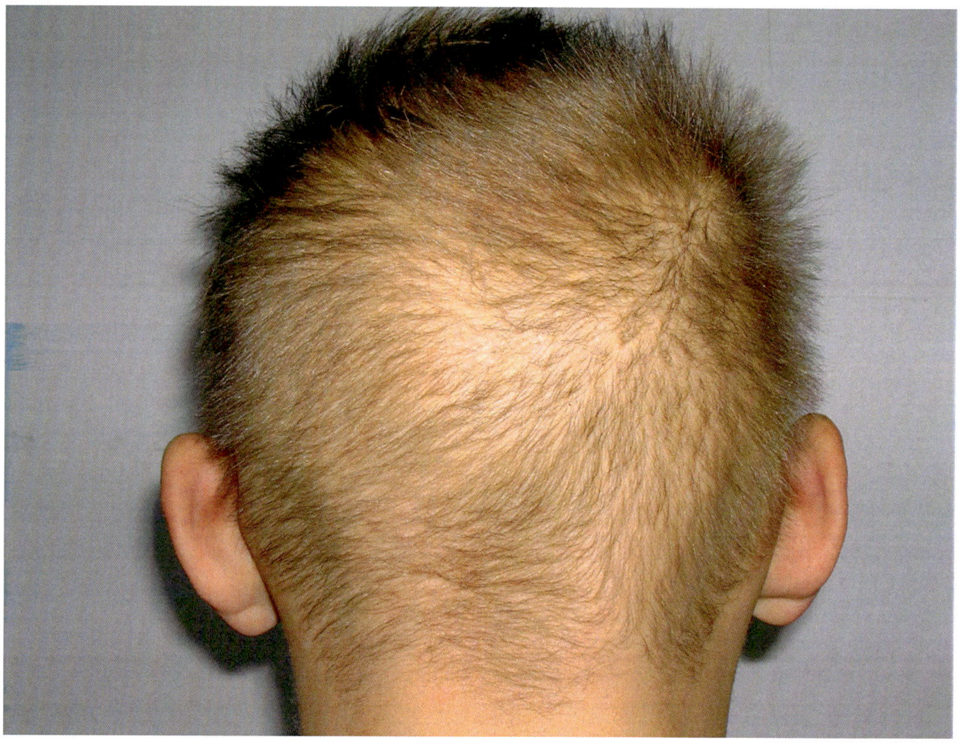

Fig. 14.1 **Trichothiodystrophy**. Clinical features of TTD vary widely in nature and severity. The single common feature in all patients is fragile hair. Scalp hairs, eyebrows, and eyelashes are brittle, unruly, and of variable lengths [11]

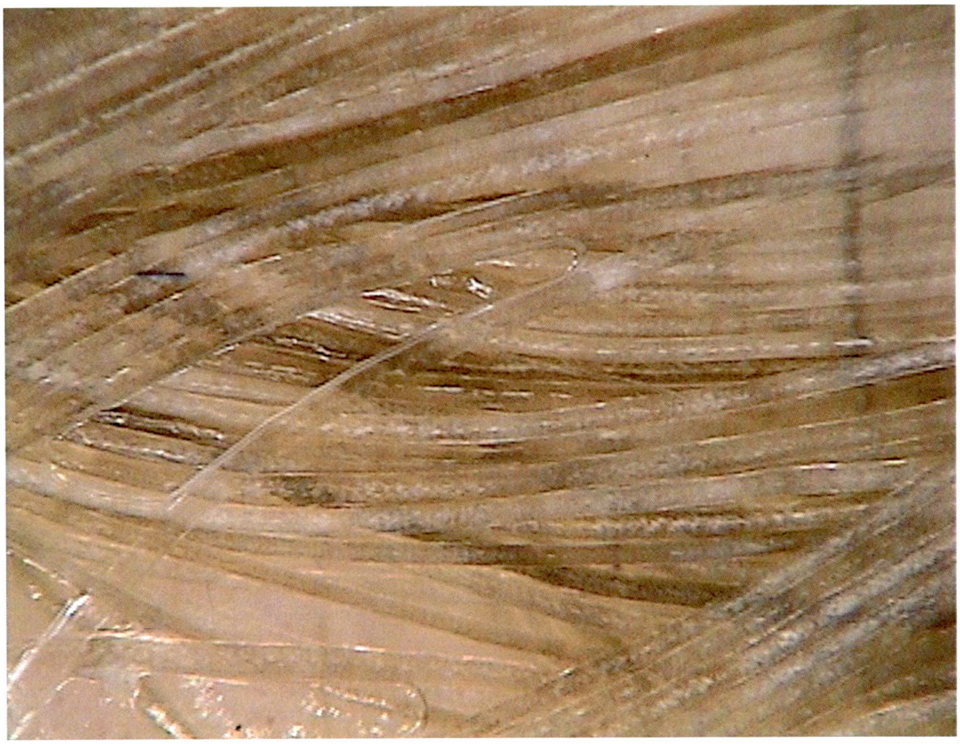

Fig. 14.2 Nonhomogenous structure of hair shafts in trichothiodystrophy. Trichoscopy does not allow visualization of the most specific feature of TTD—the "tiger tail" banding—which is observed on polarized light microscopy. The abnormalities observed on trichoscopy are significantly less characteristic. The hair shafts have a nonhomogenous structure, with an appearance resembling grains of sand [10]. The contour of the hair is very slightly wavy, which corresponds to the undulating contour observed on light microscopy [10] (×70)

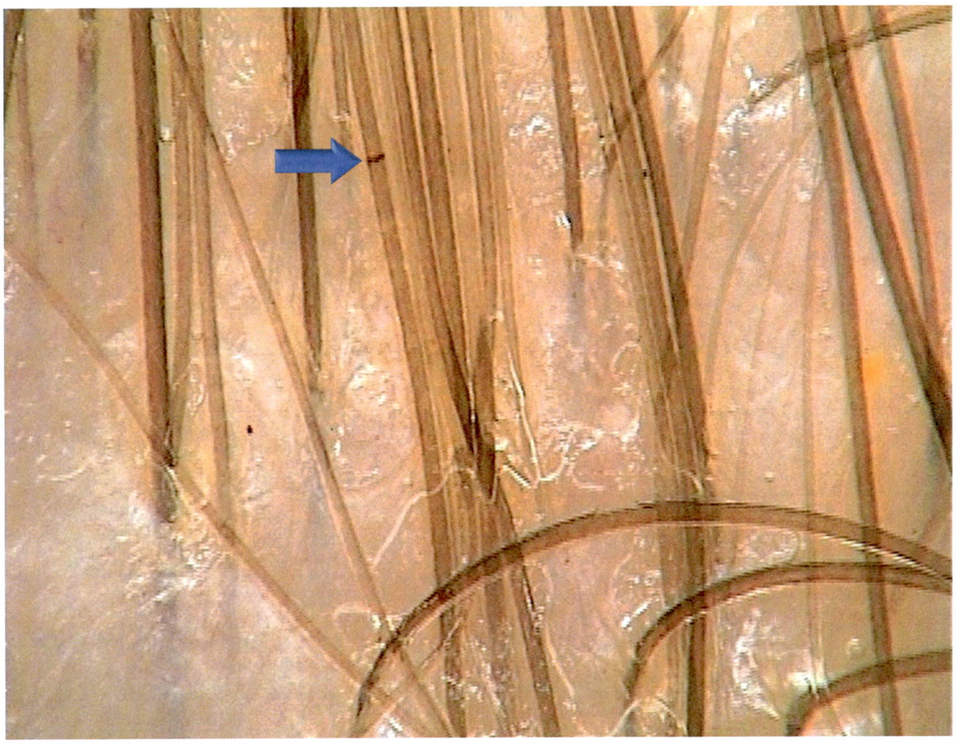

Fig. 14.3 Trichoschisis in trichothiodystrophy. Trichoschisis is a transverse fracture of the hair shaft. Fractures occur in the low-sulfur areas of the hair shaft, which lack cuticle cells [12]. Trichoschisis is characteristic of TTD but also may be observed in monilethrix and in healthy individuals when the cuticle is mechanically weakened (e.g., by excessive hairstyling procedures) [12]. The *arrow* points to trichoschisis in a patient with TTD (×70)

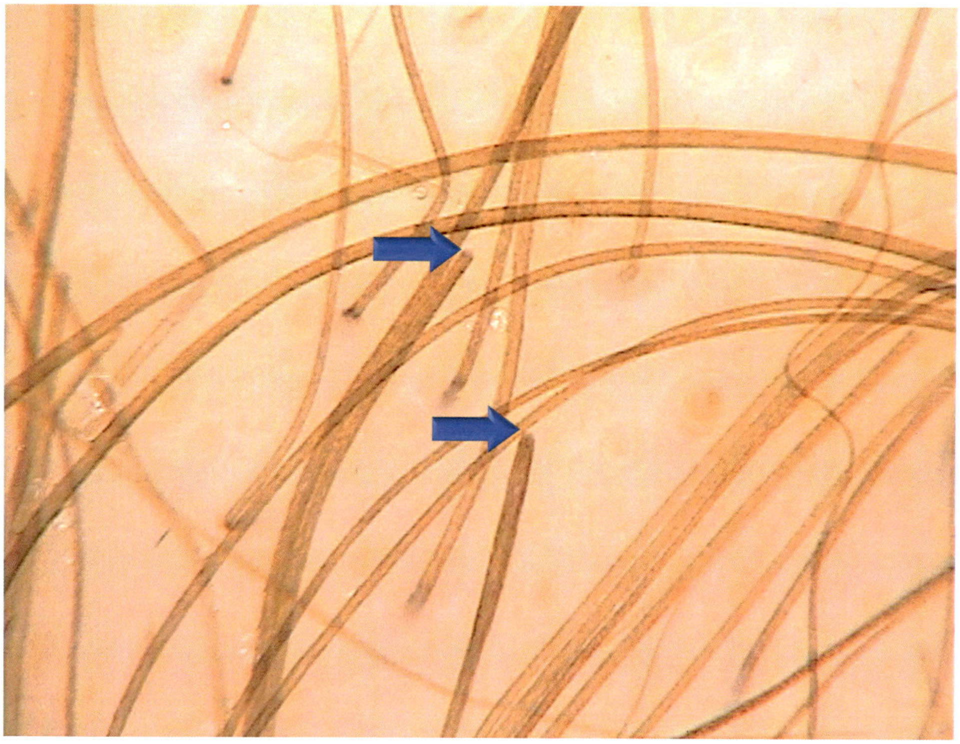

Fig. 14.4 Transversely fractured hair shaft ends in trichothiodystrophy. Trichoschisis results in detachment of the distal portion of the fractured hair. The remaining hairs are short and have a clean transverse distal end (*arrows*). This finding is characteristic of, but not specific for, TTD (×70)

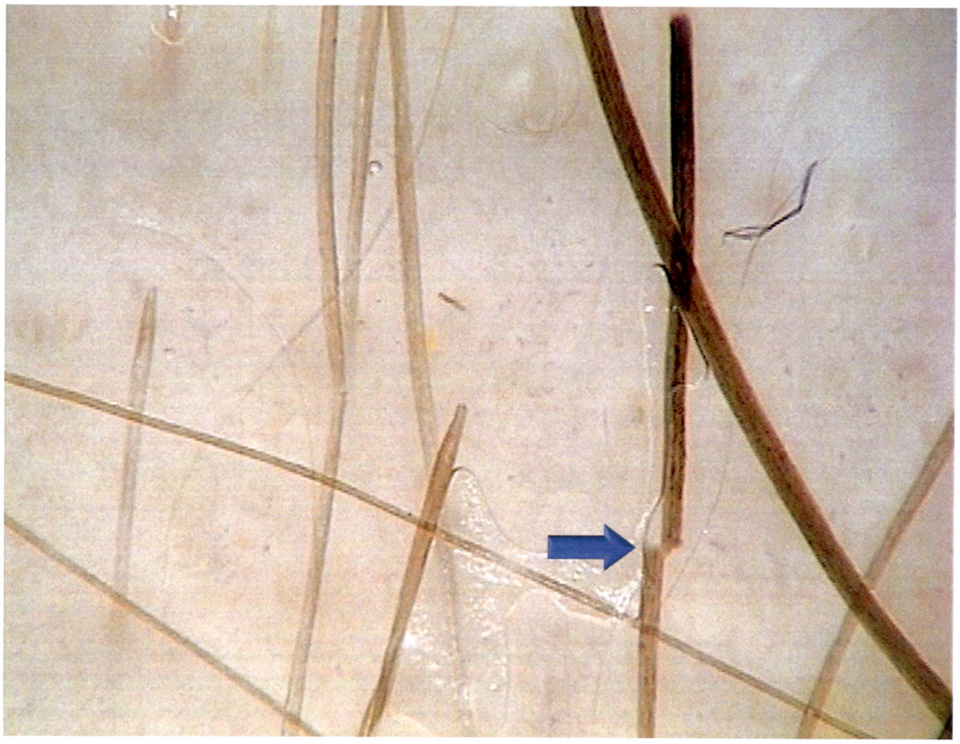

Fig. 14.5 Trichoclasis. Trichoschisis must be differentiated from trichoclasis. Trichoclasis is a transverse fracture of a hair shaft that shows irregular edges on high-magnification light microscopy. Trichoclasis occurs in hairs with an intact cuticle.On trichoscopy, trichoclasis looks similar to trichoschisis, but in trichoclasis the distal portion of the hair shaft may remain attached to the proximal portion through the intact cuticle (*arrow*) (×70)

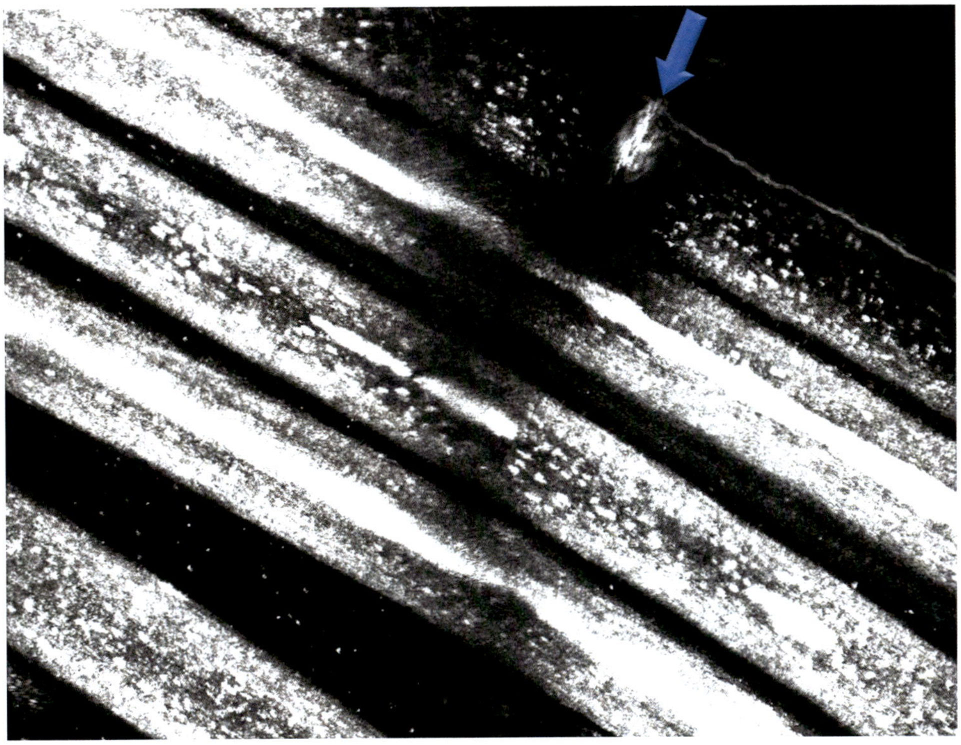

Fig. 14.6 Trichoschisis on reflectance confocal microscopy. The image shows trichoschisis (*arrow*) in a patient with TTD. Reflectance confocal microscopy does not allow differentiation between trichoschisis and trichoclasis

References

1. Itin PH, Sarasin A, Pittelkow MR. Trichothiodystrophy: update on the sulfur-deficient brittle hair syndromes. J Am Acad Dermatol. 2001;44(6):891–920; quiz 1–4.
2. Price VH, Odom RB, Ward WH, Jones FT. Trichothiodystrophy: sulfur-deficient brittle hair as a marker for a neuroectodermal symptom complex. Arch Dermatol. 1980;116(12):1375–84.
3. Morice-Picard F, Cario-Andre M, Rezvani H, Lacombe D, Sarasin A, Taieb A. New clinico-genetic classification of trichothiodystrophy. Am J Med Genet A. 2009;149A(9):2020–30.
4. Zhou X, Khan SG, Tamura D, Patronas NJ, Zein WM, Brooks BP, et al. Brittle hair, developmental delay, neurologic abnormalities, and photosensitivity in a 4-year-old girl. J Am Acad Dermatol. 2010;63(2):323–8.
5. Itin PH, Fistarol SK. Hair shaft abnormalities—clues to diagnosis and treatment. Dermatology. 2005;211(1):63–71.
6. Liang C, Kraemer KH, Morris A, Schiffmann R, Price VH, Menefee E, et al. Characterization of tiger-tail banding and hair shaft abnormalities in trichothiodystrophy. J Am Acad Dermatol. 2005; 52(2):224–32.
7. Forslind B, Andersson MK, Alsterborg E. Hereditary hair changes revealed by analysis of single hair fibres by scanning electron microscopy. Scanning Microsc. 1991;5(3):867–74; discussion 74–5.
8. de Berker D, Sinclair RD. The hair shaft: normality, abnormality, and genetics. Clin Dermatol. 2001;19(2):129–34.
9. Richetta A, Giustini S, Rossi A, Calvieri S. What's new in trichothiodystrophy. J Eur Acad Dermatol Venereol. 2001;15(1):1–4.
10. Rakowska A, Slowinska M, Kowalska-Oledzka E, Rudnicka L. Trichoscopy in genetic hair shaft abnormalities. J Dermatol Case Rep. 2008;2(2):14–20.
11. Cheng S, Stone J, de Berker D. Trichothiodystrophy and fragile hair: the distinction between diagnostic signs and diagnostic labels in childhood hair disease. Br J Dermatol. 2009;161(6):1379–83.
12. Camacho F, Montagna W. Trichology. Diseases of the pilosebaceous follicle. Farmington: S. Karger; 1998.

Part VI

Ectodermal Dysplasia and Other Genetic Syndromes Associated with Hair Loss

15 Ectodermal Dysplasia and Other Genetic Syndromes Associated with Hair Loss

Adriana Rakowska, Malgorzata Olszewska, and Lidia Rudnicka

Abstract

Hair loss is present in a wide range of genetic conditions, most of which are multiorgan diseases. When examining a child with alopecia, one must inspect for associated dental, skeletal, ocular, and other abnormalities. Genetic testing may be performed when appropriate. Although trichoscopy is not diagnostic, sparse hair with pili torti and the presence of gray hairs in a child may indicate ectodermal dysplasia.

Keywords

Alopecia areata • Aplasia cutis congenita • Atrichia • Bloch-Sulzberger syndrome Congenital skin aplasia • Congenital syndromes • Ectodermal dysplasia • Eyebrows Genodermatosis • Hypotrichosis • Incontinentia pigmenti • Komura-Guerri syndrome • Pili canaliculi • Pili torti • Satoyoshi syndrome • Trichorhinophalangeal syndrome

A wide range of genetic conditions may be associated with hair loss [1, 2]. The largest group of these conditions is made up of the ectodermal dysplasias. *Ectodermal dysplasia* is a common term for a group of more than 200 genetic disorders caused by more than 50 different genetic mutations, most commonly in ectodysplasin (*EDA1*), *EDAR*, and *EDARADD*, which encode a ligand, a receptor, and an intracellular signal mediator of a single linear pathway [3, 4]. Ectodermal dysplasias are characterized by dysplasia of two or more tissues of ectodermal origin and include abnormalities affecting the hair, teeth, nails, sweat glands, and other tissues [1, 5–7]. In patients with ectodermal dysplasias, the scalp hair often is sparse, lightly pigmented, thin, dry, brittle, and curly [8, 9]. In most patients, the number of hairs is decreased by 25–75 % [8]. It seems probable that in patients with ectodermal dysplasias, alopecia is caused by both impairment of hair follicle function and increased hair fragility [10]. Eyebrows and/or eyelashes may be sparse or absent [8, 9].

Trichogram results are normal or may show an increased percentage of telogen hairs.

Trichoscopy shows hair abnormalities in most, if not all, patients with ectodermal dysplasias. The most consistent findings are an increased percentage of follicular units with only one hair and heterogeneity in hair shaft pigmentation. Regardless of age, patients have multiple hypopigmented (gray) hairs [11]. Various hair shaft structure abnormalities may be observed, including pili torti, trichoschisis, and pili canaliculi. Trichorrhexis nodosa or monilethrix-like hairs may be present [11]. Occasionally, high-magnification trichoscopy reveals hair shafts with a nonhomogenous, grainy structure and a slightly wavy contour, which may indicate trichothiodystrophy. Although cicatricial alopecia may be present, it is extremely rare. In such cases, trichoscopy shows homogenous ivory-white areas lacking follicular openings [11].

Heterogeneity of hair shaft thickness may be observed in some patients; however, it remains unclear whether this is a

A. Rakowska
Department of Dermatology, CSK MSW, Warsaw, Poland

M. Olszewska
Department of Dermatology,
Medical University of Warsaw, Warsaw, Poland

L. Rudnicka (✉)
Faculty of Health Sciences, Medical University of Warsaw, Poland

Department of Dermatology, CSK MSW,
Woloska 137, Warsaw 02-502, Poland
e-mail: lidia.rudnicka@euderm.eu

L. Rudnicka et al. (eds.), *Atlas of Trichoscopy*,
DOI 10.1007/978-1-4471-4486-1_15,

feature related solely to ectodermal dysplasia or to coexisting androgenic alopecia [11, 12]. Trichoscopy of the eyebrows and eyelashes may show empty follicular openings, which appear brown-gray, but in many cases, no abnormalities are observed.

It is advisable to perform both dry trichoscopy and trichoscopy with immersion fluid in patients with suspected hair abnormalities in the course of ectodermal dysplasias. Dry trichoscopy allows better visualization of hair shaft structure abnormalities, especially in patients with light-colored hair. Trichoscopy with immersion fluid allows a better evaluation of the inner structure of the hair shafts and of skin surface abnormalities.

In this chapter, we also discuss the trichoscopic features of other syndromes associated with hair loss and a proven or probable genetic background.

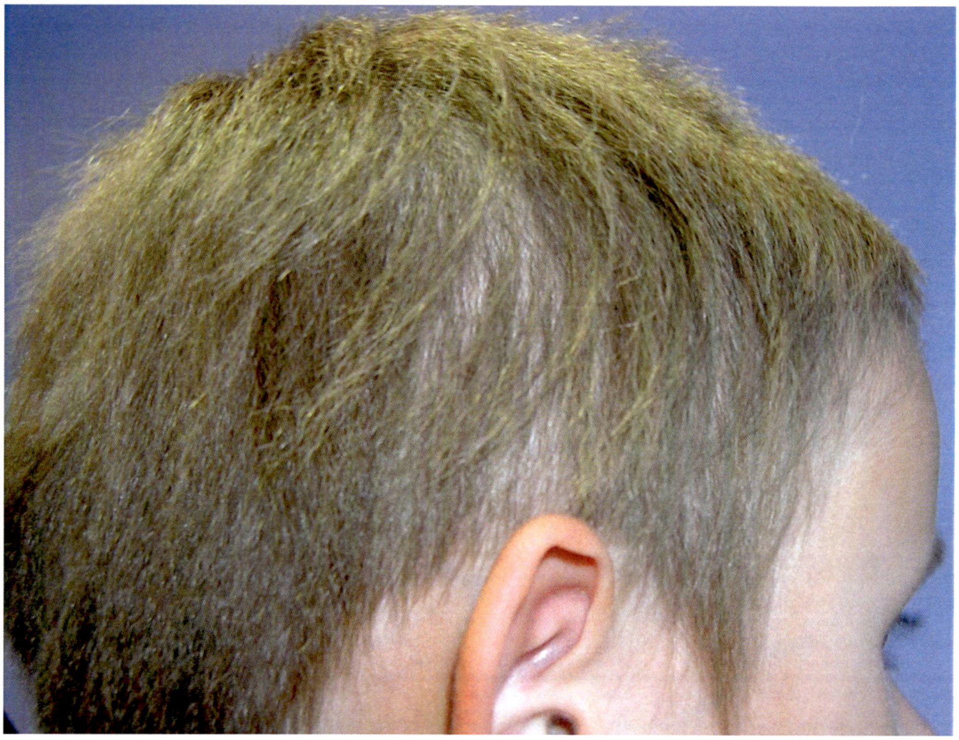

Fig. 15.1 Hair in ectodermal dysplasia. *Ectodermal dysplasia* is a common term for multiple genetic disorders caused by more than 50 different genetic mutations and showing different clinical features. In most patients with ectodermal dysplasias, the hair is sparse, thin, lightly colored, dry, and brittle [8, 9]. Occasionally, very curly hair is observed. The number of hairs usually is decreased by 25–75 % [8]. Total hair loss is rare [13]. In some patients with ectodermal dysplasia (e.g., Rapp-Hodgkin syndrome), hair loss may be accompanied by chronic dermatitis of the scalp

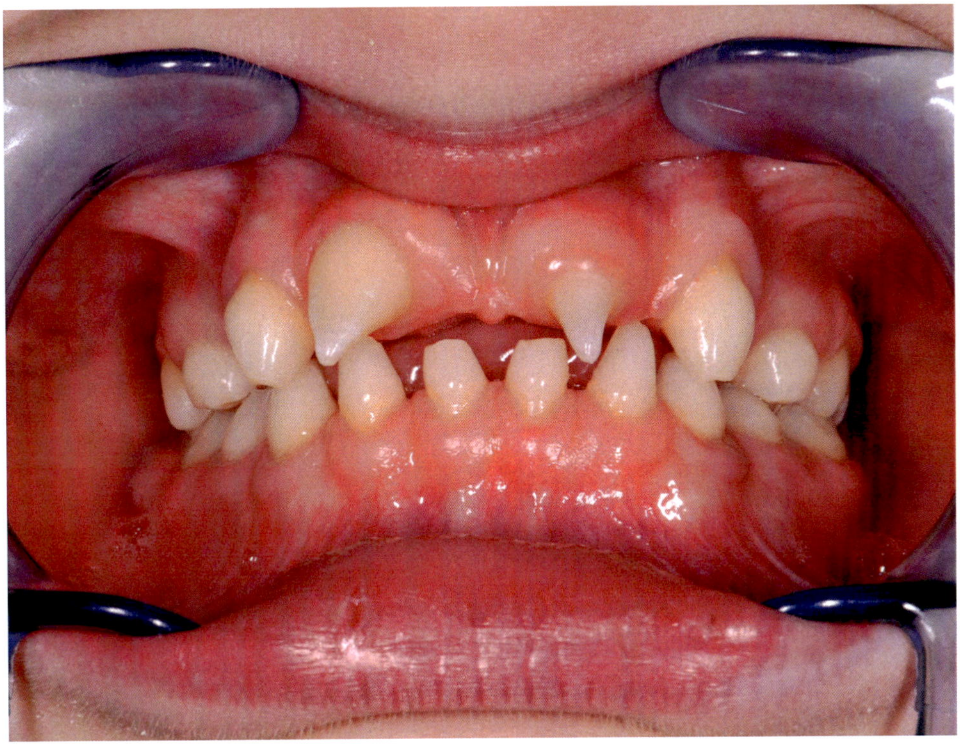

Fig. 15.2 Dental abnormalities in ectodermal dysplasia. Ectodermal dysplasias are characterized by dysplasia of two or more tissues of ectodermal origin [1, 5–7]. The basis for most classifications is the presence or absence of (1) hair anomalies, (2) dental abnormalities, (3) nail abnormalities, and (4) eccrine sweat gland dysfunction or dyshidrosis [5, 14, 15]. Finger deformities commonly are seen (e.g., in Ellis–van Creveld syndrome) but rarely are included in classifications [16]. This image shows the typical pointed teeth in a boy with hypohidrotic ectodermal dysplasia (*Photo courtesy of* Prof. Malgorzata Zadurska)

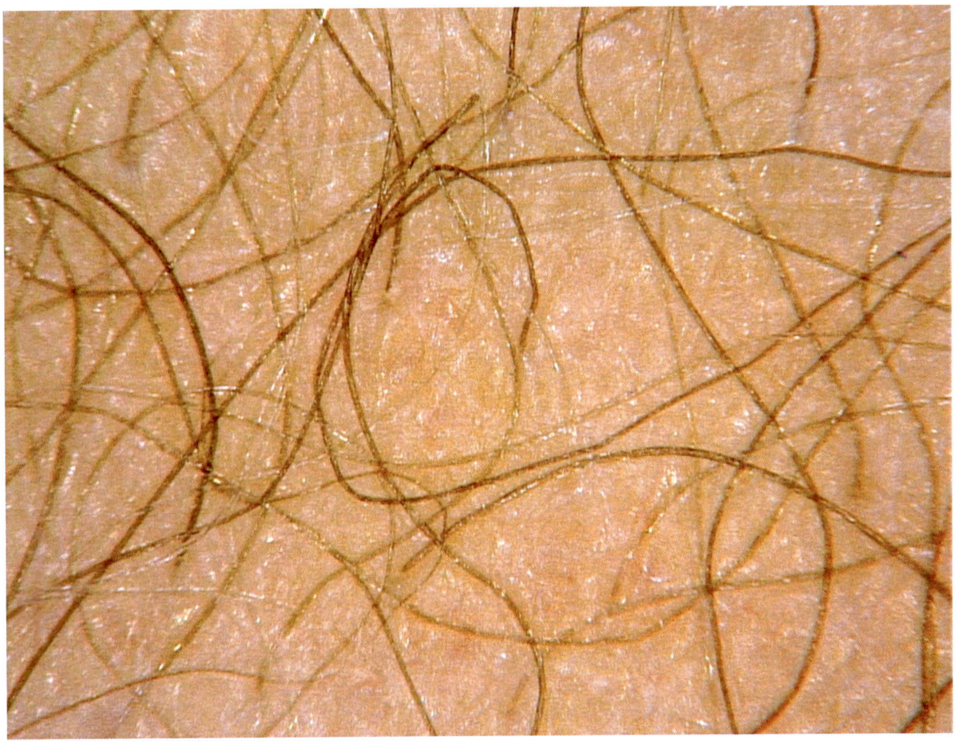

Fig. 15.3 Sparse hair and pili torti in ectodermal dysplasia. In most patients with ectodermal dysplasia, hairs are sparse and most follicular units contain only one hair. The hair shafts bend in different directions at irregular intervals, which is a typical finding on trichoscopy of pili torti [17]. Note the characteristic diversity of hair shaft pigmentation and the presence of gray hairs in this 4-year-old patient with ectodermal dysplasia (dry trichoscopy, ×20)

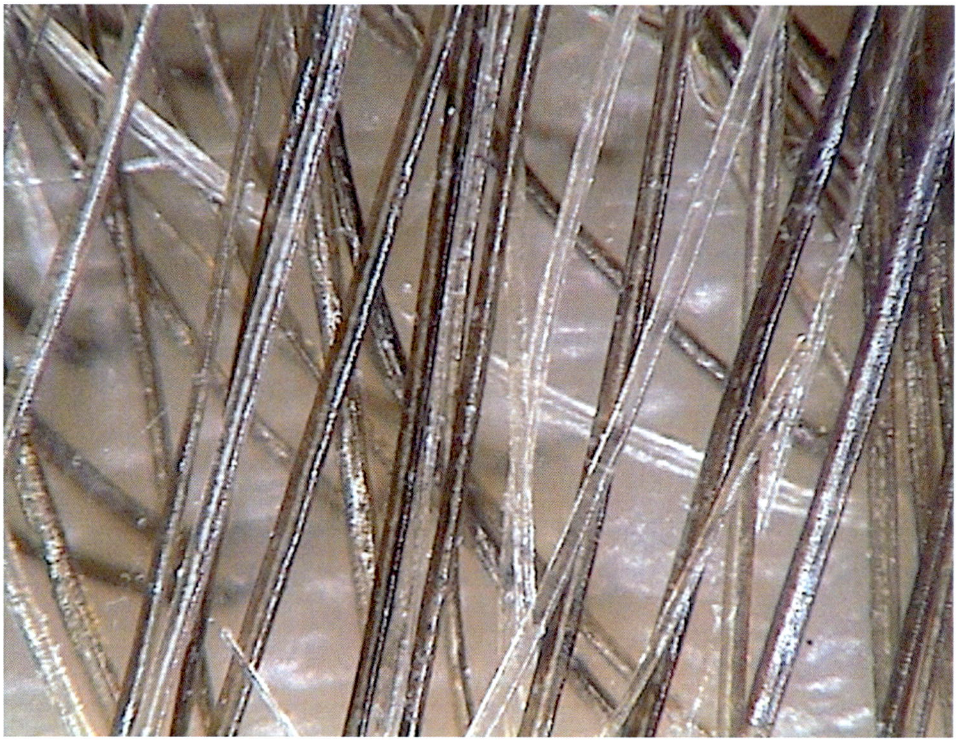

Fig. 15.4 Gray hairs in an 8-year-old girl with ectodermal dysplasia. The hair shafts show diverse pigmentation, from gray to dark brown. Diversity of hair shaft pigmentation is one of the most common trichoscopic findings in patients with ectodermal dysplasias [11, 18]. Usually, more than 10 % of hairs are gray and are visible on trichoscopy as semi-translucent hairs. Occasionally, there is a tendency for increased pigmentation toward the distal end. Longitudinal grooves are present on the surface of some hair shafts, corresponding to pili canaliculi (×70)

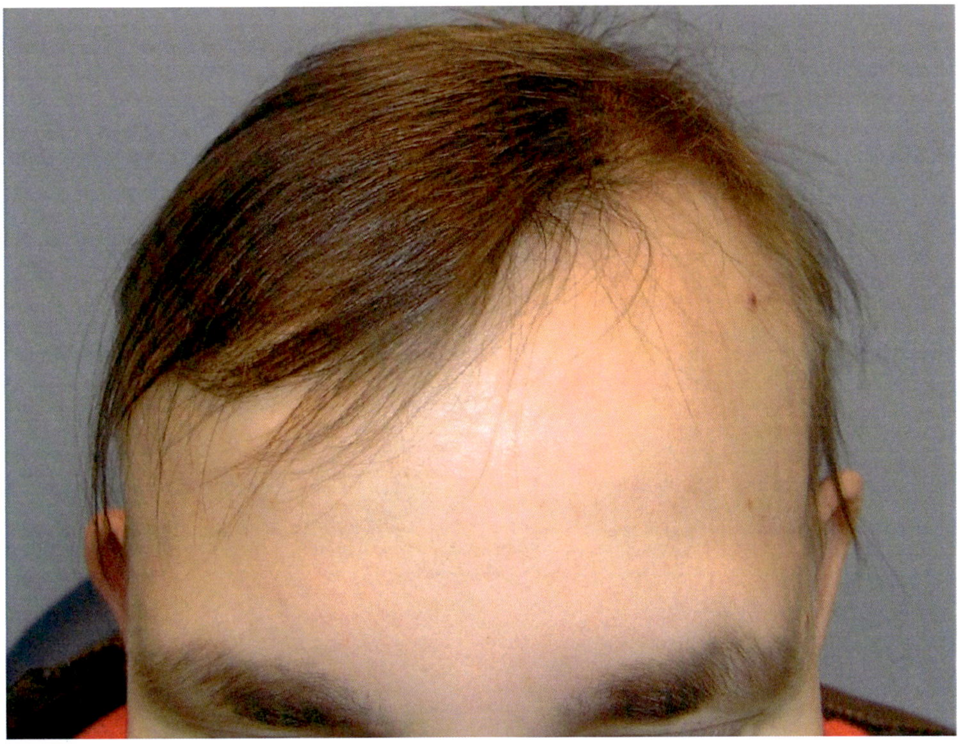

Fig. 15.5 Trichorhinophalangeal syndrome. Trichorhinophalangeal syndrome (TRPS) is a rare autosomal dominant disorder caused by a mutation in the *TRPS* gene [19]. Three clinically and molecularly distinct subtypes of TRPS have been described: type I, type II (Langer-Giedion syndrome), and type III (Sugio-Kajii syndrome). Trichologic abnormalities are similar in all subtypes and include fine, sparse, or even brittle scalp hair and diffuse alopecia, ranging from almost normal hair to severe hypotrichosis or baldness. Hairs grow slowly and reach a maximum length of only a few centimeters. The frontotemporal hairline usually is receded, clinically resembling androgenetic alopecia. A receded medio-occipital hairline also has been described. The eyebrows are very prominent in their medial part and are thinner laterally. Eyelashes may be sparse or absent. Hair sparseness also may affect the beard and axillary and pubic hair [20–22]. Trichography shows an increased percentage of telogen hairs (30–60 %) and/or dysplastic hairs. Cross-polarized light microscopy usually does not reveal hair shaft structure abnormalities. Trichorrhexis nodosa or trichoptilosis may be observed occasionally [20–24]. "Finger-end rhexis" was described in one study [25] but has not been observed in other patients with TRPS. Alterations in the cuticular pattern have been noted in detailed scanning electron microscopic studies. Seitz et al. [20] observed continuous thinning of the distal part of the hair shafts. This thinning was explained by the markedly reduced speed of hair growth, making haircuts rarely necessary, leading to thinning of the distal ends over time as a result of environmental exposure

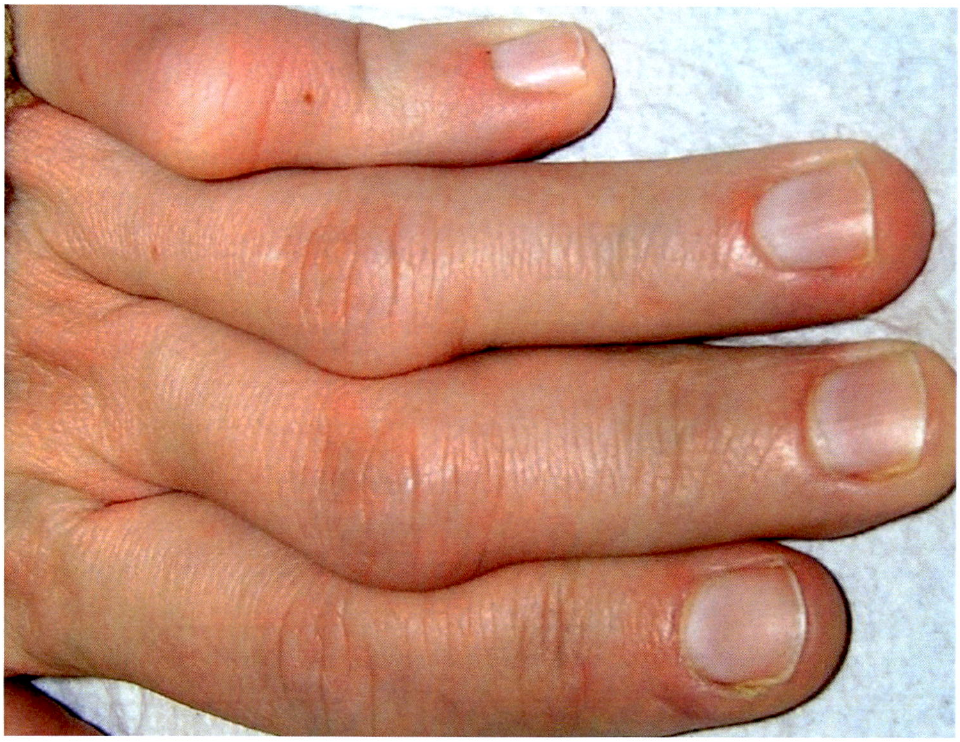

Fig. 15.6 **Trichorhinophalangeal syndrome**. Nontrichologic abnormalities in TRPS are short stature, a bulbous nasal tip, cone-shaped epiphyses, and generalized shortening of all phalanges. Other findings include a long philtrum, a thin upper lip, dental abnormalities, hypermobile joints, small feet, and short great toes [23, 24]. TRPS types I and III differ clinically from type II in their more severe skeletal abnormalities, especially brachydactyly and final height. Type II TRPS may be differentiated by the presence of exostoses [26] and significant intellectual deficits [27, 28]

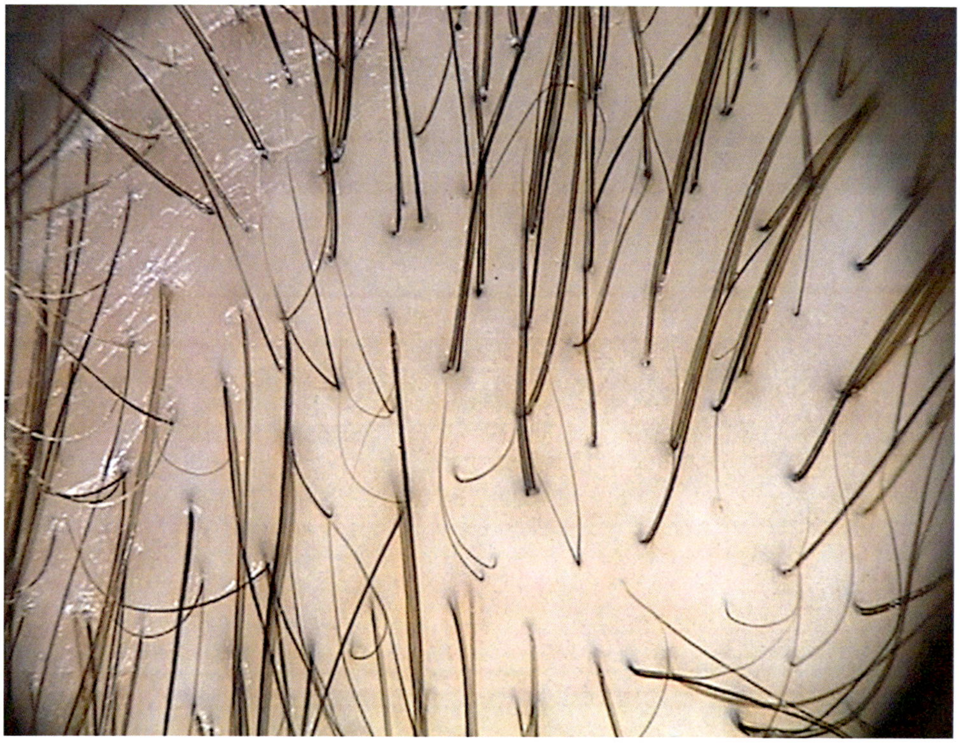

Fig. 15.7 **Trichorhinophalangeal syndrome**. This trichoscopic image from a 23-year-old patient with TRPS shows an exceptionally large proportion of short upright regrowing hairs with a pointed distal end. Some hair follicle openings are surrounded by a whitish halo. Most follicular units contain one or two hairs. In this patient, reflectance confocal microscopy showed dilated hair follicle openings and disfigured dermal papillae (×20)

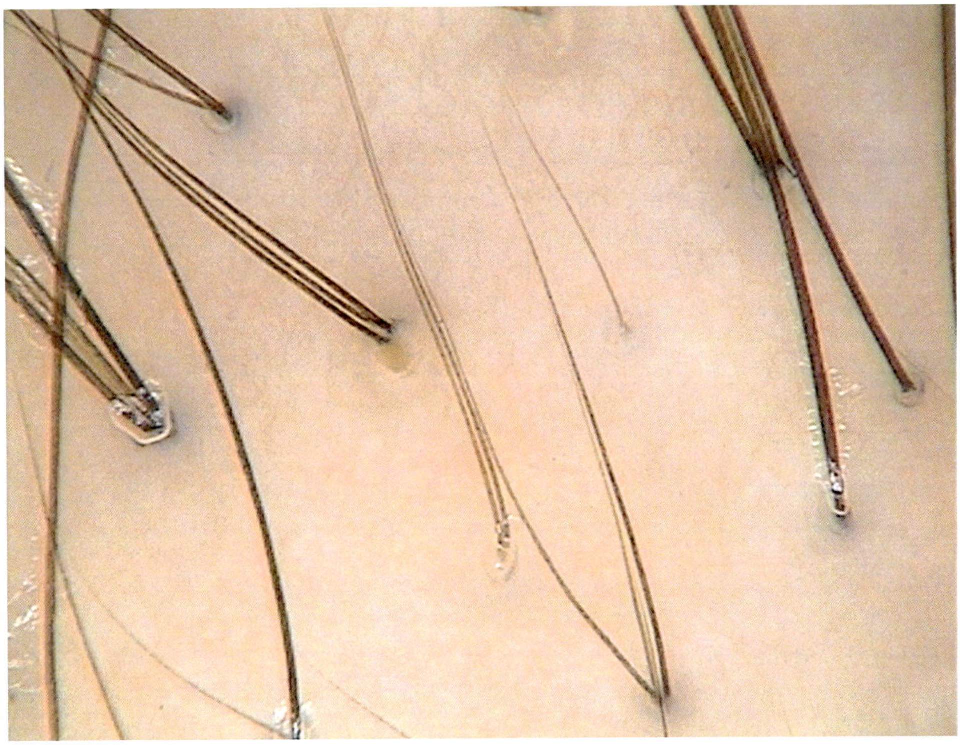

Fig. 15.8 Trichorhinophalangeal syndrome. Trichoscopy shows an exceptional number of short upright regrowing hairs with pointed distal ends. Unlike normally regrowing hairs in healthy individuals, these hairs often grow in groups of two or three hairs emerging from one follicular unit. The multiplicity of short hairs with a sharp, pointed distal end bears some resemblance to trichoscopic observations of normal eyebrows. It appears that some of these hairs never grow long enough to form long terminal hairs, resulting in the clinical appearance of sparse hairs [29] (×20)

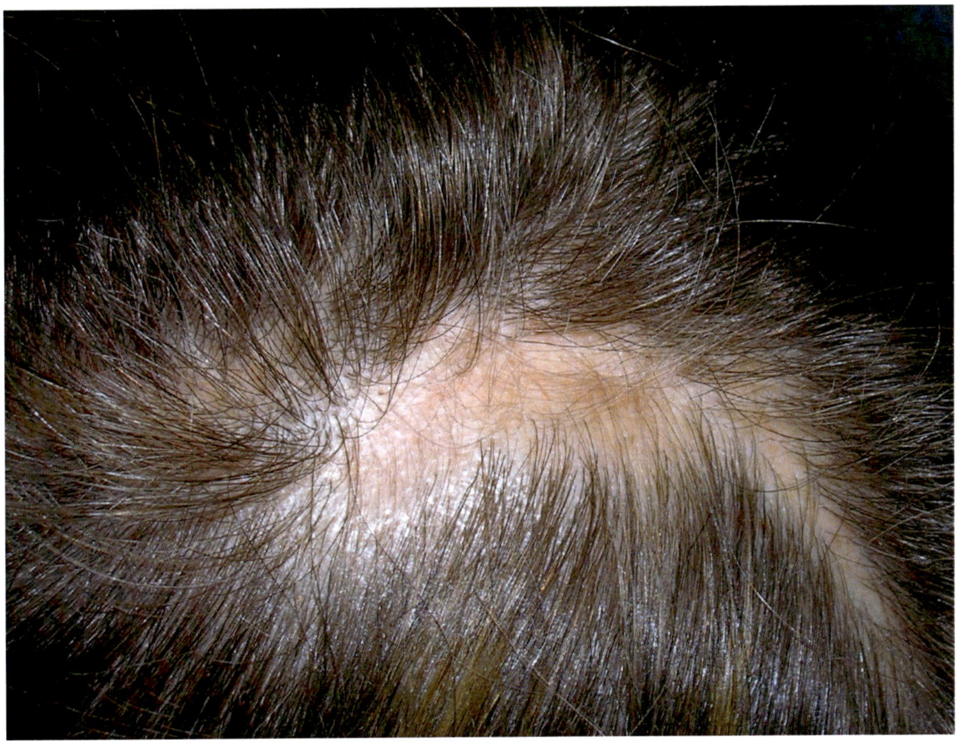

Fig. 15.9 Incontinentia pigmenti (Bloch-Sulzberger syndrome). Incontinentia pigmenti (Bloch-Sulzberger syndrome) is an inherited disorder associated with cutaneous (90–100 %), dental (65–90 %), skeletal (40 %), central nervous system (40 %), and ocular (35 %) abnormalities. It usually is seen in females, as it is an X-linked dominantly inherited disease that is lethal in males. It is a single-gene disorder caused by mutations in the gene encoding IKBKG (inhibitor of kappa-B kinase gamma). Scalp involvement is common and is associated with the presence of vesicular inflammatory lesions, which progress over months to verrucous lesions. Later, these lesions are replaced by skin atrophy with hyperpigmentation and eventually cause cicatricial alopecia. The most common late manifestation of the disease is cicatricial vertex alopecia, which occurs in 38–50 % of patients. It may be the only cutaneous sign of the disease in adult patients. There are a few reports of woolly hair in patients with incontinentia pigmenti [30–33]

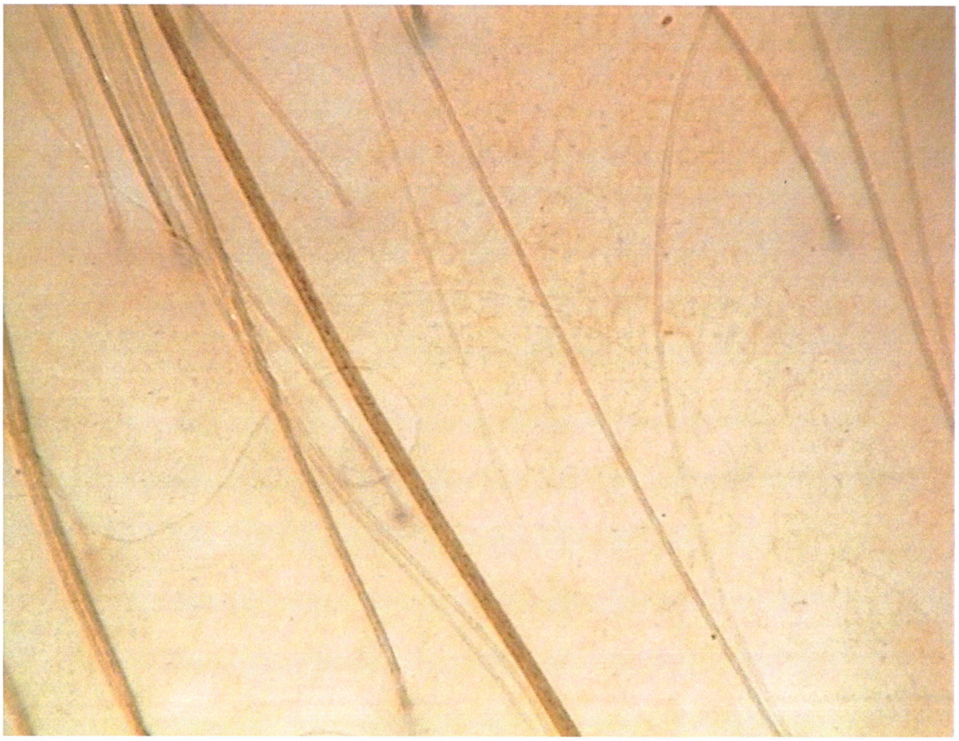

Fig. 15.10 Incontinentia pigmenti (Bloch-Sulzberger syndrome). At the hair-bearing edge of cicatricial vertex alopecia, most follicular units contain only one hair. The hair shafts are thin. Honeycomb hyperpigmentation is visible between the sparse follicular units. In the midpart of the lesion, only an ivory-white area with discrete honeycomb pigmentation is visible. The area lacks follicular openings (×40)

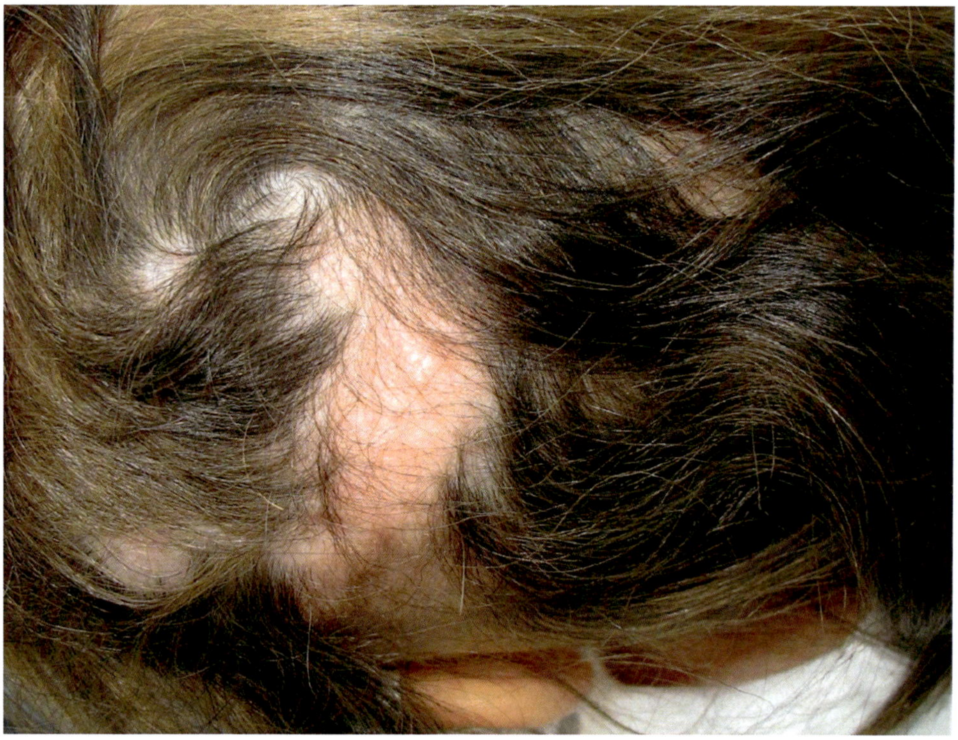

Fig. 15.11 Aplasia cutis congenita in a patient with Kabuki syndrome. Aplasia cutis congenita is the congenital, focal absence of the epidermis and dermis. Occasionally, it may extend through the bone and dura of the skull. The defect occurs most commonly in the vertex area. Clinically, neonates with aplasia cutis congenita have one or more sharply circumscribed ulcers or scars. Ulcerated lesions heal spontaneously from the periphery over the course of 1–3 months and leave a smooth, yellowish, papery atrophic area of cicatricial alopecia [1, 34–36]. Aplasia cutis congenita is classified into nine groups (types) based on the number and location of the lesions and the presence or absence of associated malformations [37, 38]. This image shows a 9-year-old female patient with type 9 aplasia cutis congenita coexisting with Kabuki syndrome

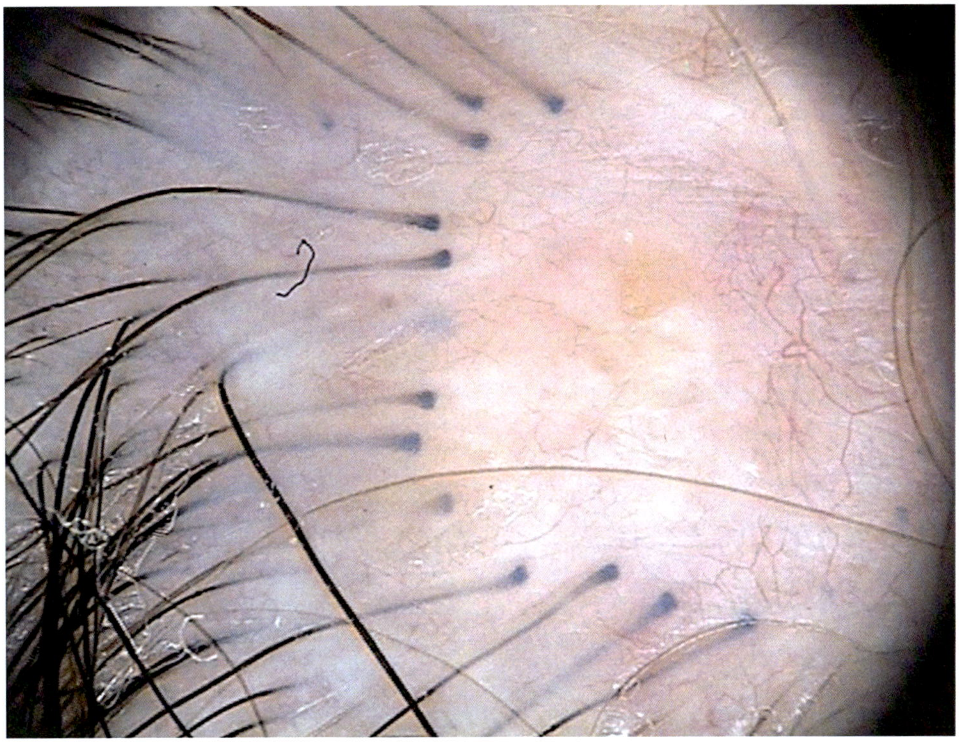

Fig. 15.12 Aplasia cutis congenita. At the hair-bearing margin, the hair shafts are arranged radially. Hair bulbs, visible through the semi-translucent epidermis, are elongated, with darkly pigmented proximal ends, which is typical of the anagen phase of the hair cycle. The midpart of the lesion shows no follicular openings. A vascular network is visible, which corresponds to skin atrophy in this area (×20)

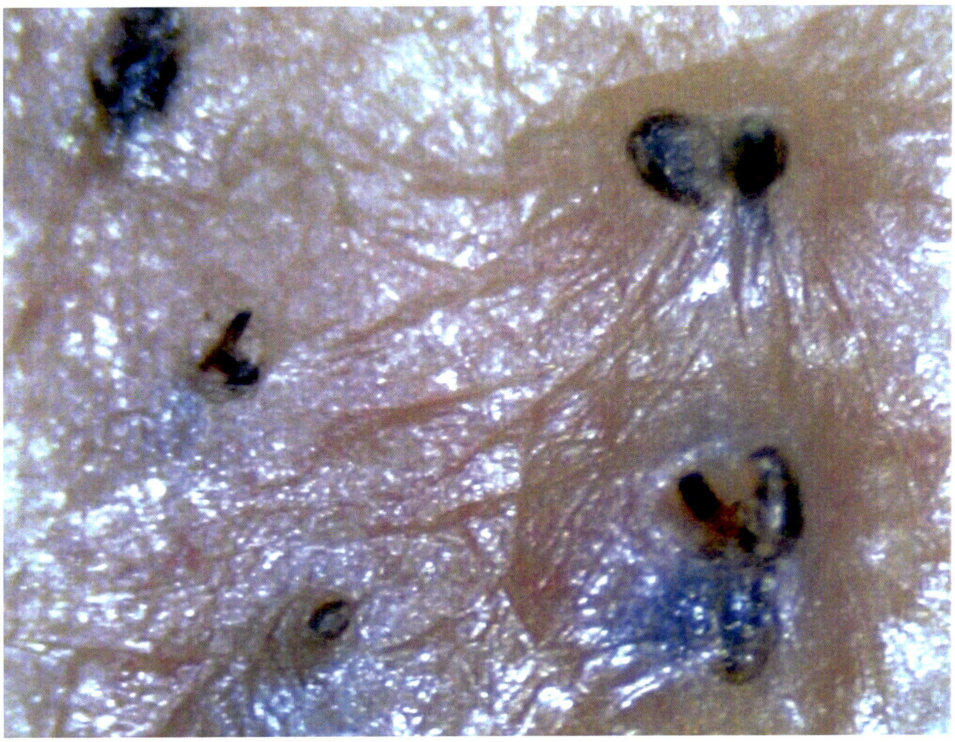

Fig. 15.13 Keratosis follicularis spinulosa decalvans. Keratosis follicularis spinulosa decalvans is a disorder associated with a missense mutation in the *MBTPS2* gene [39]. A mutation in the *SAT1* gene also has been suggested as a cause of the disease [40]. The disease is characterized by the development of hyperkeratotic follicular papules, followed by progressive cicatricial alopecia of the scalp, eyelashes, and eyebrows. Associated ocular findings include photophobia and corneal dystrophy [41–43]. In the active disease phase, trichoscopy reveals decreased hair density, dense perifollicular scaling, and follicular papules. Some papules demonstrate ingrown hairs. As the disease progresses, perifollicular scarring and starburst-like structures develop. These starburst structures differ from the hyperplastic ones seen in folliculitis decalvans in their concave, atrophic appearance. Ingrown hair residues are visible in the middle of these inverted starburst structures (×80) (*Photo courtesy of* Prof. Juan Ferrando and Prof. Ramon Grimalt)

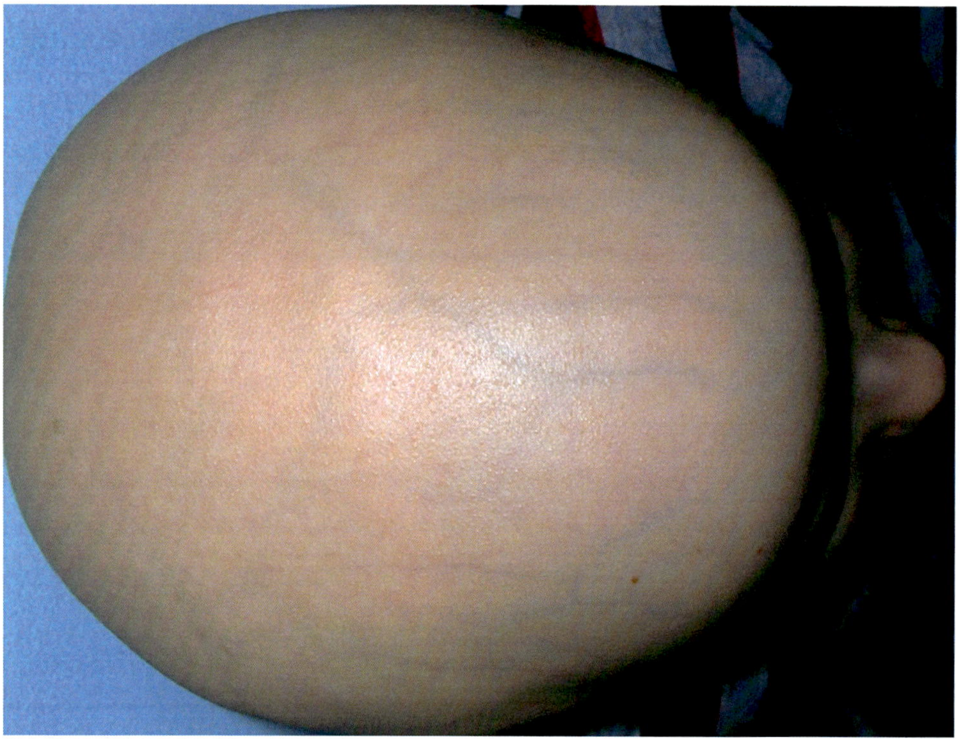

Fig. 15.14 Satoyoshi syndrome. The characteristic symptoms of Satoyoshi (Komura-Guerri) syndrome are total noncicatricial alopecia, painful muscle spasms, and diarrhea. Other clinical findings may include short stature, skeletal anomalies, and amenorrhea. Antinuclear antibodies frequently are present in high titers. Patients are asymptomatic at birth; muscle spasms start at the age of 4–19 years and usually are the initial symptom. No detailed description of hair loss is available in the literature. In the 7-year-old girl shown here, diffuse hair loss began at the age of 4 and progressed rapidly. The patient lost all her hair within 2 weeks. No alopecia areata–like focal hair loss was observed. It remains unclear whether hair loss in patients with Satoyoshi syndrome is within the spectrum of alopecia areata. So far, no hair regrowth has been reported, even in patients treated with high-dose corticosteroids and/or cyclosporine. Although several reports propose an autoimmune mechanism for the disease, others suggest that Satoyoshi syndrome may be inherited in an autosomal recessive manner [44–46]

Fig. 15.15 Satoyoshi syndrome. Trichoscopy shows regularly distributed yellow dots (hyperkeratotic plugs). The dots are arranged in groups of two or three, corresponding to the number of hairs in a follicular unit. These trichoscopic features are analogous to those observed in longstanding alopecia areata, which remains inactive over many years in adult patients. No other trichoscopic features of alopecia areata (exclamation mark hairs, black dots, regrowing hairs) were observed in this patient (dry trichoscopy, ×70)

References

1. Bennassar A, Ferrando J, Grimalt R. Congenital atrichia and hypotrichosis. World J Pediatr. 2011;7(2):111–7.
2. Wade MS, Sinclair RD. Disorders of hair in infants and children other than alopecia. Clin Dermatol. 2002;20(1):16–28.
3. Cluzeau C, Hadj-Rabia S, Jambou M, Mansour S, Guigue P, Masmoudi S, et al. Only four genes (EDA1, EDAR, EDARADD, and WNT10A) account for 90 % of hypohidrotic/anhidrotic ectodermal dysplasia cases. Hum Mutat. 2011;32(1):70–2.
4. Mikkola ML. Molecular aspects of hypohidrotic ectodermal dysplasia. Am J Med Genet A. 2009;149A(9):2031–6.
5. Salinas CF, Jorgenson RJ, Wright JT, DiGiovanna JJ, Fete MD. 2008 international conference on ectodermal dysplasias classification: conference report. Am J Med Genet A. 2009;149A(9): 1958–69.
6. Visinoni AF, Lisboa-Costa T, Pagnan NA, Chautard-Freire-Maia EA. Ectodermal dysplasias: clinical and molecular review. Am J Med Genet A. 2009;149A(9):1980–2002.
7. Simeonsson RJ. Classifying functional manifestations of ectodermal dysplasias. Am J Med Genet A. 2009;149A(9):2014–9.
8. Mehta U, Brunworth J, Fete TJ, Sindwani R. Head and neck manifestations and quality of life of patients with ectodermal dysplasia. Otolaryngol Head Neck Surg. 2007;136(5):843–7.
9. Rouse C, Siegfried E, Breer W, Nahass G. Hair and sweat glands in families with hypohidrotic ectodermal dysplasia: further characterization. Arch Dermatol. 2004;140(7):850–5.
10. Itin PH, Fistarol SK. Ectodermal dysplasias. Am J Med Genet C Semin Med Genet. 2004;131C(1):45–51.
11. Zadurska M, Rakowska A, Górska R, Rudnicka L. Hair abnormalities in patients with ectodermal dysplasia: clinical evaluation, trichogram, polarized microscopy and trichoscopy. (submitted).
12. Rudnicka L, Olszewska M, Rakowska A, Slowinska M. Trichoscopy update 2011. J Dermatol Case Rep. 2011;5(4):82–8.
13. James KA, Burkhart CN, Morrell DS. Lack of scalp and body hair on an 11-month-old girl. Pediatr Dermatol. 2010;27(6):651–2.
14. Freire-Maia N, Pinheiro M. Ectodermal dysplasias—some recollections and a classification. Birth Defects Orig Artic Ser. 1988;24(2):3–14.
15. Solomon LM, Keuer EJ. The ectodermal dysplasias. Problems of classification and some newer syndromes. Arch Dermatol. 1980;116(11):1295–9.
16. Fryns JP, Moerman P. Short limbed dwarfism, genital hypoplasia, sparse hair, and vertebral anomalies: a variant of Ellis-van Creveld syndrome? J Med Genet. 1993;30(4):322–4.
17. Rakowska A, Slowinska M, Kowalska-Oledzka E, Rudnicka L. Trichoscopy in genetic hair shaft abnormalities. J Dermatol Case Rep. 2008;2(3):14–20.
18. Zadurska M, Siemińska-Piekarczyk B, Thun-Szretter K, Rakowska A, Rudnicka L, Wysocki J. Ellis-van Creveld syndrome: case report. Pol J Environ Stud. 2010;19(6A):316–20.
19. Piccione M, Niceta M, Antona V, Di Fiore A, Cariola F, Gentile M, et al. Identification of two new mutations in TRPS 1 gene leading to the tricho-rhino-phalangeal syndrome type I and III. Am J Med Genet A. 2009;149A(8):1837–41.
20. Seitz CS, Ludecke HJ, Wagner N, Brocker EB, Hamm H. Trichorhinophalangeal syndrome type I: clinical and molecular characterization of 3 members of a family and 1 sporadic case. Arch Dermatol. 2001;137(11):1437–42.
21. Vaccaro M, Guarneri F, Barbuzza O, Gaeta M, Guarneri C. A familial case of trichorhinophalangeal syndrome type I. Pediatr Dermatol. 2009;26(2):171–5.
22. Vaccaro M, Guarneri C, Blandino A. Trichorhinophalangeal syndrome. J Am Acad Dermatol. 2005;53(5):858–60.
23. Sendi-Naderi A, Ludecke HJ, Unger S, Kern JS, Wolff G, Bruckner-Tuderman L, et al. A familial case of tricho-rhino-phalangeal syndrome type III with a novel missense mutation in exon 6 of the TRPS1 gene. J Eur Acad Dermatol Venereol. 2010;24(5): 612–4.
24. Ludecke HJ, Schaper J, Meinecke P, Momeni P, Gross S, von Holtum D, et al. Genotypic and phenotypic spectrum in tricho-rhino-phalangeal syndrome types I and III. Am J Hum Genet. 2001;68(1):81–91.
25. Lalević-Vasić BM, Nikolić MM, Polić DJ. Study of hair in type I tricho-rhino-phalangeal syndrome [in French]. Ann Dermatol Venereol. 1994;121(9):618–22.
26. Stabile M, Ametrano O, Della Bruna M, Della Monica M, Lonardo F, Strisciuglio P. Report of three cases with tricho-rhino-phalangeal syndrome type I (two cases) and type II (one case). Australas Radiol. 1988;32(3):338–42.
27. Rue M, Ludecke HJ, Sibon I, Richez C, Taine L, Foubert-Samier A, et al. Rheumatologic and neurological events in an elderly patient with tricho-rhino-phalangeal syndrome type I. Eur J Med Genet. 2011;54(4):e405–8.
28. Niikawa N, Kamei T. The Sugio-Kajii syndrome, proposed tricho-rhino-phalangeal syndrome type III. Am J Med Genet. 1986;24(4): 759–60.
29. Rudnicka L, Olszewska M, Rakowska A. Trichoscopy and reflectance confocal microscopy of the scalp in trichorhinophalangeal syndrome. J Dermatol Case Rep. 2013 (in press).
30. Okita M, Nakanishi G, Fujimoto N, Kishida M, Tanaka T. Incontinentia pigmenti with NEMO mutation in a Japanese family. J Dermatol. 2012. doi:10.1111/j.1346-8138.2011.01496.x.
31. Lin SY, Tsao PN, Hsieh WS, Hung CC, Su YN. Genetic mutation in male patients with incontinentia pigmenti. J Formos Med Assoc. 2011;110(11):726.
32. Fryssira H, Kakourou T, Valari M, Stefanaki K, Amenta S, Kanavakis E. Incontinentia pigmenti revisited. A novel nonsense mutation of the IKBKG gene. Acta Paediatr. 2011;100(1): 128–33.
33. Succi IB, Rosman FC, Oliveira EF. Do you know this syndrome? An Bras Dermatol. 2011;86(3):608–10.
34. Bakry O, Attia A, El Shafey EN. Adams-Oliver syndrome. A case with isolated aplasia cutis congenita and skeletal defects. J Dermatol Case Rep. 2012;6(1):25–8.
35. Ribuffo D, Costantini M, Gullo P, Houseman ND, Taylor GI. Aplasia cutis congenita of the scalp, the skull, and the dura. Scand J Plast Reconstr Surg Hand Surg. 2003;37(3):176–80.
36. Mihci E, Erisir S, Tacoy S, Luleci G, Alpsoy E, Oygur N. Aplasia cutis congenita: three cases with three different underlying etiologies. Turk J Pediatr. 2009;51(5):510–4.
37. Morrow D, Schelonka R, Krol A, Davies M, Kuang A. Type V aplasia cutis congenita: case report, review of the literature, and proposed treatment algorithm. Pediatr Dermatol. 2012. doi:10.1111/j.1525-1470.2012.01742.x.
38. Frieden IJ. Aplasia cutis congenita: a clinical review and proposal for classification. J Am Acad Dermatol. 1986;14(4):646–60.
39. Aten E, Brasz LC, Bornholdt D, Hooijkaas IB, Porteous ME, Sybert VP, et al. Keratosis follicularis spinulosa decalvans is caused by mutations in MBTPS2. Hum Mutat. 2010;31(10):1125–33.
40. Gimelli G, Giglio S, Zuffardi O, Alhonen L, Suppola S, Cusano R, et al. Gene dosage of the spermidine/spermine N(1)-acetyltransferase (SSAT) gene with putrescine accumulation in a patient with a Xp21.1p22.12 Duplication and keratosis follicularis spinulosa decalvans (KFSD). Hum Genet. 2002;111(3):235–41.
41. Sequeira FF, Jayaseelan E. Keratosis follicularis spinulosa decalvans in a female. Indian J Dermatol Venereol Leprol. 2011;77(3): 325–7.

42. Castori M, Covaciu C, Paradisi M, Zambruno G. Clinical and genetic heterogeneity in keratosis follicularis spinulosa decalvans. Eur J Med Genet. 2009;52(1):53–8.
43. Bellet JS, Kaplan AL, Selim MA, Olsen EA. Keratosis follicularis spinulosa decalvans in a family. J Am Acad Dermatol. 2008;58(3): 499–502.
44. Venegas-Vega CA, Rivera-Vega MR, Cuevas-Covarrubias S, Orozco J, Kofman-Alfaro S. Satoyoshi syndrome with unusual skeletal abnormalities and parental consanguinity. Am J Med Genet A. 2009;149A(11):2448–51.
45. Mukhopadhyay D, Ghosh A, Mukhopadhyay M. Satoyoshi syndrome. Indian Pediatr. 2011;48(9):729–31.
46. Heger S, Kuester RM, Volk R, Stephani U, Sippell WG. Satoyoshi syndrome: a rare multisystemic disorder requiring systemic and symptomatic treatment. Brain Dev. 2006;28(5):300–4.

Part VII

Acquired Nonscarring Alopecia

Alopecia Areata

16

Lidia Rudnicka, Malgorzata Olszewska,
Adriana Rakowska, and Joanna Czuwara

Abstract

The hallmark trichoscopic features of alopecia areata are regularly distributed yellow dots, micro–exclamation mark hairs, tapered hairs, black dots, broken hairs, and upright and regularly coiled (circle, pigtail) regrowing hairs. Trichorrhexis nodosa may be observed, especially in active, early alopecia areata. It must be emphasized that micro–exclamation mark hairs are not pathognomonic for alopecia areata. Trichoscopy of alopecia areata may differ depending on disease activity, severity, and duration.

Keywords

Alopecia areata • Black dots • Broken hairs • Cadaverized hairs • Circle hairs • Exclamation mark hairs • Micro–exclamation mark hairs • Pigtail hairs • Pohl-Pinkus constriction Regularly coiled hairs • Tapered hairs • Upright regrowing hairs • Yellow dots • Trichorrhexis nodosa • Trichotillomania • Vellus hairs

The hallmark trichoscopic features of alopecia areata are regularly distributed yellow dots, micro–exclamation mark hairs, tapered hairs, black dots (formerly called cadaverous hairs), broken hairs, and regrowing upright or regrowing coiled hairs. Trichoscopy of alopecia areata may differ depending on disease activity, severity, and duration. These differences were evaluated in several studies during recent years.

In 2004, Lacarrubba et al. [1] investigated 200 patients with alopecia areata, subdivided into acute and chronic disease. This study identified three features of acute alopecia areata: micro–exclamation marks, black dots, and vellus hairs. In chronic alopecia areata of recent onset, the scalp skin was smooth and thin, with evident follicular openings. In cases of longstanding chronic alopecia areata, the hair follicle openings appeared to be obstructed by keratotic plugs. In some patients, trichoscopy revealed hair regrowth, with a homogeneous or sparse presence of pigmented regrowing hairs. These hairs differ from delicate, hypopigmented vellus hairs in their dark pigmentation and upright position.

In a 2006 study in 58 patients with alopecia areata, Ross et al. [2] found yellow dots, exclamation mark hairs, black dots, and dystrophic hairs as the most characteristic trichoscopic features. These features were similarly expressed on trichoscopy of all investigated subgroups of alopecia areata: patchy, ophiasis, diffuse, and alopecia totalis/universalis.

Inui et al. [3] identified markers of disease activity and severity based on trichoscopy performed in 300 patients with alopecia areata. The results of this study show that the presence of black dots, tapering hairs, and broken hairs correlates positively with disease activity, whereas short vellus hairs correlate negatively. Yellow dots tend to be present more commonly in patients with inactive alopecia areata than in those with active disease.

Our experience shows that black dots are a very consistent marker of disease activity [4]. Mane et al. [5] showed that the

L. Rudnicka (✉)
Faculty of Health Sciences, Medical University of Warsaw, Poland

Department of Dermatology, CSK MSW,
Woloska 137, Warsaw 02-502, Poland
e-mail: lidia.rudnicka@euderm.eu

M. Olszewska
Department of Dermatology, Medical University of Warsaw,
Warsaw, Poland

A. Rakowska • J. Czuwara
Department of Dermatology, CSK MSW, Warsaw, Poland

L. Rudnicka et al. (eds.), *Atlas of Trichoscopy*,
DOI 10.1007/978-1-4471-4486-1_16, © Springer-Verlag London 2012

mean duration of disease in patients showing broken hairs on trichoscopy was 5.31 months. The mean disease duration in patients not showing broken hairs was 16.33 months; these findings may indicate that broken hairs tend to correlate with short disease duration. In this study, no statistically significant positive or negative correlation was found between disease severity and any trichoscopic feature. In this investigation, monilethrix-like (Pohl-Pinkus) hair shaft constrictions were observed in two of 66 patients (3 %) with alopecia areata.

In patients with diffuse alopecia areata of many years' duration, trichoscopy may not show any characteristic features, not even dots, which mark hair follicle openings [3].

Features of hair regrowth include pigmented short upright regrowing hairs [3] and regularly coiled ring (pigtail) hairs [4].

A recent study from Turkey performed with a handheld dermoscope confirmed earlier data obtained by digital videodermoscopy [6].

The most common and most difficult differential diagnosis is trichotillomania, which is characterized by decreased hair density, hairs broken at different lengths, irregularly coiled hairs, and sparse yellow dots that may or may not contain black dots [7].

Table 16.1 Trichoscopic features of alopecia areata

Feature	Patients, %[a]
Black dots	44–70
Micro–exclamation mark hairs	30–44
Tapered hairs	12–42
Broken hairs	45–58
Yellow dots	63–94
Vellus hairs	33–72
Trichorrhexis nodosa	3–16
Monilethrix-like hairs	2–3
Pohl-Pinkus constrictions	–
Upright regrowing hairs	–
Pigtail (circular) regrowing hairs	–
Zigzag hairs	–

[a]The ranges from published articles [1–10] are given for the trichoscopic features for which frequency was evaluated

Table 16.2 Trichoscopic features of alopecia areata

Active hair loss	Longstanding inactive disease	Hair regrowth
Black dots	Yellow dots	Upright regrowing hairs
Micro–exclamation mark hairs	Vellus hairs	Pigtail hairs (oval or circular)
Broken hairs	Follicular openings may not be visible	Vellus hairs
Monilethrix-like hairs		
Trichorrhexis nodosa		

Box 16.1

- Micro–exclamation mark hairs are not pathognomonic for alopecia areata
- Micro–exclamation mark hairs may be present in trichotillomania and traction alopecia

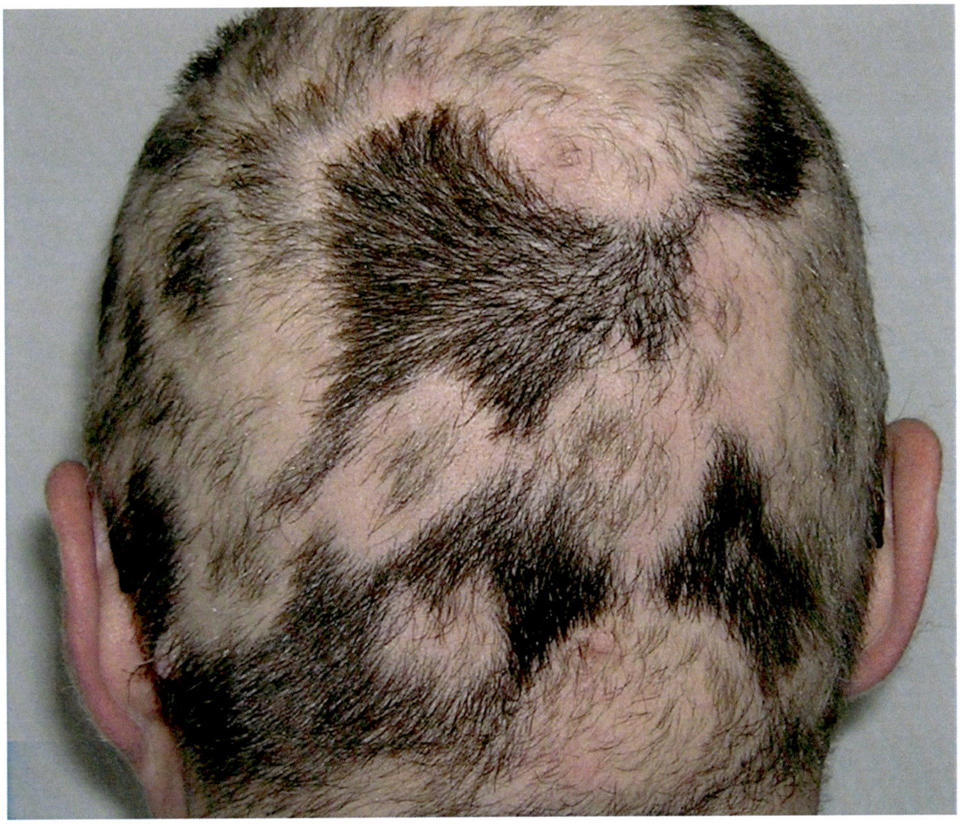

Fig. 16.1 Alopecia areata. Alopecia areata may occur on any hair-bearing area, but it affects the scalp in about 90 % of patients seen in dermatologic practice. The disease may be classified based on the extent or pattern of hair loss [11]. Trichoscopic results of alopecia areata are similar in all clinical subtypes of the disease; differences on trichoscopy depend on disease activity. This image shows a phase of partial regrowth in a patient with patchy alopecia areata treated with cyclosporine

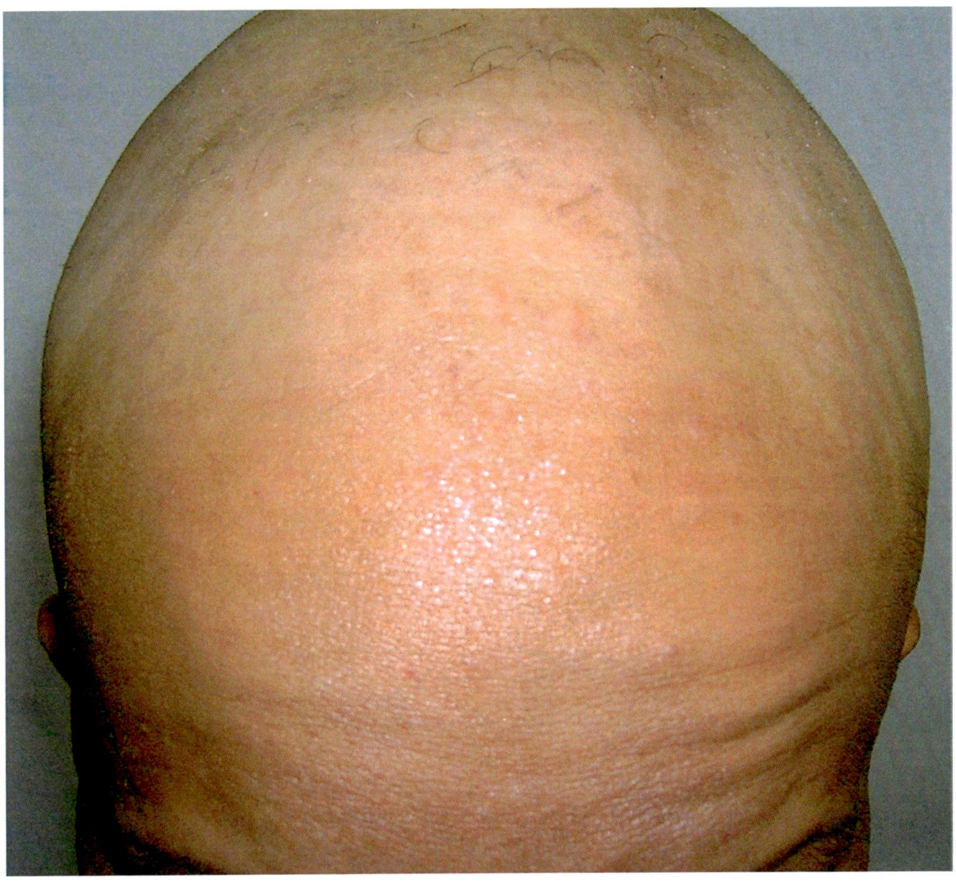

Fig. 16.2 Alopecia totalis. Alopecia totalis, in which 100 % of the scalp hair is lost, and alopecia universalis, in which there is 100 % loss of all scalp and body hair, may be difficult to diagnose by trichoscopy. A hint may be provided by the presence of regularly distributed yellow dots. However, in longstanding alopecia areata, even the yellow dots may no longer be visible. Inui and Itami [12] described a case of alopecia areata in which yellow dots reappeared after 2 months of topical corticosteroid therapy. This experience shows that repeated trichoscopic examinations may be useful in patients with an uncertain diagnosis

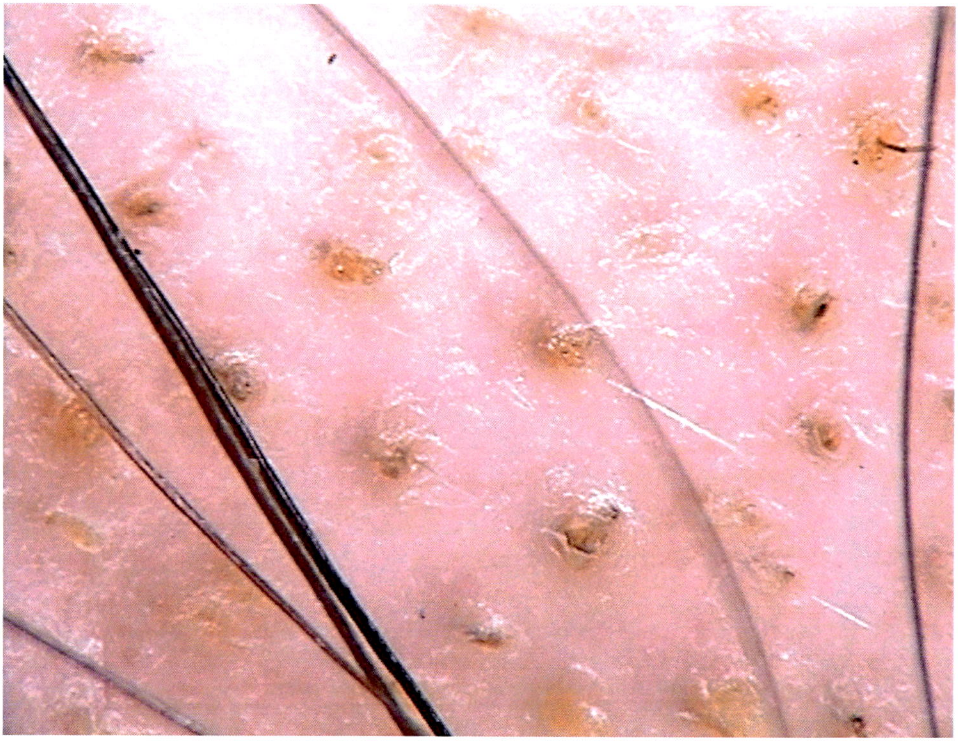

Fig. 16.3 Yellow dots in alopecia areata. Yellow dots are hyperkeratotic plugs that fill the follicular infundibula. This dry trichoscopic image shows the hyperkeratotic nature of these structures in a patient with longstanding alopecia areata. This "three-dimensional" structure may not be visible in patients who use topical therapies and when immersion fluid is used. For detailed information about yellow dots, see Chap. 3 (dry trichoscopy; ×70)

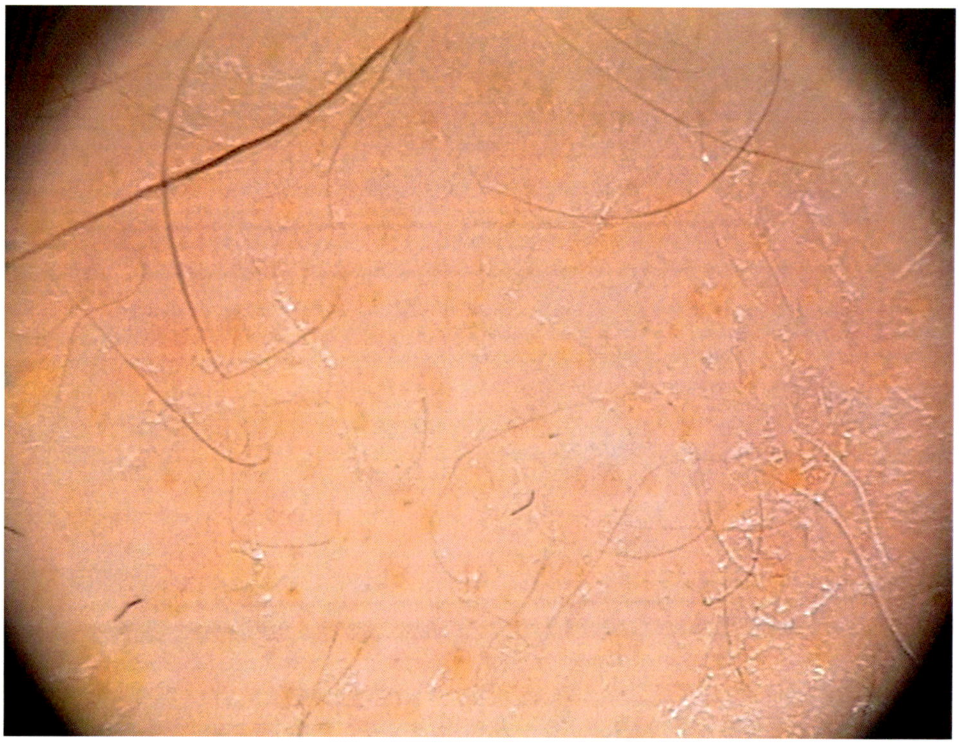

Fig. 16.4 Yellow dots in alopecia areata. A characteristic feature of yellow dots in alopecia areata is their relatively regular distribution. They are arranged in groups of two or three, reflecting the number of hair shafts per follicular unit. Accordingly, these groups may be less evident in the frontal area, where the proportion of follicular units with only one hair is usually higher. Yellow dots may be less visible in alopecia areata in Asian patients. See Chap. 38 for details about trichoscopy in Asian patients (×20)

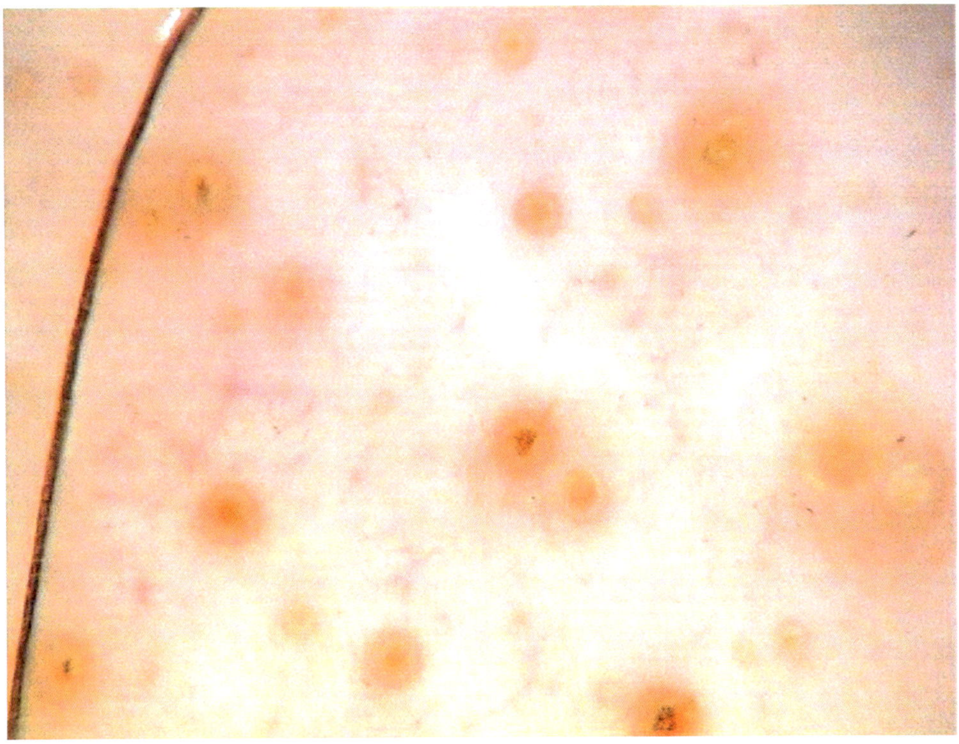

Fig. 16.5 Yellow dots in alopecia areata. High magnification shows that yellow dots may differ in size and color. A double margin may be observed in most dots. In this image, taken from the frontal area of a male patient with coexistent androgenetic alopecia, yellow dots do not appear in groups of two or three. Single yellow dots represent follicular units with only one hair (×70)

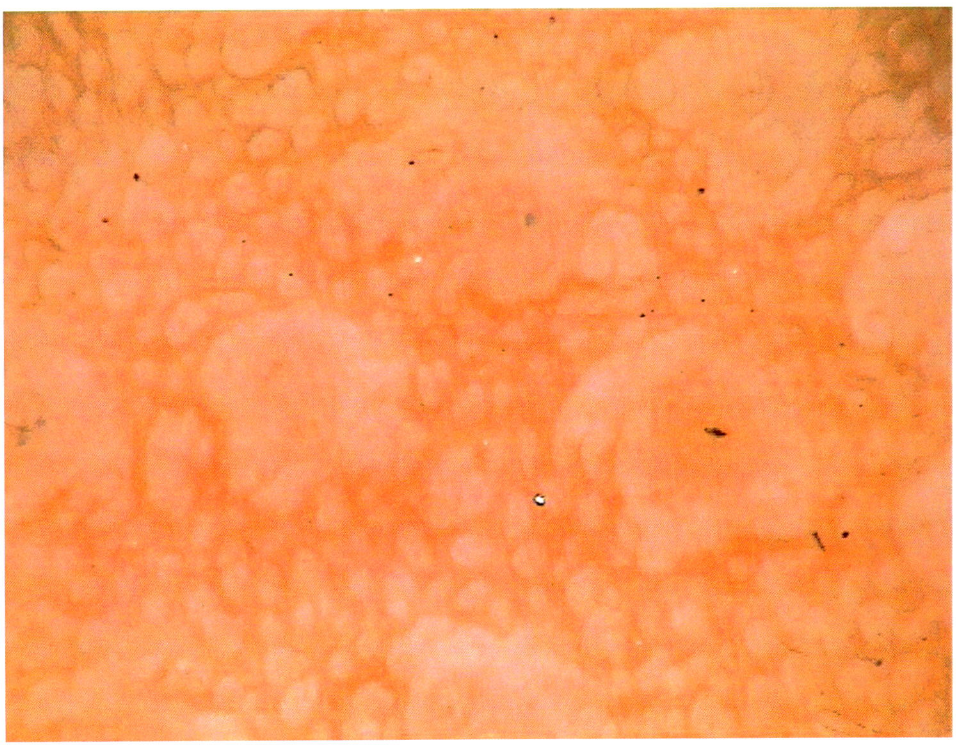

Fig. 16.6 Yellow dots in alopecia areata in sun-exposed skin. On intensely sun-exposed skin and in patients with dark skin phototypes, yellow dots may appear differently from those on untanned Caucasian skin. The background color is determined by the honeycomb pigmentation. Yellow dots must be differentiated from eccrine duct openings (small white dots) and from normal follicular openings (pinpoint white dots). Yellow dots have a yellowish color with a white halo, are regularly distributed, and are arranged in groups of two or three, as seen here. For details about trichoscopy in dark skin, see Chap. 39 (×70)

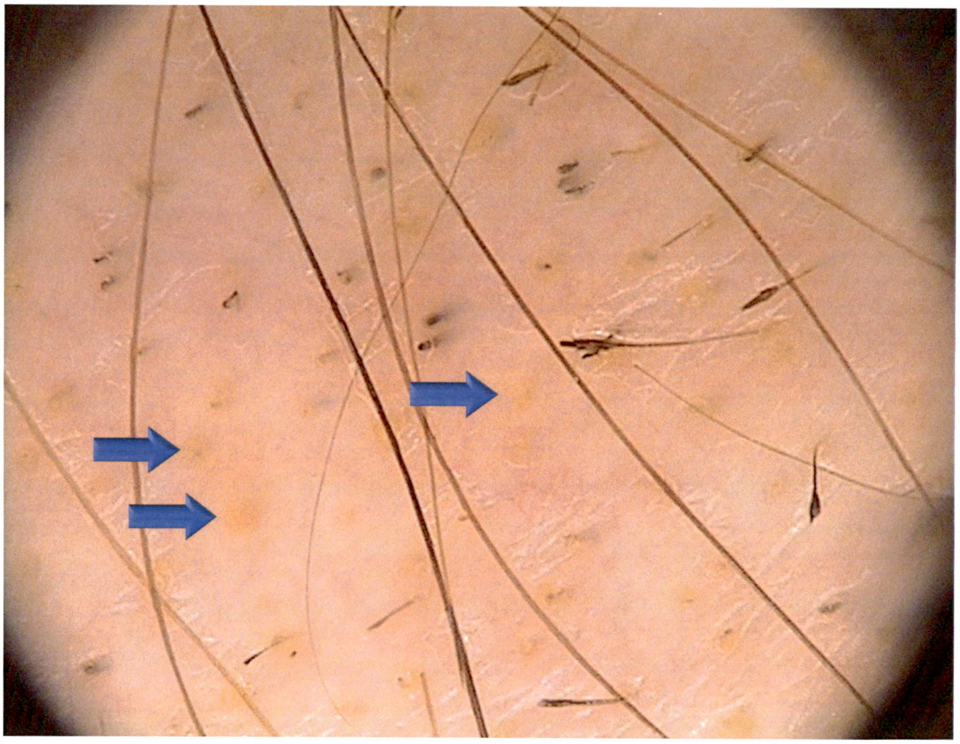

Fig. 16.7 Yellow and black dots in alopecia areata. This image shows multiple yellow dots (*arrows*). coexisting with black dots. Black dots (formerly also called "cadaverous hairs") are pigmented residues of hairs destroyed and broken at scalp level. They are present in 44–70 % of patients with alopecia areata and are a marker of active disease (×20)

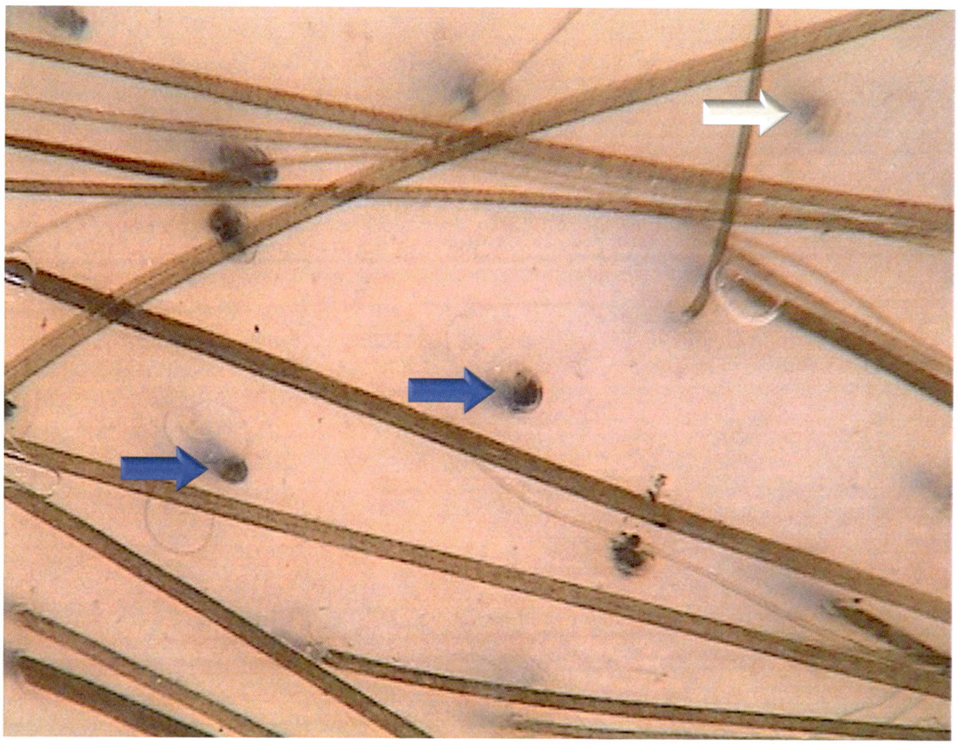

Fig. 16.8 Black dots in alopecia areata. Black dots may be clearly visible as fragments of pigmented hair shafts (*blue arrows*) but may be less noticeable when covered by the epidermis (*white arrow*). Black dots are slightly larger than the thickness of terminal hair shafts at the same location. Black dots are frequent in alopecia areata, but they are not specific. Accordingly, an image such as this one, with no other associated features of the disease, does not allow the trichoscopic diagnosis of alopecia areata to be established. Trichotillomania must be considered as the primary differential diagnosis. For detailed information about black dots, see Chap. 3 (×70)

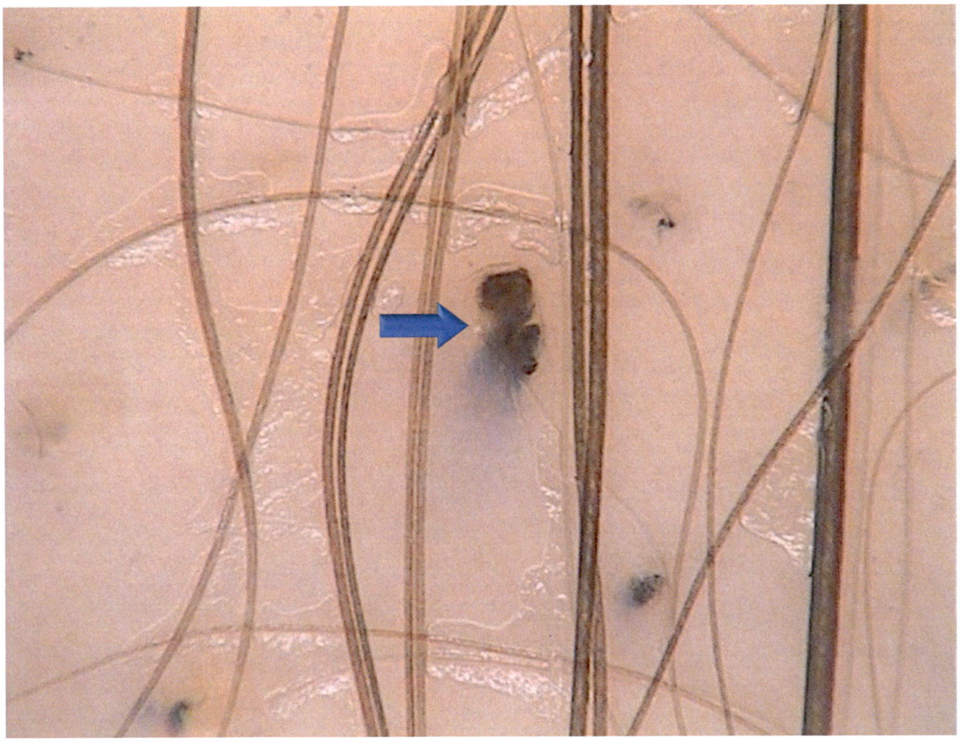

Fig. 16.9 Short damaged hair in alopecia areata. Short damaged hairs may appear as black dots on handheld trichoscopy. They are amorphous black structures emerging from the follicular openings (*arrow*). They may be significantly wider than the terminal hairs in the field of view, which probably is the result of shrinkage of the damaged hair shaft (×70)

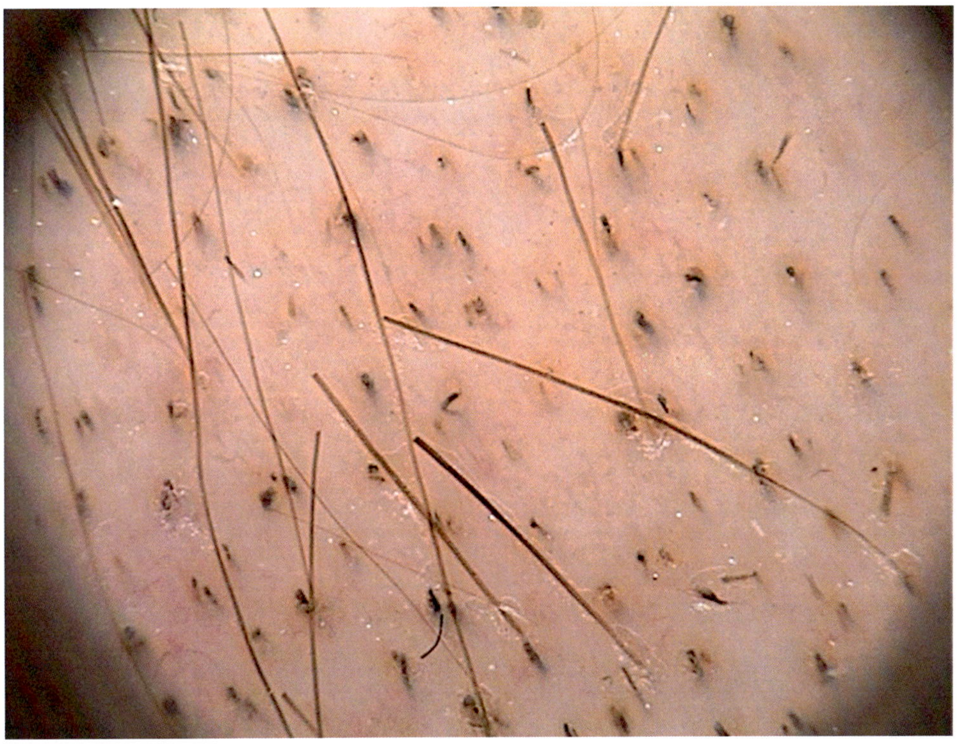

Fig. 16.10 Broken hair in alopecia areata. In alopecia areata, broken hairs may develop in two ways. One is transverse fracture of terminal hair shafts weakened by the inflammatory process. In such cases, hair fracturing may be preceded by monilethrix-like hairs (Pohl-Pinkus constriction) or by trichorrhexis nodosa in the course of the disease. The other possibility is rapid regrowth of incompletely destroyed hair shafts that previously formed the black dots. In alopecia areata, hairs usually are broken at the same level above the skin surface, whereas in trichotillomania every broken hair has a different length. Broken hairs are observed in 45–58 % of patients with alopecia areata (×20)

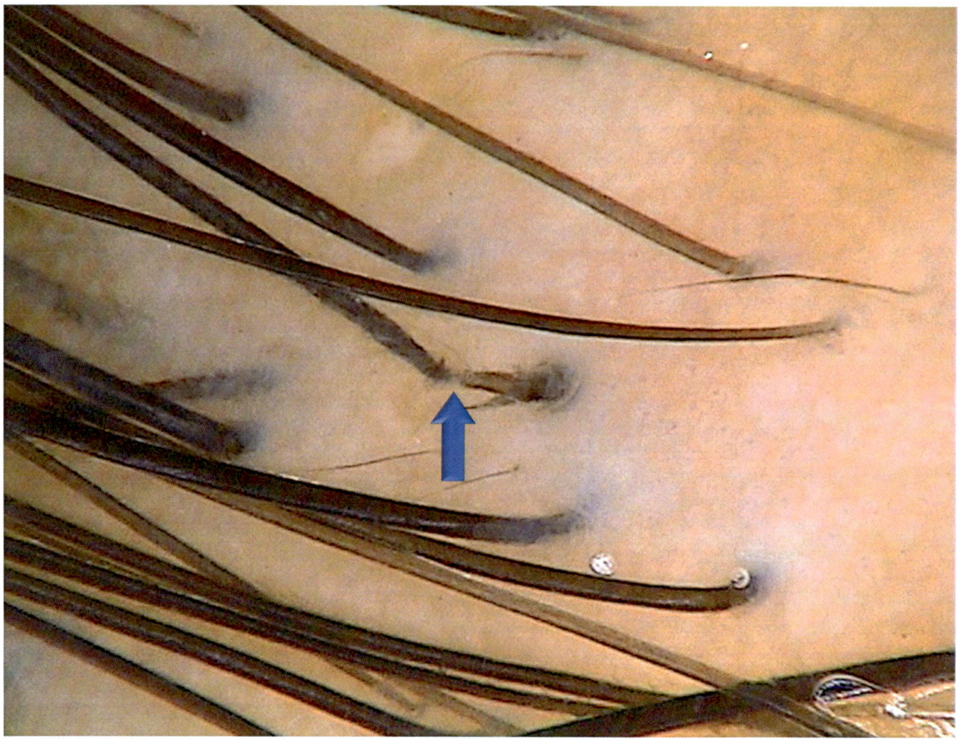

Fig. 16.11 Broken and tapered hair in alopecia areata; a Pohl-Pinkus constriction. This image shows a mechanism by which broken hairs are formed in alopecia areata. A hair shaft with a constriction in its midpart (Pohl-Pinkus constriction) breaks at its weakest point (*arrow*). Note that Pohl-Pinkus constrictions start forming in other hair shafts. The proximal end of these hairs is thinner than their distal end. These hair shafts fulfill the definition of tapered hairs. Tapered hairs may follow one of two pathways. The hair shafts may slowly regain their normal thickness. When the hairs grow, only a Pohl-Pinkus constriction will be seen as a reminder of the process. This will remain a weak point in the hair shafts, which may eventually break at constriction sites, as shown here. Another possibility is that with the ongoing inflammatory process, the hair shafts will become increasingly thinner and break at scalp level. This pathway will produce the image of black dots (×70)

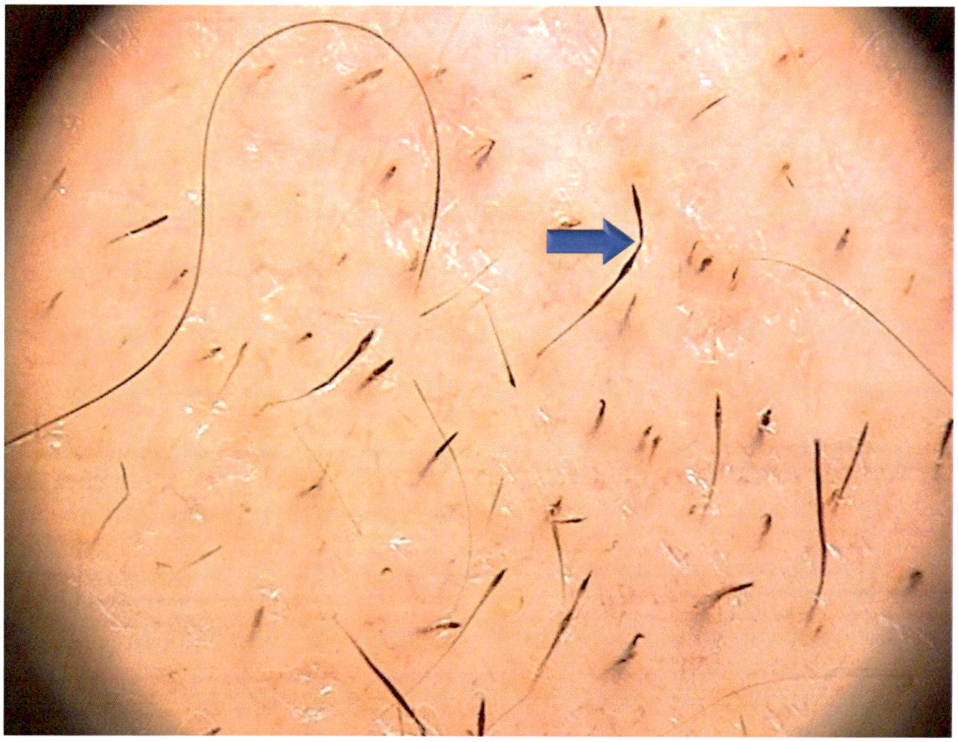

Fig. 16.12 Monilethrix-like hairs in alopecia areata. Repeated formation of Pohl-Pinkus constrictions during the course of a disease with variable activity results in the formation of monilethrix-like hairs (*arrow*). These are constrictions in the hair shaft that occur at irregular intervals. These hairs bend and then break at the constriction sites (×20)

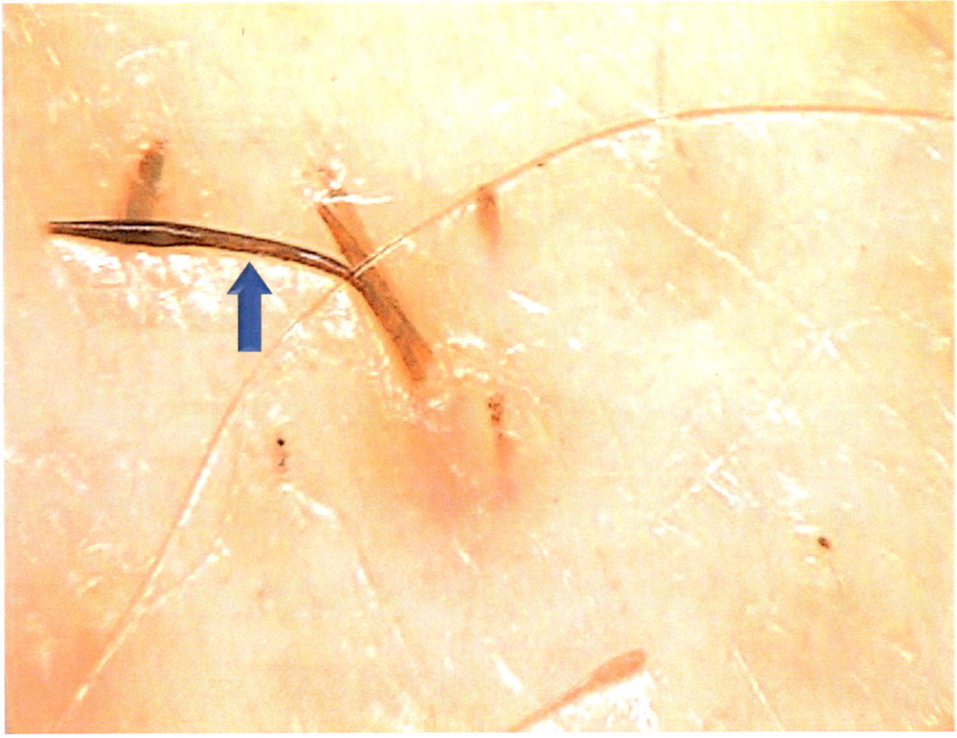

Fig. 16.13 **Monilethrix-like hairs in alopecia areata**. Shown is a high-magnification view of a monilethrix-like hair in alopecia areata that is fractured at one constriction site. Note that the constricted area (*arrow*) of the hair shaft is hypopigmented. The hair shaft has two nodosities (parts of the hair that are thicker than the constricted sites); one is thicker and longer than the other. This irregularity differentiates monilethrix-like hairs from true monilethrix (×70)

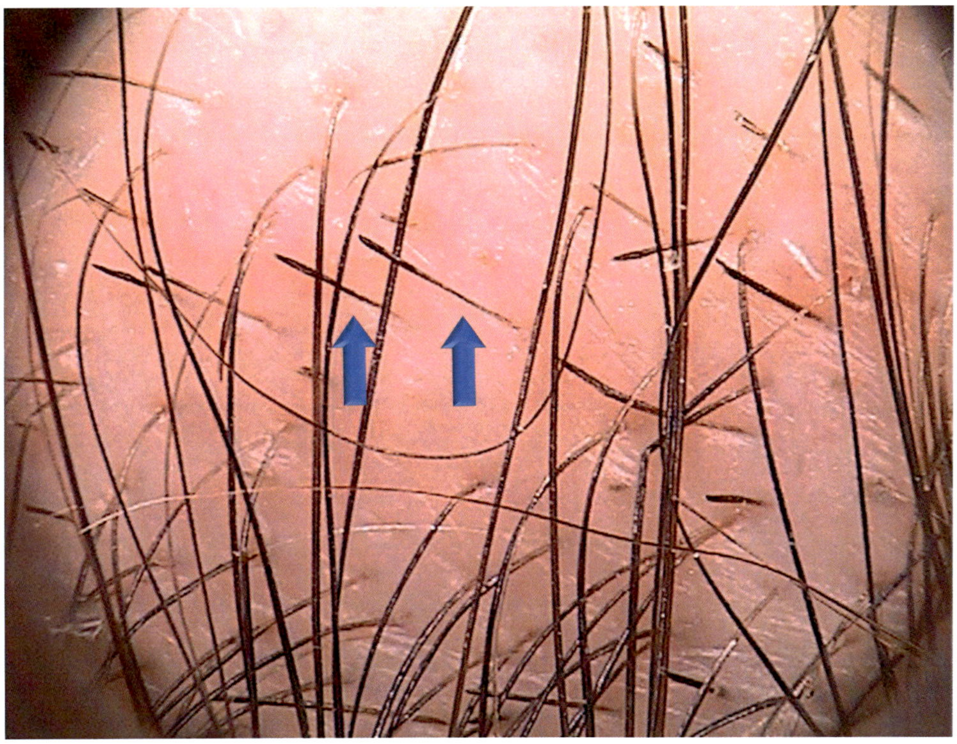

Fig. 16.14 **Micro–exclamation mark hairs in alopecia areata**. Exclamation mark hairs are hairs that are thin at the proximal end and thicker at the distal end. Exclamation mark hairs observed on trichoscopy (*arrows*) are also called micro–exclamation mark hairs. Normal exclamation mark hairs, which are visible to the naked eye, are approximately 1 cm (~ 0.5 in) long, whereas trichoscopy allows visualization of exclamation mark hairs that are 1 to 2 mm long. To differentiate between these two types of hairs, the term *micro–exclamation mark hairs* was introduced [13]. Morphologic analysis of hair follicles indicates that exclamation mark hairs in alopecia areata may result from a transient phase of cell degeneration among precortical keratinocytes and defective cortex differentiation [14] (×20)

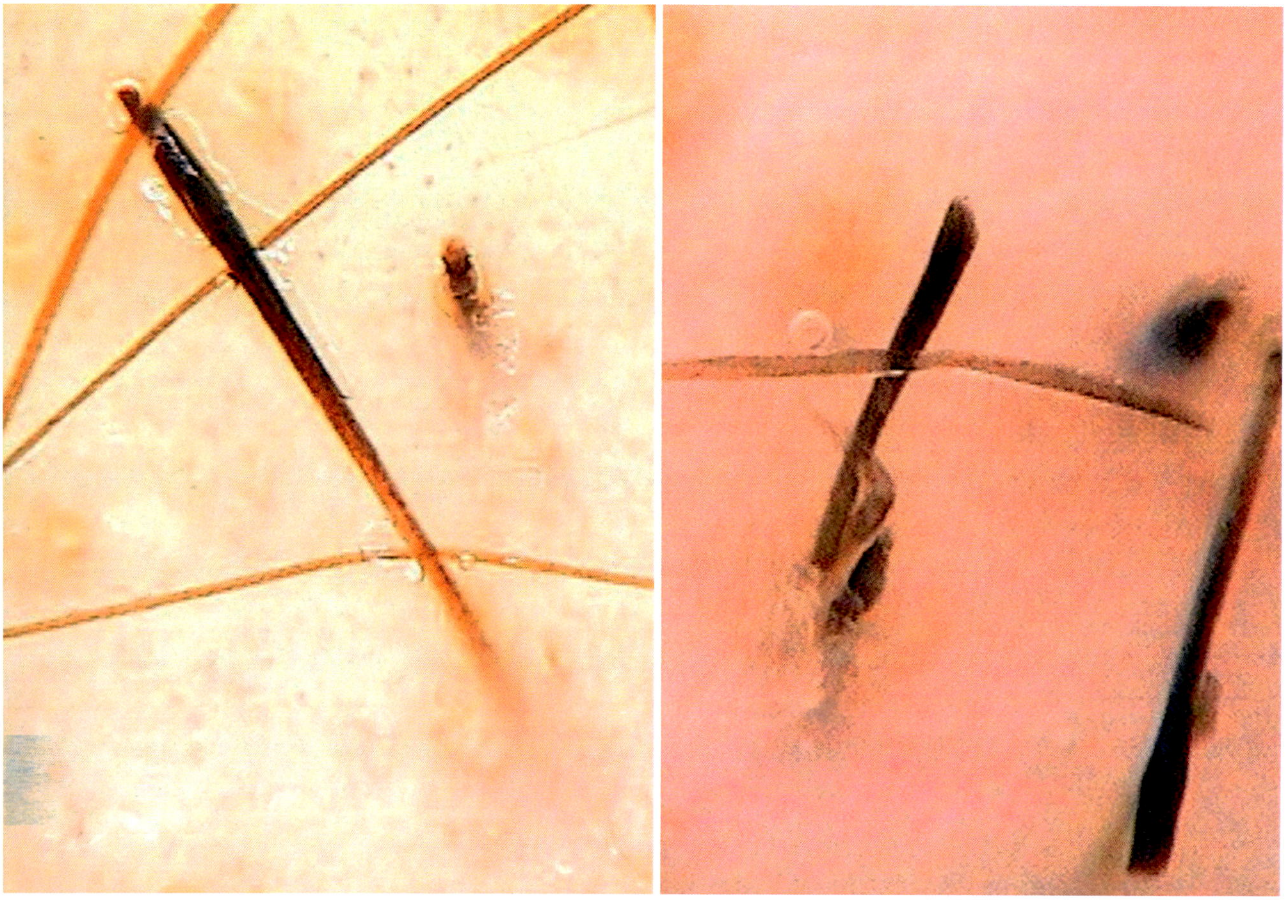

Fig. 16.15 **Micro–exclamation mark hairs in alopecia areata (*left*) and trichotillomania (*right*).** Exclamation mark hairs sometimes are wrongly interpreted as pathognomonic for alopecia areata. This may lead to misdiagnosis, because exclamation mark hairs are not uncommon in trichotillomania and other forms of traction alopecia [15, 16]. Light microscopic studies show that most exclamation mark hairs (77.8 %) in alopecia areata have irregular frayed distal ends, whereas most (82.2 %) of those in trichotillomania have blunt distal ends [15]. The authors of this study emphasize that exclamation mark hairs, even those with irregular frayed distal ends, are not pathognomonic for alopecia areata. On trichoscopy of alopecia areata, most micro–exclamation mark hairs have a hypopigmented proximal end and a pointed distal end (*left*). The pointed distal end is produced by a fracture at the site of a constriction. Most micro–exclamation mark hairs in trichotillomania do not have a clearly hypopigmented proximal end, and their distal end is flattened. The image (*right*) shows two micro–exclamation mark hairs of this type. It must be emphasized that neither type of exclamation mark hair is pathognomonic for alopecia areata or trichotillomania (×70)

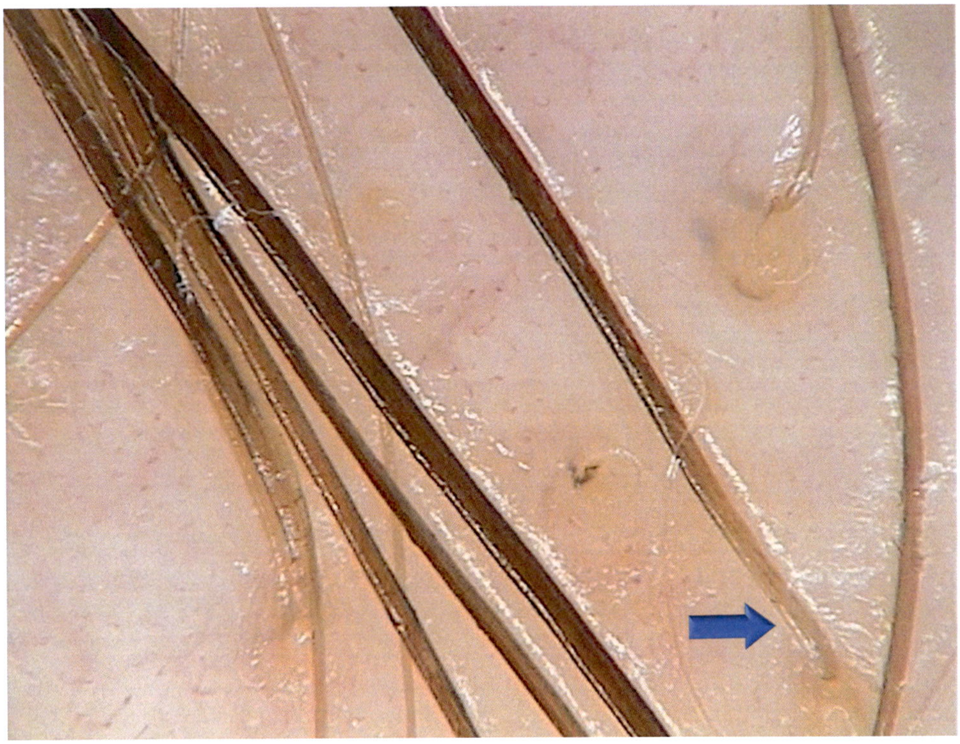

Fig. 16.16 Tapered hairs in alopecia areata. Tapered hairs (*arrow*) are very long micro–exclamation mark hairs. They are thin at the proximal end and become thicker distally, but the distal end is not visible in the dermoscopic field of view. Unlike micro–exclamation mark hairs, which are a marker of very active disease, tapered hairs slowly become thinner as they grow, which reflects low disease activity. They rarely are hypopigmented at the proximal end. Tapered hairs are not pathognomonic for alopecia areata (×70)

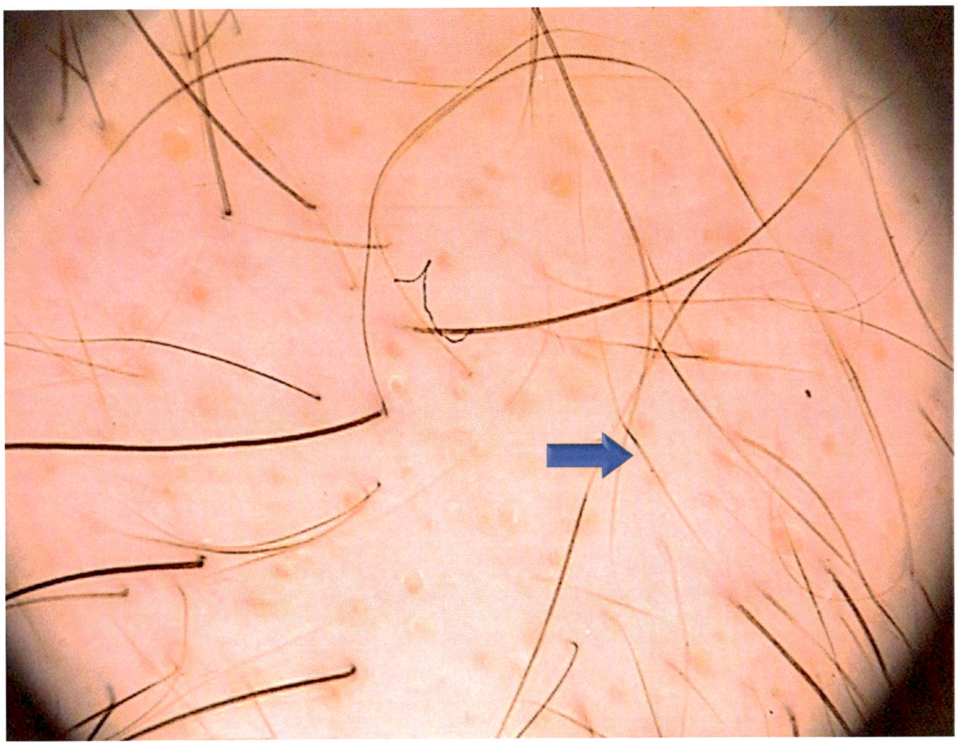

Fig. 16.17 Hair shafts of variable thickness in alopecia areata. These hairs (*arrow*) are thin at the proximal end, becoming thicker in the midpart and then thinner again toward the distal end, reflecting the variable disease activity in this patient. Some hairs tend to become thicker toward the proximal end, whereas others become thinner. This reflects the differences in inflammatory activity among the hair follicles (×20)

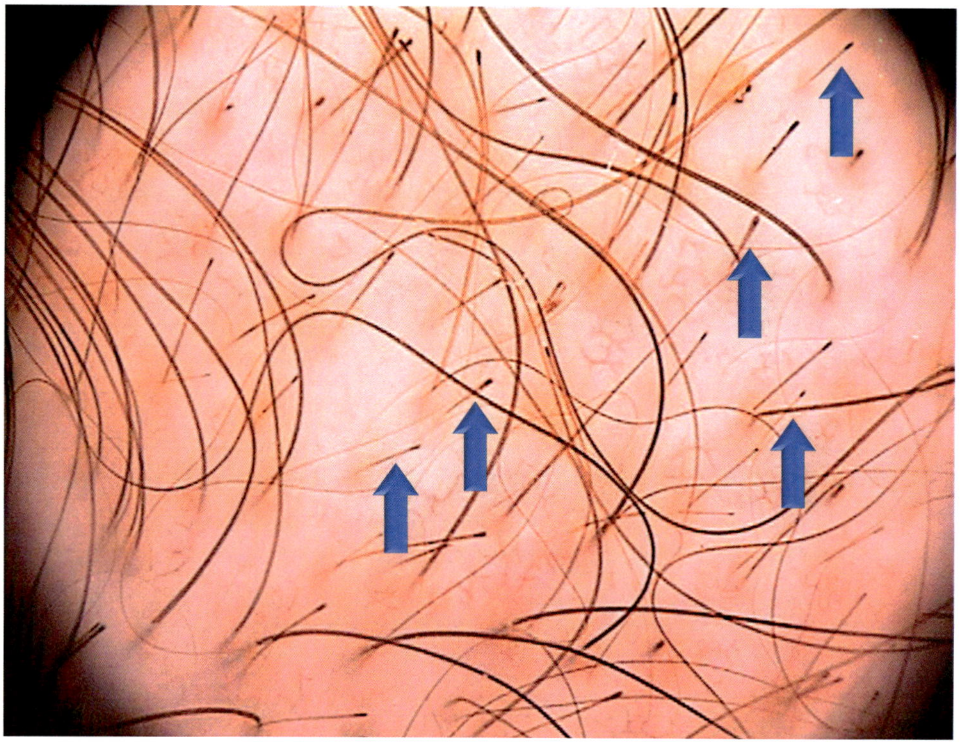

Fig. 16.18 Tulip hairs in alopecia areata. Tulip hairs (*arrows*) differ from exclamation mark hairs in that they are only slightly thinned at the proximal end and have light-colored hair shafts with only a dark distal end. The dark distal end corresponds to an area of increased pigmentation exhibiting a tulip leaf–like shape (see Chap. 2 for details). We hypothesize that this darker portion of the hair shaft corresponds to an area of oblique hair rupture. These short hairs are observed on trichoscopy of alopecia areata and trichotillomania [4] (×70)

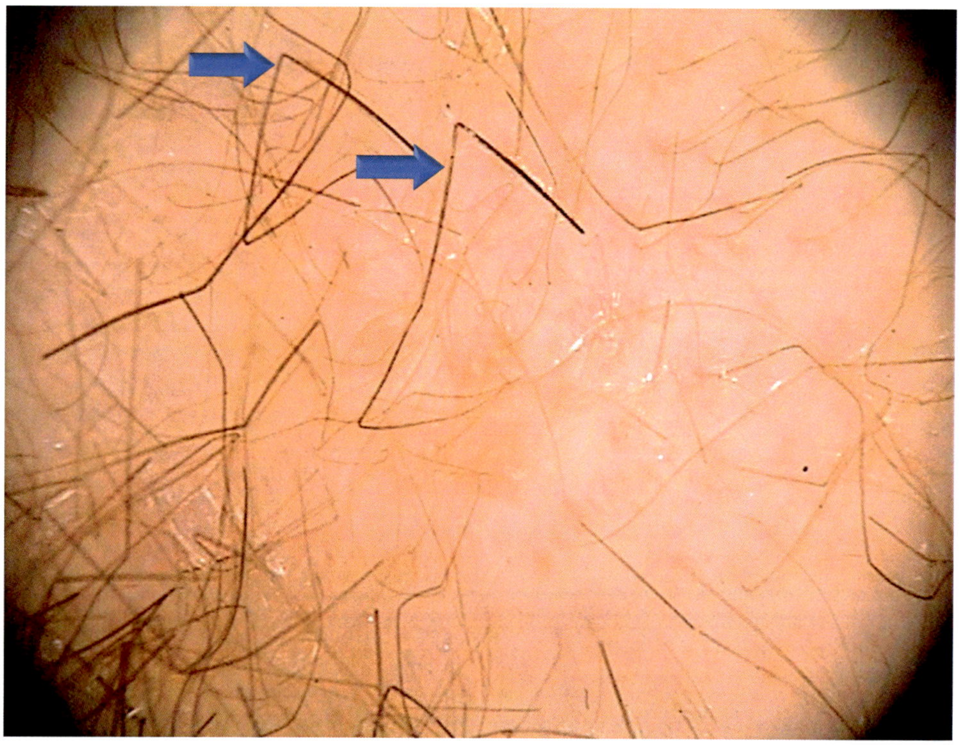

Fig. 16.19 Zigzag hairs in alopecia areata. Kinky, zigzag hairs (*arrows*) are commonly observed in active alopecia areata of recent onset. Hairs bend at sites of trichorrhexis nodosa or without visible hair shaft abnormality. This type of image should not be misdiagnosed as tinea capitis [4] (×20)

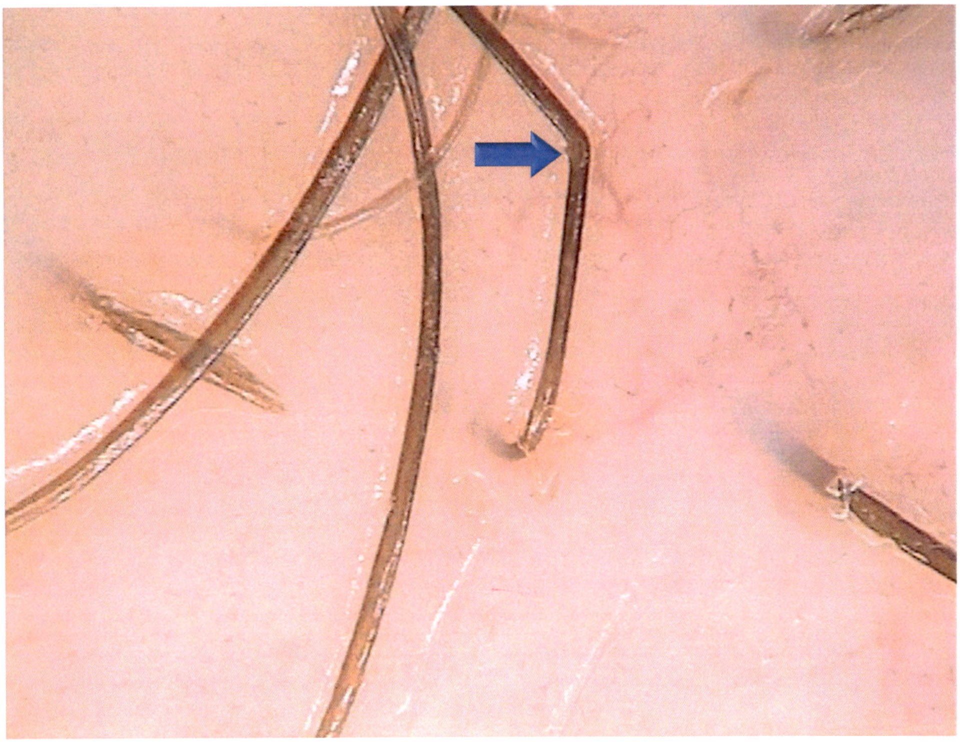

Fig. 16.20 Zigzag hairs in alopecia areata. This image shows a bent fragment of a zigzag hair and a fractured hair shaft. The flexures of zigzag hairs in alopecia areata are sites of increased hair fragility. This close-up view of the bending site shows no features of trichorrhexis nodosa, but a small indentation in the hair shaft is visible (*arrow*) (×70)

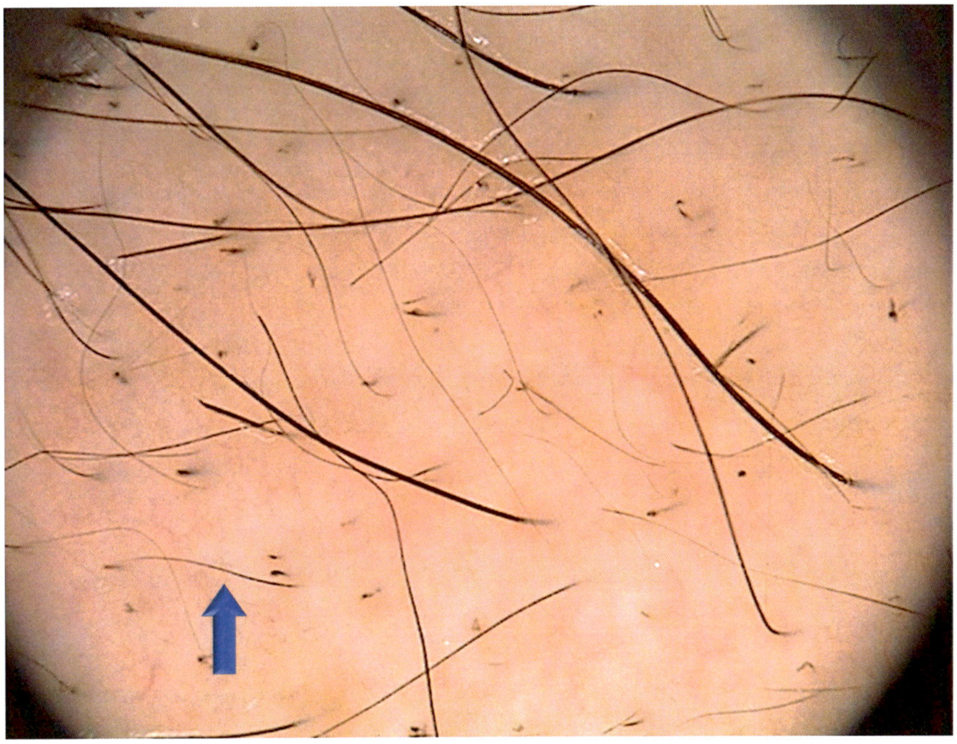

Fig. 16.21 Upright regrowing hairs in alopecia areata. Trichoscopy allows visualization of upright regrowing hairs. These anagen hairs are pigmented and sharply pointed. In this image, the regrowing hair (*arrow*) coexists with features of ongoing active disease (×20)

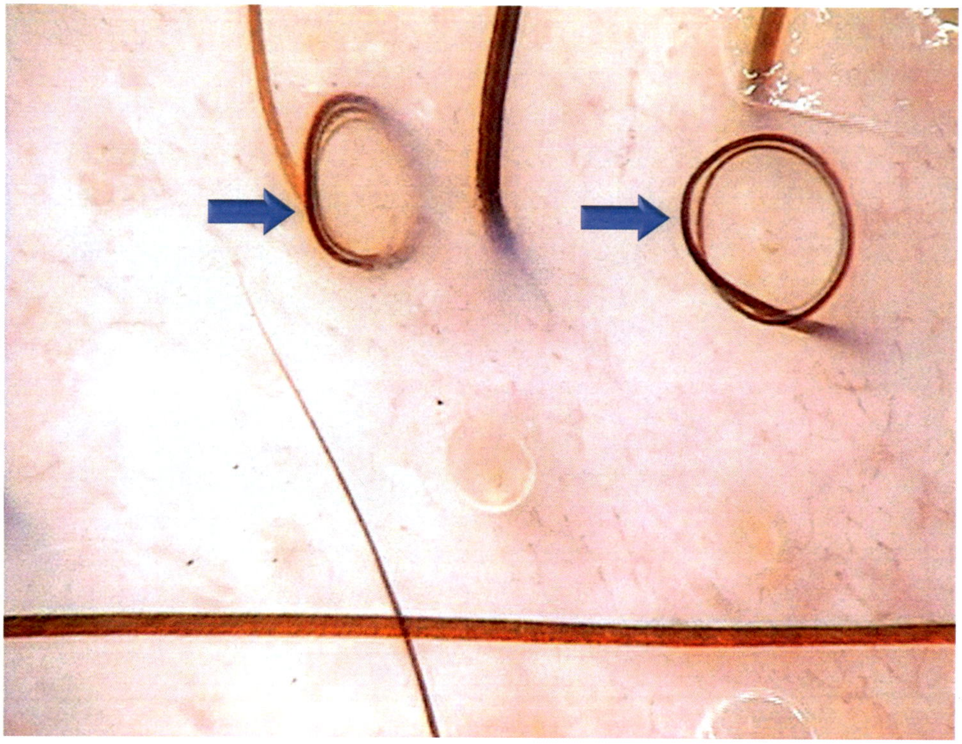

Fig. 16.22 Pigtail regrowing hairs in alopecia areata. Pigtail hairs are coiled into an oval or circular shape and have sharp ends (*blue arrows*). They demonstrate the regrowth of terminal hairs from hair follicles that are not fully intact. This feature is not specific for alopecia areata. An upright regrowing hair also is visible in this image (×70)

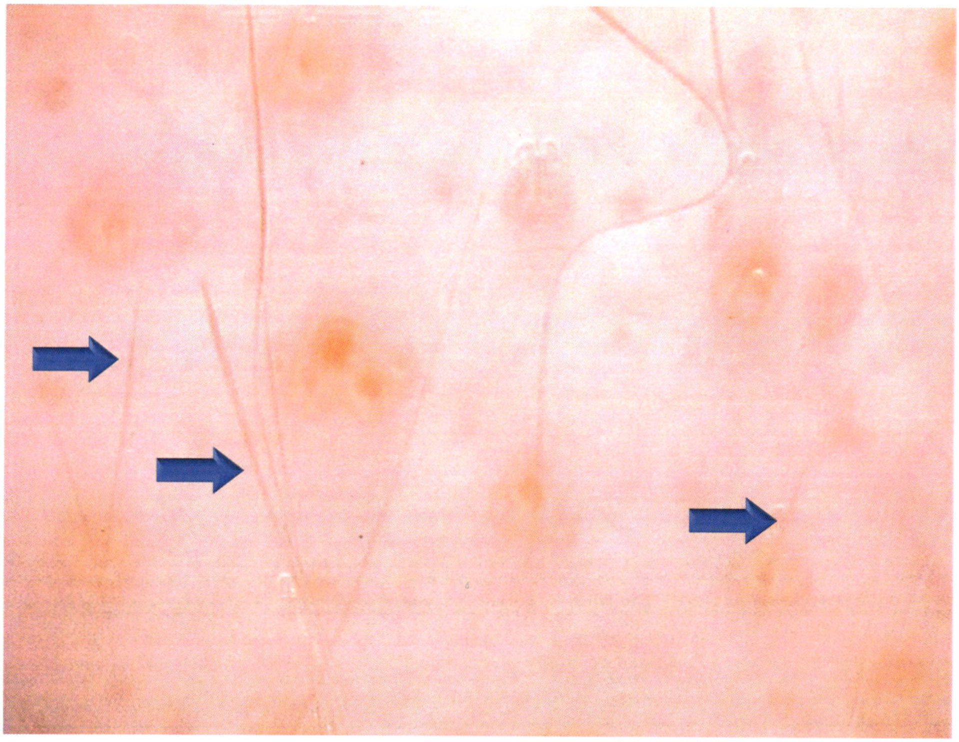

Fig. 16.23 Vellus hairs in alopecia areata. The presence of multiple regrowing short white vellus hairs (*arrows*) may be a first, weak sign of disease remission. Some authors indicate that vellus hairs are a marker of disease severity. Vellus hairs are easier to see in Asian than Caucasian patients, apparently because of the difference in background skin colors. Dry trichoscopy may be performed to enhance the visibility of vellus hairs (×70)

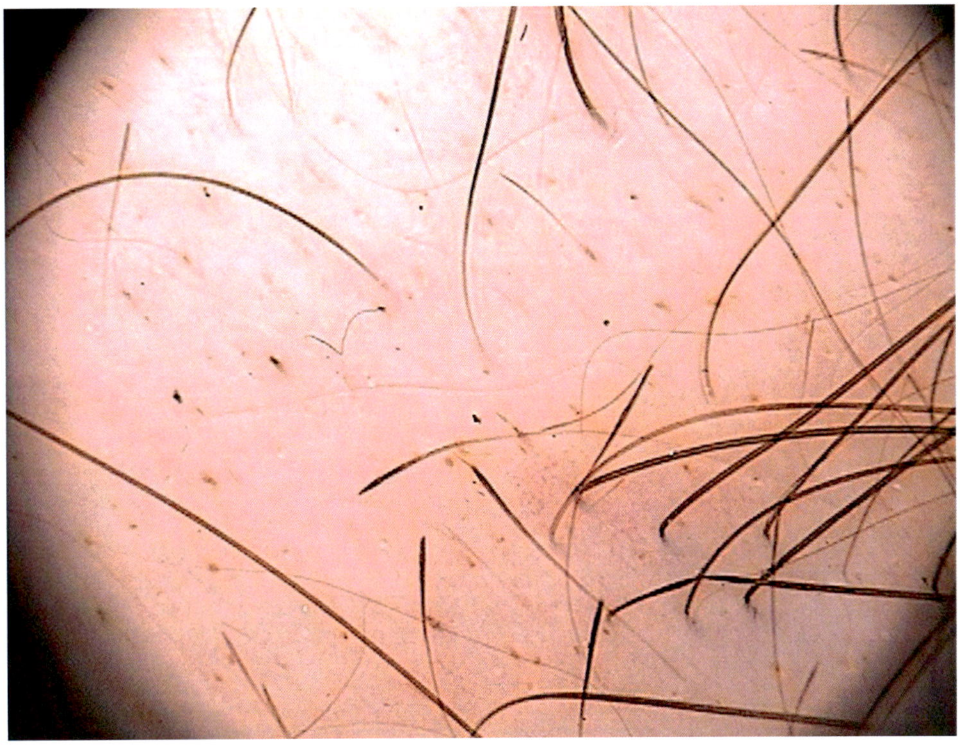

Fig. 16.24 Trichoscopic features of alopecia areata. Shown is the typical pattern of alopecia areata: multiple exclamation mark hairs, tapered hairs, black dots, and few yellow dots. This image indicates an active phase of the disease (×20)

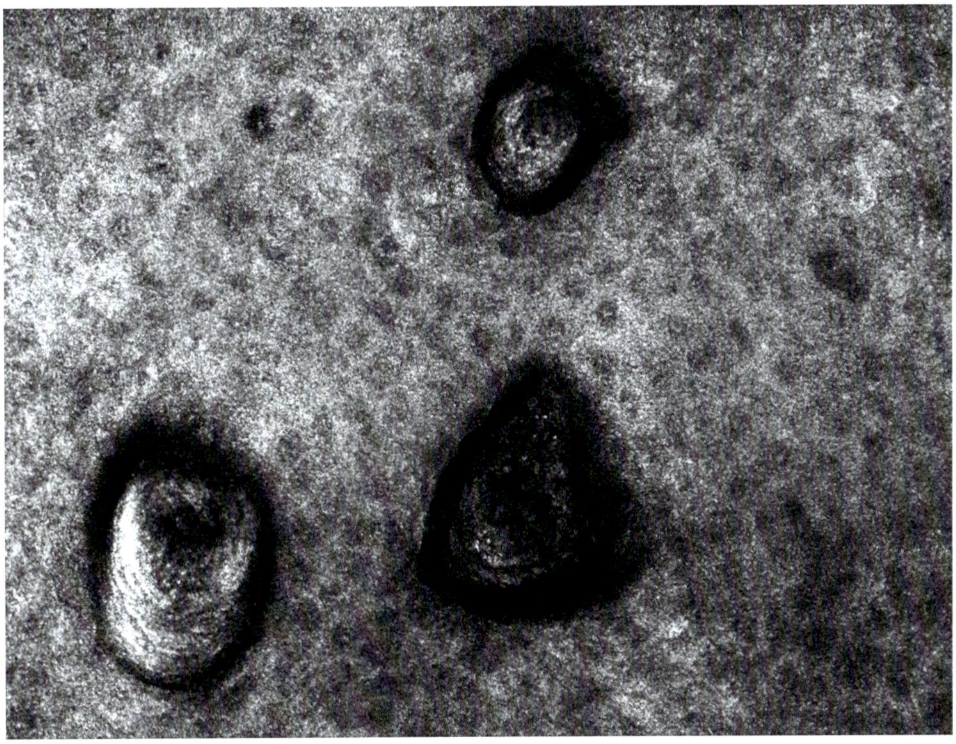

Fig. 16.25 In vivo reflectance confocal microscopy (RCM) of alopecia areata. In vivo RCM of an area with two yellow dots and one black dot observed on trichoscopy shows hair follicle openings with slightly echogenic keratosebaceous masses (corresponding to yellow dots) and one highly echogenic residual hair shaft (corresponding to the black dot). An RCM study of yellow dots in alopecia areata showed good correlation among RCM, trichoscopy, and histopathology, which show that yellow dots correspond to follicular structures containing keratotic material with or without hair residues [17]

References

1. Lacarrubba F, Dall'Oglio F, Rita Nasca M, Micali G. Videodermatoscopy enhances diagnostic capability in some forms of hair loss. Am J Clin Dermatol. 2004;5(3):205–8.
2. Ross EK, Vincenzi C, Tosti A. Videodermoscopy in the evaluation of hair and scalp disorders. J Am Acad Dermatol. 2006;55(5): 799–806.
3. Inui S, Nakajima T, Nakagawa K, Itami S. Clinical significance of dermoscopy in alopecia areata: analysis of 300 cases. Int J Dermatol. 2008;47(7):688–93.
4. Rudnicka L, Olszewska M, Rakowska A, Slowinska M. Trichoscopy update 2011. J Dermatol Case Rep. 2011;5(4):82–8.
5. Mane M, Nath AK, Thappa DM. Utility of dermoscopy in alopecia areata. Indian J Dermatol. 2011;56(4):407–11. PMCID: 3179004.
6. Karadağ Köse O, Güleç AT. Clinical evaluation of alopecias using a handheld dermatoscope. J Am Acad Dermatol. 2012;67:206–14.
7. Abraham LS, Torres FN, Azulay-Abulafia L. Dermoscopic clues to distinguish trichotillomania from patchy alopecia areata. An Bras Dermatol. 2010;85(5):723–6.
8. Inui S. Trichoscopy for common hair loss diseases: algorithmic method for diagnosis. J Dermatol. 2011;38(1):71–5.
9. Inui S, Nakajima T, Itami S. Coudability hairs: a revisited sign of alopecia areata assessed by trichoscopy. Clin Exp Dermatol. 2010; 35(4):361–5.
10. Olszewska M, Rudnicka L, Rakowska A, Kurzeja M. Postępy w diagnostyce łysienia. Przegl Dermatol. 2009;96:247–53.
11. Alkhalifah A, Alsantali A, Wang E, McElwee KJ, Shapiro J. Alopecia areata update: part I. Clinical picture, histopathology, and pathogenesis. J Am Acad Dermatol. 2010;62(2):177–88; quiz 89–90.
12. Inui S, Itami S. Emergence of trichoscopic yellow dots by topical corticosteroid in alopecia areata mimicking frontal fibrosing alopecia: a case report. J Dermatol. 2012;39(1):39–41.
13. Rudnicka L, Olszewska M, Rakowska A, Kowalska-Oledzka E, Slowinska M. Trichoscopy: a new method for diagnosing hair loss. J Drugs Dermatol. 2008;7(7):651–4.
14. Tobin DJ. Morphological analysis of hair follicles in alopecia areata. Microsc Res Tech. 1997;38(4):443–51.
15. Ihm CW, Han JH. Diagnostic value of exclamation mark hairs. Dermatology. 1993;186(2):99–102.
16. Peereboom-Wynia JD, Koerten HK, Van Joost T, Stolz E. Scanning electron microscopy comparing exclamation mark hairs in alopecia areata with normal hair fibres, mechanically broken by traction. Clin Exp Dermatol. 1989;14(1):47–50.
17. Ardigo M, Tosti A, Cameli N, Vincenzi C, Misciali C, Berardesca E. Reflectance confocal microscopy of the yellow dot pattern in alopecia areata. Arch Dermatol. 2011;147(1):61–4.

Androgenetic Alopecia

17

Adriana Rakowska, Monika Slowinska,
Malgorzata Olszewska, and Lidia Rudnicka

Abstract

Male androgenetic alopecia and female androgenetic alopecia share similar trichoscopic features, including hair shaft thickness heterogeneity, yellow dots, perifollicular discoloration (the peripilar sign), an increased proportion of thin and vellus hairs, and a large number of follicular units with only one emerging hair shaft. Thin wavy hair and honeycomb hyperpigmentation often coexist as additional, nonspecific features.

Keywords

Androgenetic alopecia • Brown perifollicular discoloration • Clinical trials • Follicular units • Hair shaft thickness • Honeycomb hyperpigmentation • Monitoring • Peripilar sign • Senescent alopecia • Senile alopecia • Vellus hairs • Wavy hair • Yellow dots

Androgenetic alopecia (AGA) is an androgen-related condition that develops in genetically predisposed individuals [1]. The disease affects up to 80 % of Caucasian men and no less than 42 % of women [1–4]. The prevalence of AGA is lower in Asian and African American men and women [5].

Male AGA (male pattern hair loss) and female AGA (female pattern hair loss) share the same histopathologic feature of hair follicle miniaturization and a similar pathogenic pathway. In susceptible hair follicles, dihydrotestosterone binds to the androgen receptor, and the hormone-receptor complex activates the genes responsible for the gradual transformation of large terminal follicles to miniaturized follicles [1–4].

Male and female AGA share similar trichoscopic features, including hair shaft thickness heterogeneity, thin hairs, yellow dots, perifollicular discoloration (the peripilar sign), an increased proportion of vellus hairs, and a large number of follicular units with only one emerging hair shaft [6–9]. Thin wavy hair and honeycomb hyperpigmentation often coexist as additional, unspecific features [7, 10].

Hair thickness heterogeneity is characterized by the simultaneous presence of hairs of different thicknesses: vellus, thin, intermediate, and thick. Hair thickness may be observed and roughly estimated with a handheld dermoscope. Some videodermoscopes have software that allows a detailed assessment of hair shaft thickness in micrometers. Although precise measurement of hair shaft thickness is not essential for diagnosis, it may be useful for monitoring treatment efficacy and in clinical trials. Hair diameter diversity has been shown to reflect follicle miniaturization in AGA [8, 11].

Trichoscopy of AGA shows an increased proportion of vellus hairs. Up to 10 % of normal human scalp hairs are vellus hairs, defined as hypopigmented, nonmedullated hairs less than 30 μm thick and less than 2–3 mm long [12, 13]. The proportion of vellus hairs in the frontal scalp area of

A. Rakowska • M. Slowinska
Department of Dermatology, CSK MSW,
Warsaw, Poland

M. Olszewska
Department of Dermatology,
Medical University of Warsaw,
Warsaw, Poland

L. Rudnicka (✉)
Faculty of Health Sciences, Medical University of Warsaw, Poland

Department of Dermatology, CSK MSW,
Woloska 137, Warsaw 02-502, Poland
e-mail: lidia.rudnicka@euderm.eu

L. Rudnicka et al. (eds.), *Atlas of Trichoscopy*,
DOI 10.1007/978-1-4471-4486-1_17,

patients with female AGA is 20.9 ± 12 % [9], which is significantly greater than the proportion of 6.15 ± 4.6 % in healthy volunteers [9].

A decreased number of hairs per follicular unit is a characteristic but nonspecific feature of AGA. In patients with female AGA, the average percentage of follicular units with only one emerging hair is 65.2 ± 19.9 % in the frontal area. The corresponding numbers are 39.0 ± 13.4 % in patients with telogen effluvium and 27.3 ± 13 % in healthy individuals.

The presence of yellow dots appears to be a variable feature of AGA. In various studies, yellow dots were observed in 66 % [9], 30.5 % [14], 10–26 % [8], and 7 % [7] of patients with AGA.

In AGA, brown perifollicular discoloration (the peripilar sign) is observed in 20–66 % of patients and in 32.4 ± 4.7 % of hair follicles [8, 9]. These numbers are significantly higher than those in healthy individuals.

Honeycomb (hyper)pigmentation results from increased sun exposure of an unprotected scalp. This feature becomes more prominent with increasing severity of AGA but may be observed in Caucasian patients with any type of nonscarring alopecia, and it is a consistent finding in healthy individuals with dark skin phototypes.

Like trichoscopy of AGA, that of senescent (senile, involutionary) alopecia reveals a predominance of follicular units with only one hair, decreased hair shaft density (honeycomb pattern pigmentation), and a slight tendency toward brown perifollicular discoloration (the peripilar sign).

In androgenetic alopecia, trichoscopic abnormalities are more pronounced in the frontal than in the occipital area.

Table 17.1 Trichoscopic features of androgenetic alopecia

Hair thickness heterogeneity
Thin hairs
Vellus hairs
Single-hair pilosebaceous units
Yellow dots
Perifollicular discoloration
Wavy hair
Honeycomb pigmentation

Table 17.2 Trichoscopic differential diagnosis of androgenetic alopecia

Telogen effluvium
Senile alopecia
Fibrosing alopecia in pattern distribution
Frontal fibrosing alopecia
Diffuse alopecia areata
Alopecia areata incognita

Box 17.1

- In androgenetic alopecia trichoscopy abnormalities are more pronounced in the frontal compared to the occipital area.

Box 17.2

- When diagnosing androgenetic alopecia with trichoscopy, be sure to exclude coexistence of other causes of hair loss.
- Androgenetic alopecia affects 42–80 % of the population. Thus, other diseases causing hair loss may be masked by features of androgenetic alopecia.
- Androgenetic alopecia most commonly coexists with telogen effluvium.

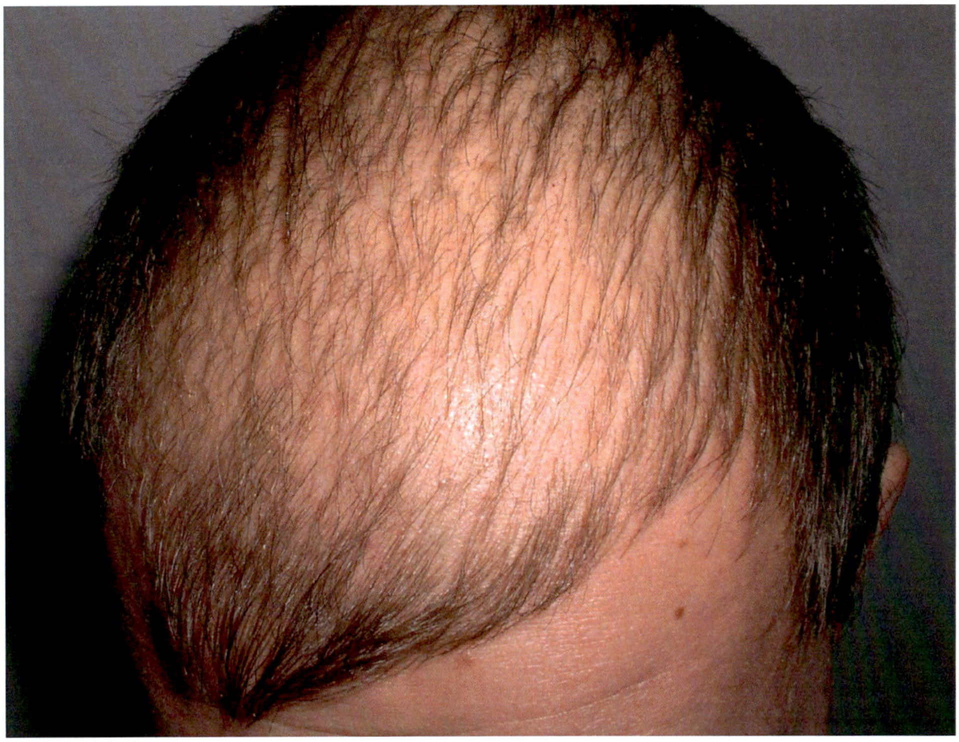

Fig. 17.1 Androgenetic alopecia (male pattern hair loss). The diagnosis of typical AGA in men usually is based on clinical evaluation. No additional diagnostic procedures are needed. Nevertheless, we recommend using the dermoscope in every patient with hair loss, even in doubtless clinical situations. Trichoscopy may help rule out diseases that mimic AGA, such as diffuse alopecia areata, trichotillomania, and hair shaft dystrophies in a pattern distribution [15]. Trichoscopy also may be used to exclude diseases that overlap AGA

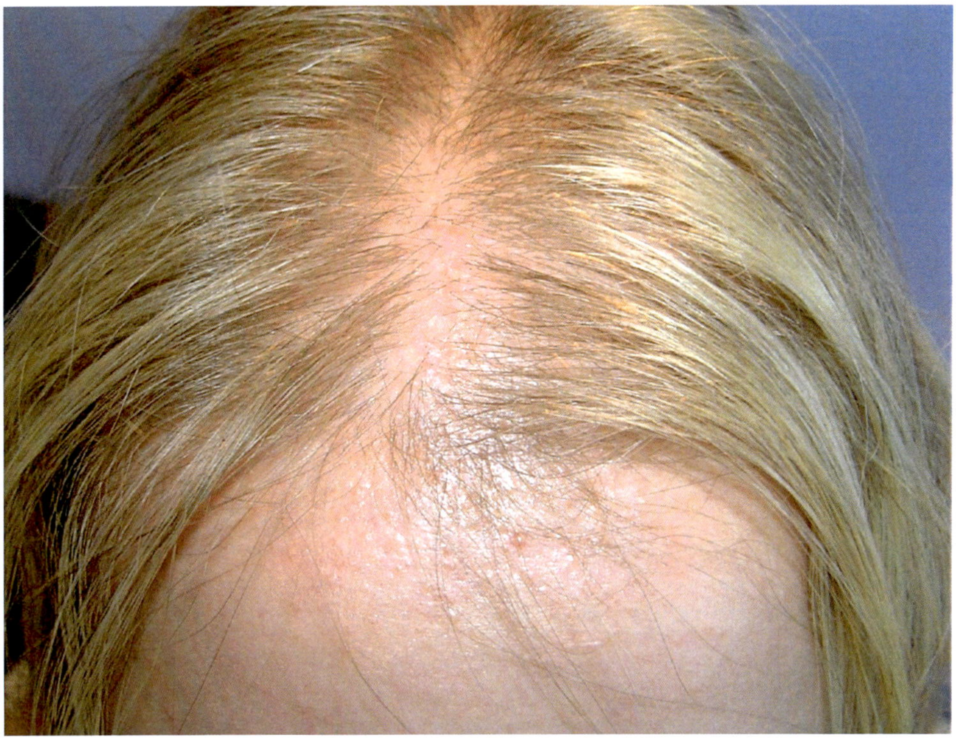

Fig. 17.2 Female androgenetic alopecia (female pattern hair loss). Differential diagnosis of early female AGA is difficult without the support of a dermoscope. In this patient, the "Christmas tree sign" may indicate female AGA. In such cases, trichoscopy may be used to confirm the diagnosis. No differences in trichoscopic observations between female and male AGA have been described. Thus, in this chapter, the abbreviation *AGA* is used for both female and male androgenetic alopecia

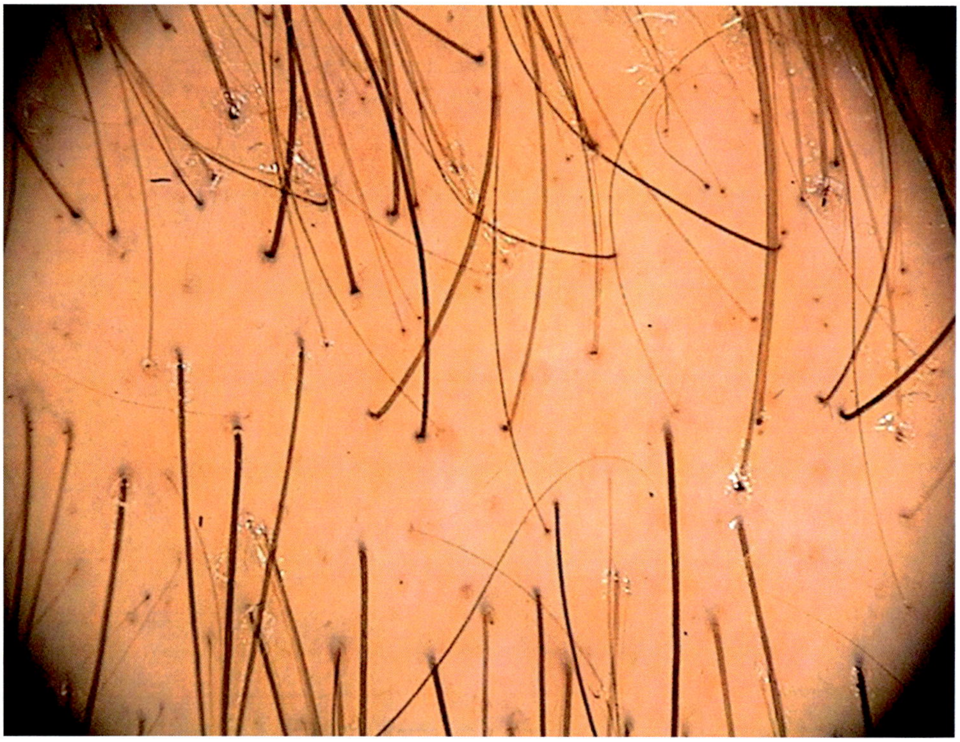

Fig. 17.3 Hair shaft thickness heterogeneity in androgenetic alopecia. Hair shaft thickness heterogeneity is the simultaneous presence of thin, intermediate, and thick hairs in one field of view. This finding is the result of hair follicle miniaturization, which affects different follicles to different degrees. Fully miniaturized follicles, which produce thin and vellus hairs, coexist with fully intact follicles, which produce terminal hairs. Hair shaft thickness heterogeneity is a hallmark of AGA [8, 9, 11] (×20)

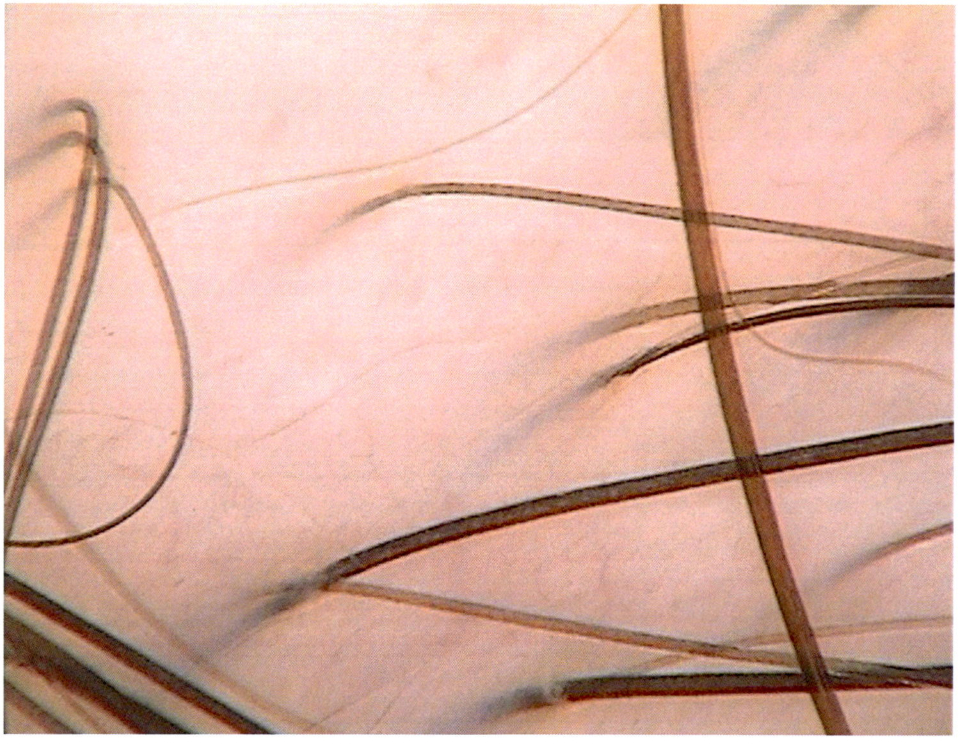

Fig. 17.4 Hair shaft thickness heterogeneity in androgenetic alopecia. The simultaneous presence of vellus, thin, intermediate, and thick hairs may be observed and roughly estimated with a handheld dermoscope. Some videodermoscopes have software that allows a detailed assessment of hair shaft thickness in micrometers. Although precise measurement of hair shaft thickness is not essential for diagnosis, it is useful for monitoring treatment efficacy and in clinical trials (×70)

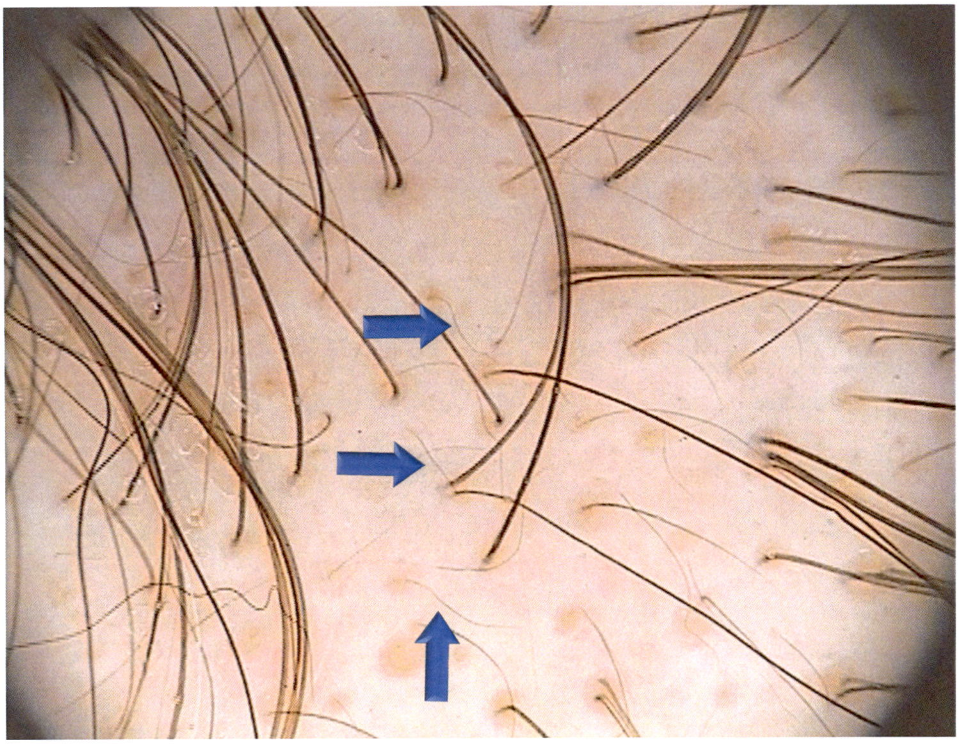

Fig. 17.5 Vellus hairs in androgenetic alopecia. Vellus hairs (*arrows*) are less than 30 μm thick and less than 2–3 mm long, and are hypopigmented and nonmedullated [12, 13]. They are produced by miniaturized hair follicles; therefore, their number is significantly increased in AGA. Shown here is a trichoscopic image of the frontal area of a male patient with AGA. Other trichoscopic features of AGA are hair shaft thickness heterogeneity, multiple follicular units with only one hair, and the peripilar sign (×20)

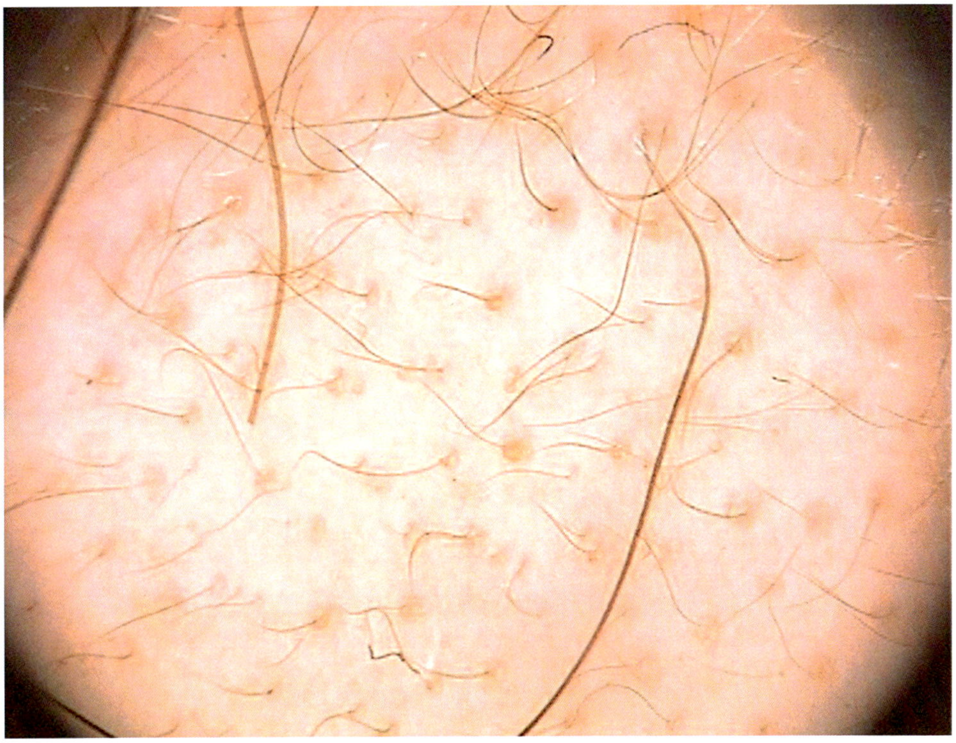

Fig. 17.6 Predominance of vellus hairs in advanced androgenetic alopecia. This trichoscopic image is from the frontotemporal region of a male patient with advanced AGA (grade V in the Norwood-Hamilton classification). Nearly all the terminal hairs were replaced by thin and vellus hairs. Vellus hairs must be differentiated from new, healthy regrowing hairs (for example in acute telogen effluvium). New regrowing hairs are also thin and short, but they differ in their upright position, pointed end, and intense pigmentation (×20)

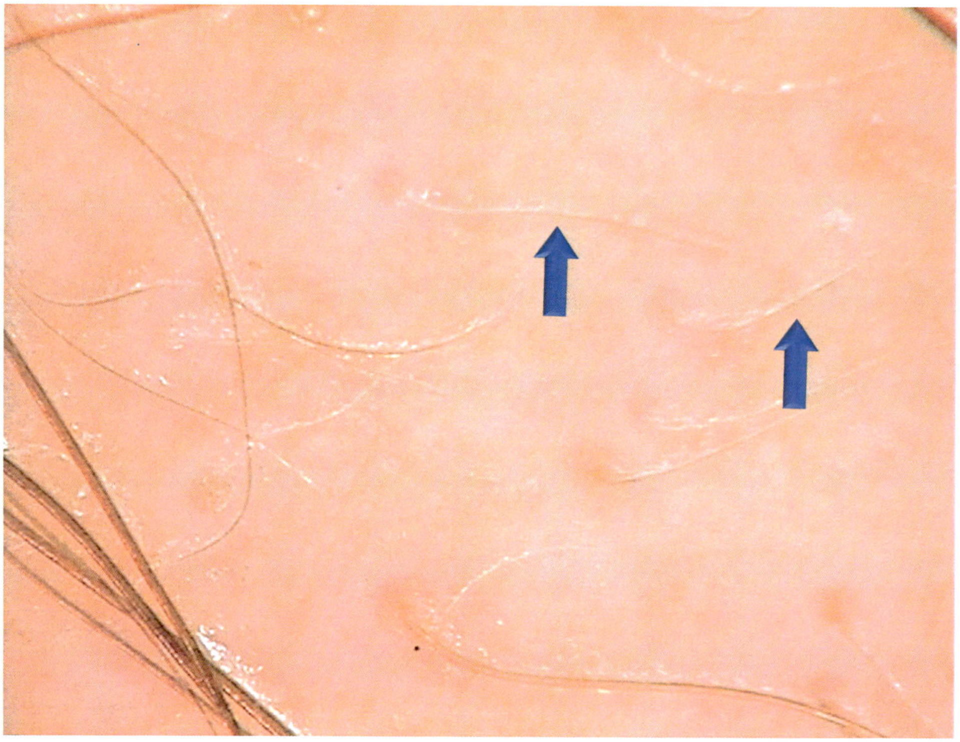

Fig. 17.7 Vellus hairs in advanced androgenetic alopecia. High-magnification trichoscopy demonstrates the faint, delicate nature of these hairs (*arrows*). Unlike upright regrowing hair, vellus hairs are bent, are hypopigmented, and have a blurred distal end (×70)

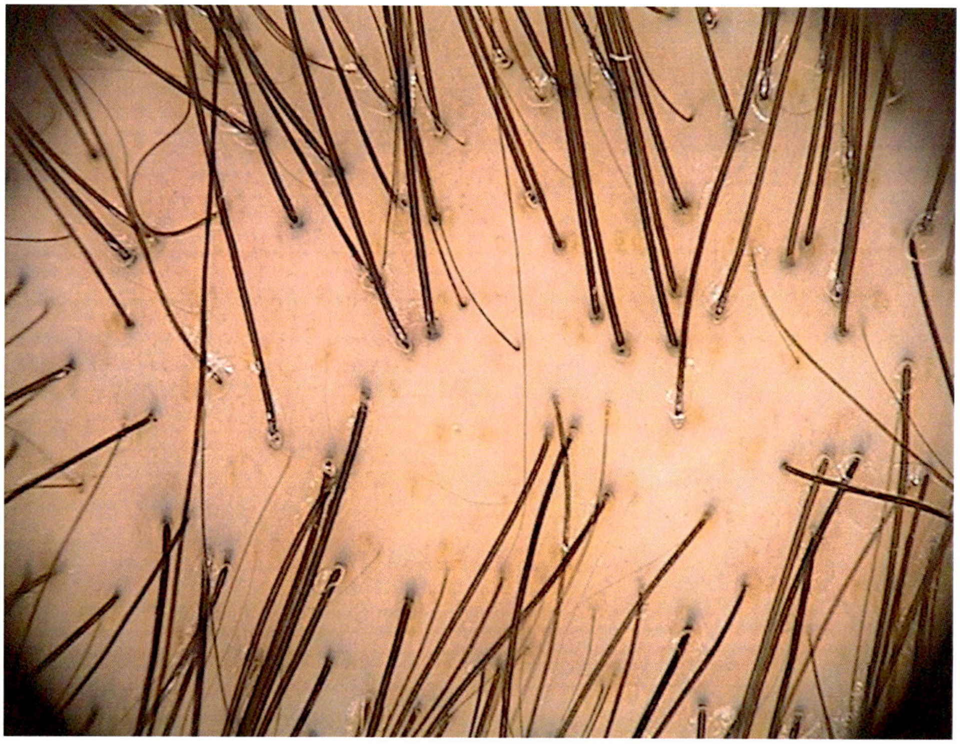

Fig. 17.8 Predominance of follicular units with only one hair in androgenetic alopecia. Usually, one to three hairs emerge from one follicular opening [13, 16]. In healthy individuals, the average number of hairs emerging from one follicular unit is 2.4 and the proportion of follicular units with only one emerging hair shaft is less than 30 % [9]. The proportion of follicular units with only one hair shaft is increased in AGA. Most follicular units in this image consist of only one hair. For detailed information about trichoscopy of follicular units, see Chap. 2 (×70)

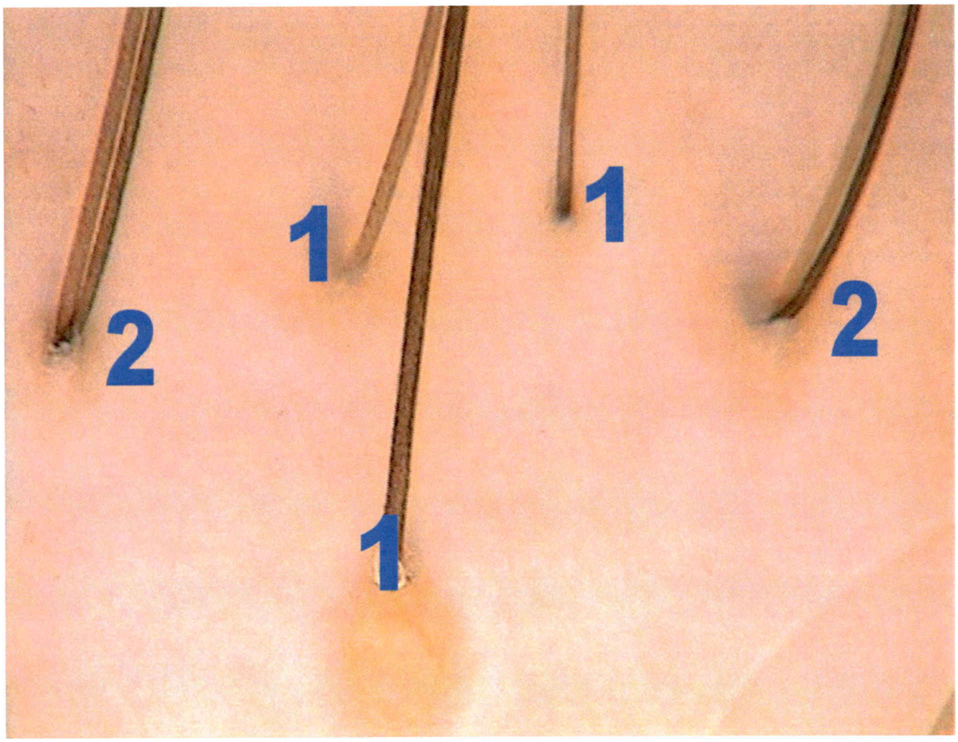

Fig. 17.9 Predominance of follicular units with only one hair in androgenetic alopecia. This image shows five follicular units, three (3/5, 60 %) of which have only one emerging hair shaft, a significantly greater percentage than that seen in healthy individuals (35 %). In clinical practice, we calculate the proportion of single-hair follicular units on the basis of four fields of view. The frontal and occipital areas are evaluated separately. The temporal area also may be evaluated for monitoring treatment efficacy or in clinical trials, but it is not diagnostically relevant. The following normal values for the frontal area in healthy Caucasian females have been established: one-hair follicular units, <35 %; two-hair units, 46–70 %; and three-hair units, >10 %. The respective numbers for the occipital area are <30 %, 45–73 %, and >10 %, and for the temporal area, <40 %, 50–75 %, and >10 % [13]. The average number of hairs per follicular unit in this image is 1.4 (from the left: 2 + 1 + 1 + 1 + 2 = 7; 7:5 = 1.4), which is significantly less than that of healthy individuals, who have an average of 2.4 hairs per follicular unit (×70)

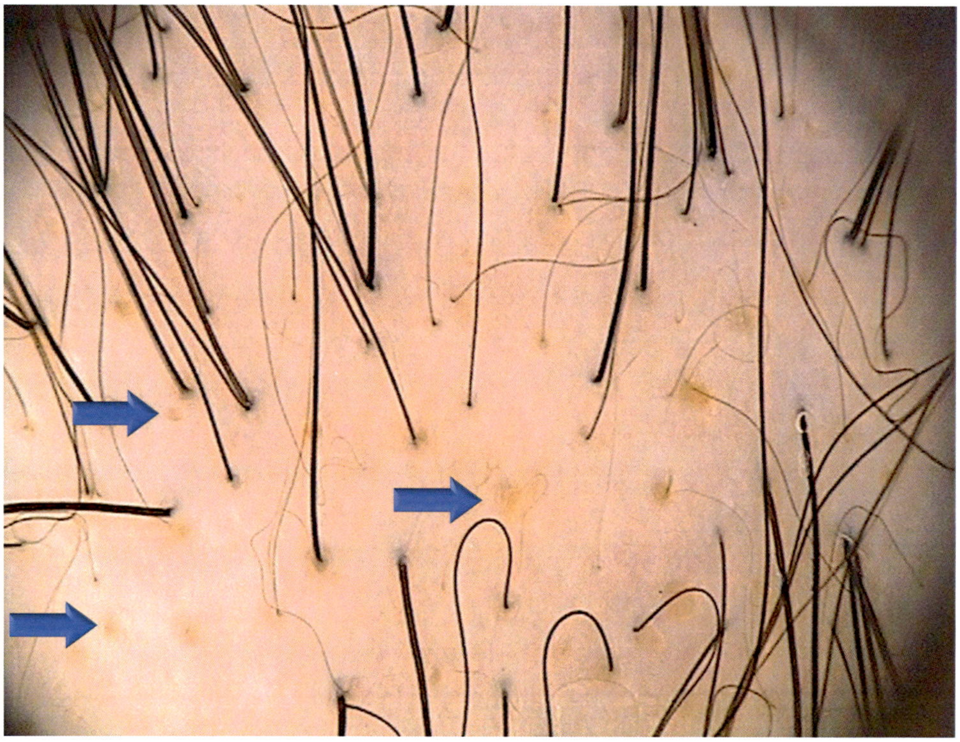

Fig. 17.10 Yellow dots in androgenetic alopecia. Yellow dots (*arrows*) are follicular openings with keratotic material and/or sebum. They were first described and are most common in alopecia areata, but their diagnostic value in AGA should not be underestimated. According to our hypothesis, presented in detail in Chap. 3, yellow dots in AGA consist mainly of sebum, which is excreted to the scalp surface by intact sebaceous glands in the absence of terminal hairs. These yellow dots contain no or only a very limited amount of keratotic material. This composition of yellow dots in AGA determines their easy disappearance during an intense hair washing. Therefore, we ask our patients not to wash their hair during the 3 days before trichoscopic examination (×20)

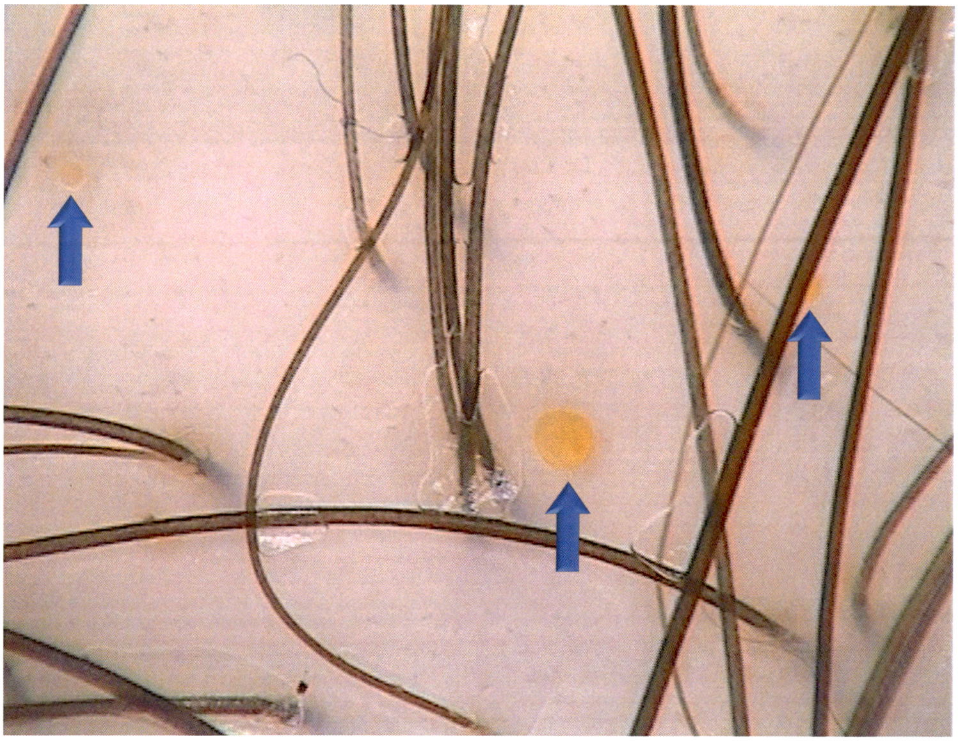

Fig. 17.11 Yellow dots in androgenetic alopecia. High magnification demonstrates the oily appearance of yellow dots (*arrows*) in a patient with AGA. Yellow dots in AGA differ from those of alopecia areata in their irregular distribution and high variability in size and shape, even in an individual patient. Unlike the yellow dots of alopecia areata, those of AGA contain mostly sebum mixed with variable amounts of keratotic material, which determines the wide variation in their inner shape, from very "oily" to "keratotic" (×70)

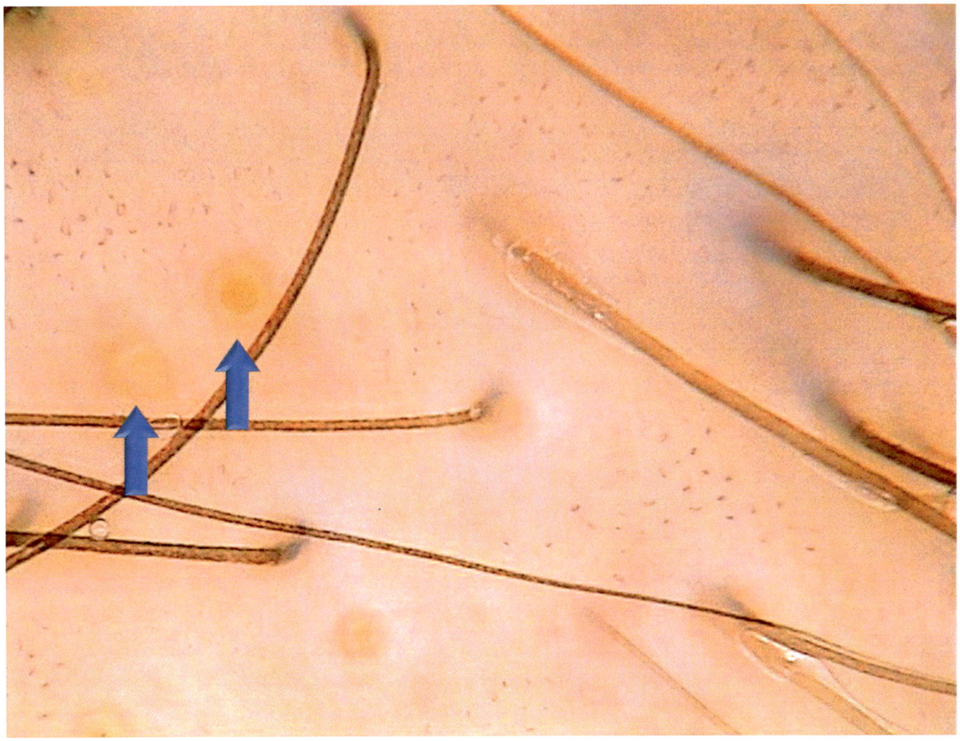

Fig. 17.12 Yellow dots in androgenetic alopecia. Yellow dots (*arrows*) containing keratinous material show a double border, and their surface may appear uneven. Note the large variation in size and shape and the irregular distribution. Yellow dots have been observed with variable frequency in different studies; they have been detected in 7–66 % of patients with AGA [7–9, 14]. The large number of patients with yellow dots in our study [9] may have resulted from our recommendation to avoid hair washing for 2–3 days before trichoscopic examination

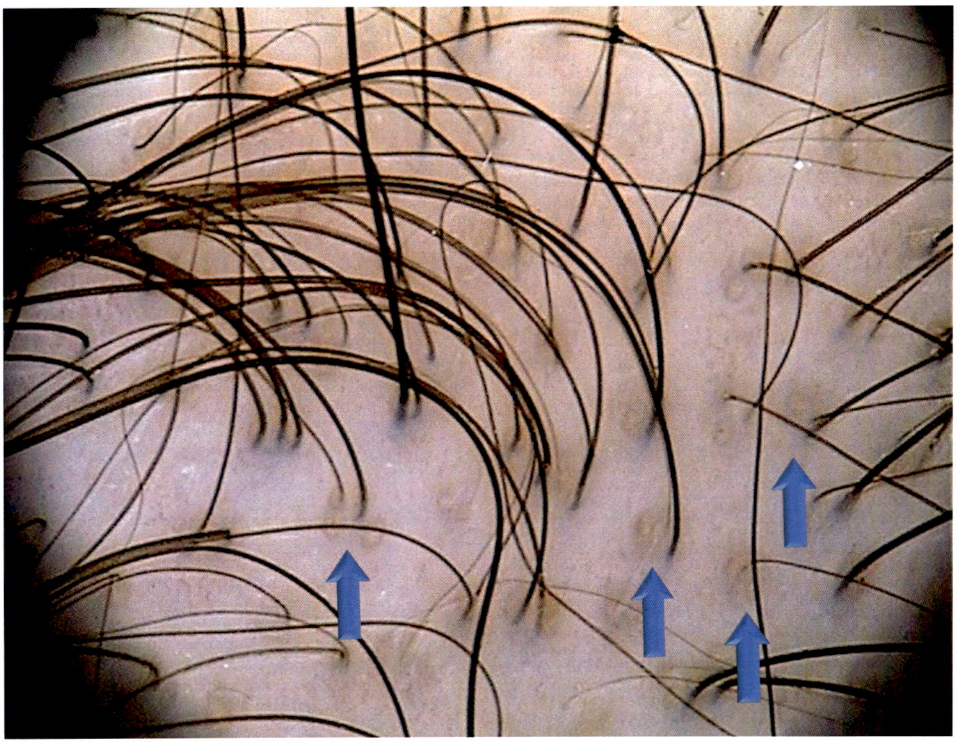

Fig. 17.13 Peripilar sign in androgenetic alopecia. The peripilar sign (*arrows*), also known as *brown perifollicular discoloration* or *perifollicular hyperpigmentation*, corresponds to the perifollicular presence of lymphocytic infiltrates. In AGA, the peripilar sign is observed in 20–66 % of patients and in 32.4 ± 4.7 % of hair follicles [8, 9]. Some authors indicate that the peripilar sign is specific for AGA [14]; however, in our experience, it is indistinguishable from a similar phenomenon observed in telogen effluvium. A limited number (<5 %) of hair follicle openings with brown perifollicular discoloration may be observed in healthy individuals [13] (×20)

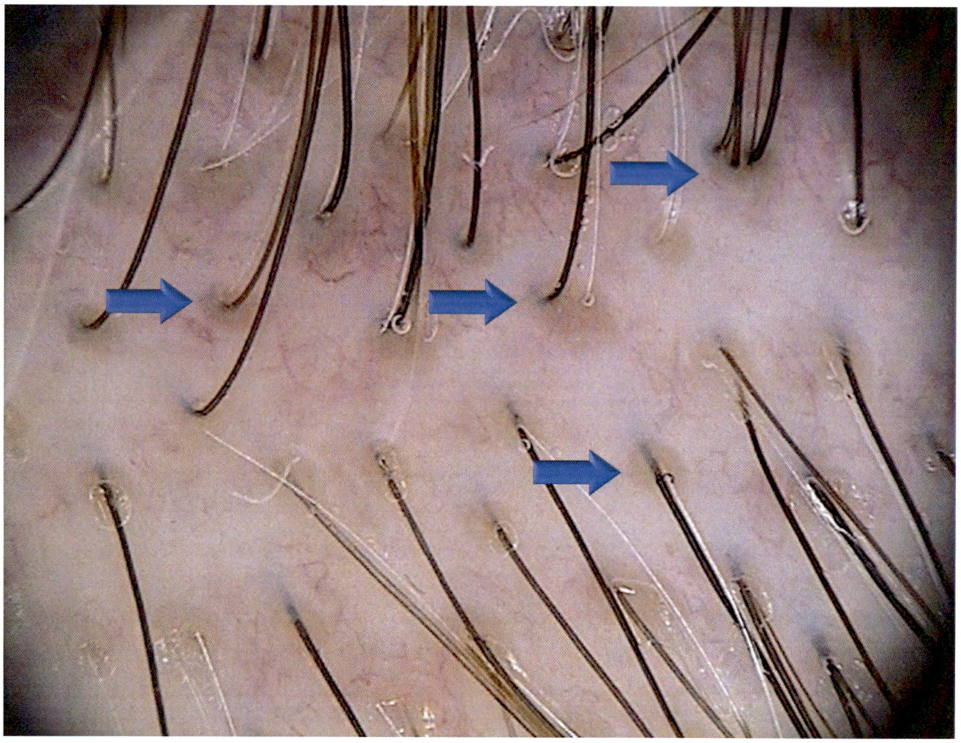

Fig. 17.14 Peripilar sign in androgenetic alopecia. Brown perifollicular discoloration (*arrows*) is present in almost all the follicular units, and individual areas of discoloration cover a larger area than in the previous image. Although the clinical relevance of the peripilar sign, the proportion of affected follicular units, and the area covered by the discoloration has not been researched yet, extensive perifollicular discoloration is believed to be a poor prognostic factor (×20)

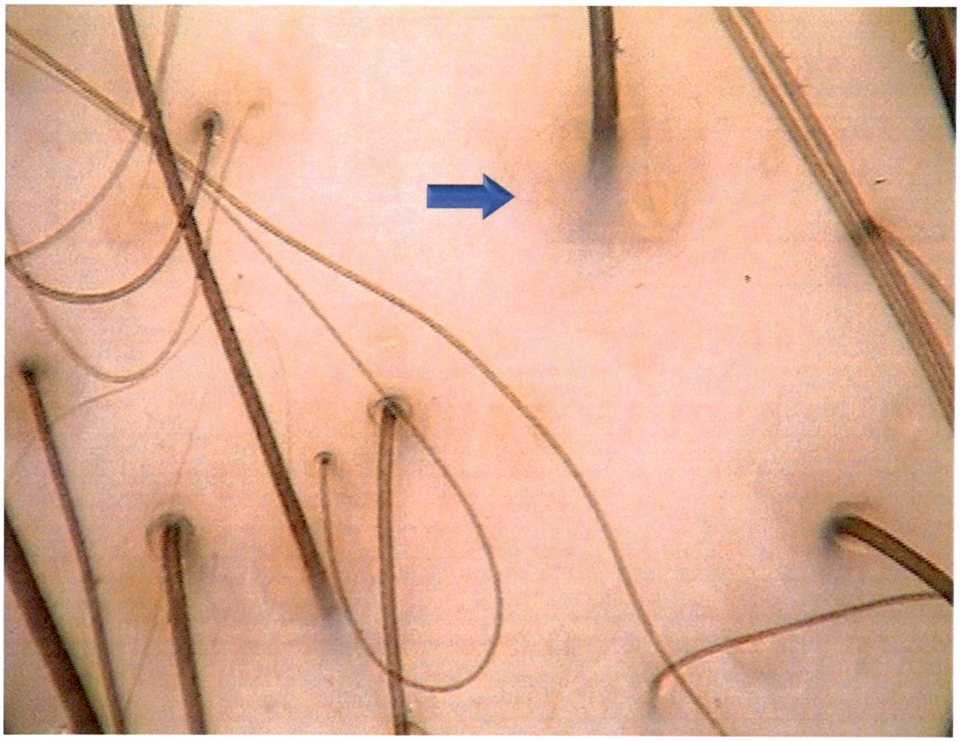

Fig. 17.15 Peripilar sign in androgenetic alopecia. The perifollicular discoloration is brown to brown-gray with unclear borders. Within a peripilar sign (*arrow*), a yellow dot with an emerging vellus hair is visible, which demonstrates a follicular unit with two hairs: one terminal and one miniaturized vellus hair. With progressive miniaturization, this vellus hair will disappear. A follicular unit with only one hair shaft will remain, which is a characteristic feature of AGA (×70)

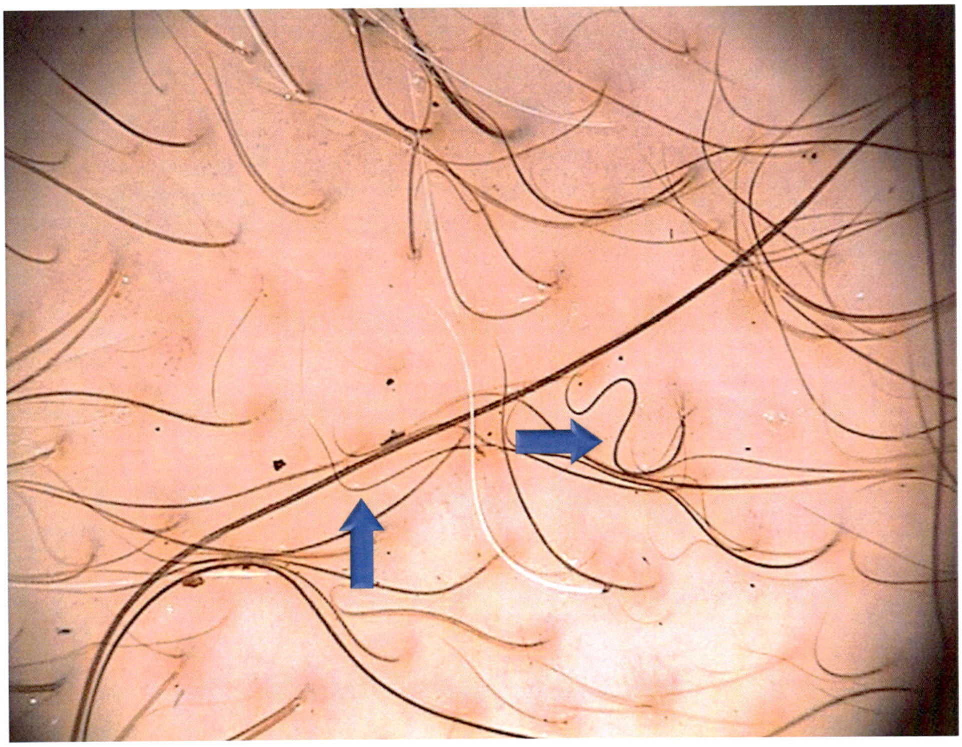

Fig. 17.16 Thin wavy hair in androgenetic alopecia. Short and thin intermittent hairs (*arrows*) with a diameter between 0.03 and 0.05 mm (a result of incomplete hair follicle miniaturization) frequently are visible on trichoscopy as wavy hairs. They are thicker and longer than typical vellus hairs, but thinner and shorter than terminal hairs. Similar hairs may be observed in a condition called *alopecia areata incognita* (×20)

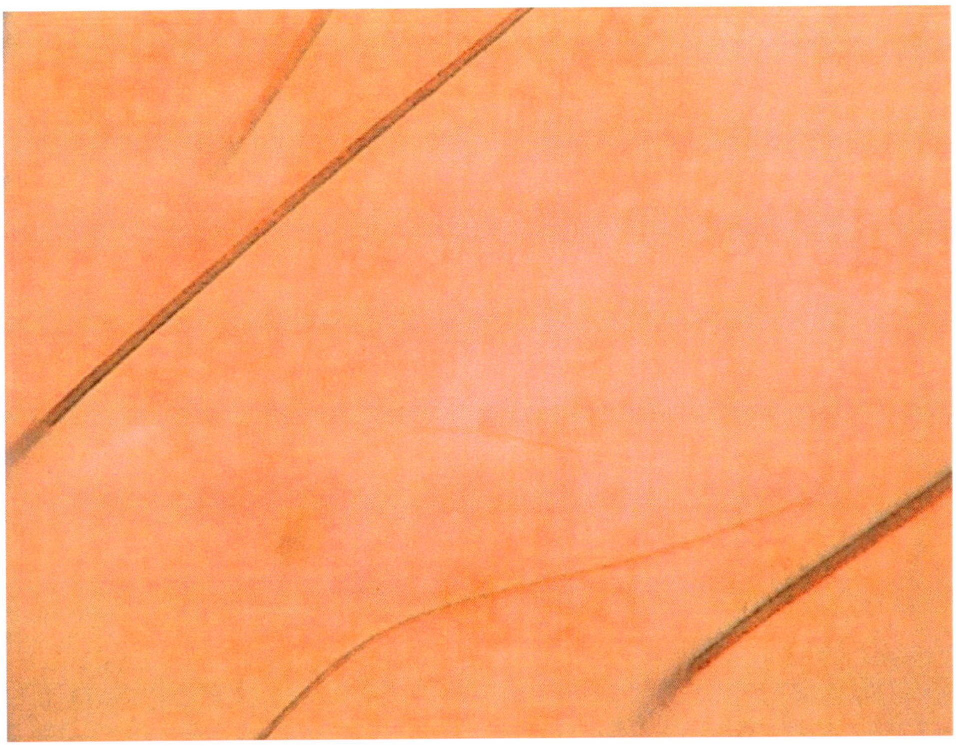

Fig. 17.17 Honeycomb pigmentation in androgenetic alopecia. Honeycomb pigmentation is a frequent finding in Caucasian patients with longstanding, advanced AGA, who do not receive sun protection from their hair. This type of pigmentation is observed on sun-exposed areas of the scalp [7]. It is a normal finding in patients with Fitzpatrick skin phototype IV, V, or VI (×70)

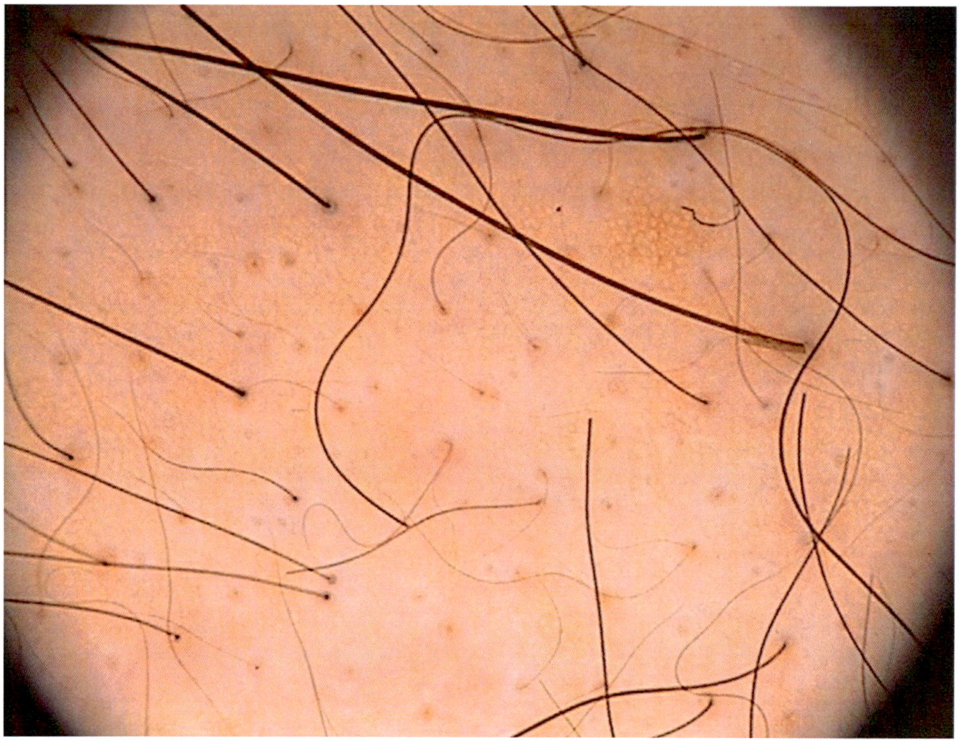

Fig. 17.18 Trichoscopic features of androgenetic alopecia. This image shows the typical pattern of AGA, with vellus hairs, hair shaft thickness heterogeneity, wavy hairs, a predominance of pilosebaceous units with only one hair, the peripilar sign, and yellow dots (×20)

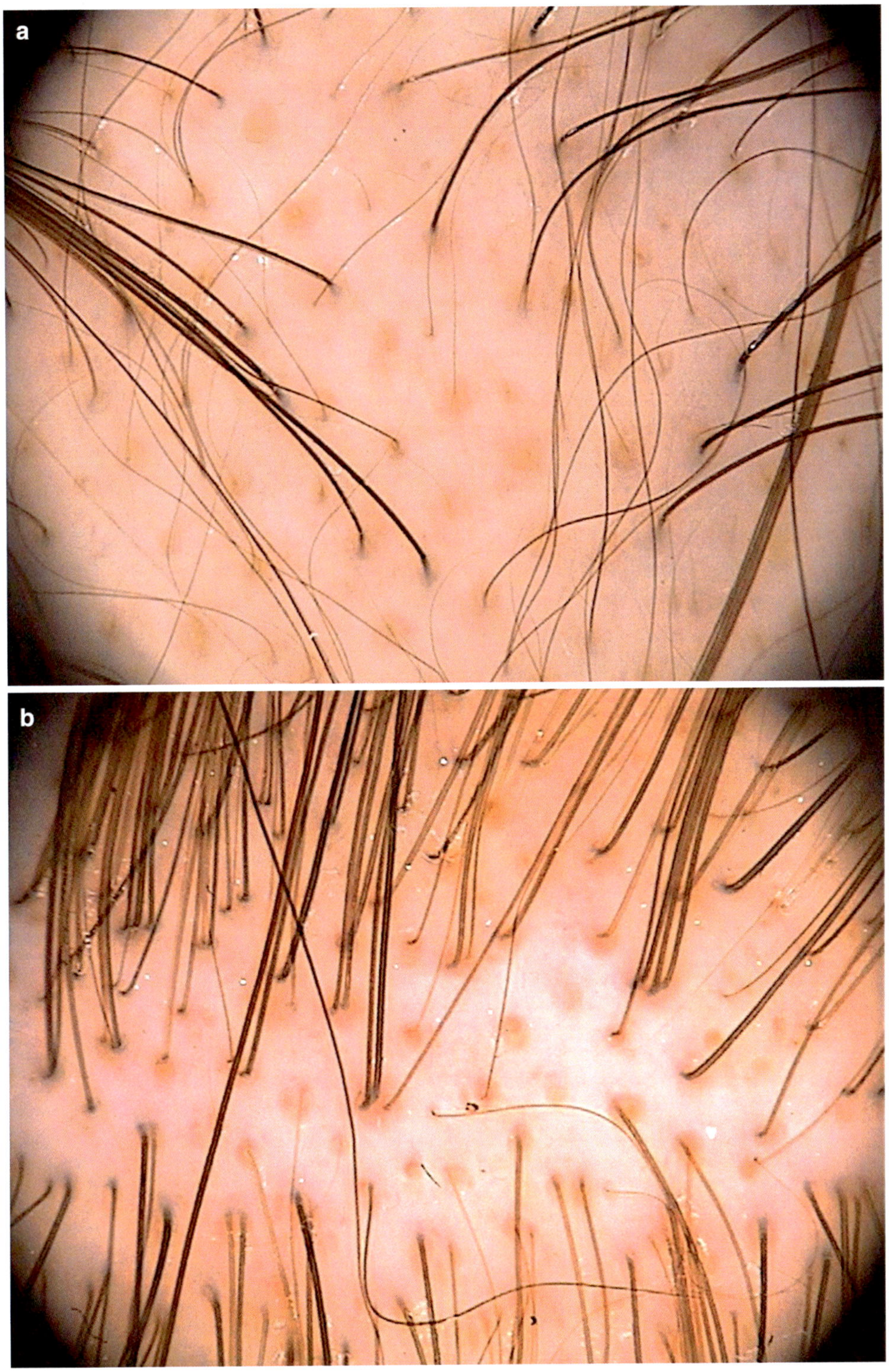

Fig. 17.19 Female androgenetic alopecia. The differences in trichoscopy between the frontal (**a**) and occipital (**b**) areas in the same patient may provide an important clue for the diagnosis of AGA in men and women. Although both the frontal and occipital areas show trichoscopic features characteristic of the disease, these features, as a rule, are more prominent in the frontal than the occipital area [9]. Abnormalities observed in the frontal area (**a**) of this patient are prominent hair shaft thickness diversity, multiple thin and vellus hairs, the peripilar sign in about 80 % of the hair follicle openings, approximately 80 % of follicular units with only one hair shaft, and yellow dots. The occipital area of this patient shows slight hair shaft thickness diversity, single thin and vellus hairs, the peripilar sign in about 70 % of hair follicle openings, approximately 50 % of follicular units with only one hair shaft, and yellow dots. The differences in abnormalities observed in the frontal area compared with those seen in the occipital area are the basis for the videodermoscopic criteria developed for female AGA [9]. The major criteria are (1) more than four yellow dots in four images (70-fold magnification) in the frontal area, (2) lower average hair thickness in the frontal area than in the occipital area, and (3) more than 10 % of thin hairs (<0.03 mm) in the frontal area. Minor criteria include an increased frontal-to-occipital ratio of (1) single-hair pilosebaceous units, (2) vellus hairs, and (3) perifollicular discoloration. Fulfillment of two major criteria or one major criterion and two minor criteria allows the trichoscopic-based diagnosis of female AGA with 98 % specificity. Details of this algorithm are presented in Chap. 40 (×20)

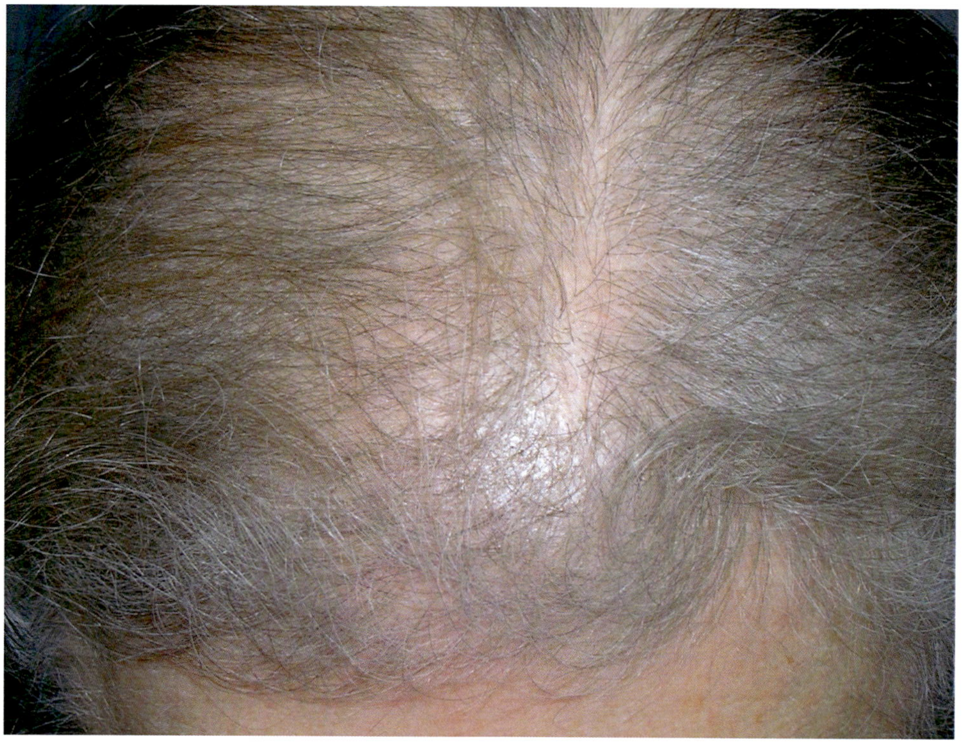

Fig. 17.20 **Senescent alopecia**. Senescent alopecia (senile, involutional alopecia) originally was thought to affect people aged 50 years or older with no family history or evidence of AGA. It was described as diffuse non–androgen-dependent hair thinning due to a programmed, age-dependent decrease in the number of thick terminal hairs. Currently, there is no consensus regarding the nature of the disease [17, 18]; however, the results of a recent histopathologic study indicate that most cases of significant hair loss in the elderly are androgen driven [18]. The results of this study and the predominant hair loss in pattern distribution in the elderly may indicate that senescent alopecia may be considered a disease in the spectrum of AGA

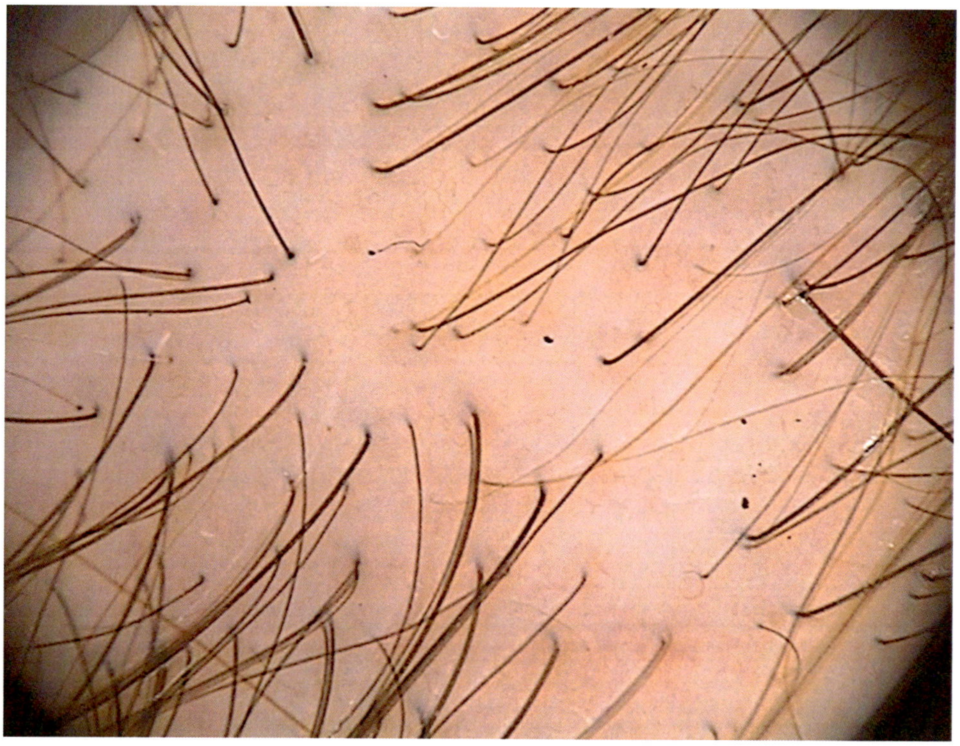

Fig. 17.21 **Senescent alopecia**. Like the trichoscopic observations in AGA, those of senescent alopecia reveal a predominance of follicular units with only one hair, decreased hair shaft density, honeycomb pattern pigmentation, and a slight tendency toward brown perifollicular discoloration (the peripilar sign). Unlike AGA, however, senescent alopecia shows a lack of evident hair shaft thickness heterogeneity, no thin or vellus hairs, and no yellow dots (×20)

References

1. Otberg N, Finner AM, Shapiro J. Androgenetic alopecia. Endocrinol Metab Clin North Am. 2007;36(2):379–98.
2. Olsen EA. Female pattern hair loss and its relationship to permanent/cicatricial alopecia: a new perspective. J Investig Dermatol Symp Proc. 2005;10(3):217–21.
3. Price VH. Androgenetic alopecia in women. J Investig Dermatol Symp Proc. 2003;8(1):24–7.
4. Trueb RM. Systematic approach to hair loss in women. J Dtsch Dermatol Ges. 2010;8(4):284–97, 298.
5. Wang TL, Zhou C, Shen YW, Wang XY, Ding XL, Tian S, et al. Prevalence of androgenetic alopecia in China: a community-based study in six cities. Br J Dermatol. 2010;162(4):843–7.
6. Lacarrubba F, Dall'Oglio F, Rita Nasca M, Micali G. Videodermatoscopy enhances diagnostic capability in some forms of hair loss. Am J Clin Dermatol. 2004;5(3):205–8.
7. Ross EK, Vincenzi C, Tosti A. Videodermoscopy in the evaluation of hair and scalp disorders. J Am Acad Dermatol. 2006;55(5): 799–806.
8. Inui S, Nakajima T, Itami S. Scalp dermoscopy of androgenetic alopecia in Asian people. J Dermatol. 2009;36(2):82–5.
9. Rakowska A, Slowinska M, Kowalska-Oledzka E, Olszewska M, Rudnicka L. Dermoscopy in female androgenic alopecia: method standardization and diagnostic criteria. Int J Trichol. 2009;1(2): 123–30.
10. Rudnicka L, Olszewska M, Rakowska A, Slowinska M. Trichoscopy update 2011. J Dermatol Case Rep. 2011;5(4):82–8.
11. de Lacharriere O, Deloche C, Misciali C, Piraccini BM, Vincenzi C, Bastien P, et al. Hair diameter diversity: a clinical sign reflecting the follicle miniaturization. Arch Dermatol. 2001;137(5):641–6.
12. Vogt A, McElwee KJ, Blume-Peytavi U. Biology of the hair follicle. In: Blume-Peytavi U, Tosti A, Whiting D, Trüeb R, editors. Hair growth and disorders. Berlin: Springer; 2008. p. 1–22.
13. Rakowska A. Trichoscopy (hair and scalp videodermoscopy) in the healthy female. Method standardization and norms for measurable parameters. J Dermatol Case Rep. 2009;3(1):14–9.
14. Karadağ Köse O, Güleç AT. Clinical evaluation of alopecias using a handheld dermatoscope. J Am Acad Dermatol. 2011;67: 206–14.
15. Jain N, Khopkar U. Monilethrix in pattern distribution in siblings: diagnosis by trichoscopy. Int J Trichol. 2010;2(1):56–9.
16. Yazdabadi A, Magee J, Harrison S, Sinclair R. The Ludwig pattern of androgenetic alopecia is due to a hierarchy of androgen sensitivity within follicular units that leads to selective miniaturization and a reduction in the number of terminal hairs per follicular unit. Br J Dermatol. 2008;159(6):1300–2.
17. Trueb RM. Aging of hair. J Cosmet Dermatol. 2005;4(2):60–72.
18. Whiting DA. How real is senescent alopecia? A histopathologic approach. Clin Dermatol. 2011;29(1):49–53.

Telogen Effluvium

18

Adriana Rakowska, Malgorzata Olszewska, and Lidia Rudnicka

Abstract

Trichoscopy has limited value in diagnosing telogen effluvium. Frequent, but not specific, findings include the presence of empty hair follicles, a predominance of follicular units with only one hair, perifollicular discoloration (the peripilar sign), and upright regrowing hairs. There is no significant difference between the findings in the frontal area and those of the occipital area, which differentiates telogen effluvium from androgenetic alopecia. However, clinicians should be aware of the frequent coexistence of both diseases.

Keywords

Androgenetic alopecia • Chronic telogen effluvium • Follicular units • Hair shaft thickness heterogeneity • Perifollicular discoloration • Peripilar sign • Telogen effluvium • Upright regrowing hairs • Yellow dots

The term *telogen effluvium*, introduced by Kligman in 1961 [1], refers to a wide range of clinical situations with the common feature of abrupt generalized shedding of telogen hairs. This peculiar type of hair loss is considered very frequent in clinical practice, but very little evidence-based knowledge is available. Two large trichology books, one by Blume-Peytavi et al. [2] and the other by Camacho and Montagna [3], devote only a few pages to telogen effluvium, reflecting the deficit in scientific information about this condition.

Available data indicate that telogen effluvium may be triggered by internal or external factors that cause a large number of hairs to enter the telogen phase at one time. These telogen hairs start shedding about 3–4 months after exposure to the triggering factor. These factors include acute febrile illness, major surgery, psychological trauma, pregnancy, thyroid diseases, discontinuation of estrogen-containing medications, crash diets, iron deficiency, medications (beta-blockers, anticoagulants, retinoids, propylthiouracil, carbamazepine, vaccines), allergic contact dermatitis, and ultraviolet exposure [4–11].

In 1996, Whiting [12] characterized the chronic form of telogen effluvium as a separate entity. Chronic telogen effluvium may represent a primary disorder or may be secondary to a variety of systemic abnormalities, including malabsorption, chronic dietary deficiencies, chronic thyroid diseases, chronic renal or liver failure, systemic lupus erythematosus, and HIV infection [4]. Of all these potential triggers, only chronic iron deficiency has been studied in detail and has had conflicting results [4].

Clinically, chronic telogen effluvium is characterized by a diffuse loss of telogen hairs involving the whole scalp and continuing for more than 6–8 months. Patients report persistent and severe hair shedding that tends to have a fluctuating course for many years. Hair loss may be associated with progressive hair thinning, which uniformly affects all the scalp hairs. Marked bitemporal recession may be present [11, 13, 14].

A. Rakowska
Department of Dermatology, CSK MSW, Warsaw, Poland

M. Olszewska
Department of Dermatology, Medical University of Warsaw, Warsaw, Poland

L. Rudnicka (✉)
Faculty of Health Sciences, Medical University of Warsaw, Poland

Department of Dermatology, CSK MSW, Woloska 137, Warsaw 02-502, Poland
e-mail: lidia.rudnicka@euderm.eu

L. Rudnicka et al. (eds.), *Atlas of Trichoscopy*,
DOI 10.1007/978-1-4471-4486-1_18,

Although telogen effluvium most commonly affects postmenopausal women, 21 % of patients with this condition are premenopausal women and 11 % are men [15].

The most accurate diagnostic aids for acute and chronic telogen effluvium are histopathology and trichogram in combination with a detailed medical evaluation to identify the cause of telogen hair loss [16].

Trichoscopy has limited value in diagnosing telogen effluvium. Frequent, but not specific, findings include the presence of empty hair follicles, a predominance of follicular units with only one hair, perifollicular discoloration (the peripilar sign), and upright regrowing hairs. There is no significant difference between the findings in the frontal area and those in the occipital area, which differentiates telogen effluvium from androgenetic alopecia. However, clinicians should be aware that both diseases frequently coexist.

Table 18.1 Trichoscopic features of telogen effluvium

- Predominance of follicular units with only one hair
- Upright regrowing hairs
- Perifollicular discoloration (peripilar sign)
- Empty hair follicles/yellow dots
- Lack of features typical of other diseases

Box 18.1

- Trichoscopy is not diagnostic for telogen effluvium
- Coexistence of telogen effluvium and female androgenetic alopecia is very common

Table 18.2 Trichoscopic features of telogen effluvium and androgenetic alopecia

Feature	Telogen effluvium	Androgenetic alopecia	Coexistence of telogen effluvium and androgenetic alopecia
Empty hair follicles (including yellow dots)	+	+	+
Follicular units with only one hair in the frontal area	+	++	++
Upright regrowing hairs	++	+/–	+
Thin terminal hairs	+	+	+
Perifollicular discoloration (peripilar sign)	+	++	++
Vellus hairs	–	+	+
Hair shaft thickness heterogeneity	–	+	+
Predominance of abnormalities in the frontal region	–	++	+

Data from Rakowska et al. [14, 17] and Slowinska [18]
+ present, ++ common, – not present

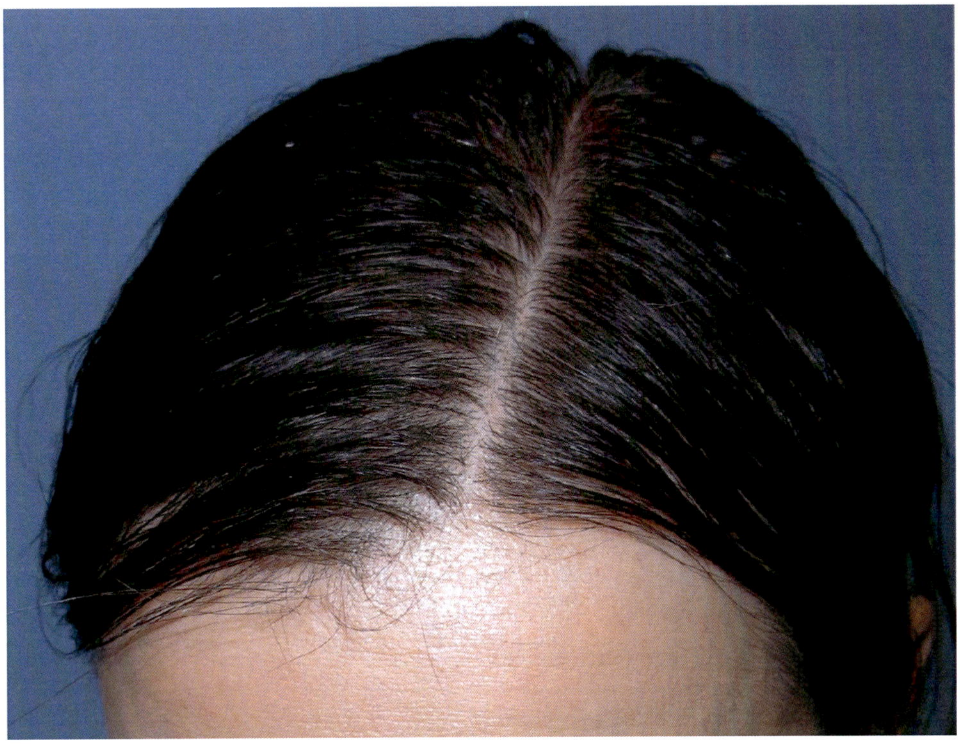

Fig. 18.1 Telogen effluvium. Telogen effluvium is characterized by the abrupt onset of hair loss involving the whole scalp. Marked bitemporal recession may be present (covered by hairs from the frontal area in this photograph). Alopecia in the temporal area results from the fact that baseline hair density in this area is normally low. In hair loss affecting the whole scalp equally, this area will appear alopecic at first. Differential diagnosis of telogen effluvium from early androgenetic alopecia may be difficult. Frequently, both diseases overlap

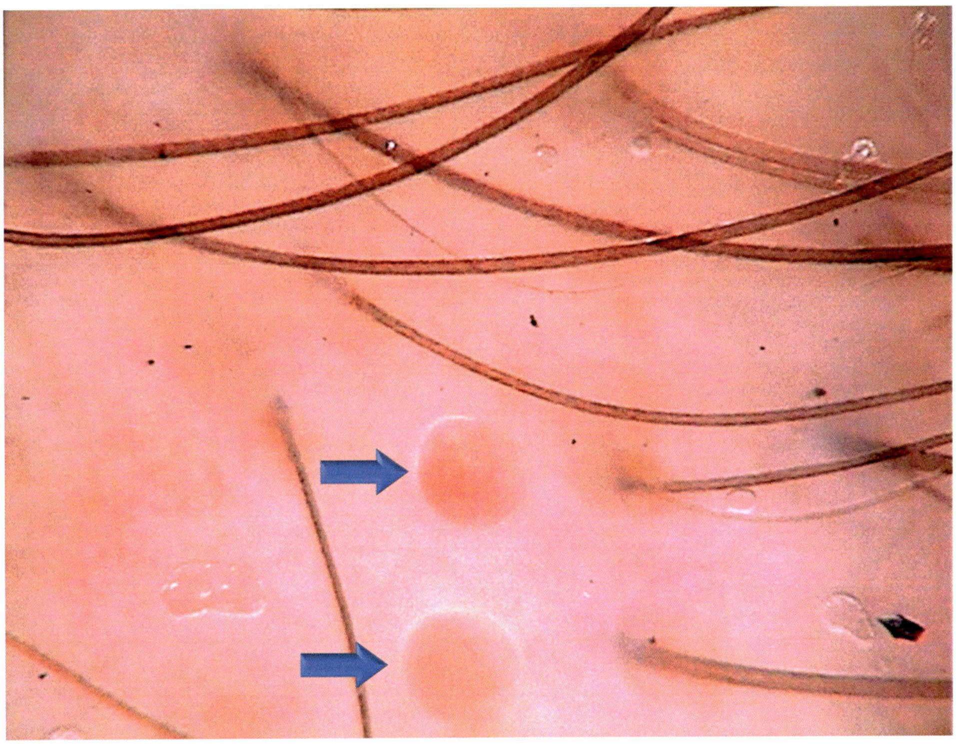

Fig. 18.2 Empty hair follicles in telogen effluvium. This feature rarely is seen in the form presented here (*arrows*) because normally, the shedding of telogen hairs (exogen phase) is followed almost immediately by the regrowth of new anagen hairs. If there is no hair regrowth, the hair follicle opening is filled with keratosebaceous material and appears as a yellow dot (×70)

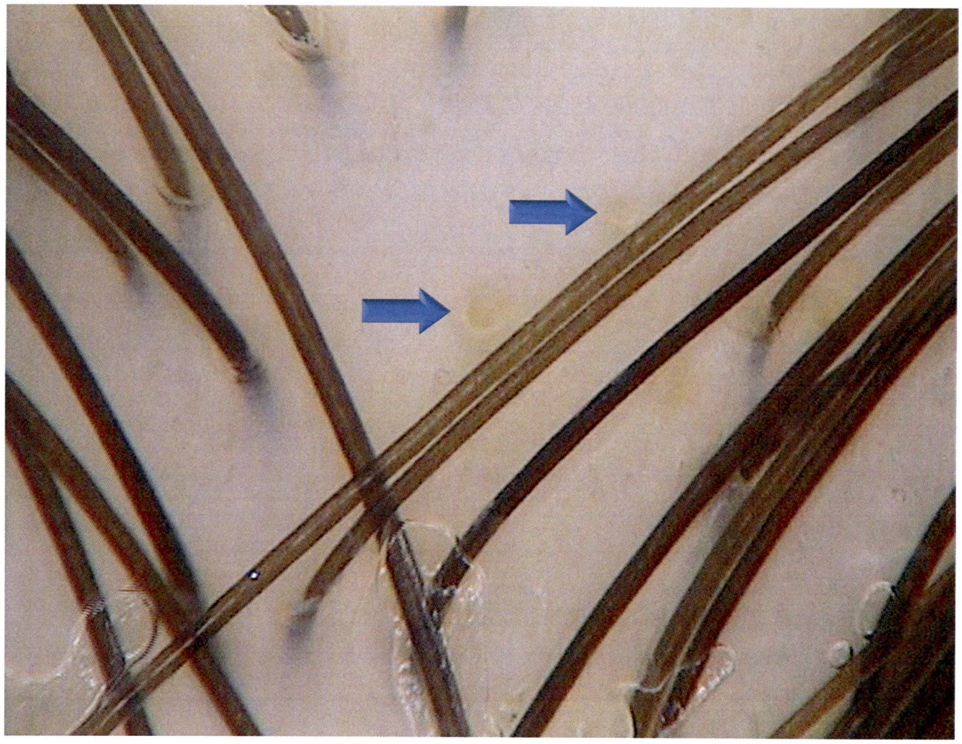

Fig. 18.3 Empty hair follicles in telogen effluvium. Shown are empty hair follicles filled with keratosebaceous material (*arrows*). They are indistinguishable from the yellow dots seen in androgenetic alopecia. Note that there are no features of androgenetic alopecia in this patient. Telogen effluvium was confirmed by trichogram (×70)

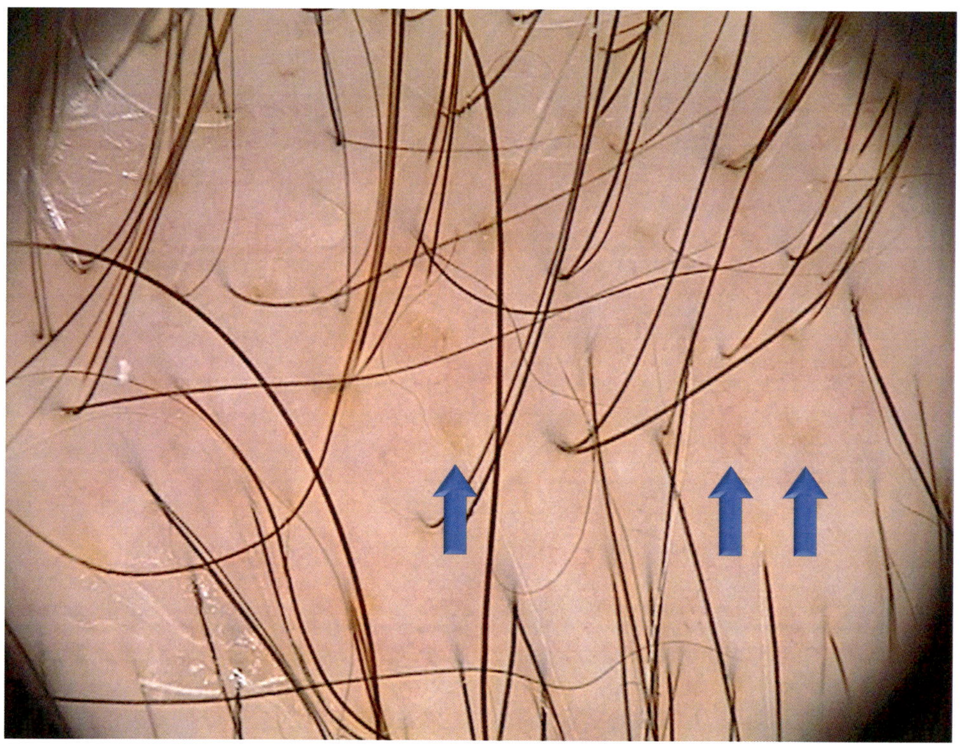

Fig. 18.4 Empty hair follicles in telogen effluvium. This image was taken from the temporal area of a patient with severe telogen effluvium due to chronic iron deficiency. Most of the empty follicular openings appear as yellow dots (*arrows*). Evaluation of the temporal area may be misleading for the beginner trichoscopist because this area generally contains the highest proportion of thin hairs and a great number of follicular units with only one hair. These characteristics may lead to the misdiagnosis of androgenetic alopecia if one tries to establish the diagnosis based on evaluation of the temporal area only (×20)

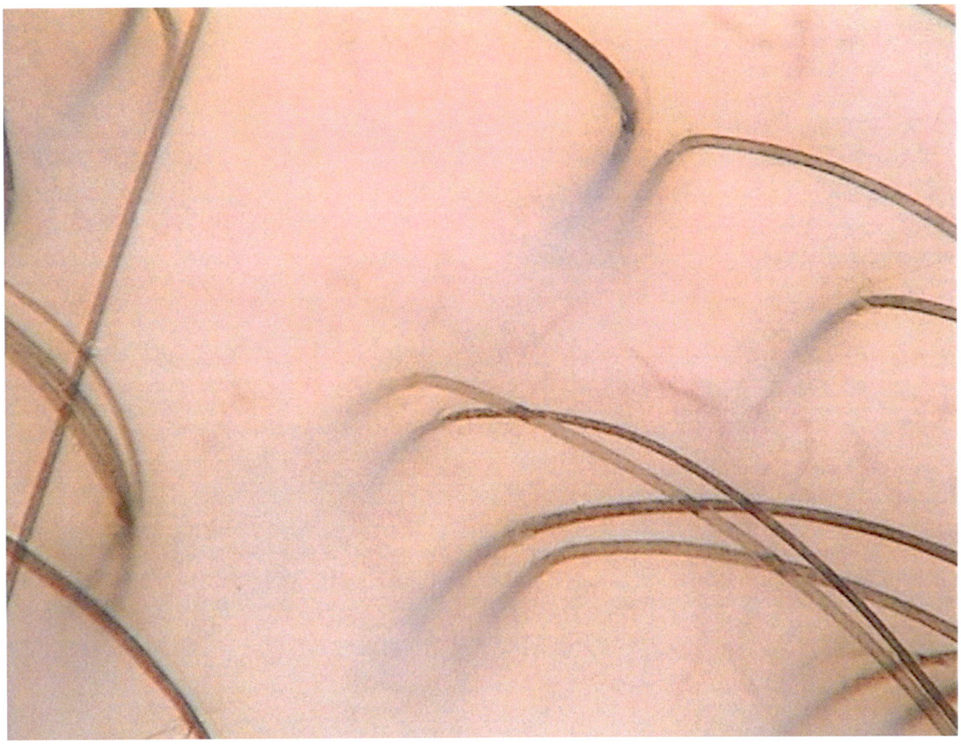

Fig. 18.5 Predominance of follicular units with only hair in telogen effluvium. Hair density is diminished during telogen effluvium. On trichoscopy, this may be seen as a predominance of follicular units with one hair and a significant decrease or absence of follicular units with three or more hairs. Note the absence of other abnormalities. Such images are highly indicative of telogen effluvium, but these findings also may be observed in other disorders, such as loose anagen hair syndrome and congenital hypotrichosis (×70)

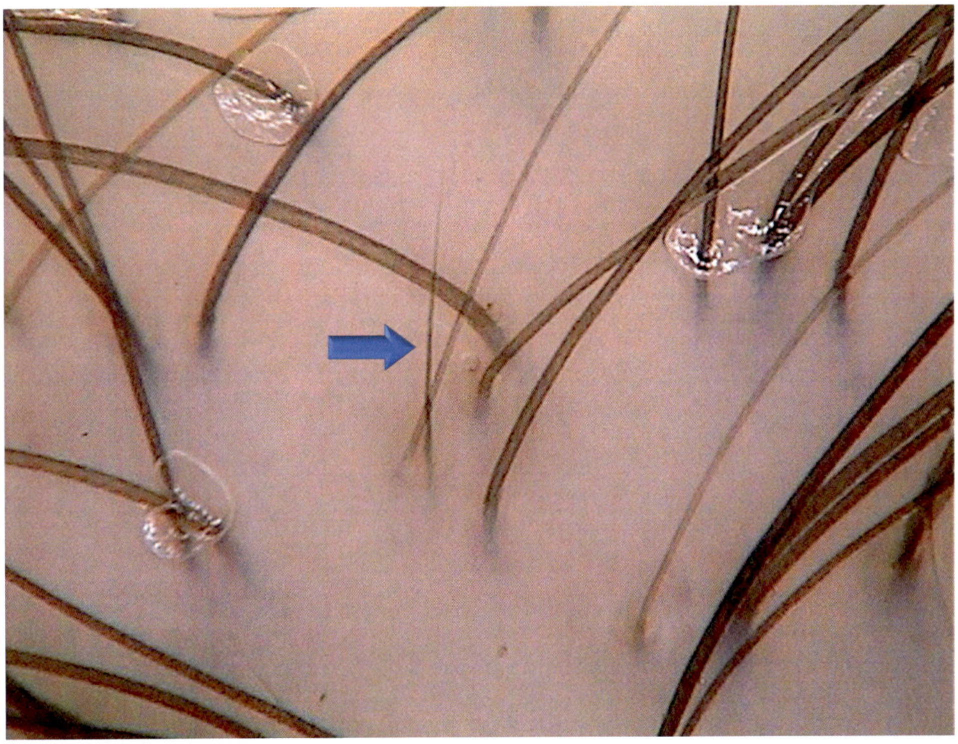

Fig. 18.6 Upright regrowing hair in telogen effluvium. In telogen effluvium, new, regrowing anagen hairs appear normal. They are firm and solid, which determines their upright position and sharp, pointed end (*arrow*). These hairs usually are pigmented similarly to terminal hairs in the area (×70)

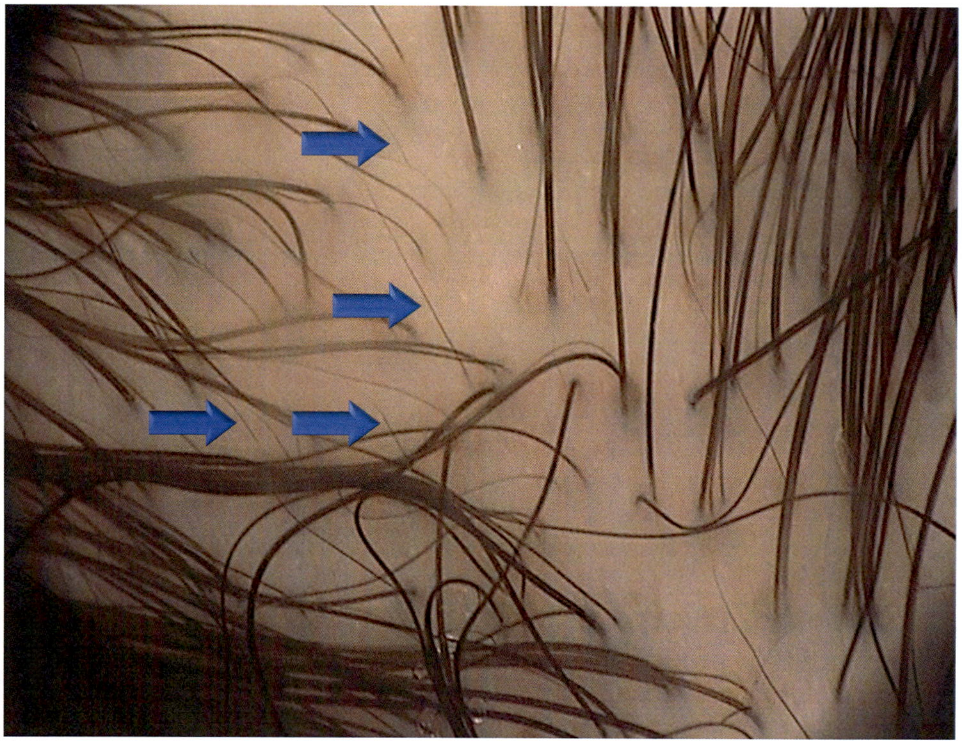

Fig. 18.7 Upright regrowing hairs in telogen effluvium. After telogen hairs shed (exogen phase), new anagen hair grows almost immediately. This regrowth is manifested by multiple upright regrowing hairs with pointed ends (*arrows*). The presence of a very large number of upright regrowing hairs is characteristic of acute, rather than chronic, telogen effluvium. Another feature differentiating acute from chronic telogen effluvium is the presence of thick terminal hairs in acute disease. In longstanding chronic telogen effluvium, the terminal hairs tend to become thinner over the years and the average hair shaft thickness is 48 μm [17], which is about 30–50 % thinner than normal terminal hairs in healthy persons (×20)

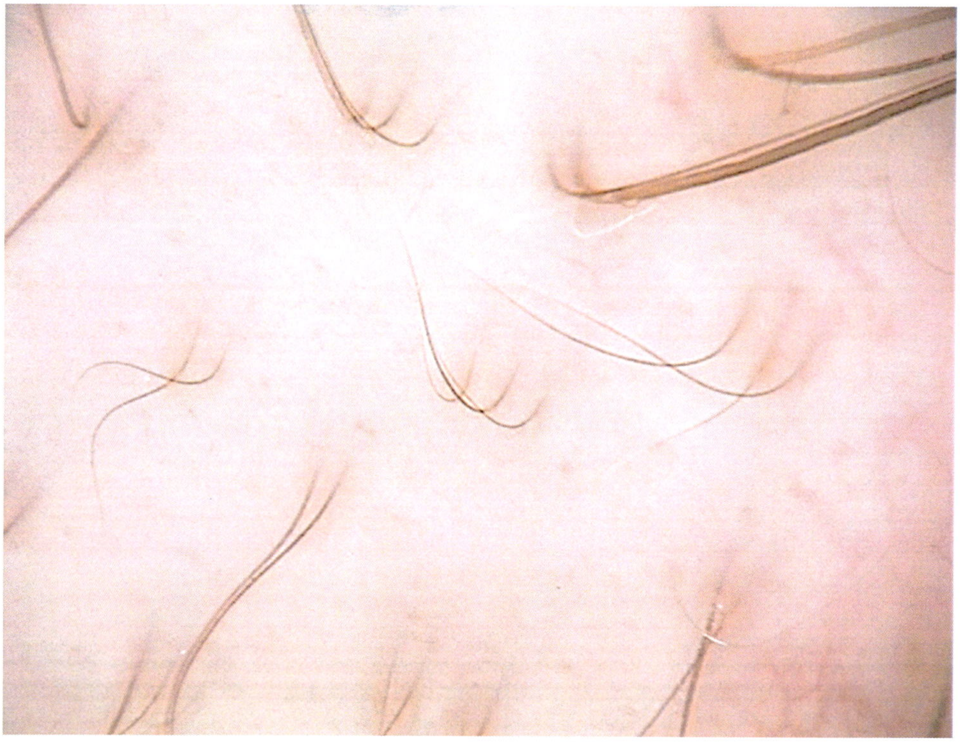

Fig. 18.8 Upright regrowing hairs in acute telogen effluvium. This image shows hair regrowth after severe hair loss in the course of acute telogen effluvium. The hairs are regrowing in follicular units of two to three hairs. These slightly bent (most probably by the dermoscope lens) hairs fulfill the criterion of upright regrowing hairs (×70)

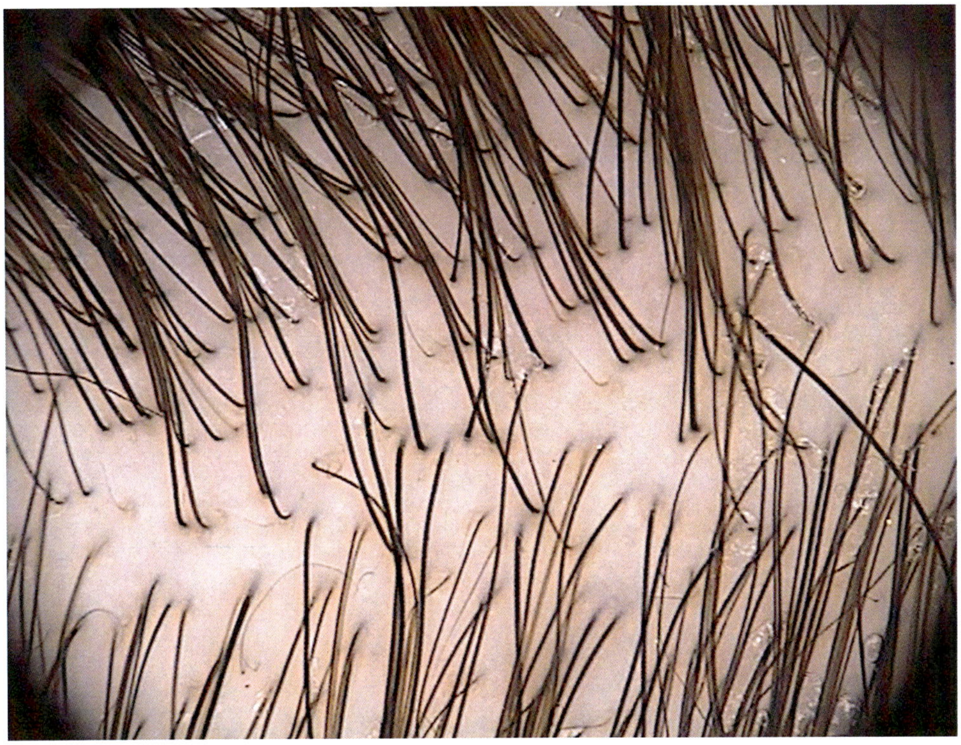

Fig. 18.9 Perifollicular discoloration (peripilar sign) in telogen effluvium. Perifollicular discoloration (the peripilar sign) is brown or brown-gray pigmentation of perifollicular skin. It is believed to reflect the presence of perifollicular lymphocytic infiltrates and was first described in androgenetic alopecia [19]. Perifollicular discoloration also is a frequent finding in telogen effluvium. Note that the terminal hairs are uniform in thickness. Sparse regrowing hairs are upright and sharply ended, which may indicate an early phase of telogen effluvium (×20)

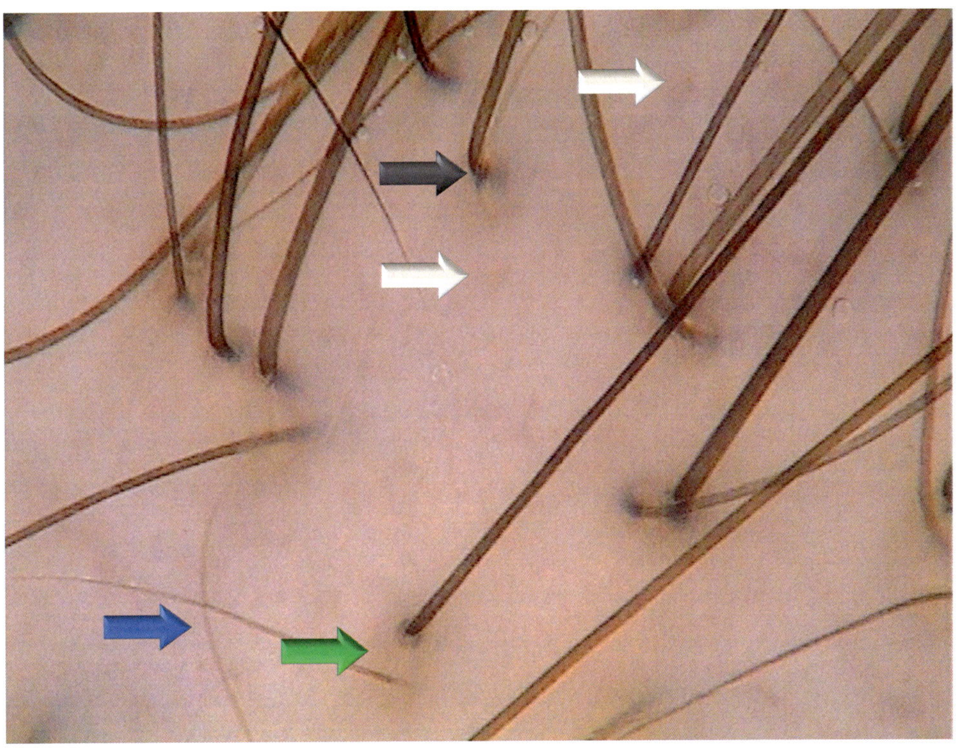

Fig. 18.10 Telogen effluvium. This image presents various trichoscopic features of telogen effluvium: short upright regrowing hairs (*blue arrow*), empty hair follicles (*white arrows*), perifollicular discoloration (*gray arrow*), and follicular units with one hair (*green arrow*) (×70)

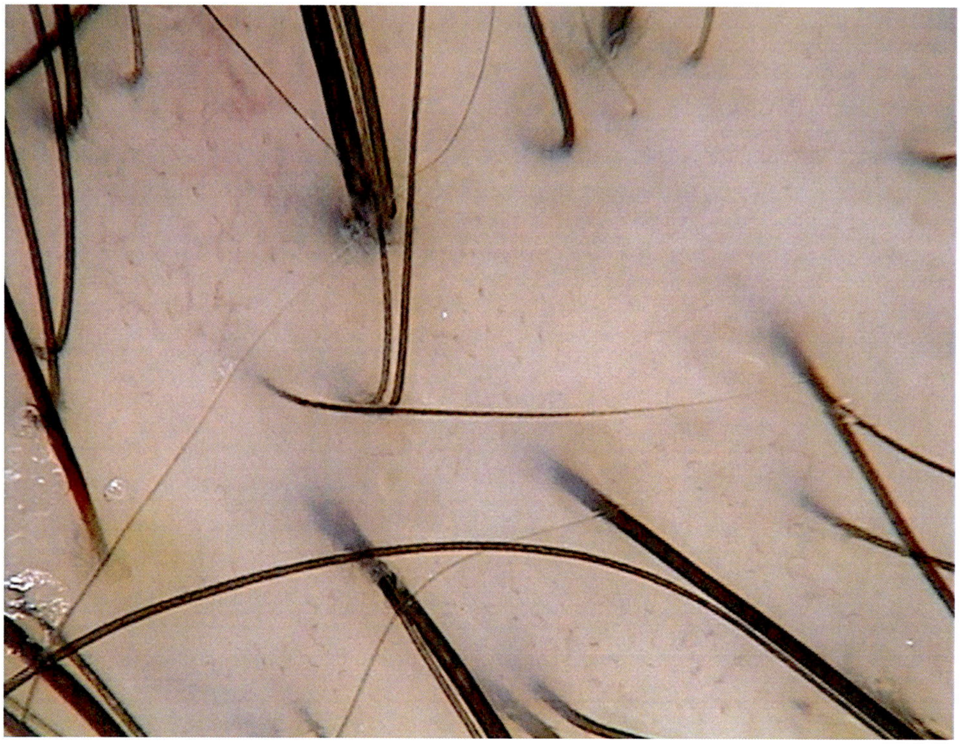

Fig. 18.11 **Trichoscopic features of telogen effluvium: short upright regrowing hairs, empty hair follicles, and perifollicular discoloration.** There is no specific vascular pattern in telogen effluvium. Areas of increased visibility of normal vessels, such as in this image, may result from the application of topical therapeutic agents (×70)

References

1. Kligman AM. Pathologic dynamics of human hair loss. I. Telogen effuvium. Arch Dermatol. 1961;83:175–98.
2. Blume-Peytavi U, Tosti A, Whiting DA, Trüeb RM, editors. Hair growth and disorders. Berlin/Heidelberg: Springer; 2008.
3. Camacho F, Montagna W, editors. Trichology: diseases of pilosebaceous follicle. Madrid: Aula Medica Group; 1997.
4. Trueb RM. Systematic approach to hair loss in women. J Dtsch Dermatol Ges. 2010;8(4):284–97, 98.
5. Mounsey AL, Reed SW. Diagnosing and treating hair loss. Am Fam Physician. 2009;80(4):356–62.
6. Durusoy C, Ozenli Y, Adiguzel A, Budakoglu IY, Tugal O, Arikan S, et al. The role of psychological factors and serum zinc, folate and vitamin B12 levels in the aetiology of trichodynia: a case-control study. Clin Exp Dermatol. 2009;34(7):789–92.
7. Katz KA, Cotsarelis G, Gupta R, Seykora JT. Telogen effluvium associated with the dopamine agonist pramipexole in a 55-year-old woman with Parkinson's disease. J Am Acad Dermatol. 2006; 55(5 Suppl):S103–4.
8. Patrizi A, Savoia F, Negosanti F, Posar A, Santucci M, Neri I. Telogen effluvium caused by magnesium valproate and lamotrigine. Acta Derm Venereol. 2005;85(1):77–8.
9. Piraccini BM, Iorizzo M, Rech G, Tosti A. Drug-induced hair disorders. Curr Drug Saf. 2006;1(3):301–5.
10. Tosti A, Piraccini BM, van Neste DJ. Telogen effluvium after allergic contact dermatitis of the scalp. Arch Dermatol. 2001;137(2):187–90.
11. Harrison S, Sinclair R. Telogen effluvium. Clin Exp Dermatol. 2002;27(5):389–95.
12. Whiting DA. Chronic telogen effluvium. Dermatol Clin. 1996; 14(4):723–31.
13. Chen W, Yang CC, Todorova A, Al Khuzaei S, Chiu HC, Worret WI, et al. Hair loss in elderly women. Eur J Dermatol. 2010;20(2): 145–51.
14. Rakowska A, Slowinska M, Kowalska-Oledzka E, Olszewska M, Rudnicka L. Dermoscopy in female androgenic alopecia: method standardization and diagnostic criteria. Int J Trichol. 2009;1(2): 123–30.
15. Garcia-Hernandez MJ, Camacho FM. Chronic telogen effluvium: incidence, clinical and biochemical features, and treatment. Arch Dermatol. 1999;135(9):1123–4.
16. Olszewska M, Warszawik O, Rakowska A, Slowinska M, Rudnicka L. Methods of hair loss evaluation in patients with endocrine disorders. Endokrynol Pol. 2010;61(4):406–11.
17. Rakowska A. Trichoscopy (hair and scalp videodermoscopy) in the healthy female. Method standardization and norms for measurable parameters. J Dermatol Case Rep. 2009;3(1):14–9.
18. Slowinska M. The value of videodermoscopy in differential diagnosis of androgenetic alopecia [doctoral thesis]. Warsaw: Medical University of Warsaw; 2010.
19. Deloche C, de Lacharriere O, Misciali C, Piraccini BM, Vincenzi C, Bastien P, et al. Histological features of peripilar signs associated with androgenetic alopecia. Arch Dermatol Res. 2004;295(10): 422–8.

Anagen Effluvium

19

Adriana Rakowska, Malgorzata Olszewska,
and Lidia Rudnicka

Abstract

Anagen effluvium is a common term for multiple conditions associated with diffuse hair loss from follicles in the anagen growth phase. This chapter focuses on trichoscopy of diverse diseases associated with anagen hair loss (e.g., chemotherapy-induced alopecia, loose anagen syndrome, short anagen syndrome). Alopecia areata incognita, which is a condition of controversial classification, also is discussed in this chapter.

Keywords

Alopecia areata incognita • Anagen effluvium • Black dots • Chemotherapy-induced alopecia • Drug-induced alopecia • Loose anagen syndrome • Monilethrix-like hair Pohl-Pinkus constriction • Short anagen syndrome

Anagen effluvium is a common term for multiple conditions associated with diffuse hair loss from follicles in the anagen growth phase. Anagen effluvium occurs most commonly when the metabolic and mitotic activity of the follicle is rapidly suppressed by a cytotoxic drug or other toxic factor [1, 2]. The most extensive anagen effluvium is observed in patients undergoing chemotherapy [1–5]. Drug-induced hair loss due to noncytotoxic agents (e.g., acitretin) also may follow an anagen pathway [6–8]. Anagen effluvium may result from exposure to radiation therapy or toxins, as well as from systemic disorders. Exposure to cigarette smoke has been indicated as another toxic factor that may induce anagen effluvium [4, 9, 10]. Trichoscopy of anagen effluvium due to toxicity is characterized by the presence of monilethrix-like hairs and black dots.

Another condition associated with anagen hair loss is loose anagen syndrome. This disease, typically seen in girls 1–6 years old, is characterized by defective (weak) anchorage of the anagen hairs to the follicle [11–13]. Hair that "does not grow" and is pulled out easily and painlessly is a typical symptom of loose anagen syndrome [11, 12]. The trichogram reveals the absence of the outer and inner root sheaths in 70 % of anagen hairs ("loose anagen hairs"). The proximal segment of the hair shaft appears disfigured and twisted, with characteristic ruffling of the cuticle. Telogen hairs may not be present [11, 14, 15]. Trichoscopy is unspecific and shows sparse hair, a decreased number of hair shafts per follicular unit, and occasionally trichorrhexis nodosa.

Loose anagen syndrome should be distinguished from short anagen syndrome. Although these two conditions share a similar name and have an analogous clinical appearance of "hair that does not grow," pathogenically they are two different entities. Short anagen syndrome is characterized by the inability of the hair to grow long because of an extremely short anagen phase. Hairs go through a full hair cycle and fall out before they grow longer then 3–6 cm [16, 17]. The trichogram shows a decreased

A. Rakowska
Department of Dermatology, CSK MSW, Warsaw, Poland

M. Olszewska
Department of Dermatology,
Medical University of Warsaw, Warsaw, Poland

L. Rudnicka (✉)
Faculty of Health Sciences, Medical University of Warsaw, Poland

Department of Dermatology, CSK MSW, Woloska 137,
Warsaw 02-502, Poland
e-mail: lidia.rudnicka@euderm.eu

L. Rudnicka et al. (eds.), *Atlas of Trichoscopy*,
DOI 10.1007/978-1-4471-4486-1_19, © Springer-Verlag London 2012

proportion of anagen hairs and an abundance of telogen hairs. The hairs have a pointed distal tip, indicating that the hair was never cut or broken [16, 17]. Trichoscopy shows normal hair density and many regrowing hairs of different lengths [18].

In recent years, a type of alopecia has been observed that does not fit current hair loss classifications [19–23]. In this condition, called *alopecia areata incognita* [23], hair loss is characterized by rapid onset, prominent hair thinning in the frontal area, and a good prognosis for regrowth. Women are predominantly affected [19–23]. This disease was first described by A. Rebora [23], who hypothesized that it is alopecia areata that develops in patients with female androgenetic alopecia. Based on trichoscopic findings, it later was suggested that the disease instead may fit into the spectrum of acute telogen effluvium, which develops in patients with subclinical female androgenetic alopecia. The term *acute hair miniaturization* has been suggested [21]. Characteristic trichoscopic features are yellow dots and numerous short regrowing hairs [20, 21].

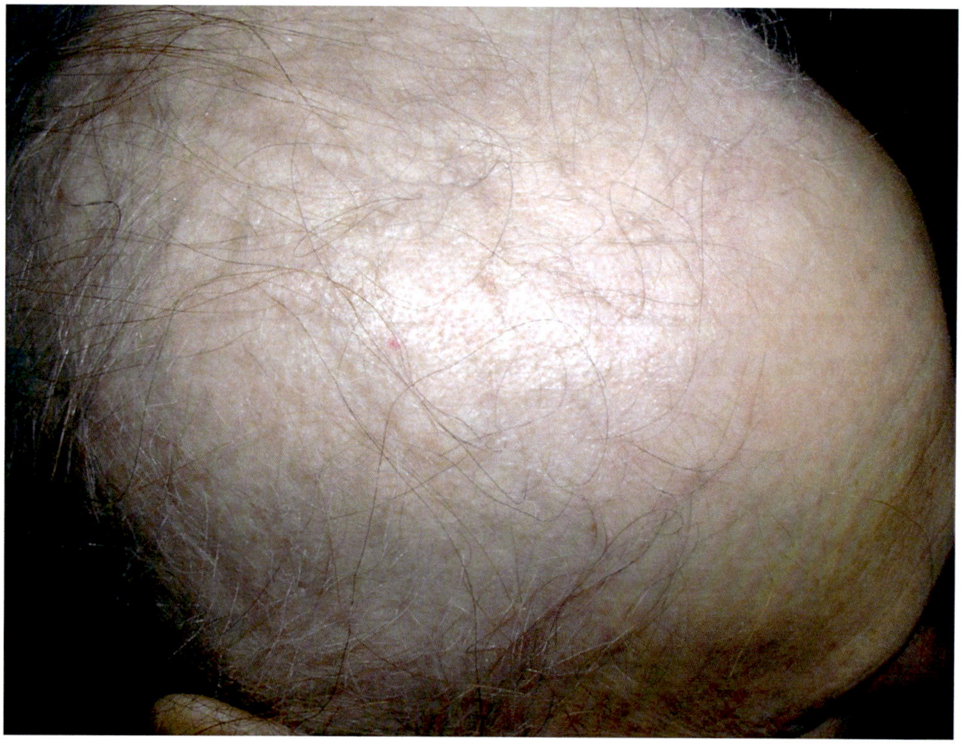

Fig. 19.1 Chemotherapy-induced alopecia. The onset of chemotherapy-induced alopecia is observed about 1–3 weeks after the first dose of chemotherapy [1]. It may be caused by a wide range of cytotoxic agents, including doxorubicin, docetaxel, daunorubicin, epirubicin, etoposide, ifosfamide, irinotecan, paclitaxel, topotecan, vindesine, and vinorelbine [1–4]. New, targeted anticancer therapies, such as sorafenib and sunitinib, also have been associated with anagen effluvium [5]. The average incidence of hair loss in patients receiving chemotherapy is about 65 %, with high variability depending on the agent. Combination therapy consisting of two or more agents produces a higher incidence of more severe hair loss compared with monotherapy [1]. Drug-induced hair loss due to noncytotoxic agents, such as acitretin, carbamazepine, fluoxetine, fluorobutyrophenone, interferon, ribavirin, risperidone, and sertraline, most likely follows both an anagen and a telogen pathway [6–8]

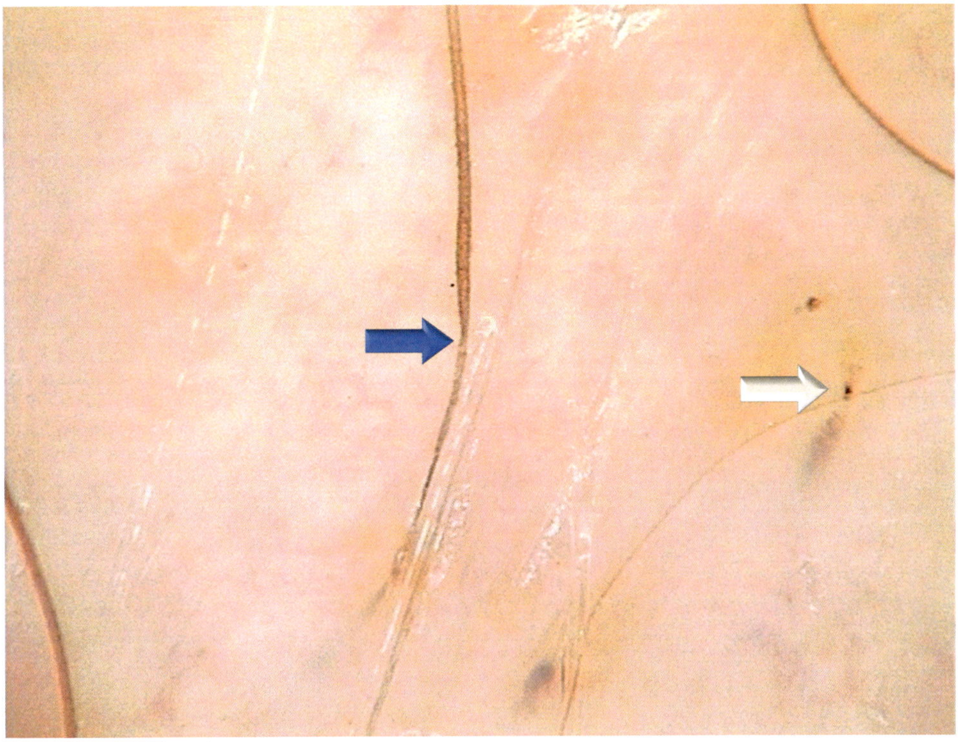

Fig. 19.2 Chemotherapy-induced alopecia. Chemotherapy-induced alopecia occurs when the mitotic activity of the follicle is rapidly suppressed. The hair shafts become thinner locally and tend to break at the thinned points. Most frequently, the fracture occurs at the scalp level. The remaining end of the fractured hair shaft appears on trichoscopy as a black dot (*white arrow*). With lower doses, there may be only segmental thinning (constriction) or narrowing, without fracture of the shaft at the point of weakness. This type of constriction is called *Pohl-Pinkus constriction* (*blue arrow*). When the drug is stopped, the follicle resumes its activity within a few weeks and the hair shaft thickens again. Another course of the drug will reproduce these changes. Multiple constrictions within the same hair give the hair shaft a monilethrix-like appearance (×70)

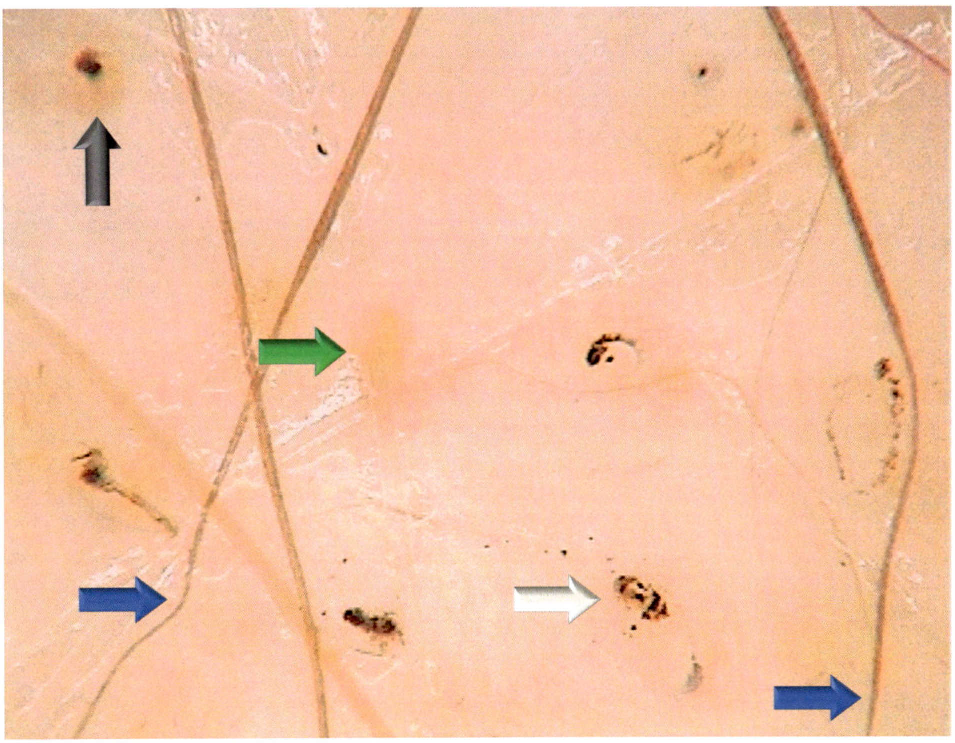

Fig. 19.3 Chemotherapy-induced alopecia. The image shows multiple hair shaft residues (*white arrow*). Note the similarity to the hair shaft residues observed in trichotillomania (see Chap. 20). Hair shafts with Pohl-Pinkus constrictions have a tapered appearance (*blue arrows*). Black dots are visible (*black arrow*). Yellow dots mark empty hair follicles (*green arrow*) (×70)

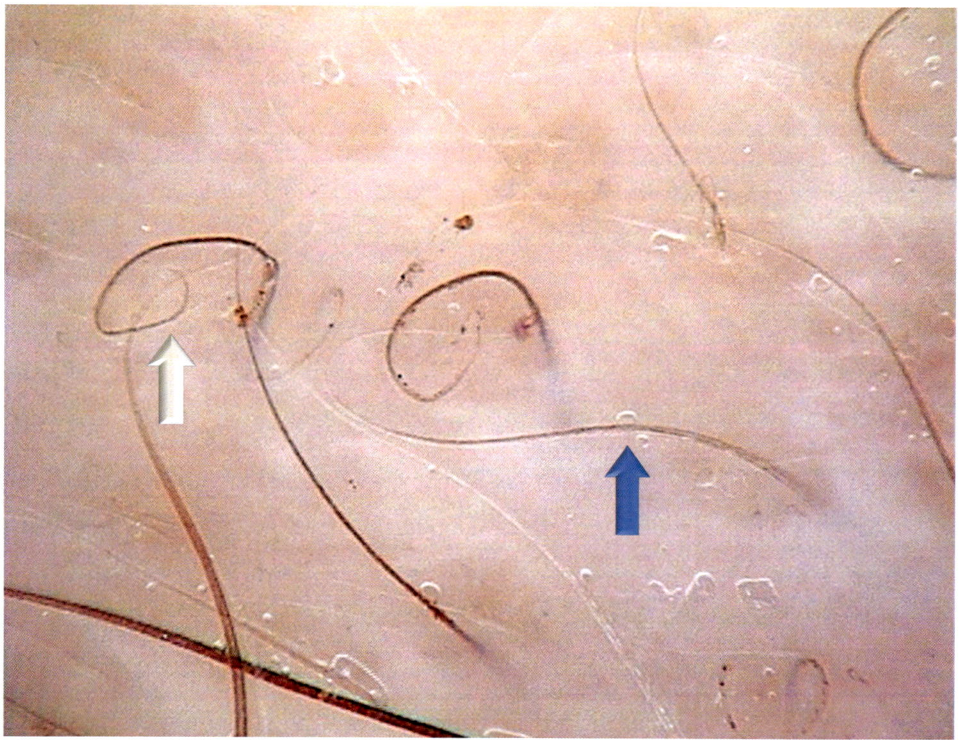

Fig. 19.4 Partial hair regrowth in chemotherapy-induced alopecia. The image shows regrowing hairs (*blue arrow*) in a patient with chemotherapy-induced alopecia. Some hairs have a pigtail appearance (*white arrow*). The grainy elements within the circular pigtail hairs indicate a defective inner structure of the distal parts of these hair shafts (×60)

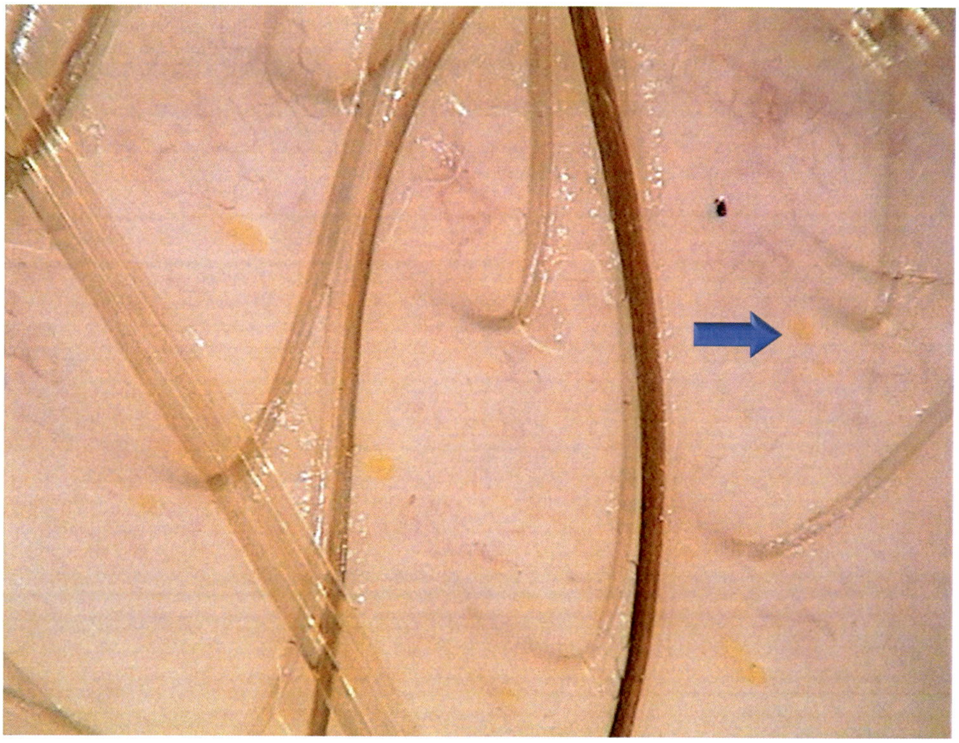

Fig. 19.5 Chemotherapy-induced alopecia. Higher magnification provides a detailed view of multiple yellow dots (*arrow*), which mark empty hair follicles. Most hair follicles contain only one hair. The hair shafts are uniform in shape and thickness (×70)

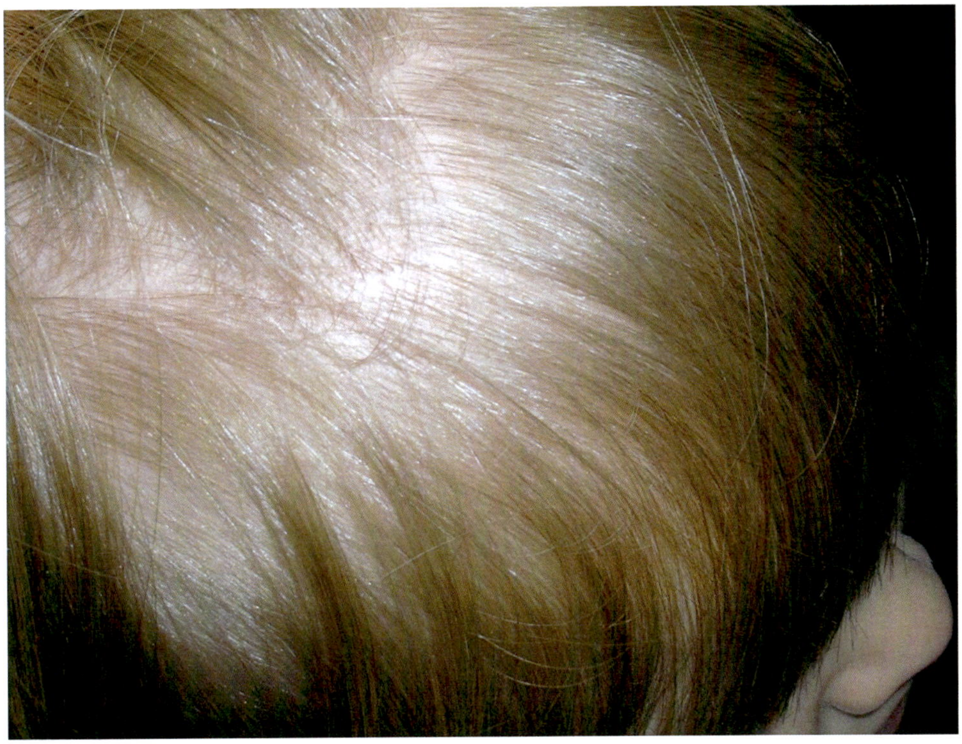

Fig. 19.6 **Loose anagen syndrome**. The most probable cause of loose anagen syndrome is premature keratinization of the inner root sheath, which causes impaired adhesion between the cuticle of the inner root sheath and that of the hair shaft. Thus, hair is pulled out easily and painlessly with minimal mechanical force, and it regrows quickly. The fast turnover of short hairs gives the impression of "short hair that does not grow." The disease predominantly affects girls (female:male = 6:1) ages 1–6 years, and the occipital area is the site of predilection. The basis for diagnosis is the trichogram, which shows a predominance of 90–100 % of anagen hairs, most of which are devoid of the outer and inner root sheath ("loose anagen hairs"). Staining with 4-dimethylaminocinnam-aldehyde, which selectively stains citrulline-containing proteins in the internal root sheath bright red, may be helpful [14, 24, 25]. The sole presence of a few loose anagen hairs is not diagnostic. A small number of loose anagen hairs also may be observed in healthy individuals, as well as in various diseases and syndromes other than loose anagen syndrome [11, 14]

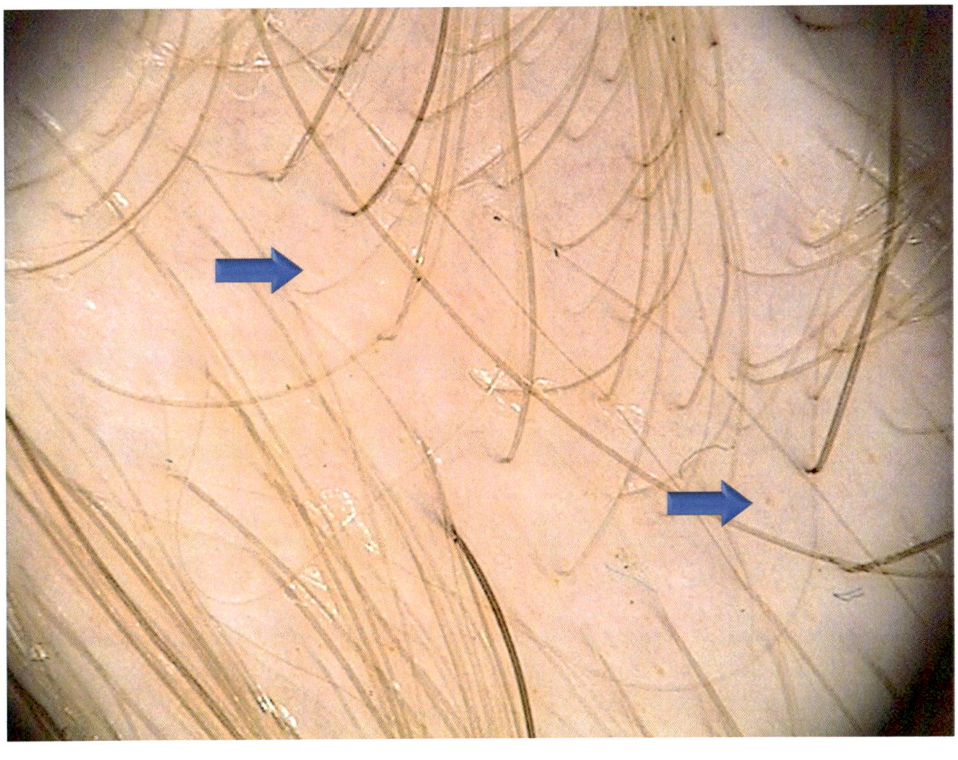

Fig. 19.7 **Loose anagen syndrome**. There are no specific trichoscopic features of loose anagen syndrome. The hair density is decreased, and most follicular units contain only one hair. Yellow dots (*arrows*) correspond to empty hair follicles (×20)

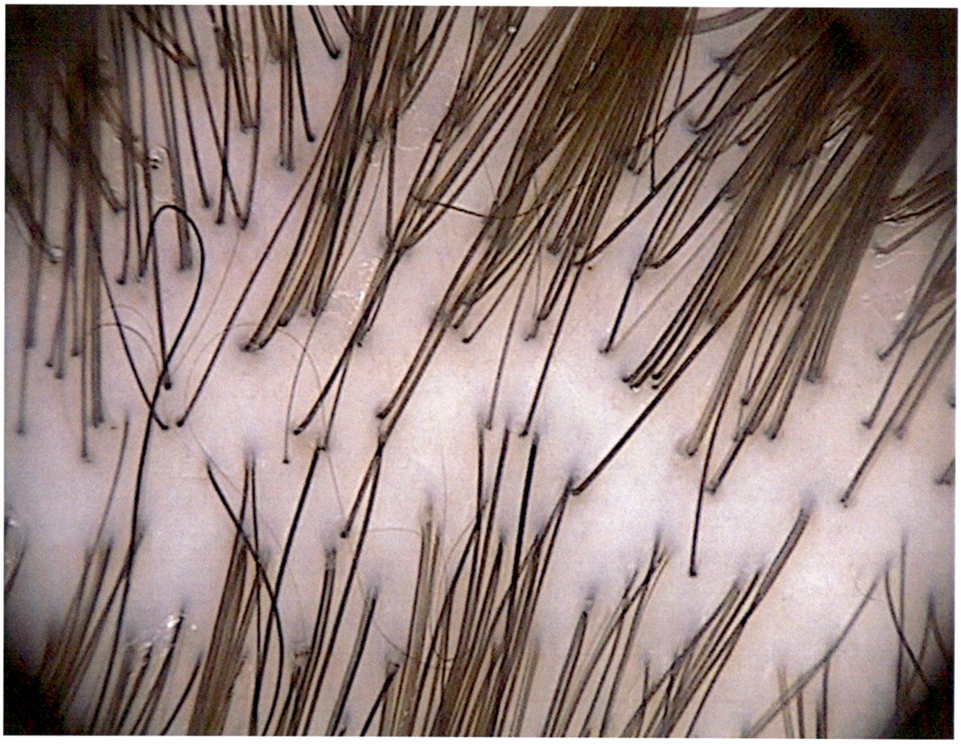

Fig. 19.8 Short anagen syndrome. In short anagen syndrome, the anagen phase is extremely short. Hairs pass through the short hair cycle and fall out before they grow longer then 3–6 cm [16, 17], giving the clinical impression of "short hair that does not grow" and "never requires a haircut." Disease onset is usually at birth or in childhood, but cases of short anagen syndrome first diagnosed in adulthood also have been described. The trichogram shows a decreased proportion of anagen hairs and a predominance of telogen hairs [16, 17]. Trichoscopy is nonspecific and shows normal hair density and numerous upright regrowing hairs of different lengths [18] (×20)

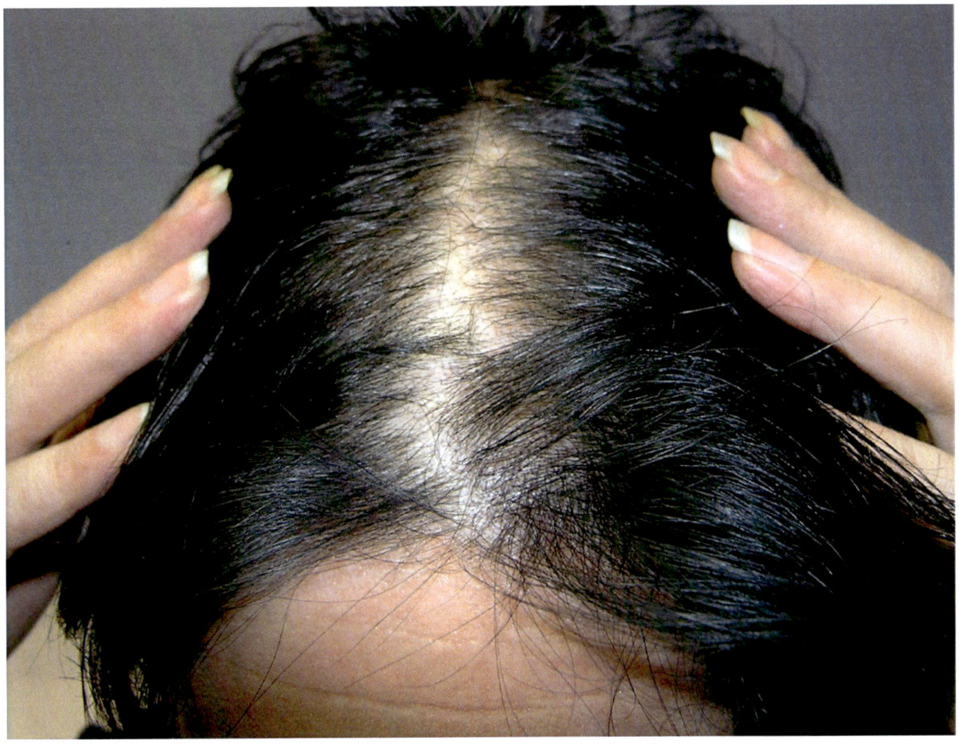

Fig. 19.9 Alopecia areata incognita. Alopecia areata incognita is acute hair loss predominantly in the frontal area and is associated with follicular miniaturization and thinning of the hair shafts. The disease is most common in middle-aged women and has a good prognosis for hair regrowth. This condition, described by Rebora in 1987 [23], became a matter of debate 20 years after the initial publication. The core issue of discussion is its similarity to alopecia areata. Rebora [23] hypothesized that alopecia areata, which develops in patients with androgenetic alopecia, causes diffuse rather than patchy hair loss; therefore he named this condition *alopecia areata incognita* [22, 26, 27]. Some authors now consider alopecia areata incognita a separate entity in the sole spectrum of alopecia areata and clearly distinguish the condition from androgenetic alopecia [20, 28, 29]. In our opinion, the condition known as *alopecia areata incognita* is most consistent with acute telogen effluvium developing in patients with female androgenetic alopecia [21]. The disease shows no features of alopecia areata, such as a young age of onset, equal incidence in females and males, a tendency to coexist with autoimmune diseases, involvement of the eyebrows and other body hair, a tendency to progress to alopecia totalis, or characteristic trichoscopic or trichogram features of alopecia areata. In contrast, the rapid onset of disease, predominant hair loss in the frontal area, good prognosis for hair regrowth regardless of therapy, increased proportion of telogen hairs, hair follicle miniaturization, and trichoscopic features indicate that, in most cases, alopecia areata incognita is in fact a subtype of acute telogen effluvium, which develops in patients with female androgenetic alopecia [21]

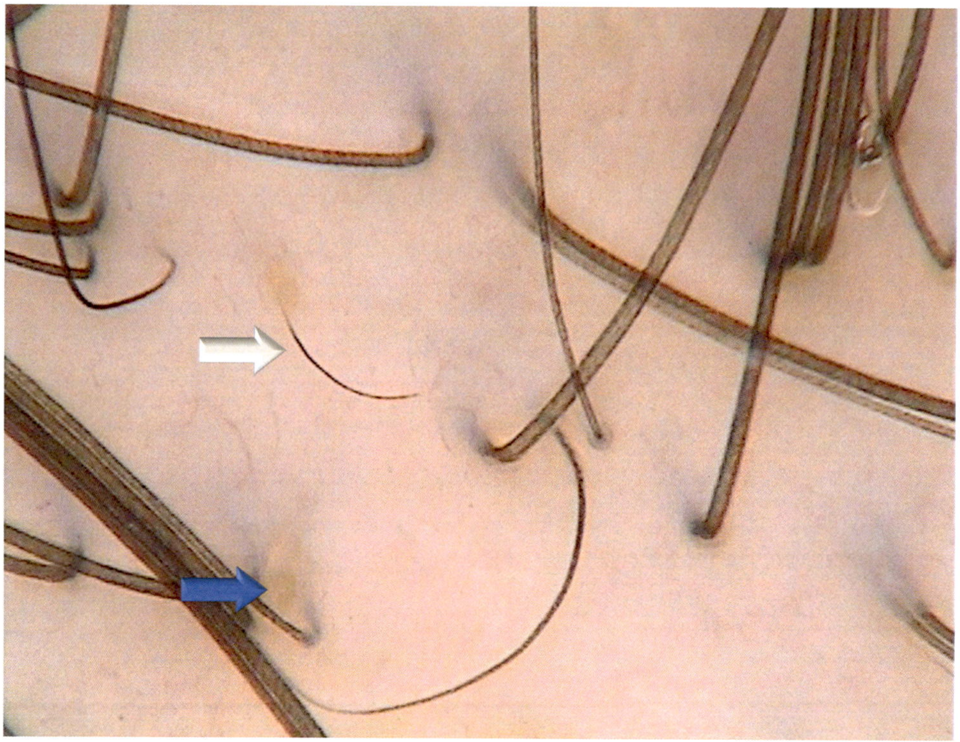

Fig. 19.10 Yellow dots and regrowing hairs in alopecia areata incognita. Trichoscopy of alopecia areata incognita shows multiple yellow dots (*blue arrow*), most abundant in "androgen-dependent" areas, and small regrowing hairs (*white arrow*). Unlike typical telogen effluvium and typical alopecia areata, in which most regrowing hairs have a pointed, upright structure, these hairs form several unusual shapes, including dark lines, S-shaped hairs, and hairs that bulge at the proximal end (tadpole-like structure) (×70)

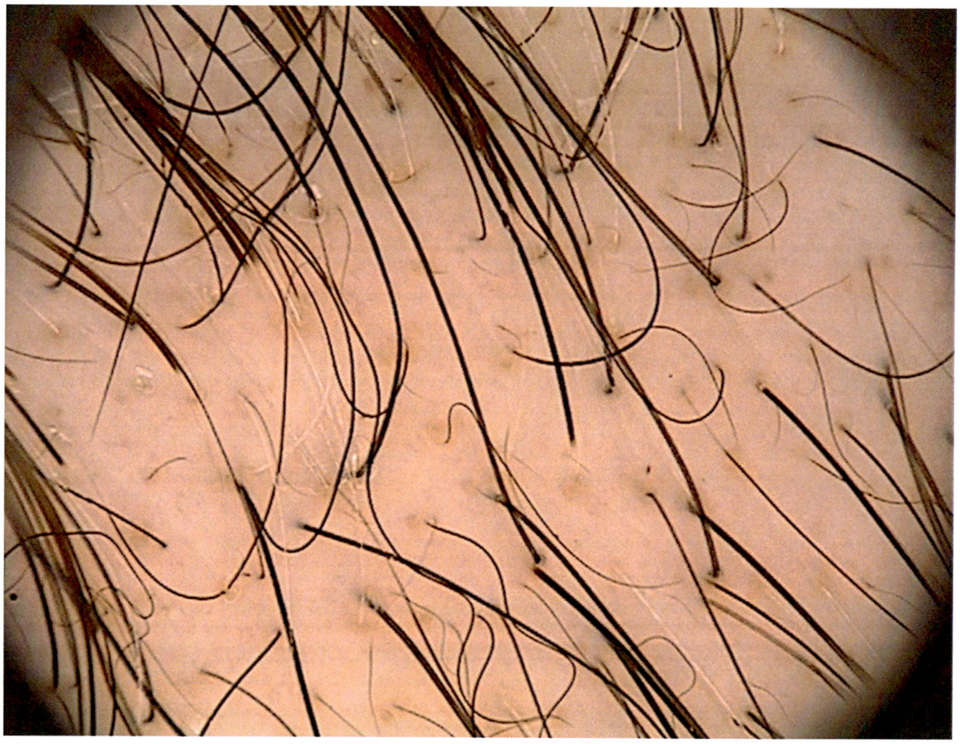

Fig. 19.11 Multiple shapes of regrowing hairs in alopecia areata incognita. Regrowing hairs in alopecia areata incognita differ in length and shape. A tendency to form S-like shapes is a common finding in most patients. A reduced number of hairs per follicular unit is visible. Note the diversity in thickness of the terminal hair shafts (×20)

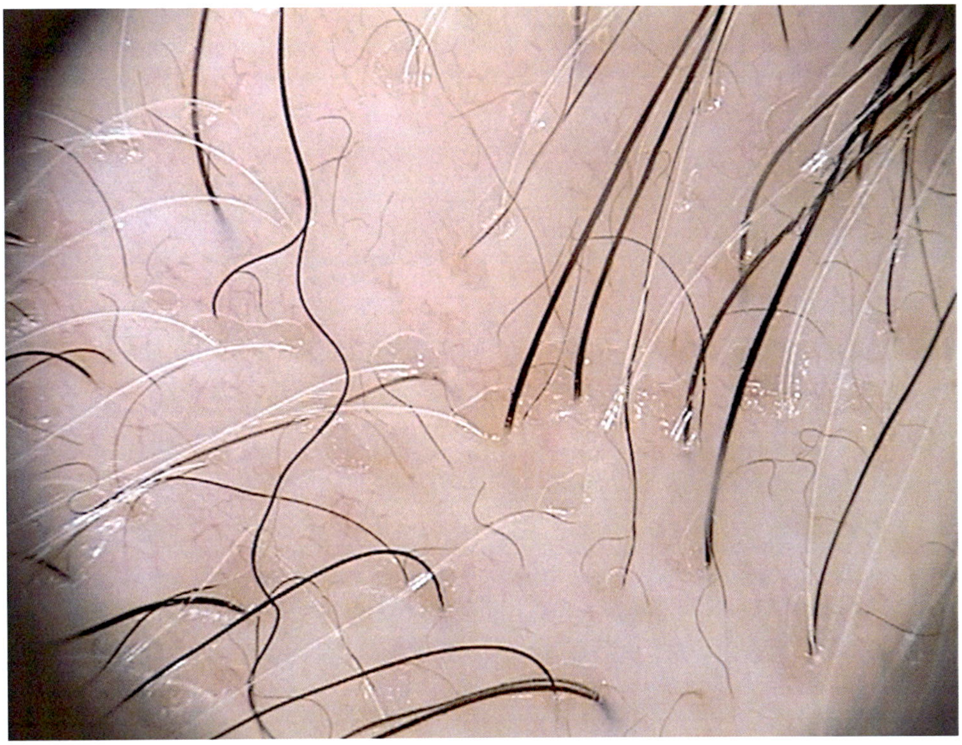

Fig. 19.12 **Dark regrowing hairs in alopecia areata incognita**. Multiple regrowing S-shaped hairs of various lengths are visible in this patient. Interestingly, in alopecia areata incognita, regrowing hairs are intensely pigmented, even in gray-haired patients (×20)

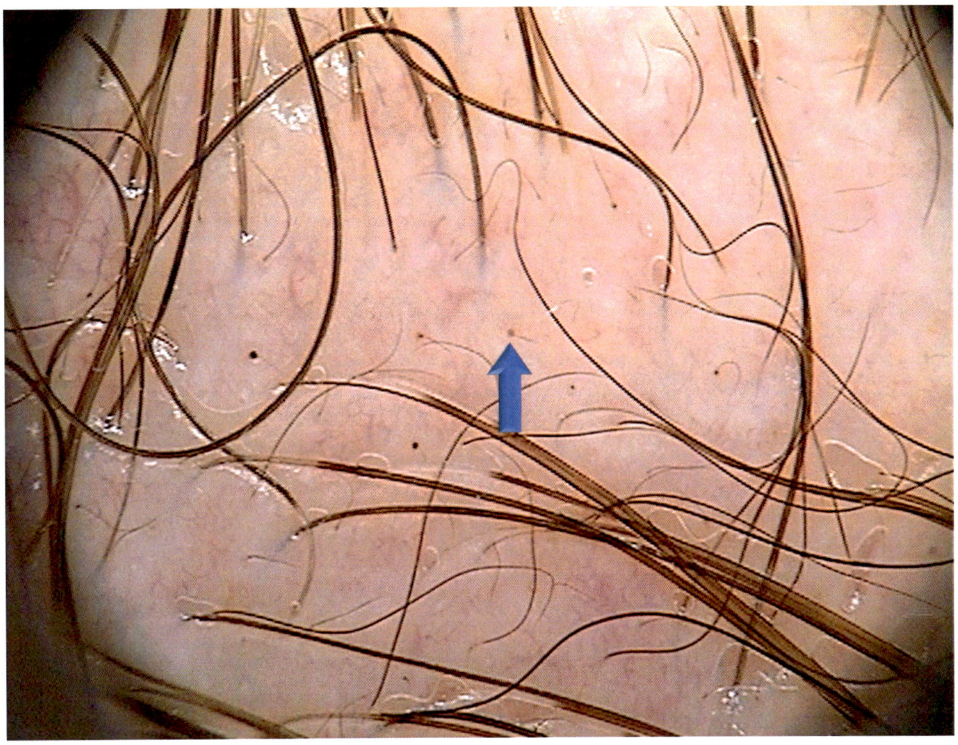

Fig. 19.13 **Tadpole-like hairs in alopecia areata incognita**. New regrowing hairs with a bulging proximal end (*arrow*) are common in alopecia areata incognita. Multiple S-shaped hairs also are visible in this image. Note that most terminal hairs are hypopigmented at the distal end, indicating hair regrowth of gray hair after colorization, whereas the small regrowing hairs are darkly colored (×20)

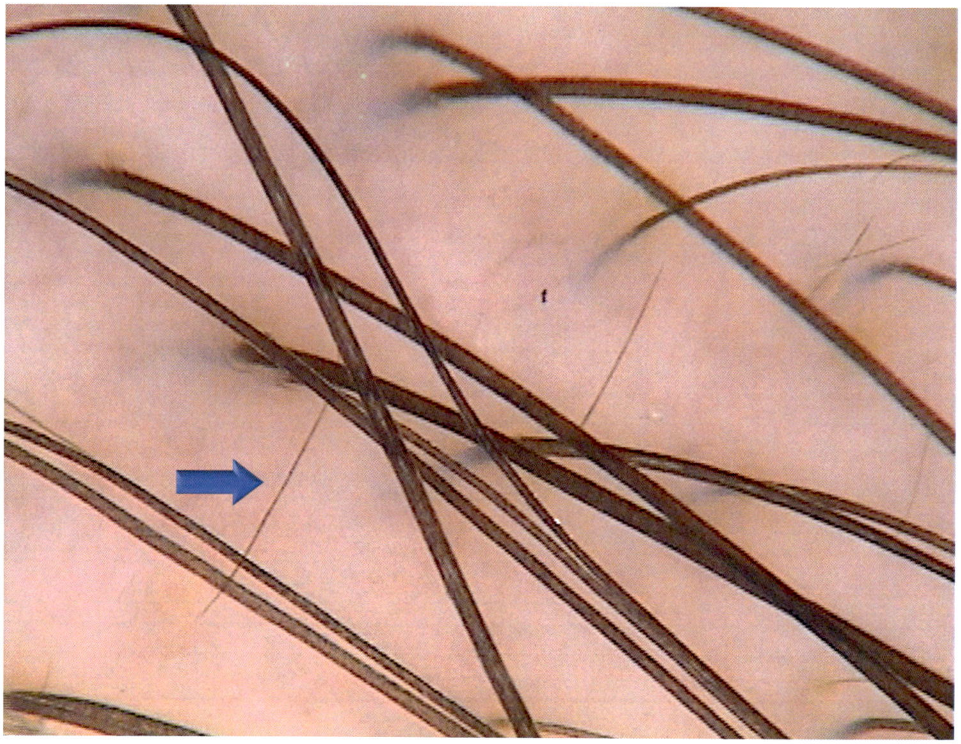

Fig. 19.14 Dark lines in alopecia areata incognita. Dark lines are regrowing hairs that are pigmented, thin, and short (*arrow*). Occasionally, they are darker than the natural color of the patient's hair. In these hairs, differentiation between proximal and distal ends often is impossible (×70)

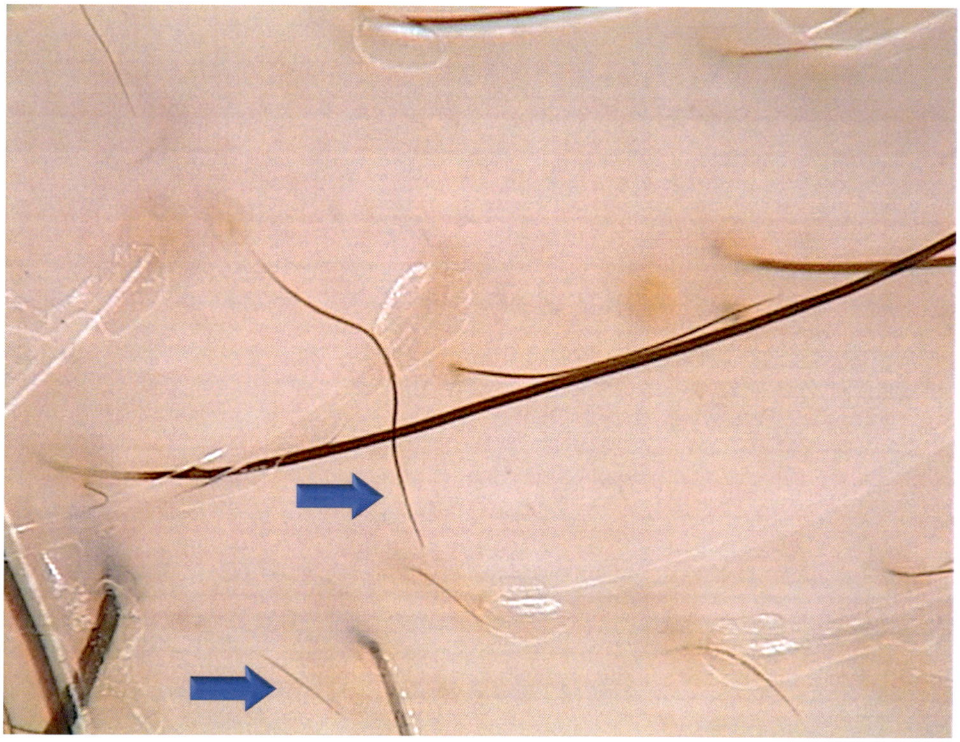

Fig. 19.15 Alopecia areata incognita. The image shows various sizes and shapes of dark lines (*arrows*) in a patient with alopecia areata incognita. Also note the presence of yellow dots, which are present both in empty hair follicles and in follicles with emerging hair shafts (×70)

References

1. Trueb RM. Chemotherapy-induced alopecia. Curr Opin Support Palliat Care. 2010;4(4):281–4.
2. Ramos-e-Silva M, Chaves Azevedo-e-Silva M, Carneiro SC. Hair, nail, and pigment changes in major systemic disease. Clin Dermatol. 2008;26(3):296–305.
3. Yeager CE, Olsen EA. Treatment of chemotherapy-induced alopecia. Dermatol Ther. 2011;24(4):432–42.
4. Guillot B, Bessis D, Dereure O. Mucocutaneous side effects of antineoplastic chemotherapy. Expert Opin Drug Saf. 2004;3(6):579–87.
5. Lee WJ, Lee JL, Chang SE, Lee MW, Kang YK, Choi JH, et al. Cutaneous adverse effects in patients treated with the multitargeted kinase inhibitors sorafenib and sunitinib. Br J Dermatol. 2009; 161(5):1045–51.
6. Tosti A, Pazzaglia M. Drug reactions affecting hair: diagnosis. Dermatol Clin. 2007;25(2):223–31, vii.
7. Piraccini BM, Iorizzo M, Rech G, Tosti A. Drug-induced hair disorders. Curr Drug Saf. 2006;1(3):301–5.
8. Trueb RM. Systematic approach to hair loss in women. J Dtsch Dermatol Ges. 2010;8(4):284–97, 298.
9. D'Agostini F, Balansky R, Pesce C, Fiallo P, Lubet RA, Kelloff GJ, et al. Induction of alopecia in mice exposed to cigarette smoke. Toxicol Lett. 2000;114(1–3):117–23.
10. Severs GA, Griffin T, Werner-Wasik M. Cicatricial alopecia secondary to radiation therapy: case report and review of the literature. Cutis. 2008;81(2):147–53.
11. Dhurat RP, Deshpande DJ. Loose anagen hair syndrome. Int J Trichol. 2010;2(2):96–100.
12. Tosti A, Piraccini BM. Loose anagen hair syndrome and loose anagen hair. Arch Dermatol. 2002;138(4):521–2.
13. Price VH, Gummer CL. Loose anagen syndrome. J Am Acad Dermatol. 1989;20(2 Pt 1):249–56.
14. Mirmirani P, Uno H, Price VH. Abnormal inner root sheath of the hair follicle in the loose anagen hair syndrome: an ultrastructural study. J Am Acad Dermatol. 2011;64(1):129–34.
15. Olsen EA, Bettencourt MS, Cote NL. The presence of loose anagen hairs obtained by hair pull in the normal population. J Investig Dermatol Symp Proc. 1999;4(3):258–60.
16. Antaya RJ, Sideridou E, Olsen EA. Short anagen syndrome. J Am Acad Dermatol. 2005;53(2 Suppl 1):S130–4.
17. Barraud-Klenovsek MM, Trueb RM. Congenital hypotrichosis due to short anagen. Br J Dermatol. 2000;143(3):612–7.
18. Giacomini F, Starace M, Tosti A. Short anagen syndrome. Pediatr Dermatol. 2011;28(2):133–4.
19. Quercetani R, Rebora AE, Fedi MC, Carelli G, Mei S, Chelli A, et al. Patients with profuse hair shedding may reveal anagen hair dystrophy: a diagnostic clue of alopecia areata incognita. J Eur Acad Dermatol Venereol. 2011;25(7):808–10.
20. Tosti A, Whiting D, Iorizzo M, Pazzaglia M, Misciali C, Vincenzi C, et al. The role of scalp dermoscopy in the diagnosis of alopecia areata incognita. J Am Acad Dermatol. 2008;59(1):64–7.
21. Rakowska A, Slowinska M, Kowalska-Oledzka E, Olszewska M, Czuwara J, Rudnicka L. Alopecia areata incognita: true or false? J Am Acad Dermatol. 2009;60(1):162–3.
22. Rebora A. Alopecia areata incognita: a comment. Clinics (Sao Paulo). 2011;66(8):1481–2.
23. Rebora A. Alopecia areata incognita: a hypothesis. Dermatologica. 1987;174(5):214–8.
24. Baden HP, Kubilus J, Baden L. A stain for plucked anagen hairs. J Am Acad Dermatol. 1979;1(2):121–2.
25. Cantatore-Francis JL, Orlow SJ. Practical guidelines for evaluation of loose anagen hair syndrome. Arch Dermatol. 2009;145(10):1123–8.
26. Rebora A. Alopecia areata incognita. J Am Acad Dermatol. 2011; 65(6):1228.
27. Rebora A. A comment regarding 'follicular Swiss cheese' in the diagnosis of alopecia areata. J Cutan Pathol. 2012;39(2):307–8.
28. Molina L, Donati A, Valente NS, Romiti R. Alopecia areata incognita. Clinics (Sao Paulo). 2011;66(3):513–5.
29. Muller CS, El Shabrawi-Caelen L. 'Follicular Swiss cheese' pattern—another histopathologic clue to alopecia areata. J Cutan Pathol. 2011;38(2):185–9.

Trichotillomania and Traction Alopecia

20

Lidia Rudnicka, Malgorzata Olszewska, and Adriana Rakowska

Abstract

Trichoscopy of trichotillomania is characterized by a chaotic pattern of diverse features related to hair fracturing. The most characteristic features are hairs broken at different lengths, short hairs with trichoptilosis ("split ends"), irregular coiled hairs, amorphous hair residues, and black dots. Micro–exclamation mark hairs are rare in trichotillomania, but they may be a diagnostic pitfall and lead to misdiagnosis of alopecia areata. Trichoscopic features of traction alopecia and traumatic cicatricial marginal alopecia are described briefly in this chapter.

Keywords

Alopecia areata • Alopecia groenlandica • Black dots • Broken hairs • Cicatricial alopecia • Cicatricial marginal alopecia • Coiled hairs • Exclamation mark hairs • Flame hairs • Micro–exclamation mark hairs • Tinea capitis • Traction alopecia • Tulip hairs • Trichoptilosis • Trichotillomania • Yellow dots

Trichotillomania is a form of traction alopecia resulting from habitual, repetitive removal of one's own hair [1–3]. From a psychiatric point of view, this term encompasses an entire syndrome of pathologic hair pulling. According to the American Psychiatric Association's *Diagnostic and Statistical Manual of Mental Disorders*, 4th edition (DSM-IV), the diagnostic criteria for trichotillomania are (a) the recurrent pulling out of one's own hair, resulting in noticeable hair loss; (b) an increasing sense of tension immediately before pulling out the hair or when attempting to resist the behavior; (c) pleasure, gratification, or relief when pulling out the hair; (d) hair pulling that cannot be better accounted for by another mental disorder; and (e) significant distress or impairment in social, occupational, or other important areas of functioning [4]. This definition describes a mental disorder that perhaps should be called *trichotillomania syndrome*. Accordingly, the validity of the DSM-IV criteria recently was questioned by several authors [4, 5].

From a dermatologist's point of view, trichotillomania is self-induced hair loss due to the repetitive pulling of one's own hair [6, 7]. Most patients fulfill no other DSM-IV criteria.

The condition most frequently affects children between the ages of 9 and 13 years [6]. There is a female predominance of 70–93 % [6]. Adult-onset trichotillomania may be secondary to underlying psychiatric disturbances and has a long-lasting course [6].

Clinically, patients present with patches of irregular-length hair or hairless areas. Commonly, the vertex is affected. Hair loss in this area creates the characteristic "tonsure trichotillomania," or the "Friar Tuck sign" [8]. Pull test is negative. Patients may pull hair at multiple sites, including the eyebrows, eyelashes, face, arms, legs, and pubic area [6, 7].

L. Rudnicka (✉)
Faculty of Health Sciences, Medical University of Warsaw, Poland

Department of Dermatology, CSK MSW, Woloska 137, Warsaw 02-502, Poland
e-mail: lidia.rudnicka@euderm.eu

M. Olszewska
Department of Dermatology, Medical University of Warsaw, Warsaw, Poland

A. Rakowska
Department of Dermatology, CSK MSW, Warsaw, Poland

L. Rudnicka et al. (eds.), *Atlas of Trichoscopy*,
DOI 10.1007/978-1-4471-4486-1_20, © Springer-Verlag London 2012

Trichoscopy shows decreased hair density, hairs broken at different lengths, short hairs with trichoptilosis ("split ends"), irregular coiled hairs, upright regrowing hairs, and black dots [9–11]. Yellow dots generally are not observed in trichotillomania [9]. Inui et al. [12] observed yellow dots in one patient with this condition. These dots differ from yellow dots in other diseases in that they contain a black dot in their central part [12].

Micro–exclamation mark hairs are rare in trichotillomania [13, 14], but they may be a diagnostic pitfall and lead to the misdiagnosis of alopecia areata.

Alopecia areata may be the initial trigger for trichotillomania, and these two conditions may coexist [6], making trichoscopic differential diagnosis even more challenging.

Traction alopecia, which is most commonly caused by hairstyling procedures, shows similar trichoscopic features. Occasionally, hair casts may be present. So far, no differences in trichoscopic results between trichotillomania and traction alopecia have been described. Traumatic cicatricial marginal alopecia, a late manifestation of traction alopecia, is characterized by decreased hair density, hair thinning, and white dots or white areas lacking follicular openings.

Table 20.1 Trichoscopic differential diagnosis of trichotillomania

Feature	Trichotillomania	Alopecia areata	Tinea capitis
Broken hairs	++	+	+
Coiled hairs (irregular)	+	–	–
Short hairs with trichoptilosis (split ends)	+	–	–
Upright regrowing hairs (<3 mm)	+	+	+
Micro–exclamation mark hairs	+	++	–
Tapered hairs	+	++	–
Flame hairs	+	–	–
Tulip hairs	++	+/–	–
V-sign	++	+/–	–
Amorphous hair residues	+	+/–	+
Hair powder (sprinkled hairs)	+	–	–
Black dots	+	++	+
Yellow dots	+/–	++	–
Yellow dots with black peppering	+	–	–
Regrowing pigtail hairs (circular or oval)	–	++	–
Block hairs	+/–	–	++
i-Hairs	+/–	–	+
Hypopigmented vellus hairs	–	+	–
Comma hairs	–	–	+
Corkscrew hairs	–	–	+
Zigzag hairs	–	+/–	+
No hairs in field of view	–	+	–

– not present, + present, ++ common

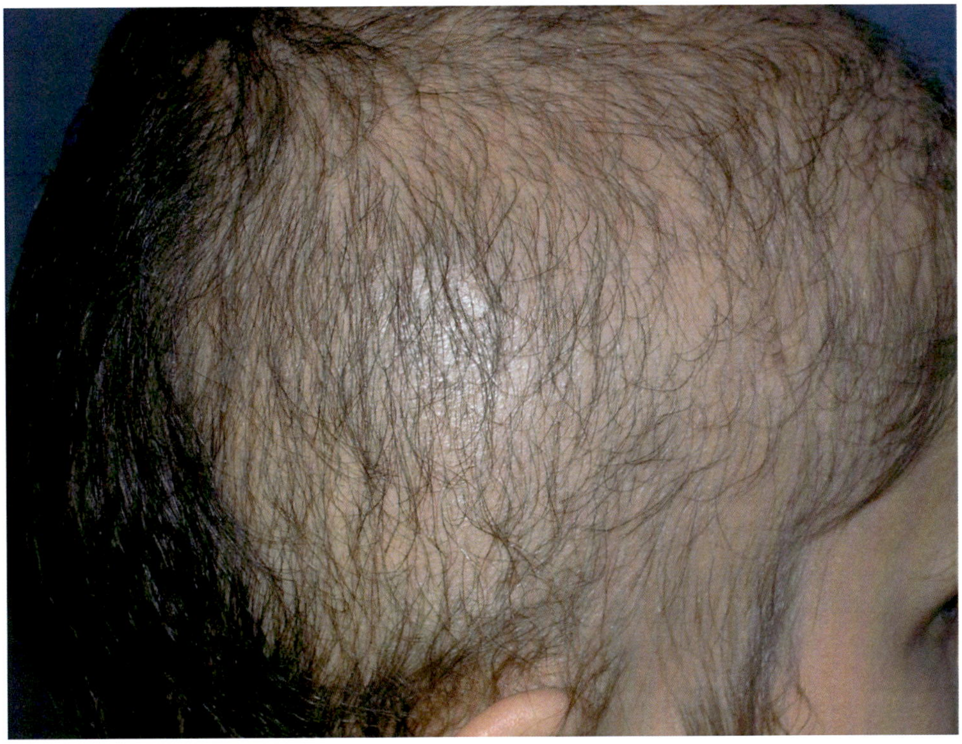

Fig. 20.1 Trichotillomania. Clinically, trichotillomania is characterized by patches of decreased hair density and irregular hair length. Totally hairless areas are rare because patients tend to pull only the long hairs. Usually, the midoccipital area is spared because it is out of easy reach of the hands. In this patient, the hair pulling is limited to the range of her right hand. Some patients may not remember pulling their hair

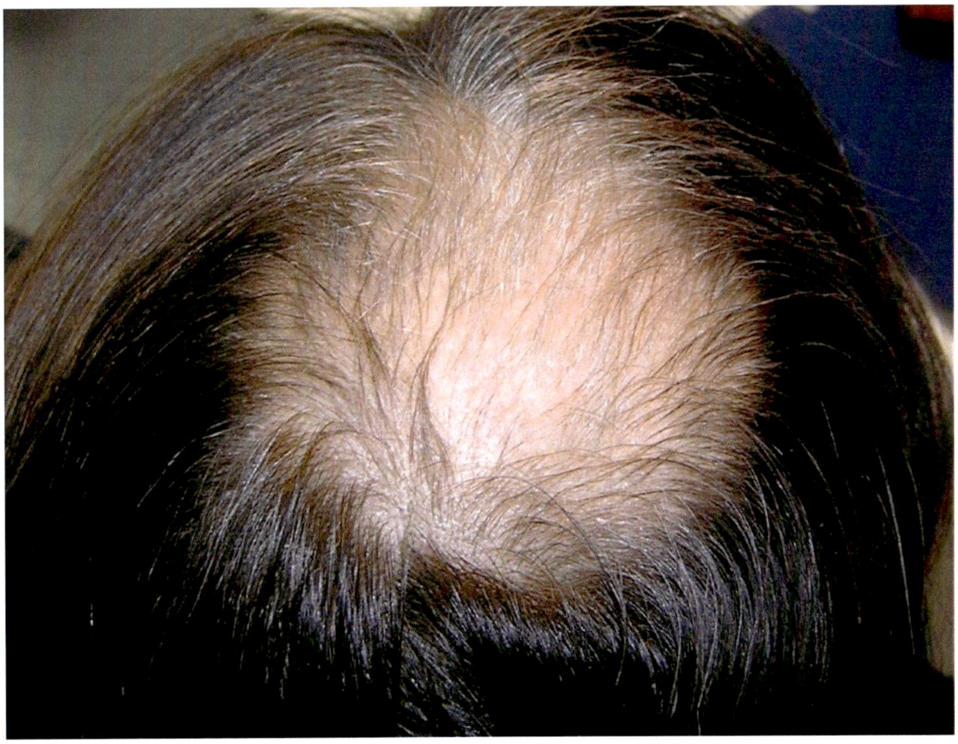

Fig. 20.2 Trichotillomania: the Friar Tuck sign. Shown is a patient with hair loss in the vertex area. Hair loss due to compulsive hair pulling in or beyond this area creates the characteristic tonsure trichotillomania, also known as the Friar Tuck sign, which refers to the traditional Christian practice of shaving the midscalp hair and leaving a peripheral circle of hairs unshaved [8]. This image shows a characteristic Friar Tuck sign in a 16-year-old female patient with trichotillomania

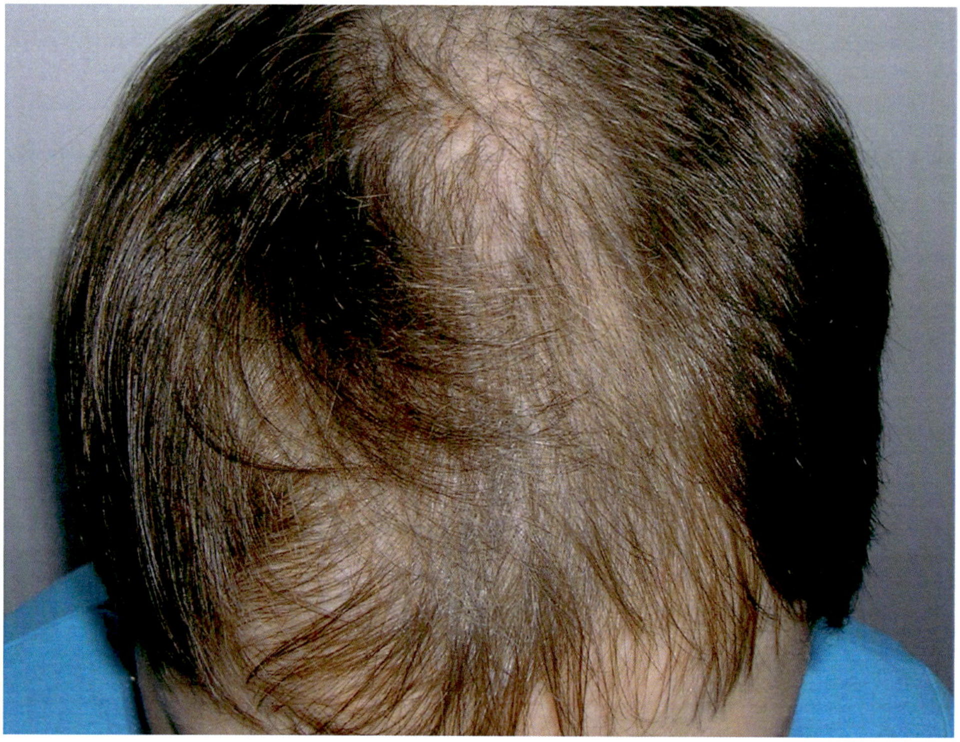

Fig. 20.3 Trichotillomania in an "androgenetic" distribution. In this 22-year-old patient with trichotillomania, clinical evaluation showed partial hair loss in an androgenetic (pattern) distribution, which may indicate the diagnosis of androgenetic alopecia. In this case, however, trichoscopy showed features of trichotillomania. Therefore, it appears that trichoscopy is most useful as a diagnostic aid in clinically atypical cases of trichotillomania. This method also may be of special value in patients with two overlapping causes of hair loss. Recently, Neila Iglesias et al. [15] reported a case of trichotillomania coexisting with monilethrix in which trichoscopy provided a valuable hint for diagnosis

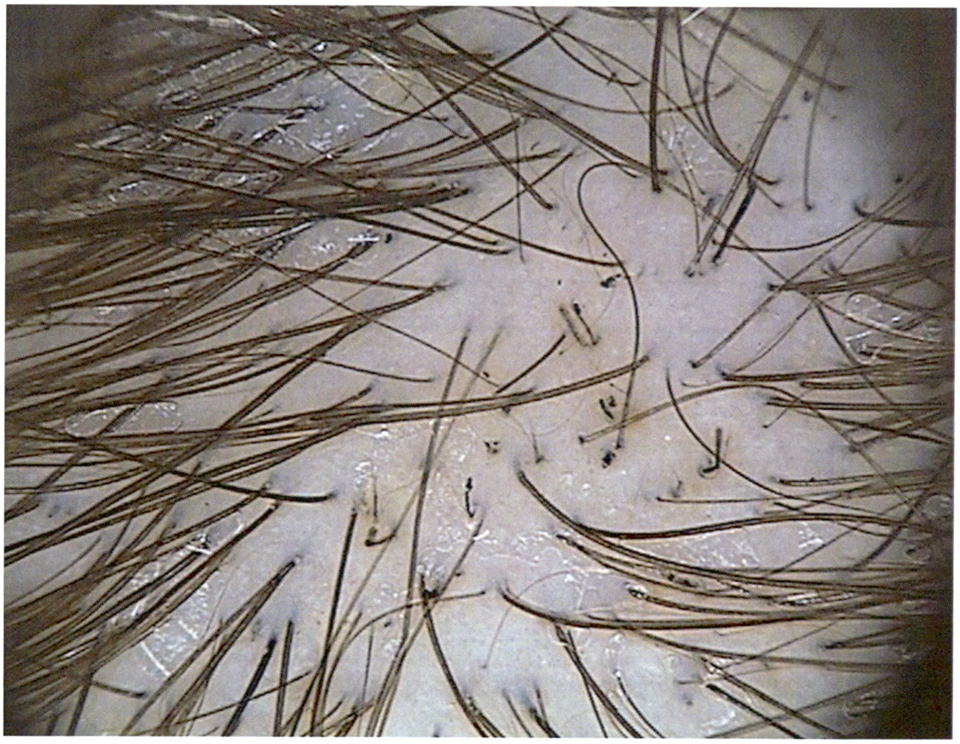

Fig. 20.4 Broken hairs in trichotillomania. Trichoscopy of trichotillomania shows a multicomponent image of chaotic destruction that may be focal (as in this image) or encompass the whole field of view. The presence of multiple hairs broken at different lengths is the most consistent finding in trichotillomania. These hairs show extreme variability in morphology. The images in this chapter show several variants of these hairs. Some may be seen in greater detail on high-magnification trichoscopy. The presence of broken hairs is not specific for trichotillomania. They also may be observed in alopecia areata, tinea capitis, and trichorrhexis nodosa; however, in all these diseases, the hairs do not show a high variability in length and shape as do those seen in trichotillomania (×20)

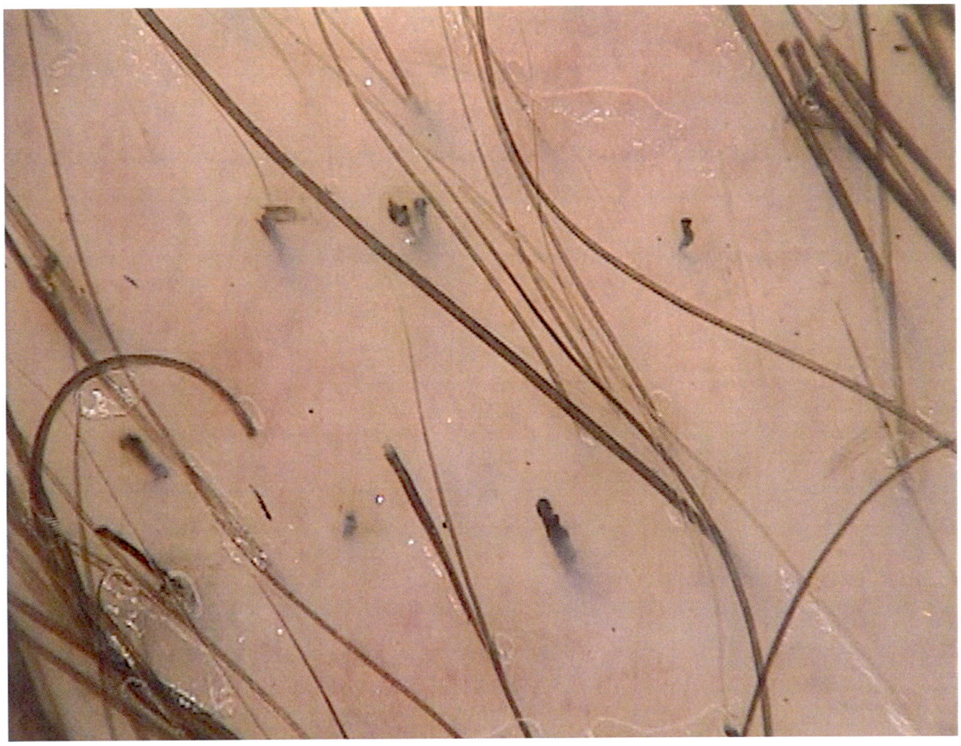

Fig. 20.5 Broken hairs in trichotillomania. Several broken hairs are visible in the central part of this image. This photograph shows in greater detail that every broken hair has a different length and morphology (×40)

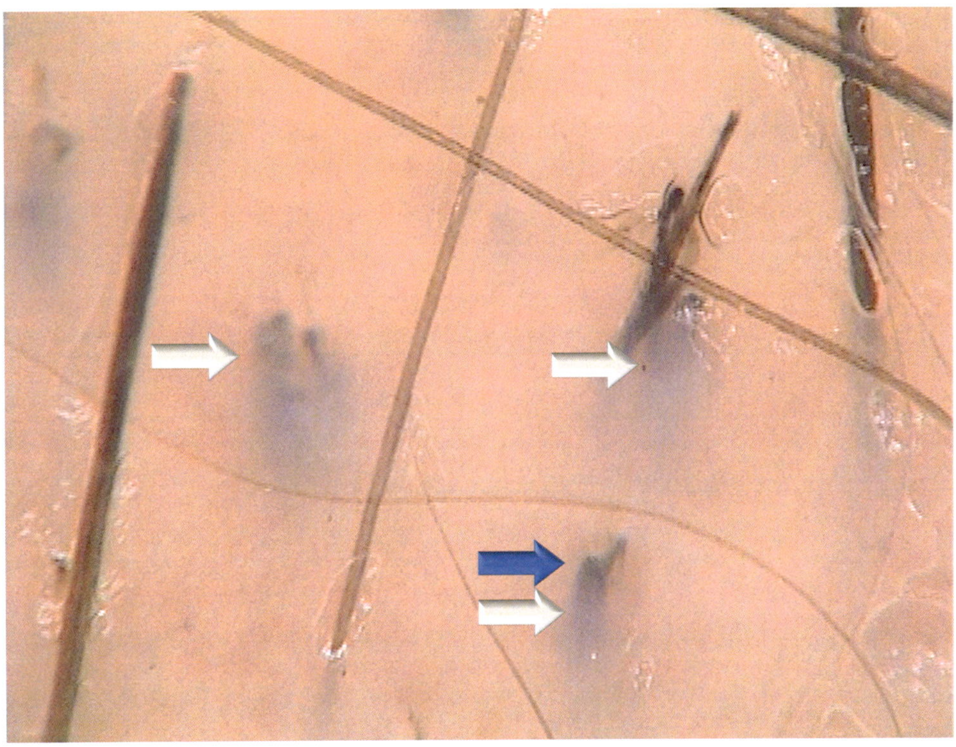

Fig. 20.6 Broken hairs in trichotillomania. In trichotillomania, hairs may have a near-transverse fracture with only part of the cuticle broken at a different length (*blue arrow*). Hairs pulled by mechanical force frequently are broken below the skin surface (*white arrows*); they are visible through the intact epidermis (×70)

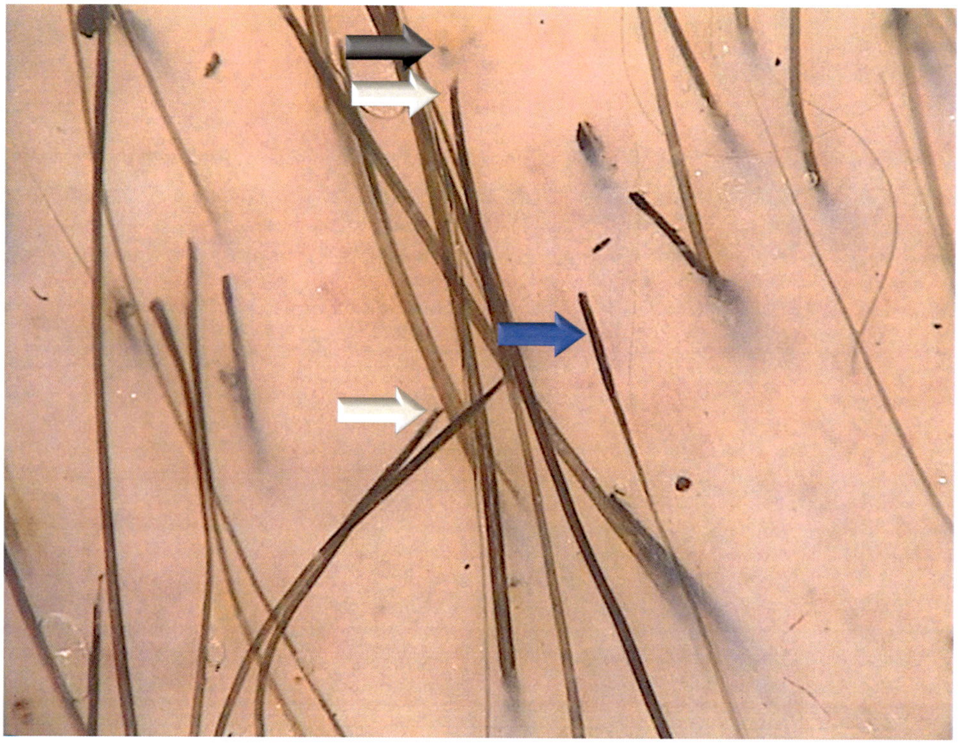

Fig. 20.7 Various types of broken hairs in trichotillomania. A characteristic micro–exclamation mark hair (*blue arrow*) with a thin proximal end and a thick, flat distal end is visible. Some hairs show trichoptilosis at the distal end (*white arrows*). The *gray arrow* points to a black dot (×70)

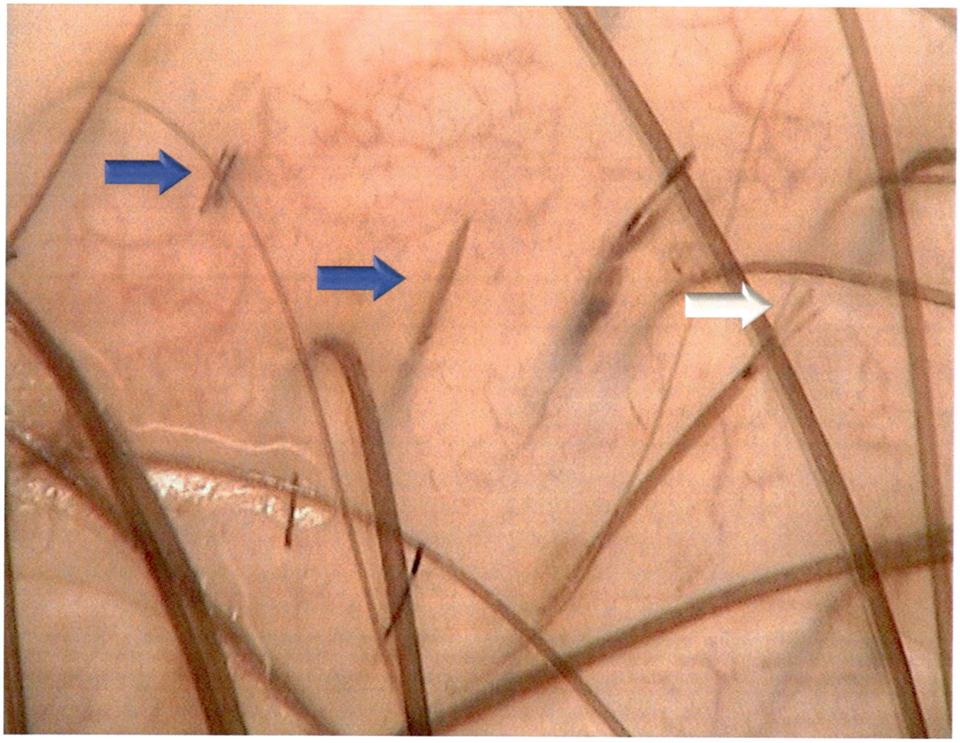

Fig. 20.8 Broken hairs and trichoptilosis (split ends) in trichotillomania. Typical short broken hairs (*blue arrows*) are located between normal terminal hairs at the hair-bearing margin of a patch of alopecia due to trichotillomania. Characteristically, the ends of these hairs are irregular and uneven. Trichoptilosis (*white arrow*) is a frequent finding in trichotillomania (×70)

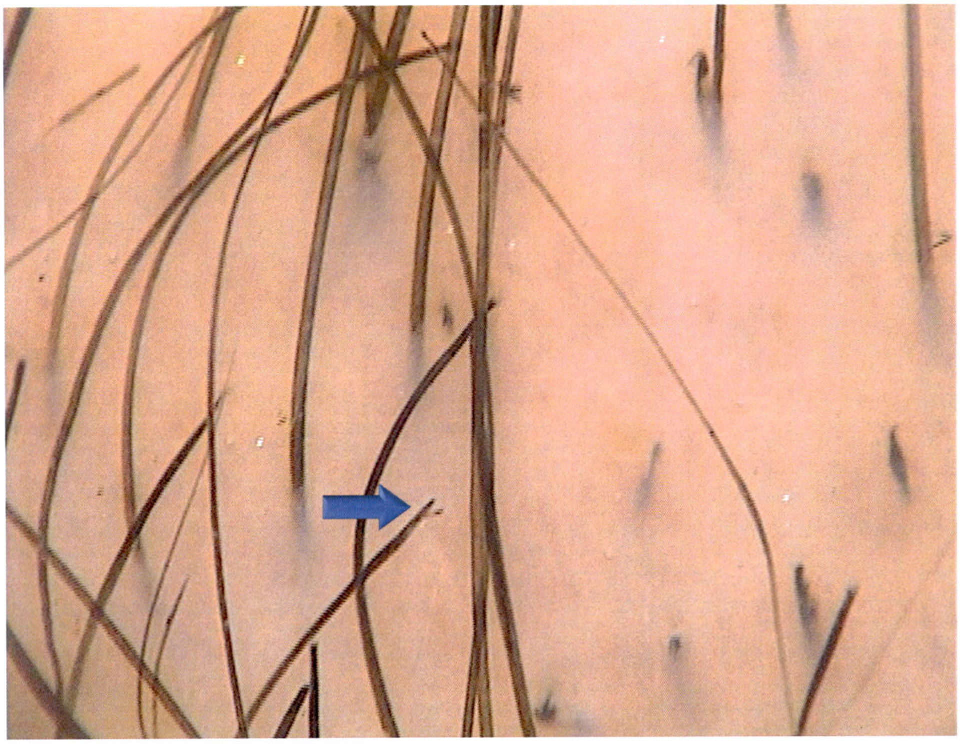

Fig. 20.9 Trichoptilosis (split ends) in trichotillomania. In healthy individuals, trichoptilosis (split ends; *arrow*) is a frequent finding. It commonly affects the distal ends of long hairs that have not been cut for a while. The difference in trichotillomania is that trichoptilosis affects short hairs. Note that this trichoscopic photograph, taken at a 70-fold magnification, reflects a scalp area of about 3.5 × 2.6 mm. Accordingly, hairs shorter than the height of this image are shorter than 2.6 mm. Thus, when evaluating trichoptilosis in trichotillomania, it must be kept in mind that this is a feature of (very) short hairs (×70)

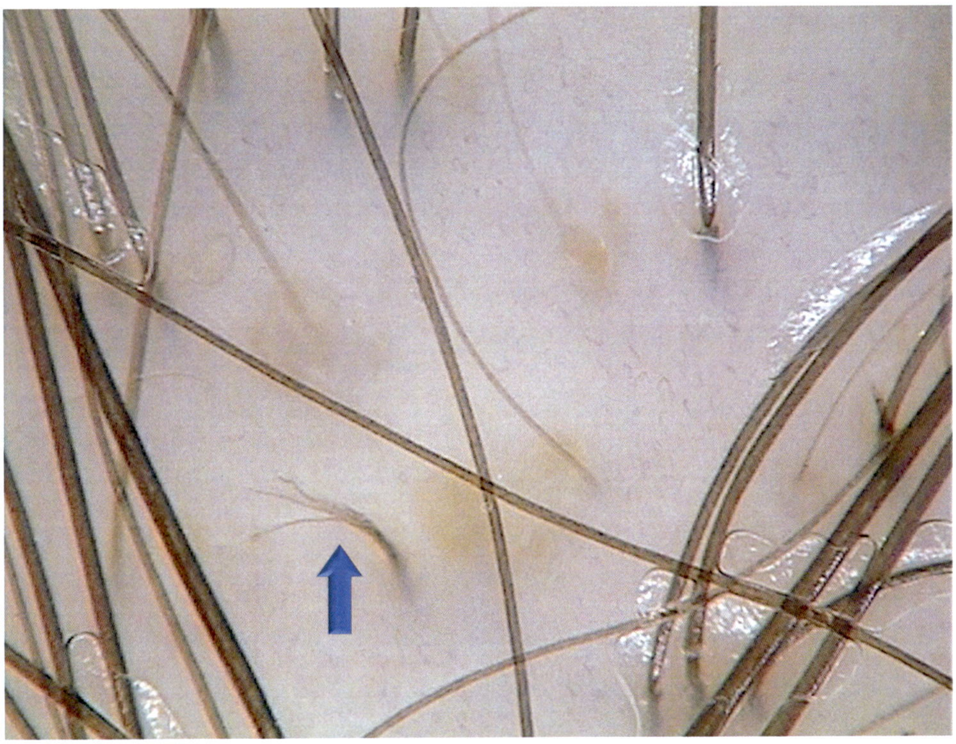

Fig. 20.10 Trichoptilosis (split ends) in trichotillomania. The *arrow* points to a hair with split ends. These hairs must be differentiated from broom hairs [14]. In the literature, broom hairs also are called *brush hairs* (German: *Pinselhhare*), *twin hair* (German: *Zwillingshaare*), *multiple hairs* (*Flemming-Giovannini*), and *pili multigemini* [16]. Pinkus [16] described these hairs in detail in 1951. These terms partly refer to two or more hair shafts emerging from one follicular unit. New data, particularly trichoscopic observations, show that a phenomenon previously called *multiple hairs* partly refers to a normal situation of two to four terminal hairs emerging from one follicular unit. Thus, the terms *broom hairs* and *broom fibers* have been suggested for the abnormal presence of multiple thin *hairs or "hair fibers"* emerging from one follicular opening. This image also shows sebaceous yellow dots, which resulted from androgenetic alopecia coexisting in this patient with trichotillomania (×70)

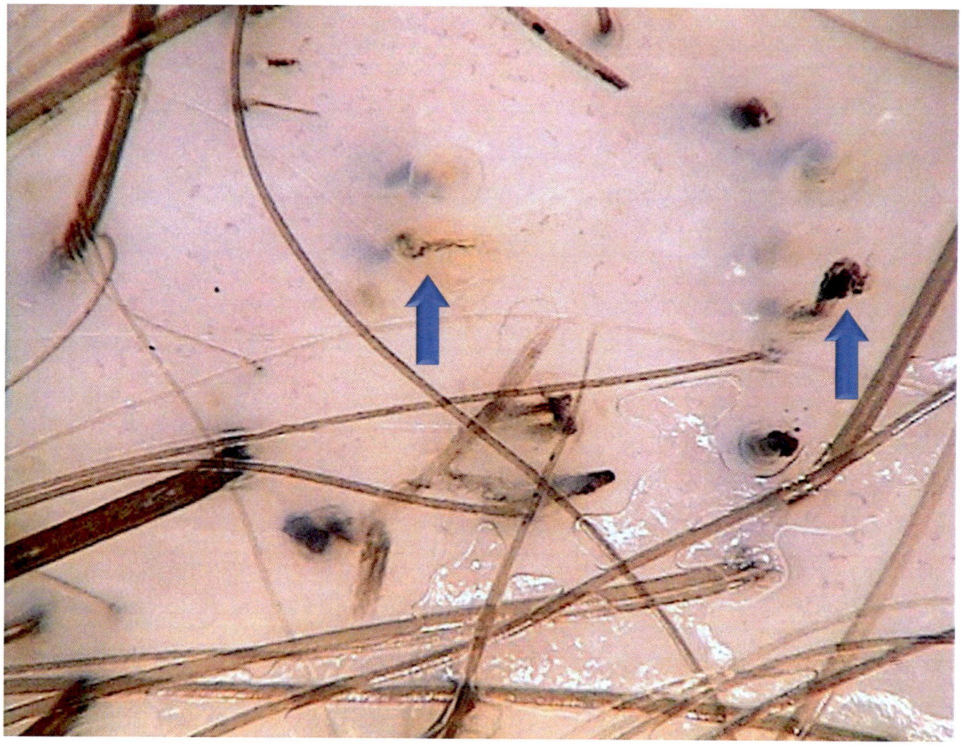

Fig. 20.11 Flame hairs in trichotillomania. Severe mechanical trauma due to hair pulling may result in hair residue that is semitransparent, wavy, and cone shaped (*arrows*). Because of their characteristic shape, these hairs are called *flame hairs*. This finding is highly characteristic of trichotillomania (×70)

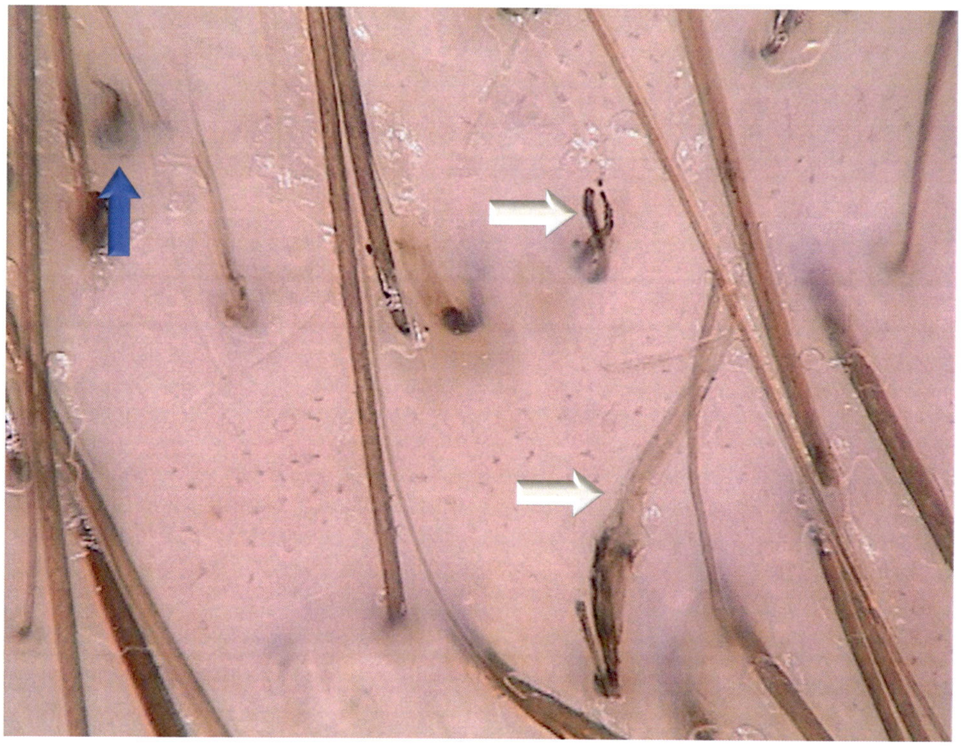

Fig. 20.12 Variants of flame hairs in trichotillomania. The most characteristic flame hair is indicated by the *blue arrow*, but a few other hairs in this image (*white arrows*) also may fulfill the definition of wavy hairs (×70)

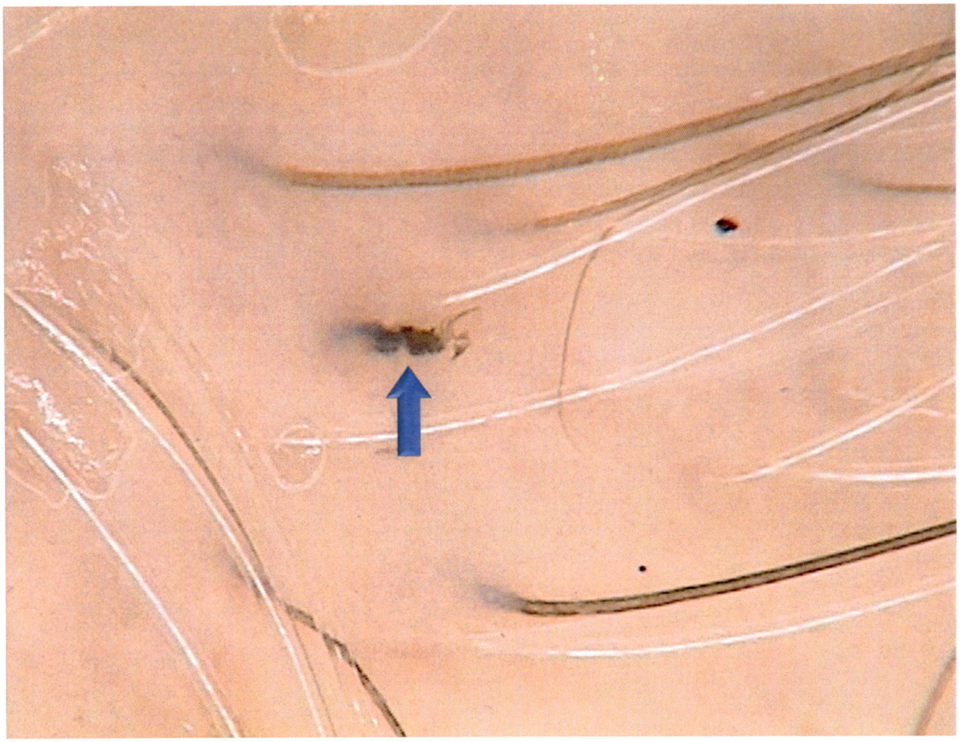

Fig. 20.13 Flame hairs in trichotillomania. A flame-like hair is visible among normal pigmented and gray terminal hairs. This image shows that, occasionally, a flame hair may appear thicker and more intensely pigmented compared with other hairs (×70)

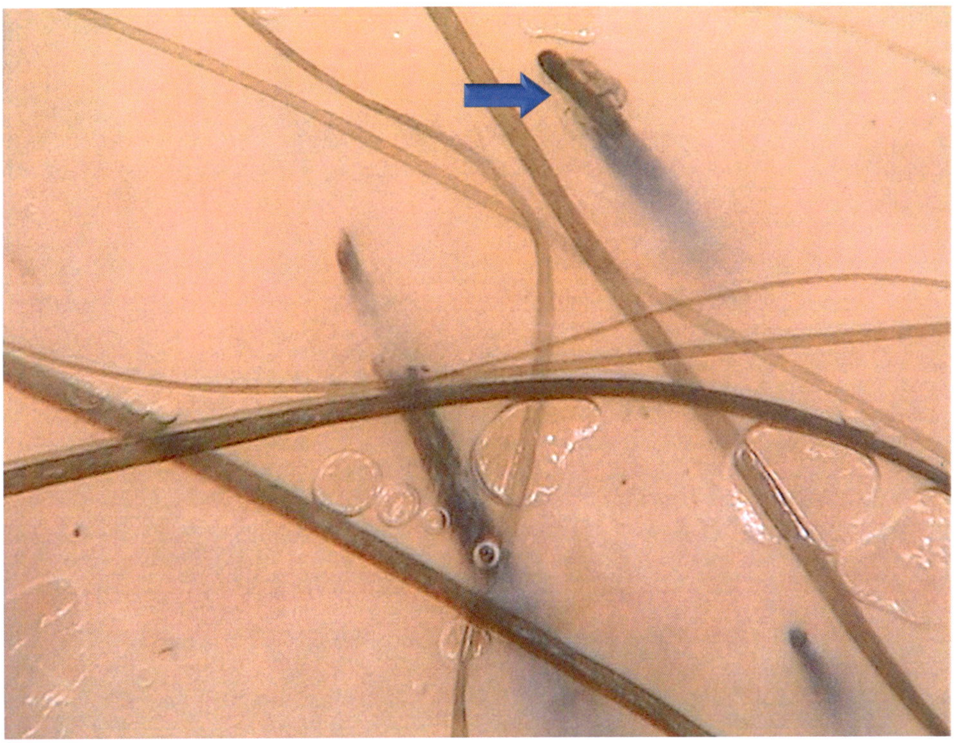

Fig. 20.14 Flame-like hair elements in trichotillomania. The *arrow* points to a broken hair with a semitransparent, wavy, and cone-shaped element, which fulfills the definition of a flame hair. This may indicate that a flame hair is composed of hair cuticle; however, this hypothesis requires confirmation (×70)

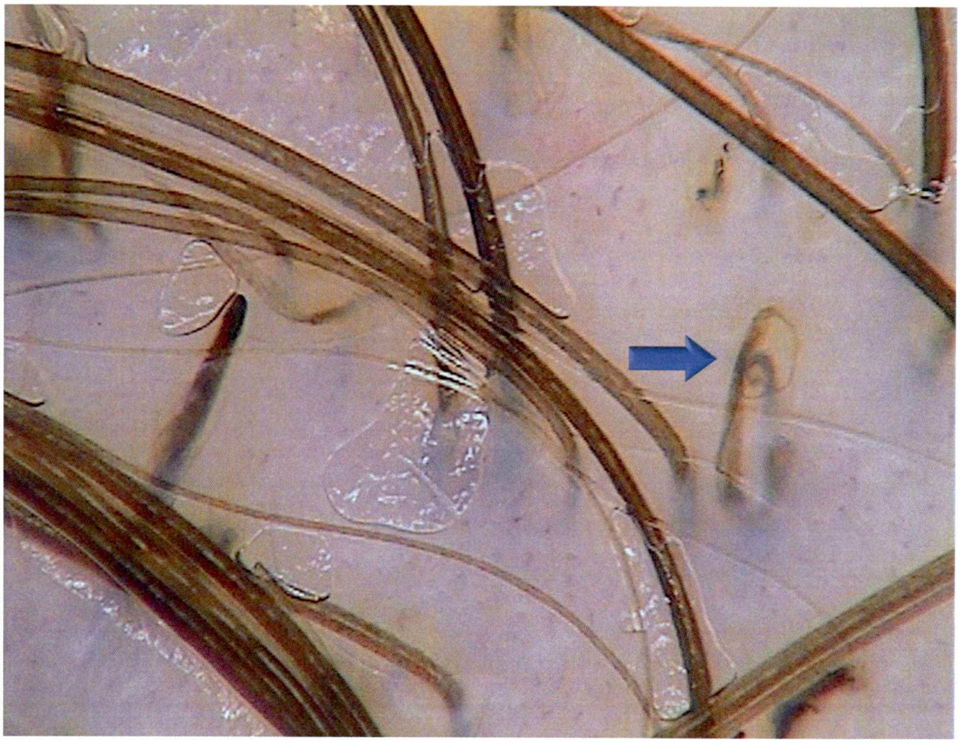

Fig. 20.15 Coiled hairs in trichotillomania. In response to a pulling force, a hair shaft fractures and the remaining, distal part, which is fixed to the scalp, may contract and coil (*arrow*). This produces coiled hairs, which are irregularly shaped and frequently have features of trichoptilosis (split ends). These coiled hairs are highly characteristic of trichotillomania/traction alopecia (×70)

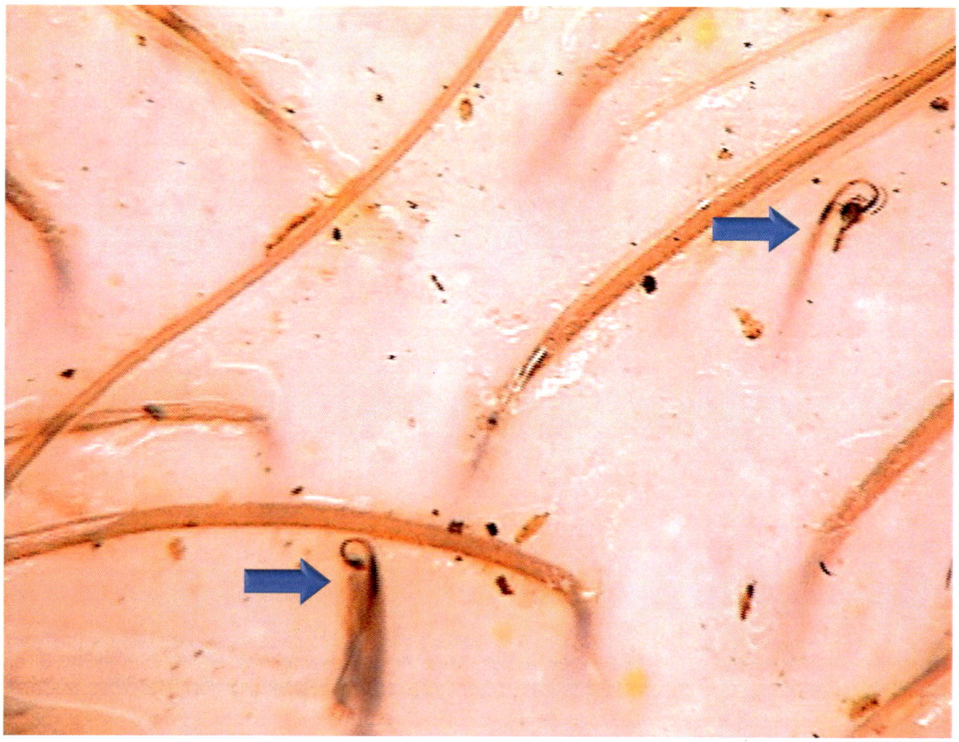

Fig. 20.16 Coiled hairs in trichotillomania. In this child with trichotillomania, two irregularly coiled hairs are visible (*arrows*). These fractured coiled hairs must be differentiated from circular or oval "pigtail" hairs. Pigtail hairs are new, regrowing hairs present in various diseases with hair follicle abnormalities. These hairs also are coiled, but they are uniform in thickness and color and regular in shape. The presence of multiple "dirty dots" may indicate the young age of this patient (×70)

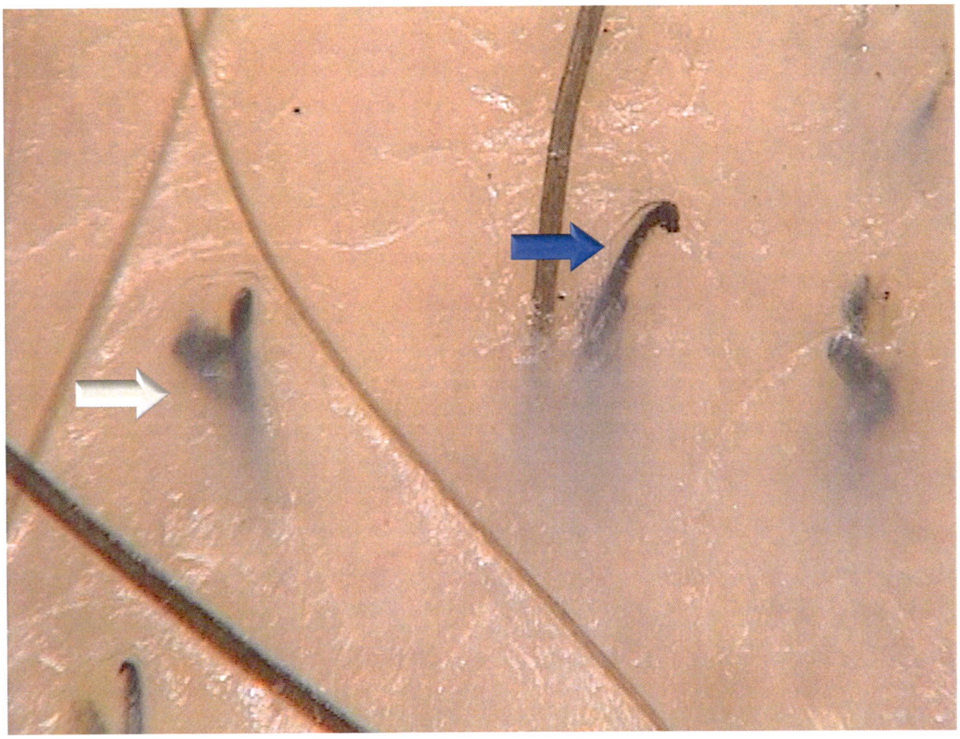

Fig. 20.17 Coiled hairs and the V-sign in trichotillomania. Partial coiling of the distal part of fractured hairs results in a hook-like appearance (*blue arrow*), which is highly characteristic of trichotillomania/traction alopecia. These partially coiled hairs also have been called *hook hairs* or *question mark hairs*. A V-sign is visible in this image (*white arrow*) (×70)

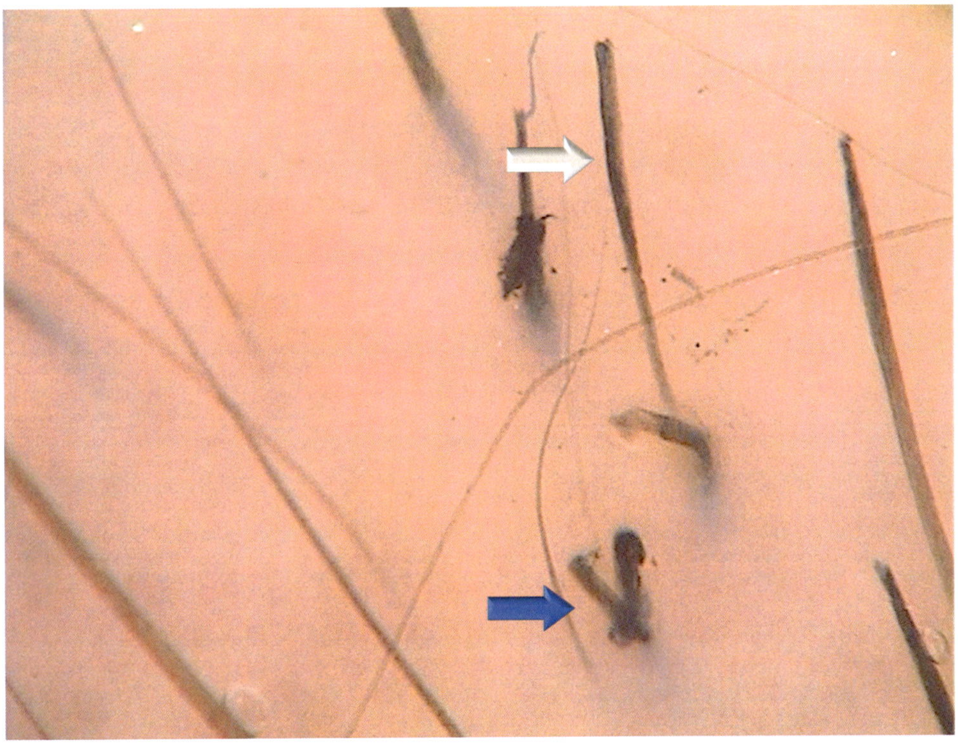

Fig. 20.18 V-sign and micro–exclamation mark hair in trichotillomania. A V-sign is created when two or more hairs emerging from one follicular unit are pulled simultaneously and break at the same length above the scalp surface (*blue arrow*). This feature must be distinguished from healthy regrowing terminal hair in a person who shaves her/his scalp. In a healthy person, all hairs in the field of view are similar in length, whereas in a patient with trichotillomania, the V-sign is surrounded by long terminal hairs. The *white arrow* points to a micro–exclamation mark hair. Differential diagnosis of diseases associated with the presence of micro–exclamation mark hairs requires special caution. In trichotillomania, micro–exclamation mark hairs more commonly tend to have a flat distal end and a pigmented proximal end. However, micro–exclamation mark hairs with uneven, ragged, distal ends and hypopigmented proximal ends occasionally may be observed in trichotillomania. In doubtful cases, the environment of the micro–exclamation mark hair must be observed. In this image, variable broken hairs may be seen (×70)

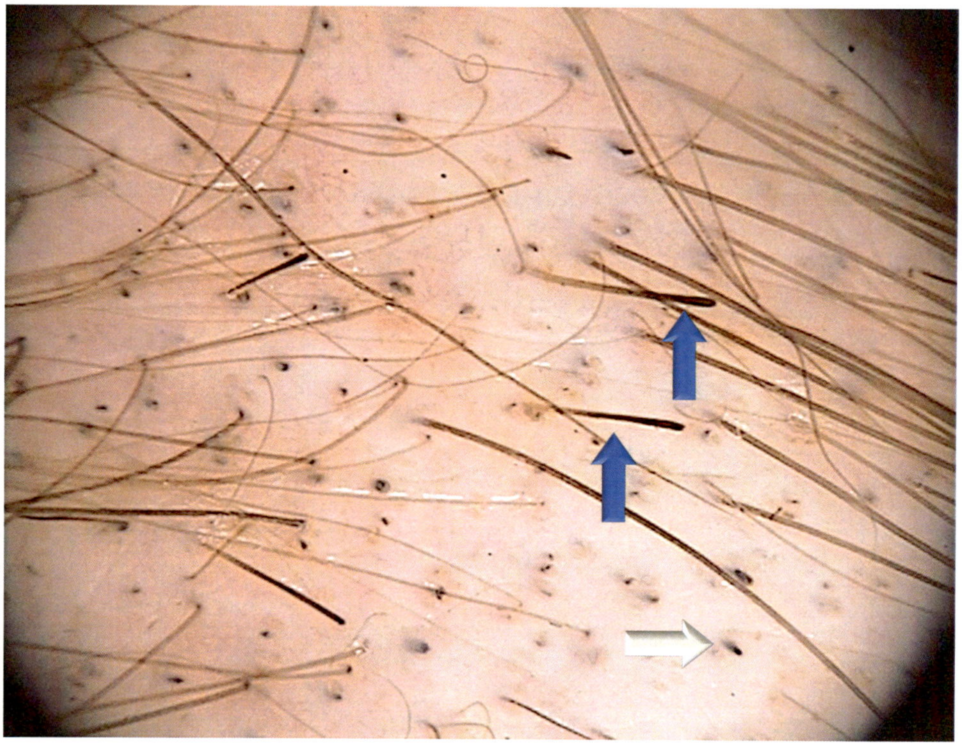

Fig. 20.19 Micro–exclamation mark hairs and amorphous hair residues in trichotillomania. Multiple micro–exclamation mark hairs are visible in this image (*blue arrows*). Note that all have a flat distal end. Small amorphous hair shaft residues are almost indistinguishable from black dots (*white arrow*). Multiple broken hairs are visible (×20)

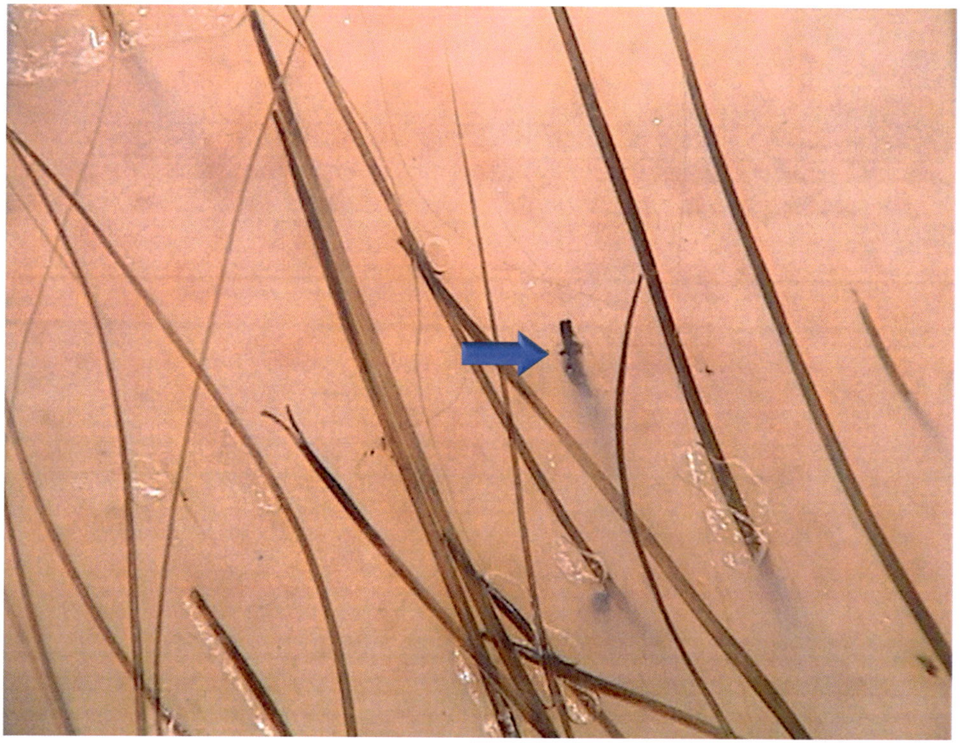

Fig. 20.20 Amorphous hair residues in trichotillomania. Higher magnification reveals that hair residues are very short, broken, dystrophic hairs protruding from the follicular openings (*arrow*). A hair with trichoptilosis and a few broken hairs also are visible in this image (×70)

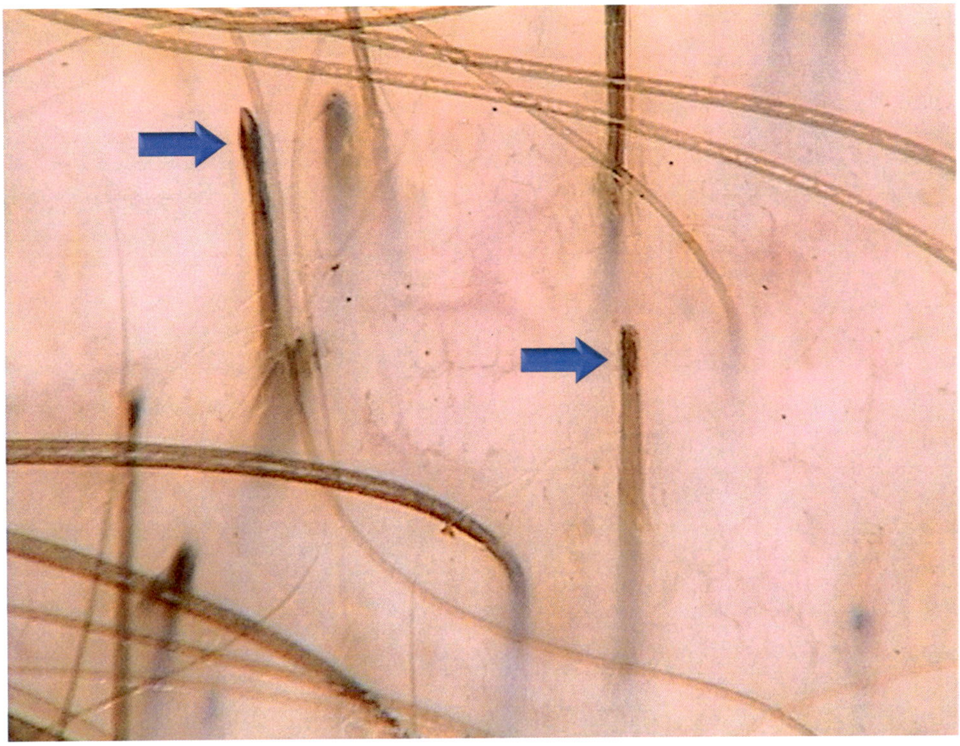

Fig. 20.21 Tulip hairs in trichotillomania. Tulip hairs are short hairs with darker, tulip-shaped ends (*arrows*). The distal ends of the hair shafts appear "empty" inside. These hairs are characteristic of trichotillomania but also may be observed in other diseases. We hypothesize that these are hairs in which pulling caused a diagonal fracture (×70)

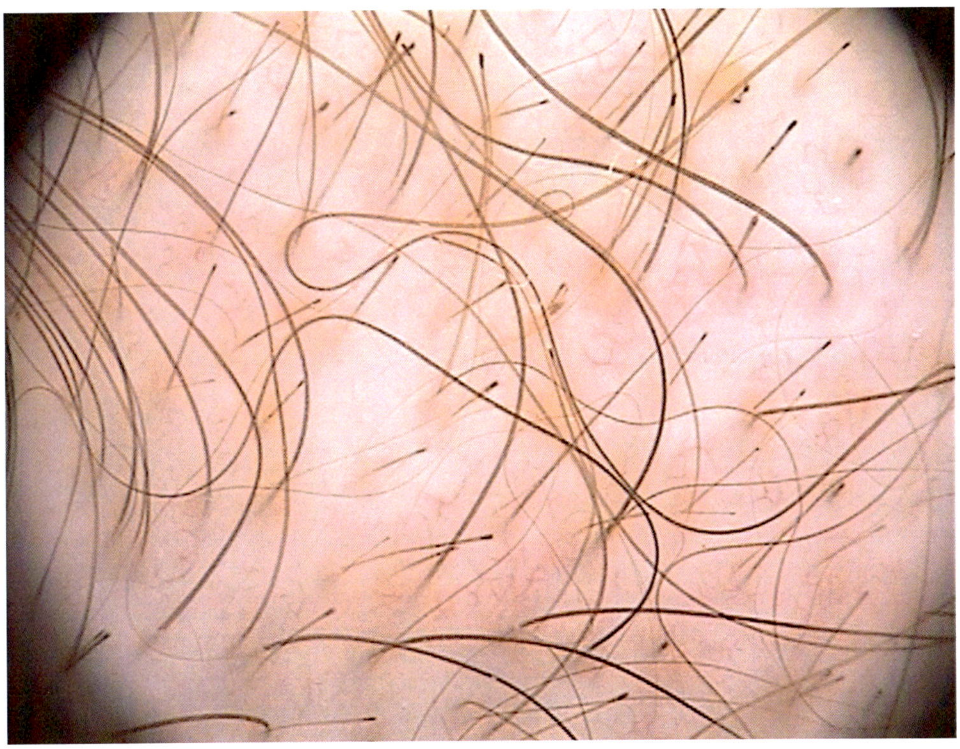

Fig. 20.22 Tulip hairs in trichotillomania. Multiple tulip hairs of similar length are observed at lower magnification. Without other, coexisting features of trichotillomania, trichoscopic diagnosis is difficult. Traction alopecia and alopecia areata should be considered the most probable differential diagnoses (×20)

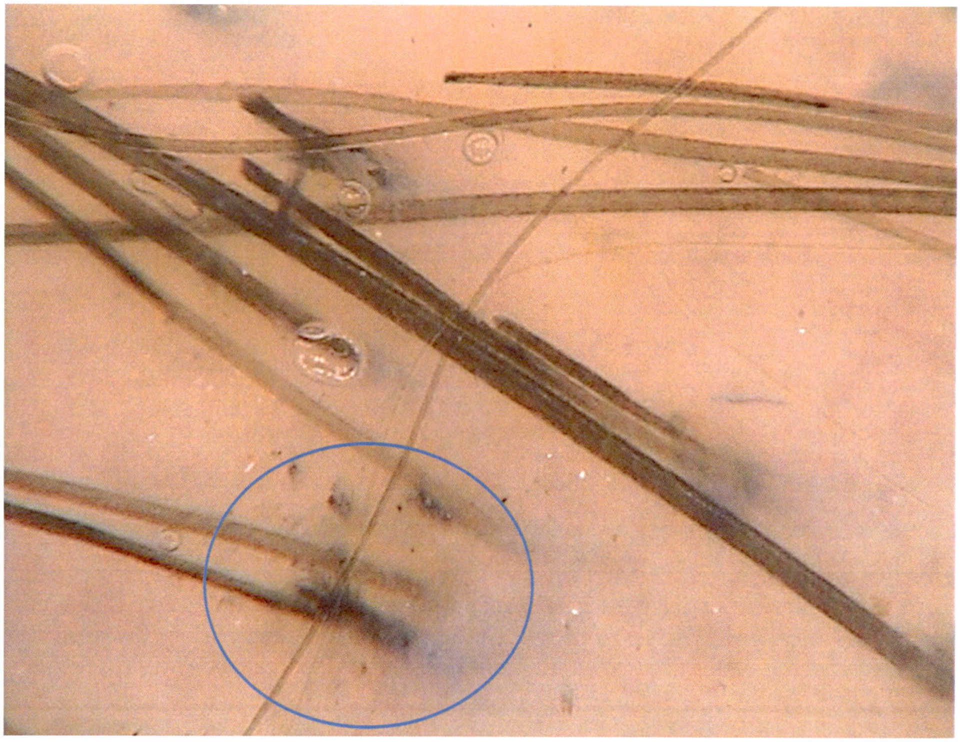

Fig. 20.23 **Hair powder in trichotillomania**. In trichotillomania, the hair shafts may be totally damaged by mechanical manipulation and only a sprinkled "hair powder" may be visible (*blue circle*). Hair powder may be distinguished from "dirty dots"[17] observed in healthy children by its uniform color, fine pulverization, and direct proximity to hair shafts with other features of hair damage. In the midpart of the *blue circle*, an amorphous residue of a hair shaft is visible (×70)

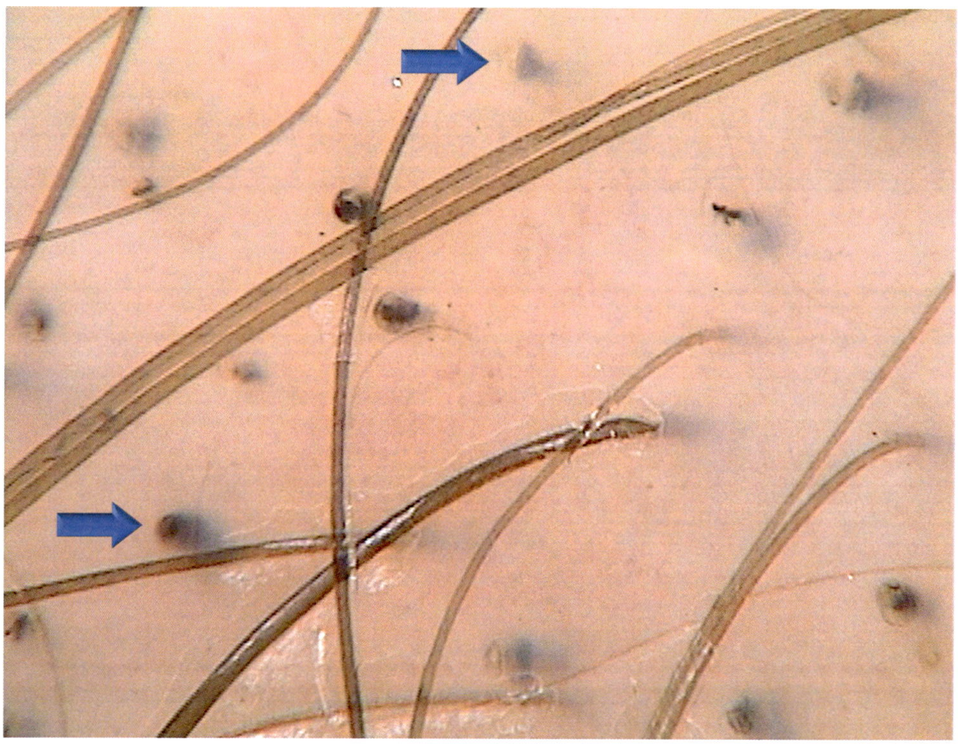

Fig. 20.24 **Black dots in trichotillomania**. When pulled hairs fracture at the level of the scalp surface, they appear as black dots (*arrows*) on trichoscopy. These black dots are indistinguishable from those observed in other diseases, such as alopecia areata, tinea capitis, chemotherapy-induced alopecia, and monilethrix (×70)

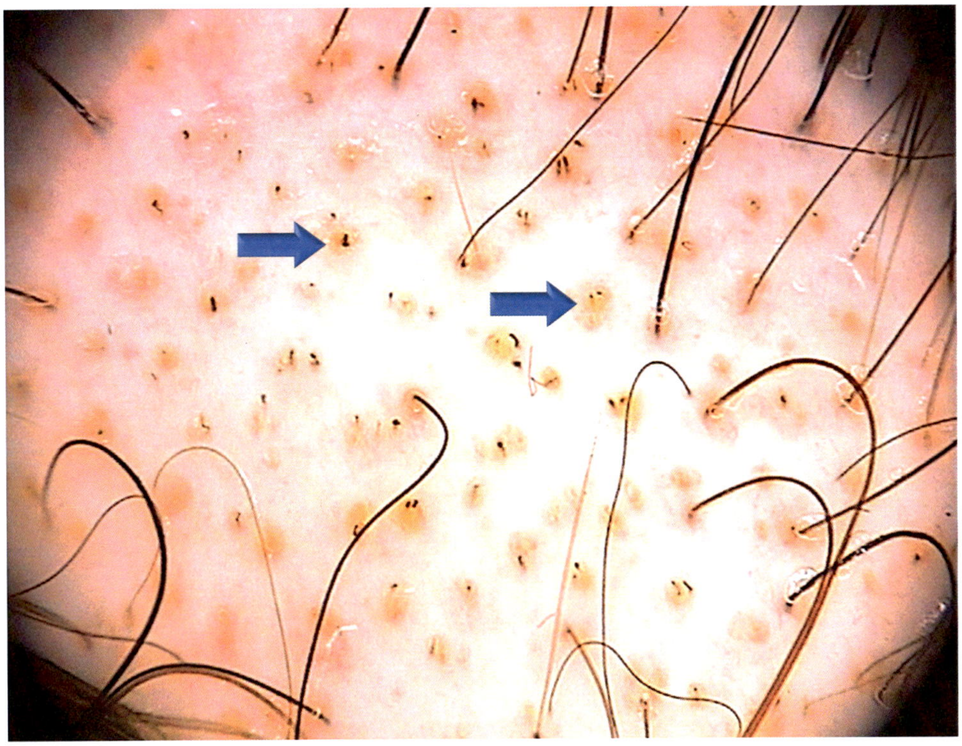

Fig. 20.25 Yellow dots in trichotillomania. Yellow dots are a rare finding in trichotillomania [18]. If present, they contain a black dot or characteristic black peppering inside (*arrows*). The mechanism leading to this abnormality remains unclear. It also must be considered that trichotillomania may coexist with hair loss of another cause associated with the presence of yellow dots (×20)

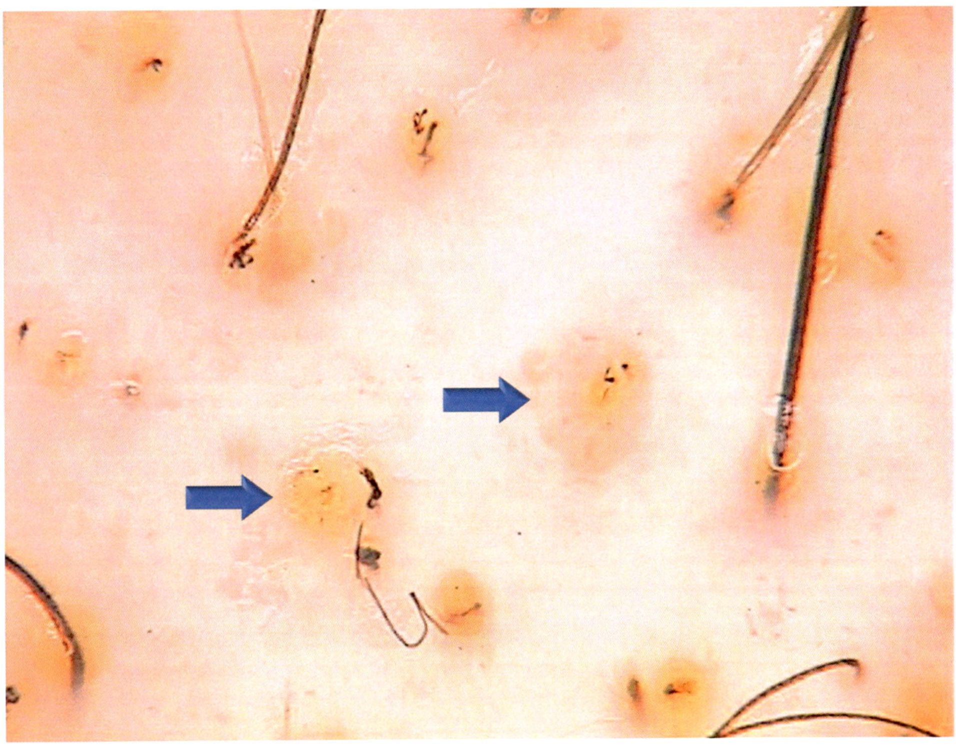

Fig. 20.26 Yellow dots in trichotillomania. Higher magnification shows that yellow dots (*arrows*) contain small hair residues, which may occur in groups of two or three. Some of these dots are surrounded by an erythematous halo. This image requires differential diagnosis with alopecia areata (×70)

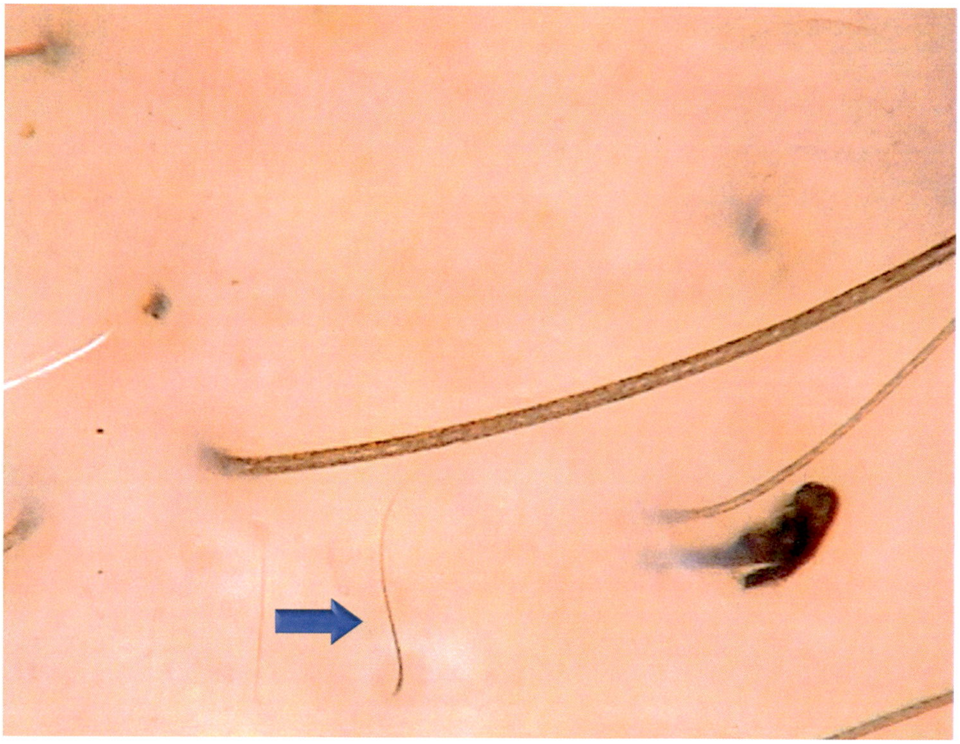

Fig. 20.27 **Upright regrowing hair in trichotillomania**. An upright regrowing hair (*arrow*) coexists with features of ongoing hair pulling, such as an amorphous hair residue and two black dots. The presence of upright regrowing hairs is a natural process in all diseases in which hair regrowth occurs (×70)

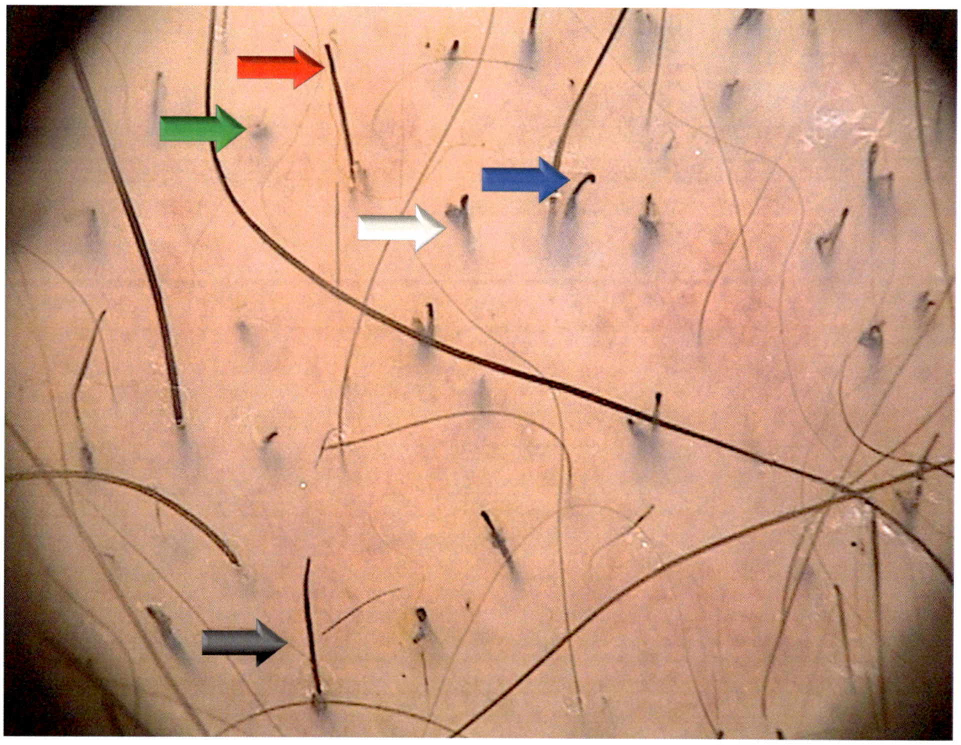

Fig. 20.28 **Trichotillomania**. This image shows a typical chaotic, multicomponent trichoscopic pattern of trichotillomania. A partly coiled hair (*blue arrow*), V-sign (*white arrow*), broken hair (*gray arrow*), black dot (*green arrow*), and micro–exclamation hair (*red arrow*) are visible. Additional findings include amorphous hair residues and areas with hair powder near the hair residues (×20)

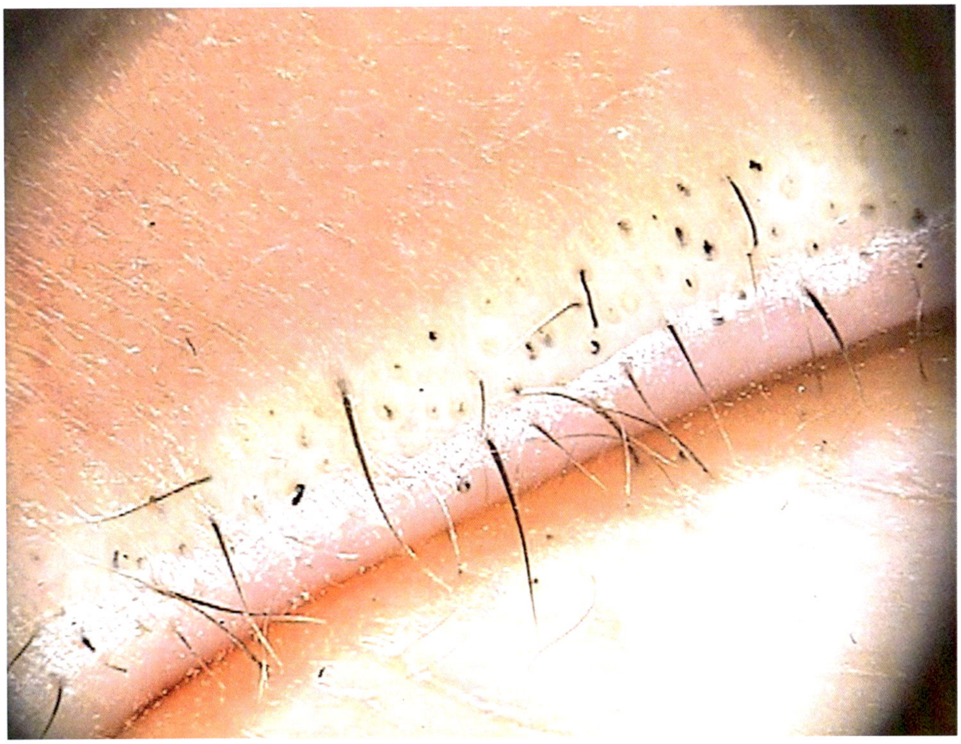

Fig. 20.29 Trichotillomania of the eyelashes. Madarosis (loss of eyelashes) is a diagnostic challenge in clinical practice. Differential diagnosis also is difficult with trichoscopy. The presence of eyelashes broken at different lengths and black dots, as in this image, may indicate trichotillomania but does not exclude alopecia areata. In performing trichoscopy of the eyelashes, one should remember not to use alcohol as an immersion fluid. We usually use sterile 0.9 % NaCl or perform dry trichoscopy (×20)

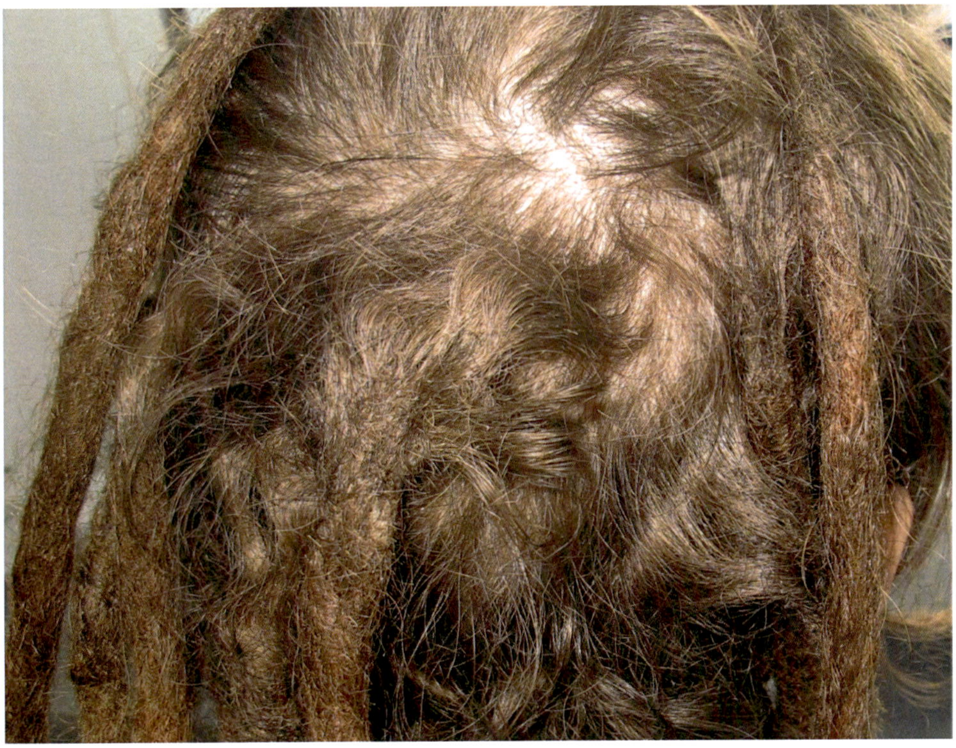

Fig. 20.30 **Traction alopecia**. Traction alopecia (formerly also called *alopecia groenlandica*) is traumatic hair loss secondary to the stretching of scalp hair. In this condition, hair pulling is unintentional and may result from cultural, social, or hairstyling practices [19]. Traction alopecia due to traumatic hair care practices is most frequent in African American women and children. The most common causes are ponytails, tight buns, weaves, braids, dreadlocks, cornrows, clips on hair extensions, turbans, and sleeping in rollers. Clinically, marginal and nonmarginal traction alopecia may be distinguished. The term *marginal traction alopecia* refers to hair loss that is most prominent at the hair-bearing margin. Traction alopecia usually follows a predictable progression of clinical manifestations. Early features are perifollicular erythema, hair thinning, and a focal decrease in hair density. With prolonged traction, perifollicular scarring and cicatricial alopecia develop. When cicatricial patches develop at the hair-bearing margin of the scalp, the disease is called *cicatricial marginal alopecia* or, more precisely, *traumatic cicatricial marginal alopecia* [19, 20]

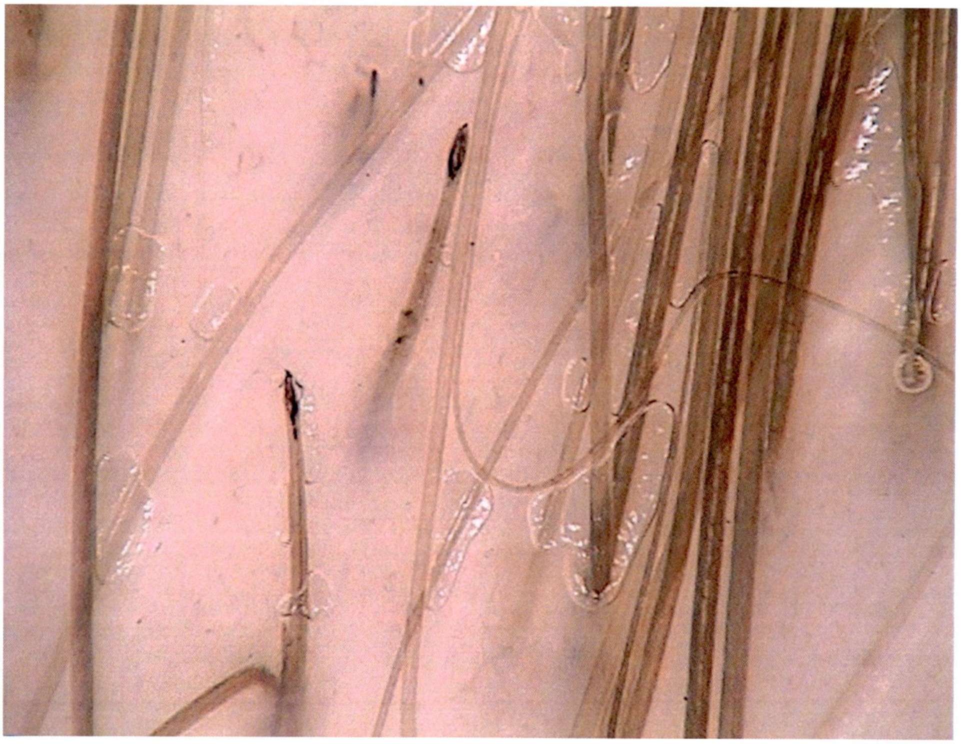

Fig. 20.31 **Tulip hairs in traction alopecia**. Our experience shows that the trichoscopic features of traction alopecia are often similar to those of trichotillomania. These features include decreased hair density, thinned hairs, broken hairs, and tulip hairs. The general picture tends to be less chaotic in traction alopecia than in trichotillomania. Flame hairs and coiled hairs are less common, probably because the mechanical force applied to the hair is not as great in traction alopecia. Adequate studies comparing trichoscopy of unintentional, noncicatricial traction alopecia to that of trichotillomania have not been performed yet. In some patients with traction alopecia, hair casts (fine white keratin cylinders) form and may be seen both clinically and trichoscopically [19, 21]. These hair casts are freely movable along the hair shaft and range from 3 to 7 mm in diameter. Figure 39.7 presents an example of a hair cast in traction alopecia. Hair casts are a nonspecific finding in traction alopecia; they also may be associated with lichen planopilaris and other hyperkeratotic scalp disorders (×70)

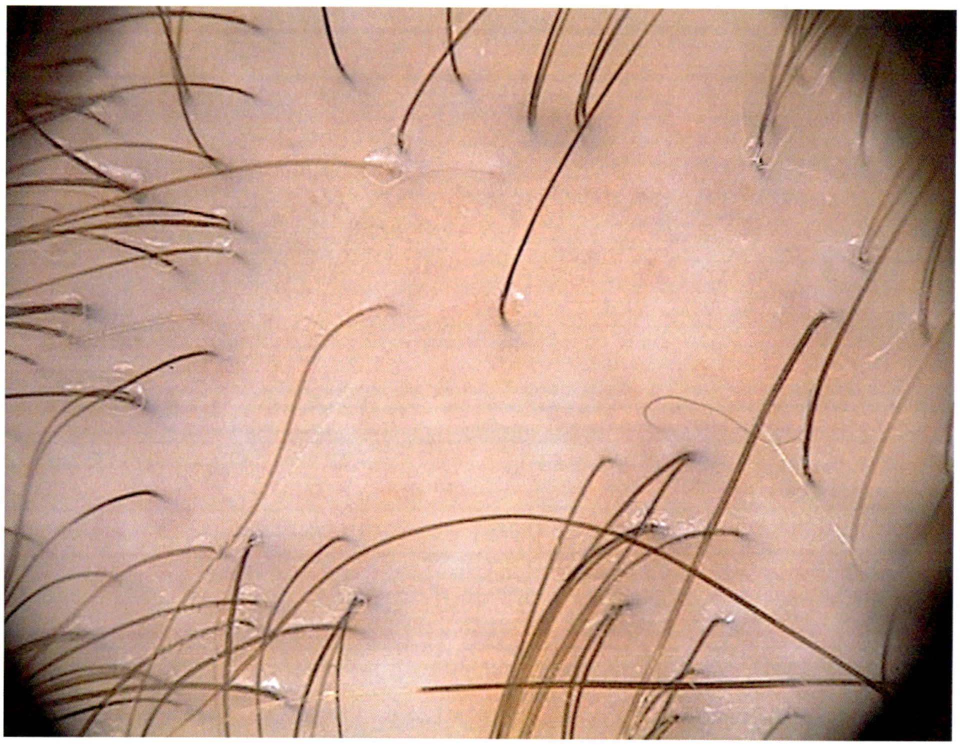

Fig. 20.32 **Cicatricial marginal alopecia**. Trichoscopy of cicatricial marginal alopecia shows low hair density, a predominance of follicular units with only one hair, and the absence of follicular openings [22]. Fibrotic white dots may be present as a manifestation of perifollicular fibrosis. In patients with straight hair, thin and wavy hair shafts may emerge from fibrotic white dots. Trichoscopy of advanced cicatricial marginal alopecia does not share common features with noncicatricial traction alopecia or trichotillomania. The main differential diagnosis is lichen planopilaris, which differs from cicatricial marginal alopecia in its prominent perifollicular scaling, tubular scaling, and abnormal vascular network (×20)

References

1. Witkowski AM, Schwartz RA, Janniger CK. Trichotillomania: an important psychocutaneous disorder. Cutis. 2010;86(1):12–6.
2. Szepietowski JC, Salomon J, Pacan P, Hrehorow E, Zalewska A. Frequency and treatment of trichotillomania in Poland. Acta Derm Venereol. 2009;89(3):267–70.
3. Franklin ME, Zagrabbe K, Benavides KL. Trichotillomania and its treatment: a review and recommendations. Expert Rev Neurother. 2011;11(8):1165–74.
4. Lochner C, Stein DJ, Woods D, Pauls DL, Franklin ME, Loerke EH, et al. The validity of DSM-IV-TR criteria B and C of hair-pulling disorder (trichotillomania): evidence from a clinical study. Psychiatry Res. 2011;189(2):276–80.
5. Stein DJ, Grant JE, Franklin ME, Keuthen N, Lochner C, Singer HS, et al. Trichotillomania (hair pulling disorder), skin picking disorder, and stereotypic movement disorder: toward DSM-V. Depress Anxiety. 2010;27(6):611–26.
6. Sah DE, Koo J, Price VH. Trichotillomania. Dermatol Ther. 2008; 21(1):13–21.
7. Hautmann G, Hercogova J, Lotti T. Trichotillomania. J Am Acad Dermatol. 2002;46(6):807–21; quiz 22–6.
8. Dimino-Emme L, Camisa C. Trichotillomania associated with the "Friar Tuck sign" and nail-biting. Cutis. 1991;47(2):107–10.
9. Abraham LS, Torres FN, Azulay-Abulafia L. Dermoscopic clues to distinguish trichotillomania from patchy alopecia areata. An Bras Dermatol. 2010;85(5):723–6.
10. Gallouj S, Rabhi S, Baybay H, Soughi M, Meziane M, Rammouz I, et al. Trichotemnomania associated to trichotillomania: a case report with emphasis on the diagnostic value of dermoscopy [in French]. Ann Dermatol Venereol. 2011;138(2):140–1.
11. Lee DY, Lee JH, Yang JM, Lee ES. The use of dermoscopy for the diagnosis of trichotillomania. J Eur Acad Dermatol Venereol. 2009; 23(6):731–2.
12. Inui S, Nakajima T, Nakagawa K, Itami S. Clinical significance of dermoscopy in alopecia areata: analysis of 300 cases. Int J Dermatol. 2008;47(7):688–93.
13. Ihm CW, Han JH. Diagnostic value of exclamation mark hairs. Dermatology. 1993;186(2):99–102.
14. Rudnicka L, Olszewska M, Rakowska A, Slowinska M. Trichoscopy update 2011. J Dermatol Case Rep. 2011;5(4):82–8.
15. Neila Iglesias J, Rodriguez Pichardo A, Garcia Bravo B, Camacho Martinez F. Masquerading of trichotillomania in a family with monilethrix. Eur J Dermatol. 2011;21(1):133.
16. Pinkus H. Multiple hairs (Flemming-Giovannini; report of two cases of pili multigemini and discussion of some other anomalies of the pilary complex. J Invest Dermatol. 1951;17(5):291–301.
17. Fu JM, Starace M, Tosti A. A new dermoscopic finding in healthy children. Arch Dermatol. 2009;145(5):596–7.
18. Inui S. Trichoscopy for common hair loss diseases: algorithmic method for diagnosis. J Dermatol. 2011;38(1):71–5.
19. Hantash BM, Schwartz RA. Traction alopecia in children. Cutis. 2003;71(1):18–20.
20. Goldberg LJ. Cicatricial marginal alopecia: is it all traction? Br J Dermatol. 2009;160(1):62–8.
21. Tosti A, Miteva M, Torres F, Vincenzi C, Romanelli P. Hair casts are a dermoscopic clue for the diagnosis of traction alopecia. Br J Dermatol. 2010;163(6):1353–5.
22. Tosti A, Torres F, Misciali C, Vincenzi C, Duque-Estrada B. The role of dermoscopy in the diagnosis of cicatricial marginal alopecia. Br J Dermatol. 2009;161(1):213–5.

Part VIII

Primary Cicatricial Alopecia

Classic Lichen Planopilaris and Graham Little Syndrome

21

Malgorzata Olszewska, Adriana Rakowska, Monika Slowinska, and Lidia Rudnicka

Abstract

Classic lichen planopilaris may be suspected based on trichoscopy only in the active phase of the disease. Characteristic trichoscopic features include perifollicular scaling, with scales entangling hair shafts in a tubular manner up to a few millimeters above the scalp surface. Blood vessels are elongated and commonly arranged concentrically around a hair follicle opening. In long-lasting, inactive lichen planopilaris, trichoscopy shows large irregular white dots, which become confluent and form milky red areas with a characteristic strawberry ice cream color. In Graham Little syndrome, scalp trichoscopic findings do not differ from those of classic lichen planopilaris. Trichoscopy of the axillae and pubic area shows very sparse, thin terminal hairs with no features of fibrosis.

Keywords

Blood vessels • Graham Little syndrome • Folliculitis decalvans • Hair casts • Lichen planopilaris • Perifollicular scaling • Tubular scaling • Tufted hairs • Violaceous areas White dots

Lichen planopilaris is the most frequent cause of adult primary scarring alopecia [1–3]. Three variants of the disease may be distinguished: classic lichen planopilaris, frontal fibrosing alopecia [4], and Lassueur–Graham Little–Piccardi, called also Graham Little syndrome. Some authors consider fibrosing alopecia in a pattern distribution a fourth variant of the disease [5, 6].

The classic form of lichen planopilaris most commonly involves the vertex, but any region of the scalp may be affected.

M. Olszewska
Department of Dermatology, Medical University of Warsaw, Koszykowa 82A, Warsaw 02-008, Poland
e-mail: malgorzata.olszewska@wum.edu.pl

A. Rakowska • M. Slowinska
Department of Dermatology, CSK MSW, Woloska 137, Warsaw 02-507 , Poland

L. Rudnicka (✉)
Faculty of Health Sciences, Medical University of Warsaw, Poland

Department of Dermatology, CSK MSW, Woloska 137, Warsaw 02-502, Poland
e-mail: lidia.rudnicka@euderm.eu

Lichen planopilaris rarely involves other hair-bearing areas. Early lesions are characterized by a violaceous follicular erythema and perifollicular keratotic lesions. Perifollicular inflammation or hyperkeratosis may be very subtle in some cases, which makes the clinical diagnosis more difficult. When inflammatory changes resolve, they are replaced by perifollicular areas of atrophic scarring, which merge to form an atrophic scar. This corresponds to the end stage of any cicatricial alopecia. Some hairs affected by the inflammatory process may persist in the center of the bald area [2, 5].

The most characteristic trichoscopic features of lichen planopilaris are perifollicular scaling, perifollicular inflammation, violaceous areas, and elongated, parallel-oriented blood vessels.

The most characteristic trichoscopic feature of active lichen planopilaris is perifollicular scaling. The scales migrate along the hair shaft and form a tubular structure, which covers the proximal portion of the emerging hair shaft. This structure is called "collar-like" or "tubular" perifollicular hyperkeratosis [7, 8]. The hair shaft may be covered with scales up to a few millimeters above the scalp surface. This feature is believed to be a

L. Rudnicka et al. (eds.), *Atlas of Trichoscopy*,
DOI 10.1007/978-1-4471-4486-1_21, © Springer-Verlag London 2012

consequence of changes in the outer hair follicle root sheath, which result in excessive perifollicular scaling. This feature is characteristic of but not pathognomonic for lichen planopilaris.

Round perifollicular blue-gray or violaceous areas surrounding empty hair follicle openings in a targetoid pattern have been described in patients with dark phototypes [9]. This observation most probably corresponds to subepidermal melanin, produced in hair follicles, that entered the catagen phase before definite involution, resulting in end-stage fibrotic tracts.

White dots in lichen planopilaris are considered a residue of conduced perifollicular fibrosis [9–11]. These are irregularly shaped whitish areas lacking follicular openings. They usually are greater than 100 μm in diameter and tend to become confluent and form ivory-white or milky red areas. They must be distinguished from small pinpoint white dots, which represent empty follicular ostia in patients with dark skin phototypes IV, V, and VI [12]. White dots and milky red areas are late manifestations of lichen planopilaris. The sole presence of white dots and milky red areas lacking follicular openings is nonspecific and may be observed in other types of folliculocentric scarring alopecia [9, 10].

Acquired pili torti may be observed at the periphery of fibrotic lesions [13]. Elongation of blood vessels adjacent to emerging hairs occurs in 78.9 % of patients with lichen planopilaris [8].

In Graham Little syndrome, trichoscopic results do not differ from those of classic lichen planopilaris. In the axillae and pubic area, trichoscopy shows sparse, hypopigmented, thin but long hair shafts and occasionally barely visible yellow dots [7].

Table 21.1 Trichoscopic features of classic lichen planopilaris

Active lesions
Perifollicular scaling
Scales entangling hair shafts up to 2–3 mm above the scalp surface in a tubular manner
Hair casts
Elongated linear blood vessels
Violaceous areas
Inactive lesions
Irregular, large white dots (fibrotic white dots)
White areas
Milky red areas (strawberry ice cream color)
Tufted hairs

Table 21.2 Trichoscopic differential diagnosis of classic lichen planopilaris

Frontal fibrosing alopecia
Folliculitis decalvans
Discoid lupus erythematosus
Dissecting cellulitis
Scalp psoriasis
Seborrheic dermatitis
Monoclonal gammopathy
Cicatricial pemphigoid

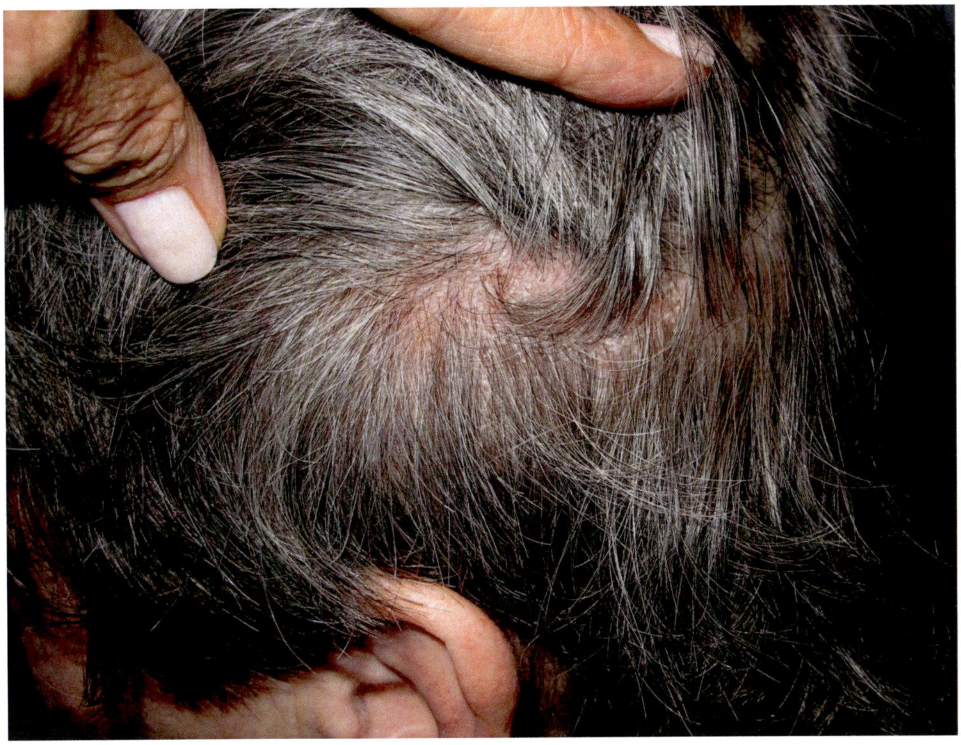

Fig. 21.1 **Lichen planopilaris**. Clinical image of early lichen planopilaris showing mild erythema and scaling. An excoriation in the midpart of the lesion results from scratching. Itching may be constant and intense in lichen planopilaris

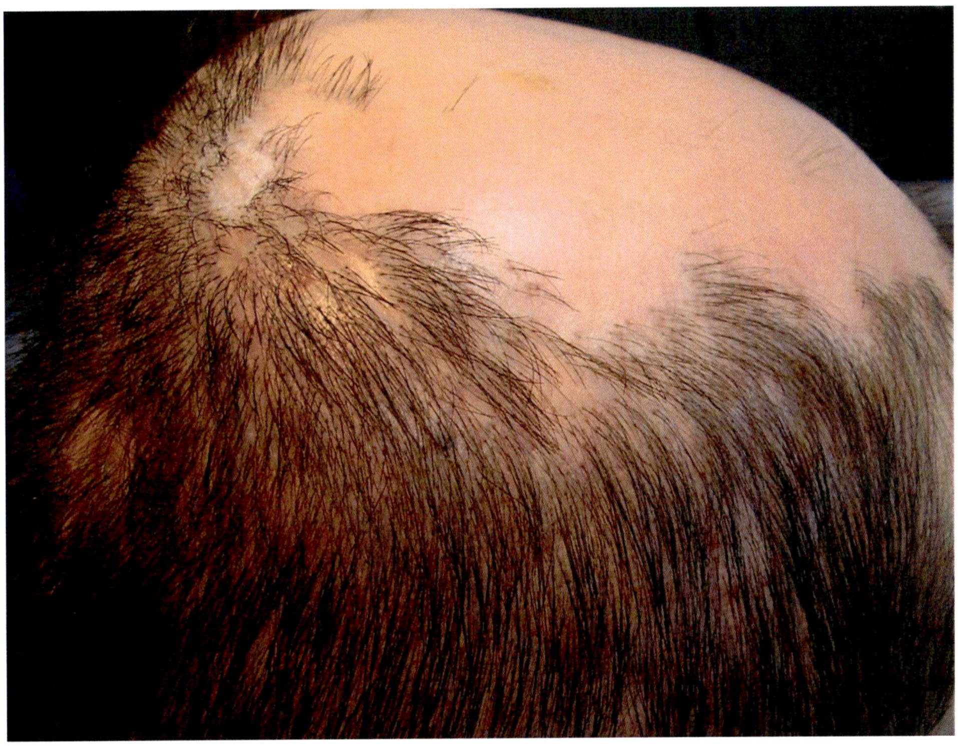

Fig. 21.2 **Late-stage lichen planopilaris mimicking androgenetic alopecia**. Clinical image of advanced hair loss in the course of classic lichen planopilaris. Alopecia is seen in the frontal and vertex areas ("patterned alopecia"), with a hairline consisting of multifocal patches of hair loss. Some thick terminal hairs persist in the center of the bald area, which is characteristic of classic lichen planopilaris [2, 5] but also may be observed in other lichen planopilaris variants [14]. Mild perifollicular erythema at the hair-bearing margin may indicate lichen planopilaris. In patients with focal hair loss, trichoscopy, similar to biopsy, should be performed at the hair-bearing margin of the lesion

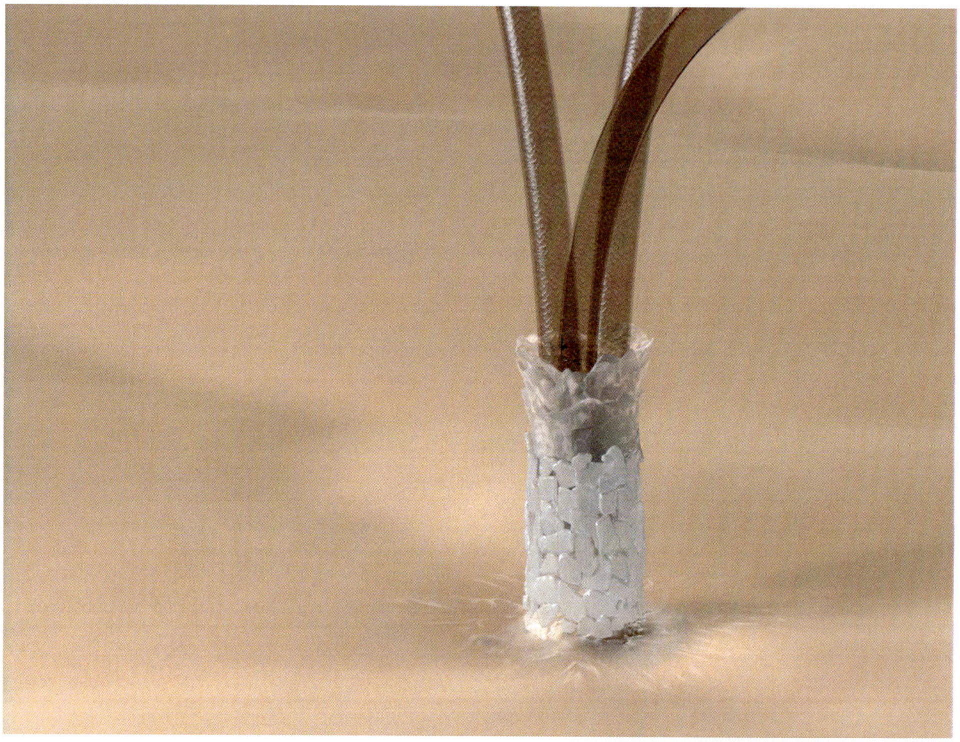

Fig. 21.3 Perifollicular scaling in lichen planopilaris. Perifollicular collar scaling is a hallmark of lichen planopilaris. Scales form silver-white tubular structures around the emerging hair shafts, usually reaching about 1–3 mm above the scalp surface (*Graphic by* Dr. Wawrzyniec Podrzucki)

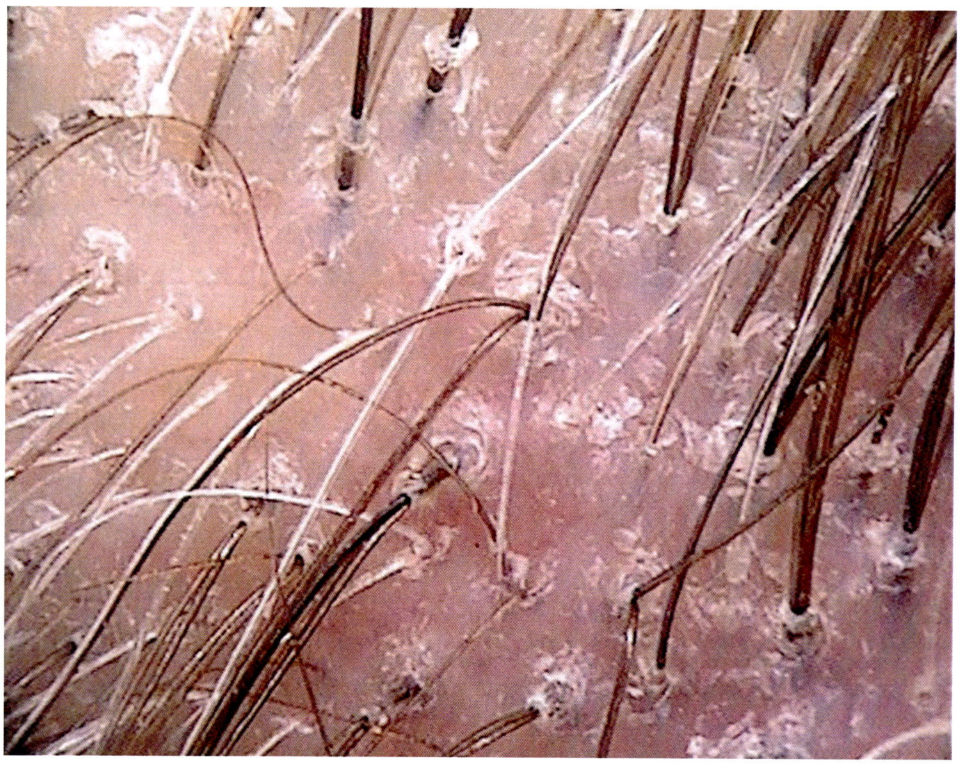

Fig. 21.4 Perifollicular scaling in lichen planopilaris. The scales are white or silver-white and form tubular structures around the emerging hair shafts. This feature is best observed by dry trichoscopy. The background (interfollicular area) is smooth and slightly glossy on dry trichoscopy (×20; dry trichoscopy)

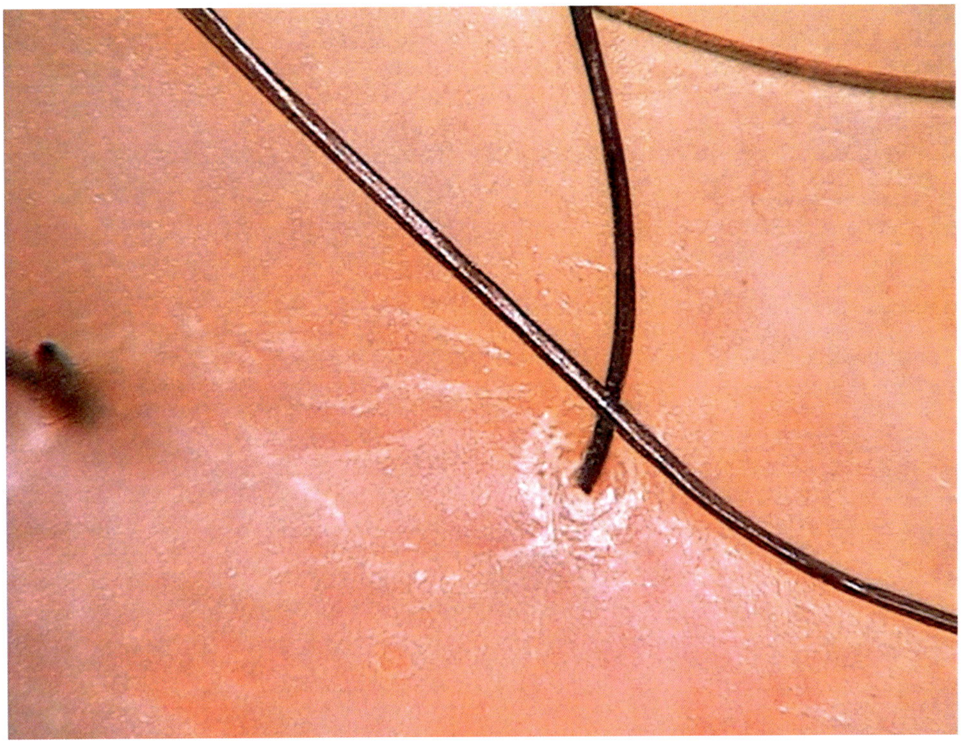

Fig. 21.5 Perifollicular scaling in lichen planopilaris. Mild silver-white perifollicular scaling surrounds a pilosebaceous unit with a single hair in a patient with long-lasting disease of medium activity. The smooth reflective pink of the surrounding skin reflects cicatricial changes of recent onset. The term *strawberry ice cream* is used by some authors to describe the color of early cicatricial alopecia [7]. Trichoscopy of frontal fibrosing alopecia may show similar white scaling, but the background color usually is ivory-white, which results from less inflammatory activity in these patients (×70; dry trichoscopy)

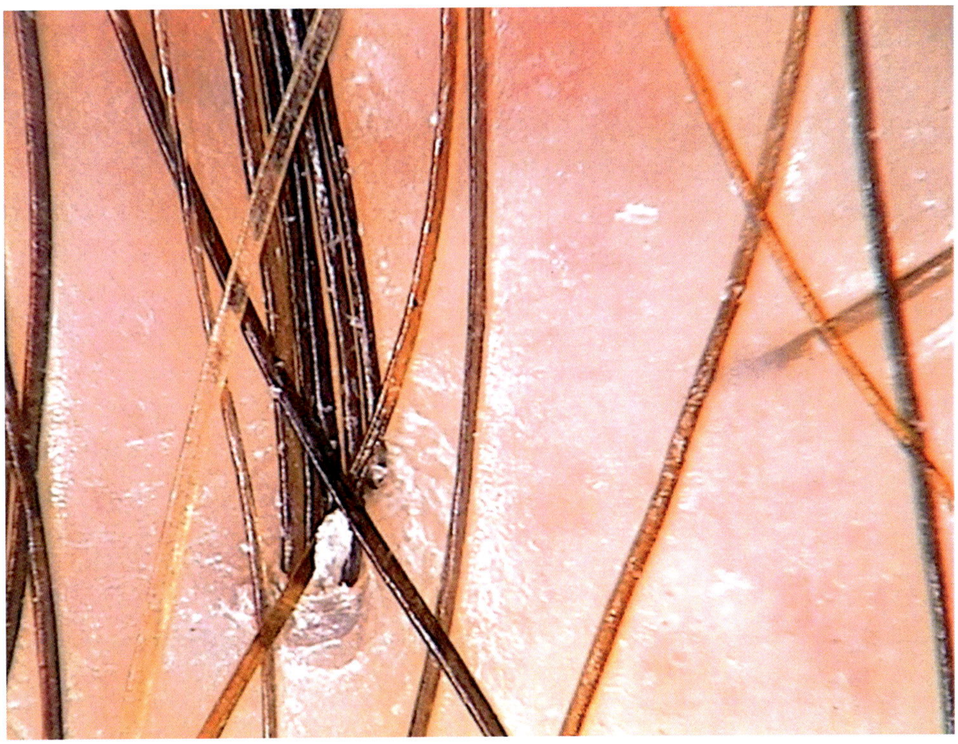

Fig. 21.6 Perifollicular scaling and tufted hairs in lichen planopilaris. Tufted hairs (five or more hairs emerging from one follicular opening) are observed in only 5 % of patients with lichen planopilaris. Usually, these are small tufts of five to seven hairs, which differs from what is observed in folliculitis decalvans, with about ten or more hairs per tuft. In lichen planopilaris, the hair tufts are walled with silver-white scales. Similar scaling observed in folliculitis decalvans is usually yellowish from the yellow purulent content. In lichen planopilaris less commonly than in folliculitis decalvans, the scaly tube is rolled out at the distal end (×70; dry dermoscopy)

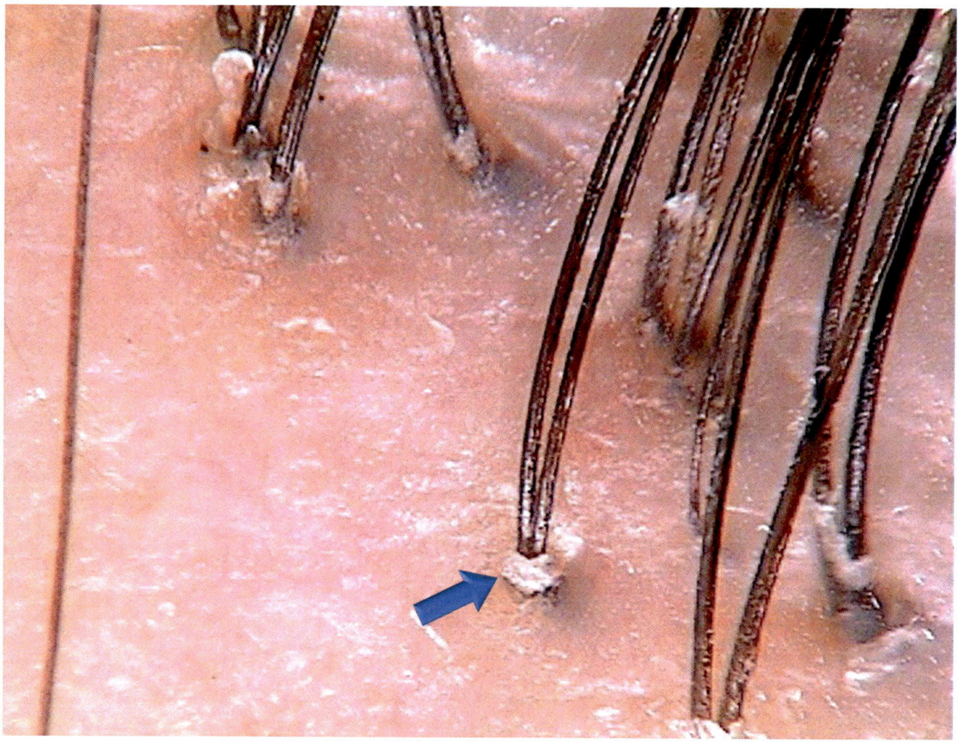

Fig. 21.7 Perifollicular scaling and areas lacking follicular openings in lichen planopilaris. In the hair-bearing margin, trichoscopy shows perifollicular inflammation and scaling in all pilosebaceous units. They form silver-white tubular structures attached to the hair shafts. Occasionally, the scales roll out at the distal end and form a wide collar around the hair shaft (*arrow*). There is less tendency for these collar-like structures to form in lichen planopilaris compared with folliculitis decalvans. The left part of the image shows adjacent skin lacking follicular openings, which corresponds to completed fibrosis (×70; dry trichoscopy)

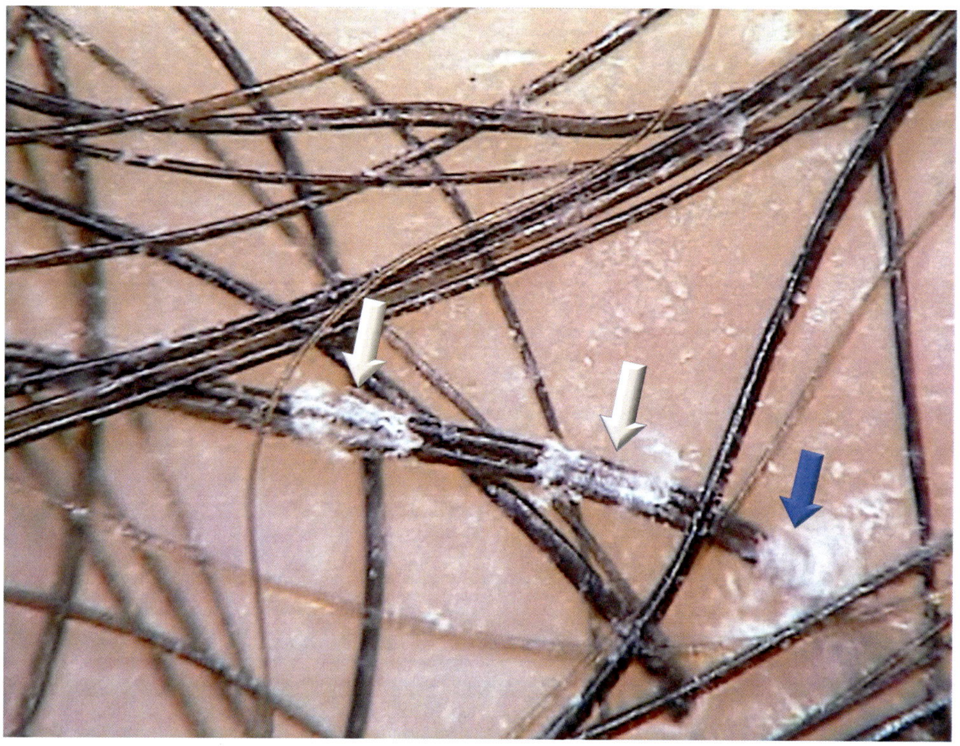

Fig. 21.8 Tubular silver-white hair casts in lichen planopilaris. Hair casts are small white keratinous structures that completely wrap the hair shaft. They are characterized by freely movable, tubular masses distributed along the scalp hair. This symptom has been associated with various diseases, including seborrheic dermatitis, psoriasis, pediculosis, white piedra, and monoclonal gammopathy [7, 15, 16]. In lichen planopilaris, the tubular perifollicular scales, which surround the hair shaft occasionally, detach from the base and remain attached to the hair shaft as the hair grows. This results in tubular silver-white hair casts. The image shows typical perifollicular scaling of lichen planopilaris (*blue arrow*) in the proximal portion of the hair and two hair casts (*white arrows*), each about 4 mm long. This feature is visualized best on dry trichoscopy (×70; dry trichoscopy)

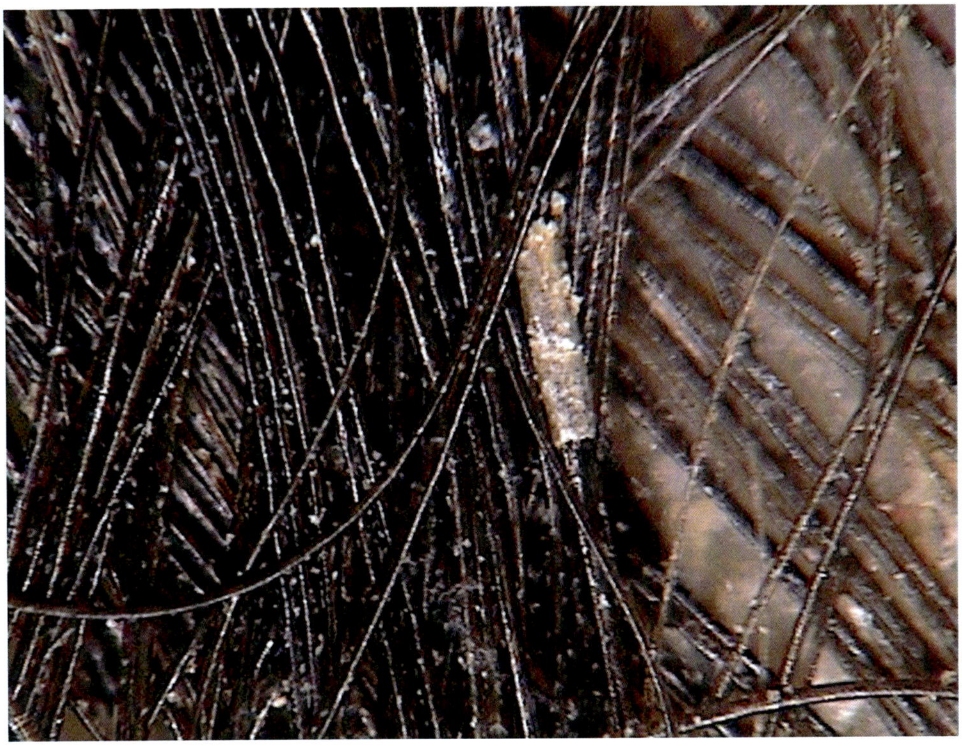

Fig. 21.9 **Tubular silver-white hair cast in lichen planopilaris**. The silver-white scales that detach from the perifollicular epidermis create shapes determined by hair shaft structure. These tubular hair casts may be attached very firmly to the hair shaft and persist despite multiple hair washings. This image shows an approximately 6 mm–long hair cast growing around two hair shafts and moving distally with the growth of these hairs. These uniform tubular structures observed in lichen planopilaris do not fulfill the classic definition of a *hair cast*, which indicates that a cast has a conical proximal end and a tapered or funnel-shaped distal end [16], resembling a pilar infundibulum (×70)

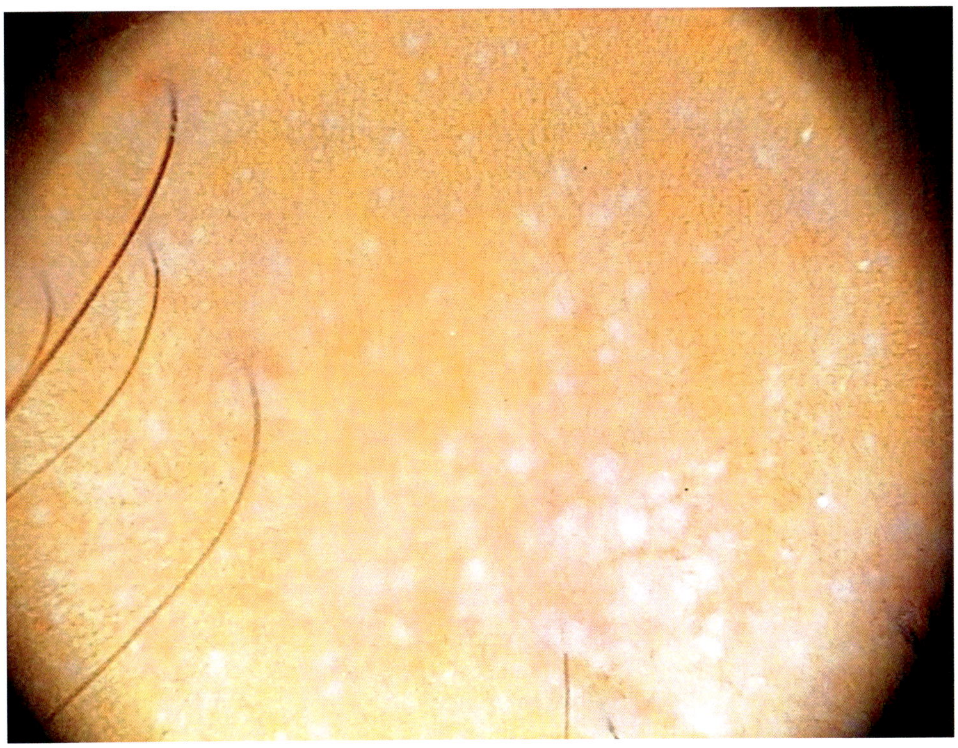

Fig. 21.10 **White dots in lichen planopilaris**. Two types of white dots are visible in this image. The *upper part* of the image shows pinpoint white dots corresponding to eccrine sweat gland and follicular openings on sun-exposed skin. This feature is visualized best in patients with dark skin phototypes and in those with lighter phototypes after intense suntanning (*see* Chap. 3 for details). The *lower part* of the picture shows larger white irregular dots with blunt borders and the tendency to become confluent. These white dots correspond to follicular fibrosis in the course of lichen planopilaris (×70)

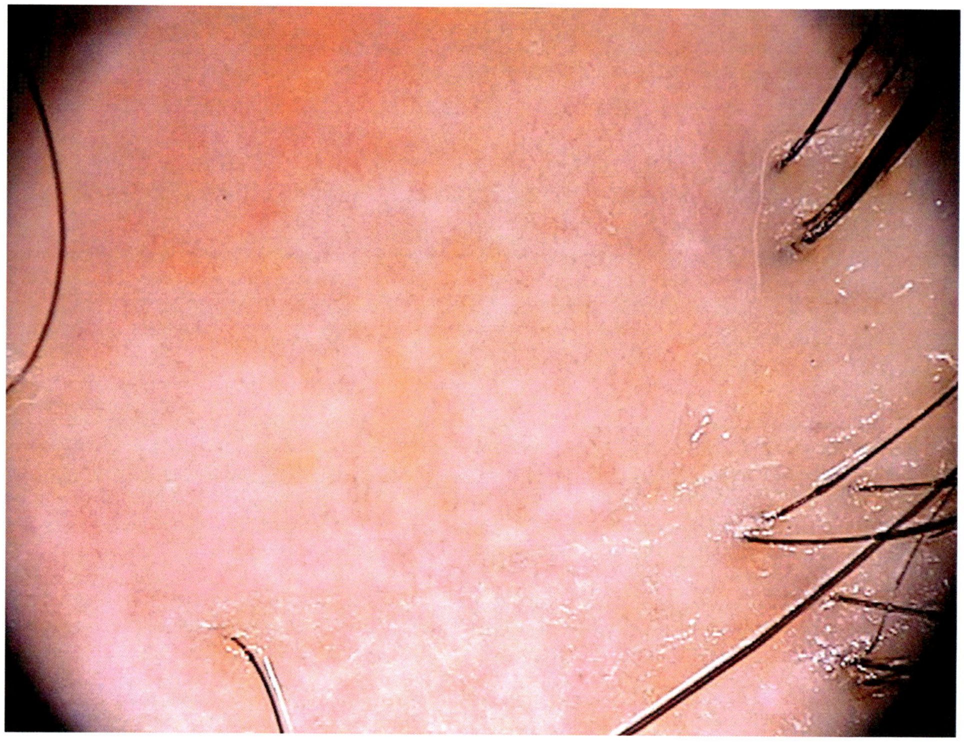

Fig. 21.11 Strawberry ice cream pattern with milky red areas and white dots in lichen planopilaris. In lichen planopilaris, white dots tend to merge and become confluent. They form white or milky red areas lacking follicular openings. This finding corresponds to fibrosis. Some trichoscopists refer to the milky red areas as a "strawberry ice cream pattern" because of their color. This pattern is characteristic of fibrosis of recent onset in cicatricial alopecia. The color fades over time and changes to ivory white or white (×20)

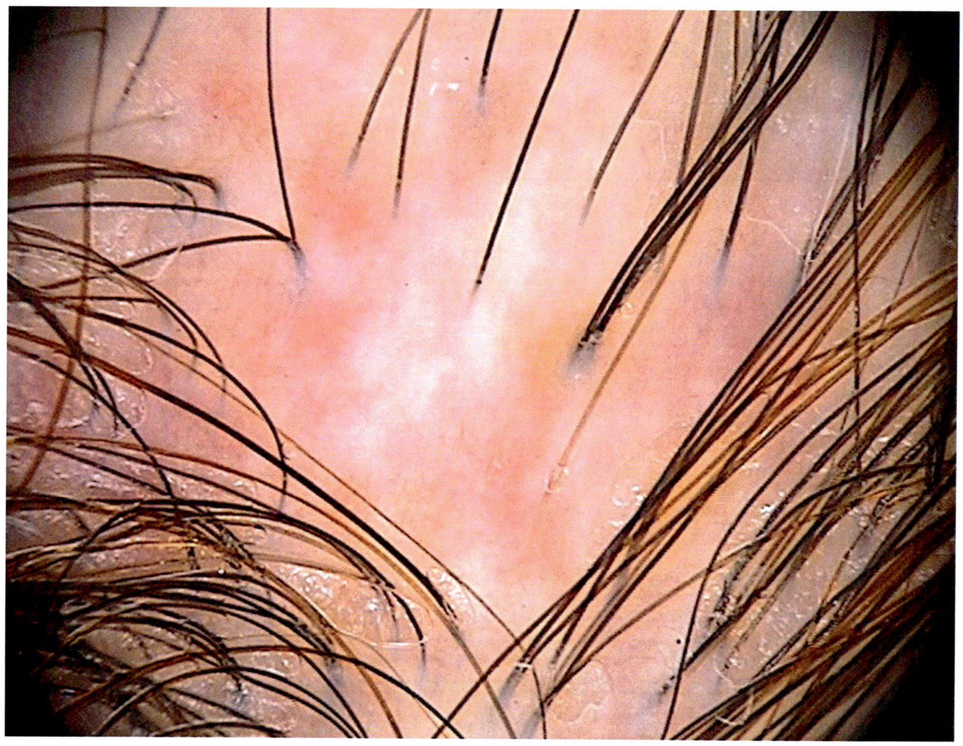

Fig. 21.12 White dots and white areas lacking follicular openings in lichen planopilaris. Trichoscopy of hair-bearing margins shows white halos surrounding the emerging hair shafts, corresponding to perifollicular fibrosis. When this process continues, the hair follicle is replaced by fibrotic tissue and appears on trichoscopy as large irregular white dots, which merge into white or milky red areas (×20)

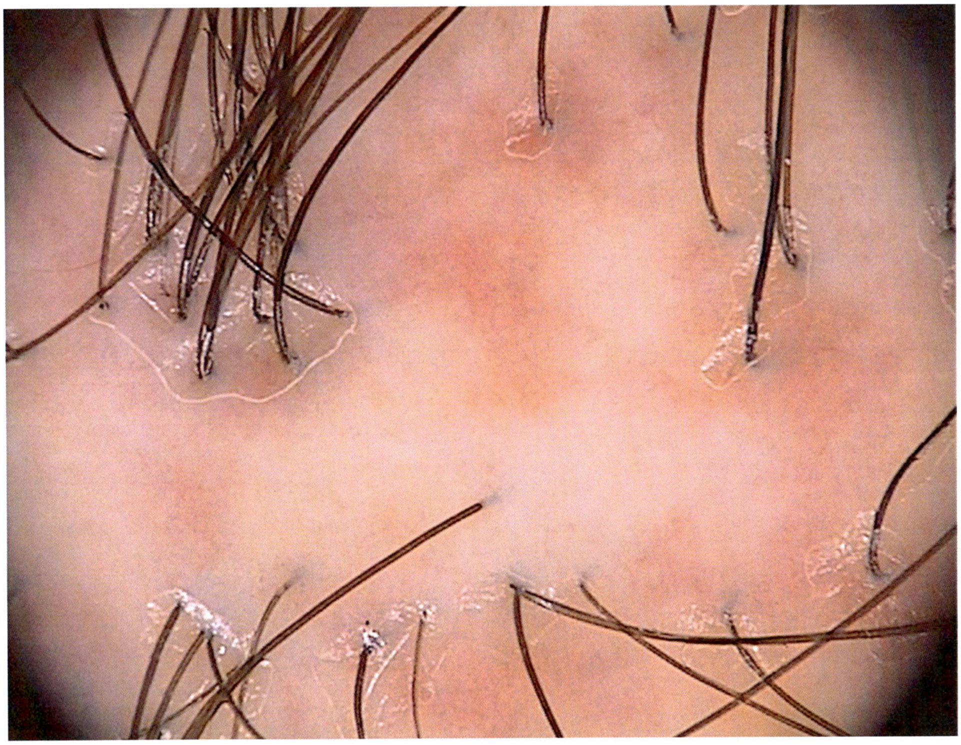

Fig. 21.13 White areas in lichen planopilaris. Fibrosis appears on trichoscopy as interfollicular confluent white areas on a milky red background. These areas lack follicular openings. Red halos around hair-bearing follicles correspond to perifollicular inflammation (×20)

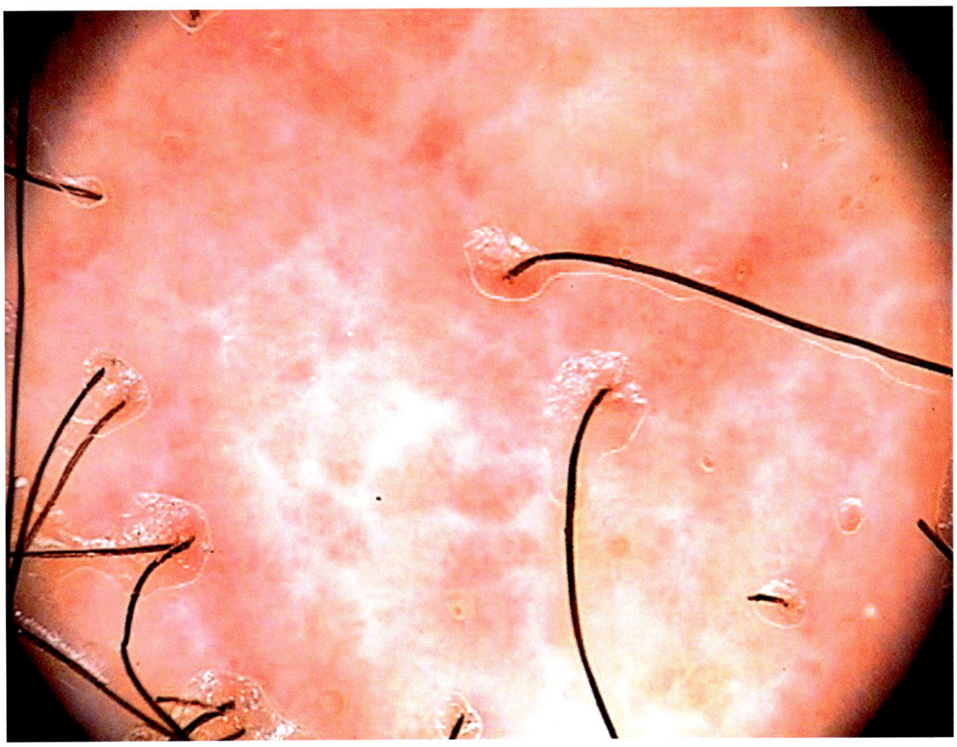

Fig. 21.14 Wickham striae in lichen planopilaris. Wickham striae represent a white net of lines on a reddish background visible in papules of cutaneous lichen planus and reflect hypergranulosis. They are visualized easily on dermoscopy [17]. This feature is very rare in lichen planopilaris of the scalp, observed in less than 5 % of patients (×20)

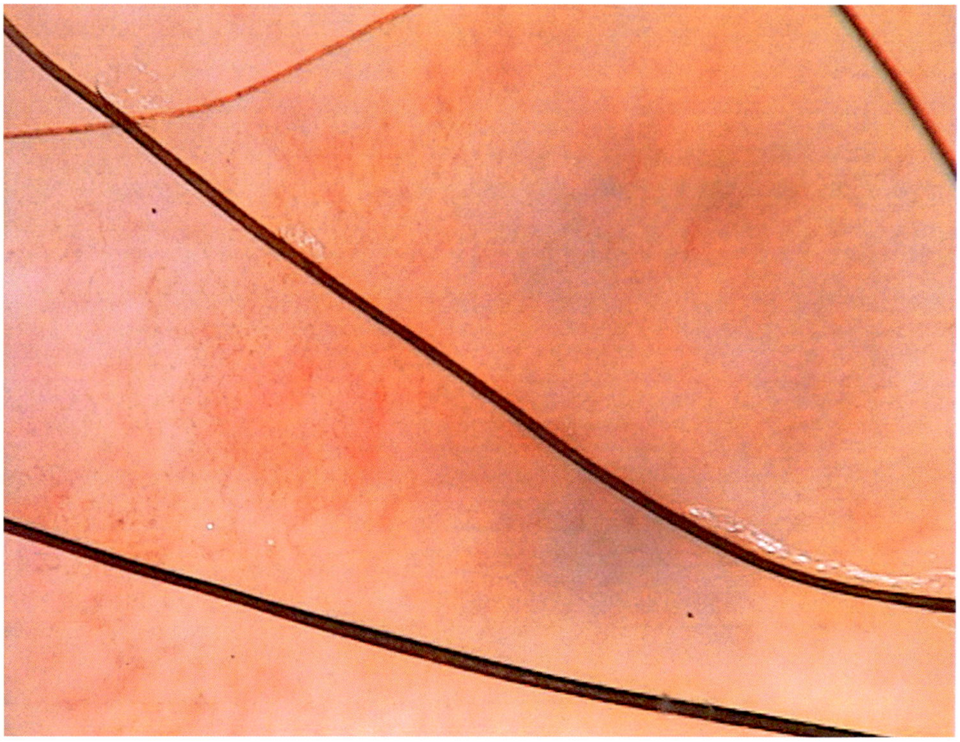

Fig. 21.15 Violaceous areas in lichen planopilaris. Violaceous or violet-brown areas are common in inflammatory lesions of lichen planopilaris. They are most common in active lesions and correspond to the pigment incontinence seen on histopathology (×70)

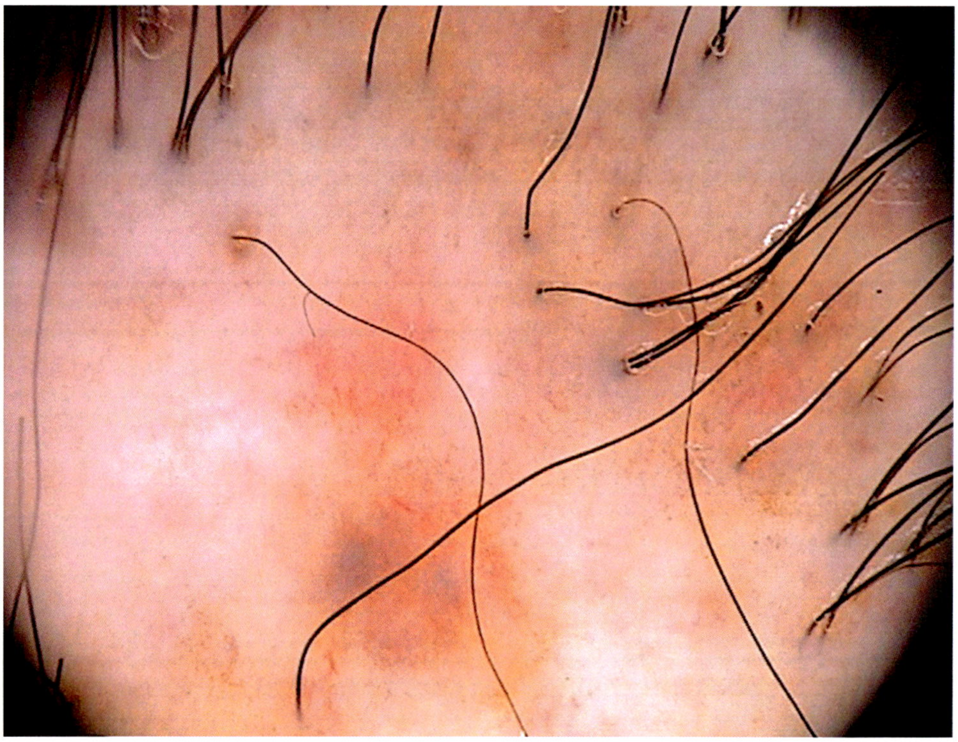

Fig. 21.16 Violaceous areas and acquired hair shaft dystrophy in lichen planopilaris. In the midpart of this patch of cicatricial alopecia, a violaceous area is visible. From the fibrotic areas, few hairs emerge. The hair shafts show an irregular crooked, kinked structure. Such abnormalities are common, especially in the hair-bearing margin of fibrotic areas in lichen planopilaris and cicatricial alopecia of other origins. Acquired hair shaft dystrophy results from perifollicular fibrosis, which changes the structure of the hair follicle (×20)

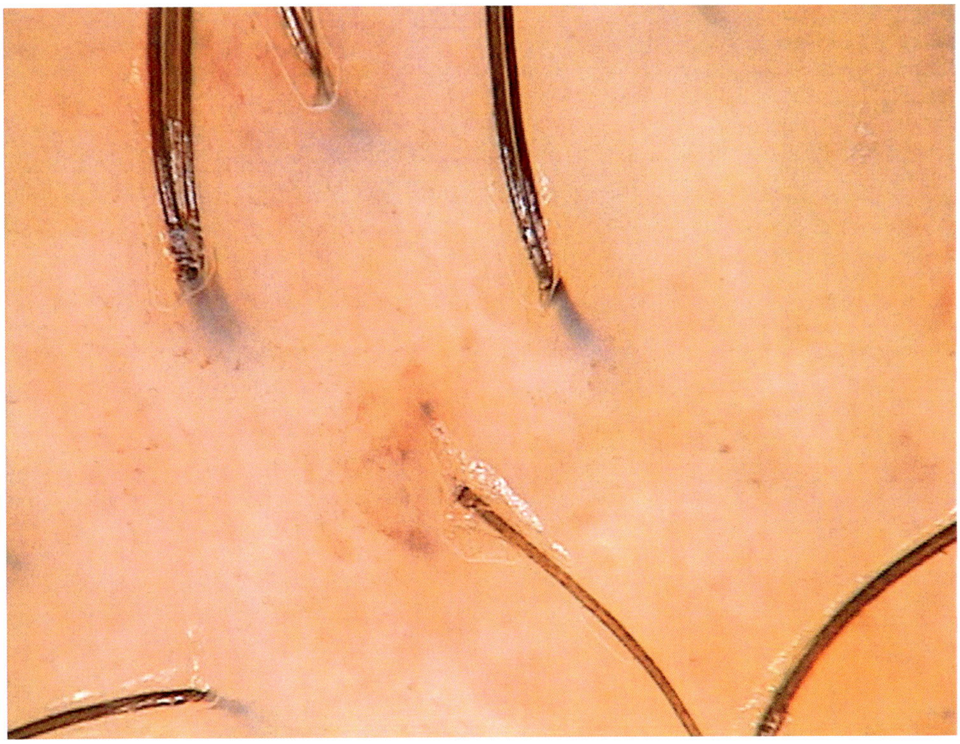

Fig. 21.17 Scattered brown skin discoloration in lichen planopilaris. Scattered brown skin discoloration is rare in lichen planopilaris. This finding, which corresponds to a superficial location of melanin or to pigment incontinence coexisting with atrophic epidermis, is most common in discoid lupus erythematosus (×70)

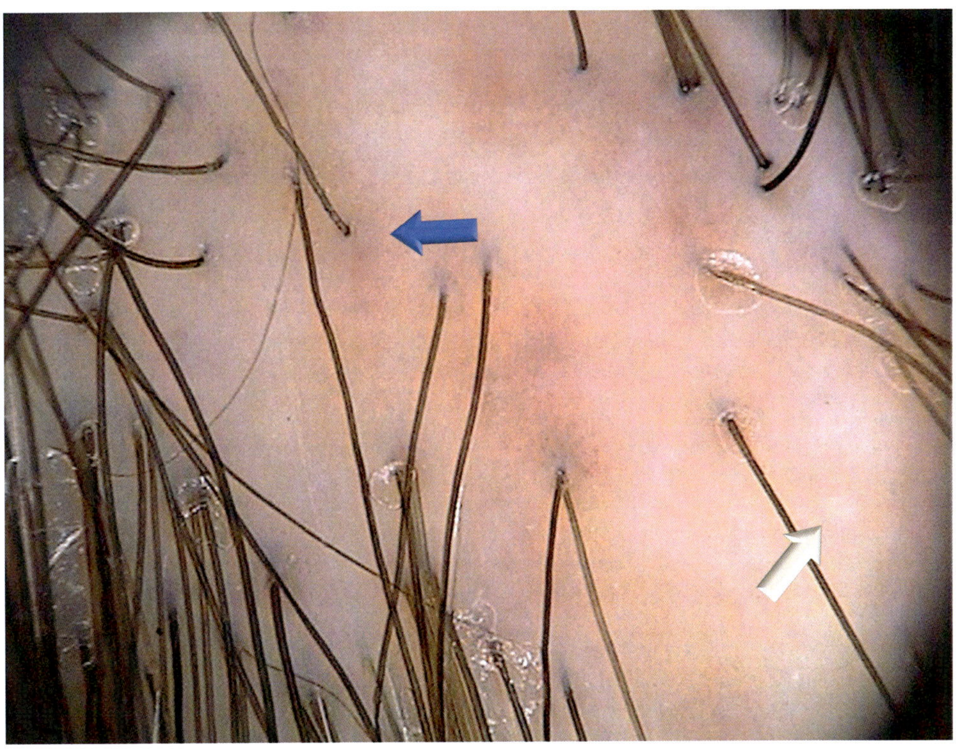

Fig. 21.18 Perifollicular violaceous skin discoloration in lichen planopilaris. Bluntly demarcated violaceous, blue-gray, and brown-gray areas (*blue arrow*) correspond to pigment incontinence in areas of epidermal acanthosis. They differ from perifollicular hyperpigmentation in androgenic alopecia in their violaceous tint, bigger size, and irregular blunt borders. White dots (*white arrow*) merge into white areas of fibrosis, which lack follicular openings (×20)

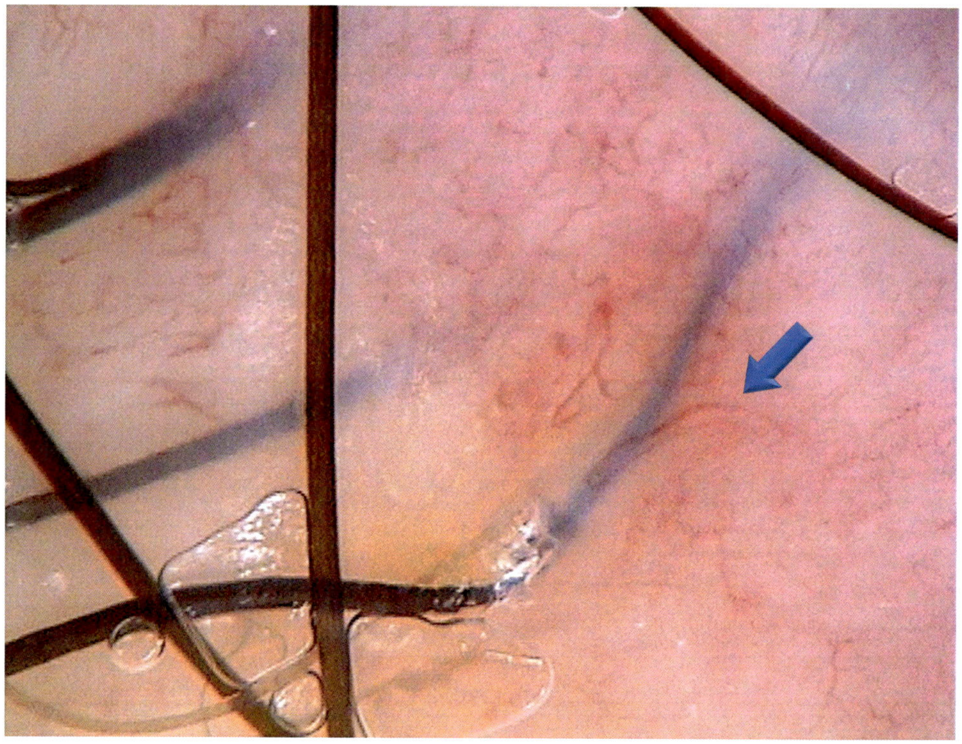

Fig. 21.19 Elongated blood vessels in lichen planopilaris. Examination of hair-bearing margins of scarring alopecia reveals a vascular network with multiple elongated blood vessels close to the hair follicle. The elongated vessels form a *V* with the corresponding emerging hair shaft (*arrow*). Frequently, elongated vascular loops form a concentric pattern around the hair follicle opening (×70)

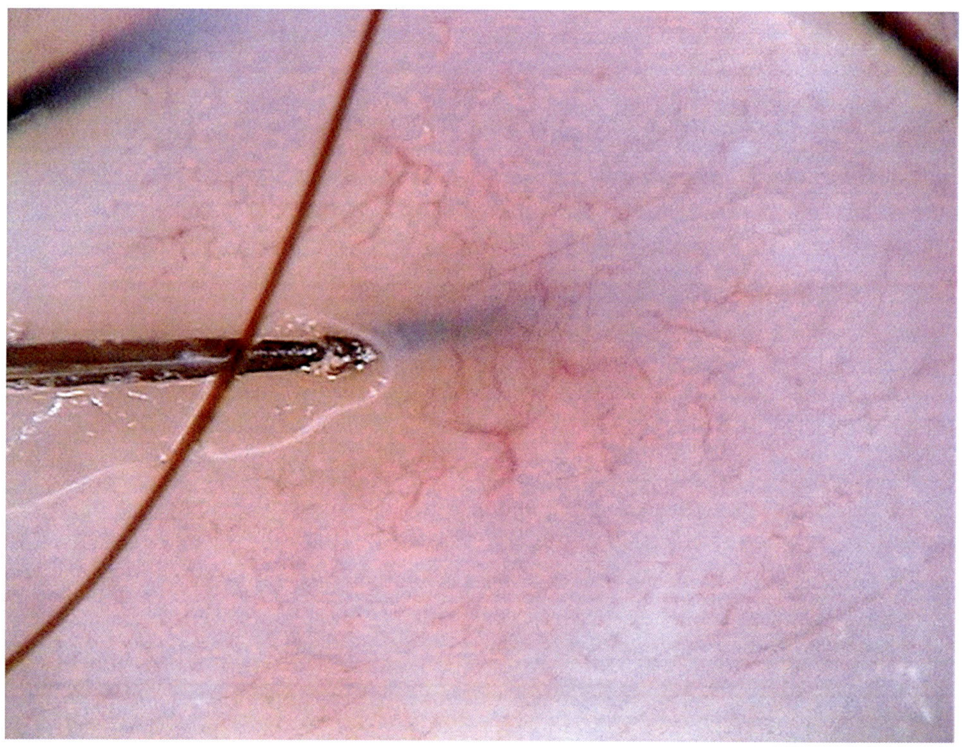

Fig. 21.20 Elongated blood vessels in lichen planopilaris forming a concentric pattern around a hair follicle opening. A perifollicular vascular network is seen at the hair-bearing margins of a lichen planopilaris patch. Multiple thin elongated linear vessels and arborizing vessels form a concentric pattern around a hair follicle opening with an emerging hair shaft. Some elongated vessels form a *V* with the corresponding emerging hair shaft. This appearance is characteristic of active perifollicular inflammation in the reversible phase of the disease (×70)

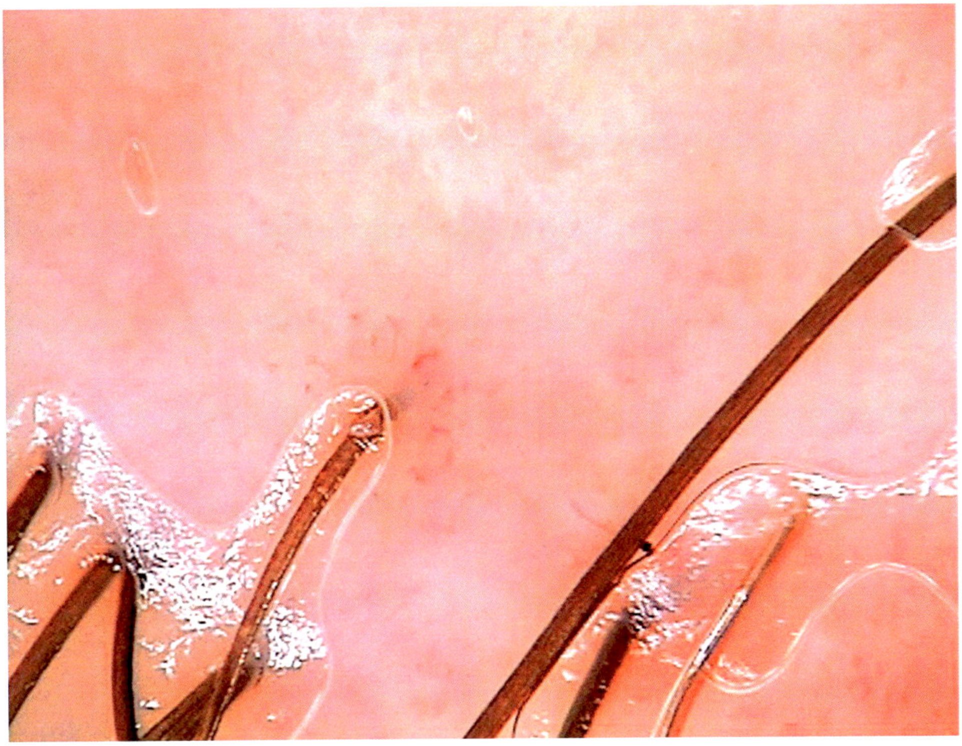

Fig. 21.21 Concentric perifollicular blood vessels in lichen planopilaris. A perifollicular concentration of blood vessels is characteristic of the early, reversible phase of lichen planopilaris. Small perifollicular vessels can be visualized only with immersion fluid and application of mild pressure with the dermoscope lens at the hair-bearing margin of lichen planopilaris patches. Visualization of small blood vessels may be easier with ultrasound gel rather than alcohol or water. The disadvantage of gel is easier formation of air bubbles, as may be seen in the *lower part* of the image (×70)

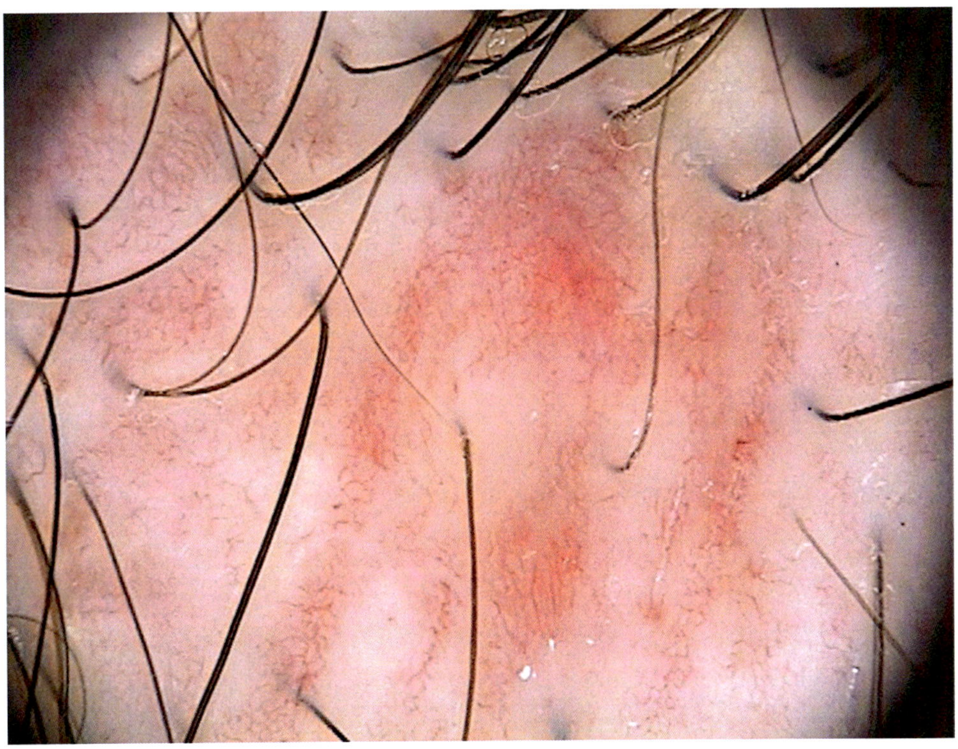

Fig. 21.22 Blood vessels and white areas in lichen planopilaris. Large white dots with blunt borders and white halos surrounding hair shafts correspond to perifollicular fibrosis. Multiple elongated blood vessels are seen in a patient with lichen planopilaris treated with potent topical glucocorticosteroids. Long-term glucocorticosteroid use causes skin atrophy and increased visibility of multiple blood vessels (×20)

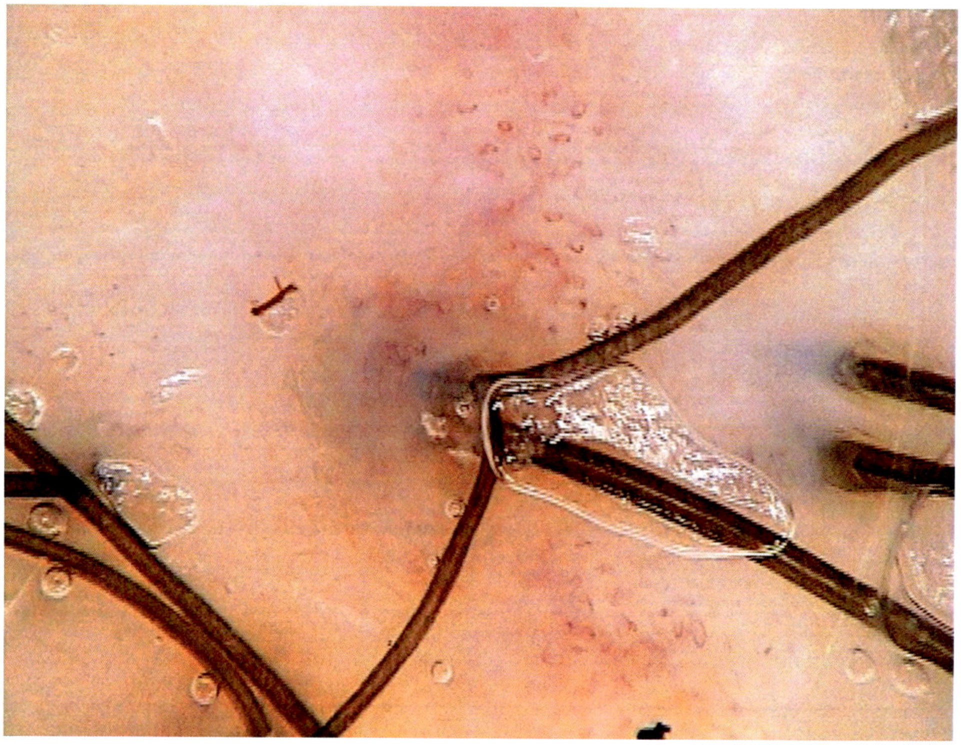

Fig. 21.23 Blood vessels, violaceous perifollicular areas, and white areas in lichen planopilaris. Multiple coiled and dotted blood vessels with a whitish halo are arranged in a perifollicular manner. Pinpoint vessels with a whitish halo are rare in lichen planopilaris and require differential diagnosis with dissecting cellulitis and other diseases. However, the perifollicular arrangement of these vessels, violaceous areas surrounding the hair follicle opening, and white interfollicular areas are indicative of lichen planopilaris (×70)

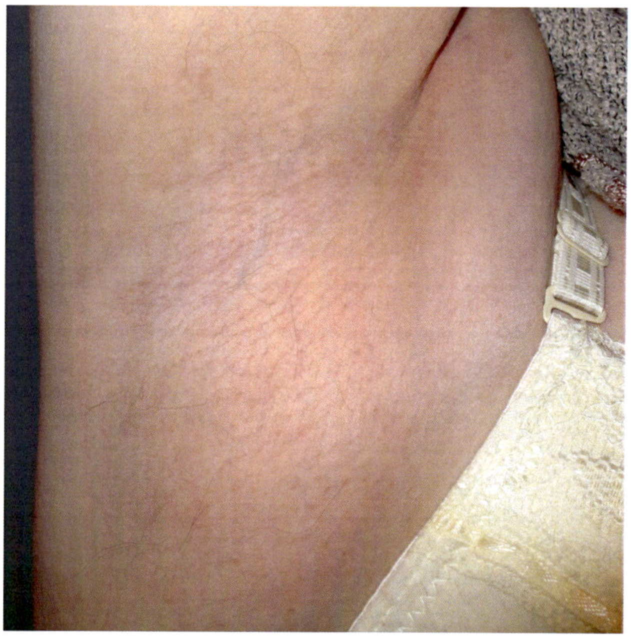

Fig. 21.24 Nonscarring loss of axilla hair in a patient with Graham Little syndrome. Graham Little syndrome (also called Graham Little–Piccardi or Graham Little–Piccardi–Lasseur syndrome) is characterized by a triad of (1) patchy scarring alopecia of the scalp, (2) noncicatricial alopecia of the axillae and pubic area, and (3) follicular lichen planus on glabrous skin [18]

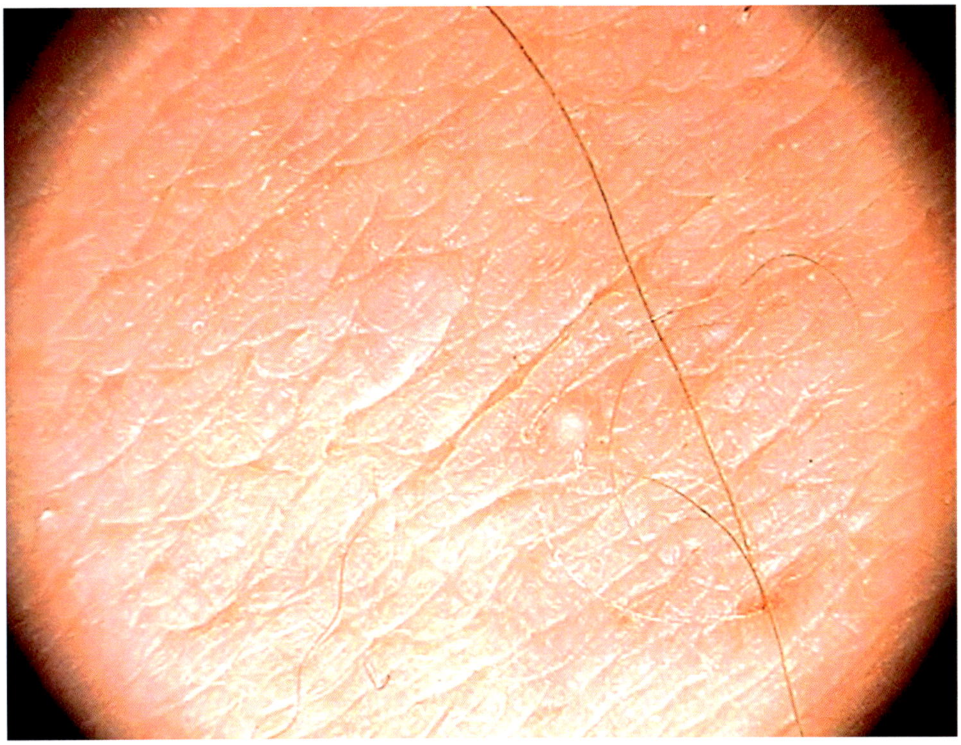

Fig. 21.25 Noncicatricial alopecia of the axillae in Graham Little syndrome. Trichoscopy shows sparse, thin terminal hairs and areas of skin folds and crevices lacking hairs but no features of fibrosis, such as white dots or smooth white to ivory-white areas. Trichoscopy of the pubic area shows comparable, nonspecific features corresponding to noncicatricial alopecia. Trichoscopy of scalp lesions in Graham Little syndrome does not differ from that of classic lichen planopilaris (×20)

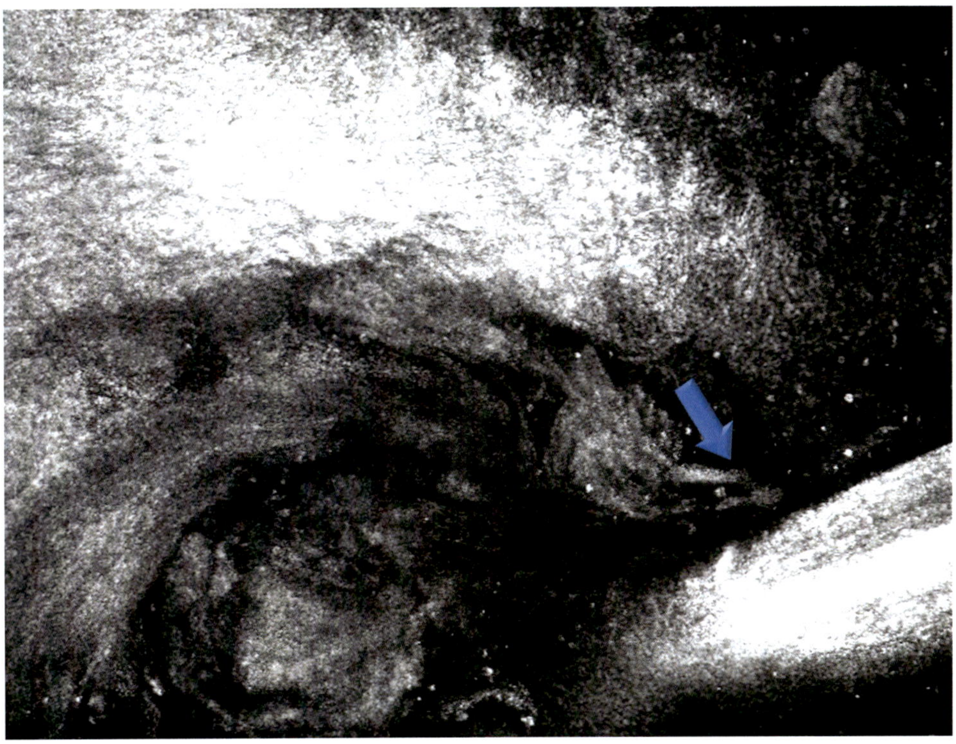

Fig. 21.26 Reflectance confocal microscopy of lichen planopilaris. Reflectance confocal microscopy shows enlarged hair follicle openings filled with keratotic material. The scales adhere to the outer part of the hair shaft and cover its proximal part (*arrow*). The granular layer of the infundibulum and adjacent epidermis is accentuated. Hair shafts show no abnormality

References

1. Ochoa BE, King Jr LE, Price VH. Lichen planopilaris: annual incidence in four hair referral centers in the United States. J Am Acad Dermatol. 2008;58(2):352–3.
2. Otberg N, Kang H, Alzolibani AA, Shapiro J. Folliculitis decalvans. Dermatol Ther. 2008;21(4):238–44.
3. Price V, Mirmirani P, editors. Cicatricial alopecia: an approach to diagnosis and management. New York: Springer; 2011.
4. Abbas O, Chedraoui A, Ghosn S. Frontal fibrosing alopecia presenting with components of Piccardi-Lassueur-Graham-Little syndrome. J Am Acad Dermatol. 2007;57(2 Suppl):S15–8.
5. Assouly P, Reygagne P. Lichen planopilaris: update on diagnosis and treatment. Semin Cutan Med Surg. 2009;28(1):3–10.
6. Wiseman MC, Shapiro J. Scarring alopecia. J Cutan Med Surg. 1999;3 Suppl 3:S45–8.
7. Rudnicka L, Olszewska M, Rakowska A. Trichoscopy update 2011. J Dermatol Case Rep. 2011;5(4):82–8. doi:10.3315/jdcr.2011.1083.
8. Rakowska A, Slowinska M, Kowalska-Oledzka E, Olszewska M, Rudnicka L. Trichoscopy in cicatricial alopecia. J Drugs Dermatol. 2012;11(6):753–8.
9. Duque-Estrada B, Tamler C, Sodre CT, Barcaui CB, Pereira FB. Dermoscopy patterns of cicatricial alopecia resulting from discoid lupus erythematosus and lichen planopilaris. An Bras Dermatol. 2010;85(2):179–83.
10. Ross EK, Vincenzi C, Tosti A. Videodermoscopy in the evaluation of hair and scalp disorders. J Am Acad Dermatol. 2006;55(5):799–806.
11. Rudnicka L, Olszewska M, Rakowska A, Kowalska-Oledzka E, Slowinska M. Trichoscopy: a new method for diagnosing hair loss. J Drugs Dermatol. 2008;7(7):651–4.
12. Abraham LS, Pineiro-Maceira J, Duque-Estrada B, Barcaui CB, Sodre CT. Pinpoint white dots in the scalp: dermoscopic and histopathologic correlation. J Am Acad Dermatol. 2010;63(4):721–2.
13. Trueb RM. Systematic approach to hair loss in women. J Dtsch Dermatol Ges. 2010;8(4):284–97, 98.
14. Tosti A, Miteva M, Torres F. Lonely hair: a clue to the diagnosis of frontal fibrosing alopecia. Arch Dermatol. 2011;147(10):1240.
15. Miller JJ, Anderson BE, Ioffreda MD, Bongiovanni MB, Fogelberg AC. Hair casts and cutaneous spicules in multiple myeloma. Arch Dermatol. 2006;142(12):1665–6.
16. Whiting DA, Dy LC. Office diagnosis of hair shaft defects. Semin Cutan Med Surg. 2006;25(1):24–34.
17. Vazquez-Lopez F, Alvarez-Cuesta C, Hidalgo-Garcia Y, Perez-Oliva N. The handheld dermatoscope improves the recognition of Wickham striae and capillaries in Lichen planus lesions. Arch Dermatol. 2001;137(10):1376.
18. Zegarska B, Kallas D, Schwartz RA, Czajkowski R, Uchanska G, Placek W. Graham-Little syndrome. Acta Dermatovenerol Alp Panonica Adriat. 2010;19(3):39–42.

Frontal Fibrosing Alopecia

22

Adriana Rakowska, Malgorzata Olszewska, and Lidia Rudnicka

Abstract
The trichoscopic features of frontal fibrosing alopecia include loss of follicular openings and minor perifollicular scaling. Lonely hair and, occasionally, perifollicular erythema may be observed. The background is ivory white to ivory beige. In the eyebrow area, trichoscopy shows regularly distributed red or gray dots.

Keywords
Cicatricial alopecia • Eyebrows • Frontal fibrosing alopecia • Gray dots • Ivory-white areas
Lichen planopilaris • Perifollicular scaling • Red dots

Frontal fibrosing alopecia (FFA) is a primary lymphocytic cicatricial alopecia within the spectrum of lichen planopilaris [1, 2]; it usually, but not exclusively, affects postmenopausal women [3, 4]. According to a literature review by Chew et al. [3], only 7.6 % of all reported patients with FFA were premenopausal women and 1.9 % were men.

The disease is characterized clinically by slowly progressive symmetric hairline recession in the frontotemporal and/or frontoparietal region. Disease progression is variable; the usual rate of hairline recession is 0.3–1.7 mm per month [5]. Eyebrow loss is observed in 50–83 % of patients. Characteristically, eyebrow loss begins at the lateral third of the brow and uncommonly progresses to total eyebrow loss. Body hair loss may be associated with FFA in 27–77 % of patients and usually affects the axilla, pubic area, and occasionally the upper or lower limbs [5–7].

Usually, the diagnosis is based on characteristic clinical appearance. Histopathology and trichoscopy may aid in the differential diagnosis.

Trichoscopic findings in FFA include a lack of follicular openings and minor perifollicular scaling [8–12]. Occasionally, perifollicular erythema may be observed. There is a strong predominance of follicular openings with only one hair at the hair-bearing margin. Lonely hair may be observed. Arborizing vessels were described in one study [13], but they have not been confirmed by other authors [8, 9].

In contrast to classic lichen planopilaris, in which the background may be milky red in the early fibrotic phase of the disease, the background in patients with FFA is usually ivory white to ivory beige [8, 9].

In the eyebrow area, trichoscopy shows regularly distributed red or gray dots throughout the course of the disease, with some tendency toward a loss of follicular openings in advanced disease [10].

Although the eyebrow area appears noninflammatory and nonscarring on trichoscopy, most authors indicate that histopathologic examination of the scalp and eyebrows shows similar features, with a reduced number of hair follicles, perifollicular lymphoid cell infiltrates, and fibrosis [5–7].

A. Rakowska
Department of Dermatology, CSK MSW, Warsaw, Poland

M. Olszewska
Department of Dermatology, Medical University of Warsaw, Warsaw, Poland

L. Rudnicka (✉)
Faculty of Health Sciences, Medical University of Warsaw, Poland

Department of Dermatology, CSK MSW, Woloska 137, Warsaw 02-502, Poland
e-mail: lidia.rudnicka@euderm.eu

L. Rudnicka et al. (eds.), *Atlas of Trichoscopy*,
DOI 10.1007/978-1-4471-4486-1_22, © Springer-Verlag London 2012

Table 22.1 Trichoscopic features of frontal fibrosing alopecia

Scalp
Lack of follicular openings
Homogenous ivory-colored background
Minor perifollicular scaling
Perifollicular erythema
Follicular openings with only one hair at the hair-bearing margin
Perifollicular brown or brown-violet areas (in dark-skinned patients)
Eyebrows
Multiple regularly distributed red dots (early phase of disease)
Multiple regularly distributed red or gray to gray-brown dots (advanced disease)

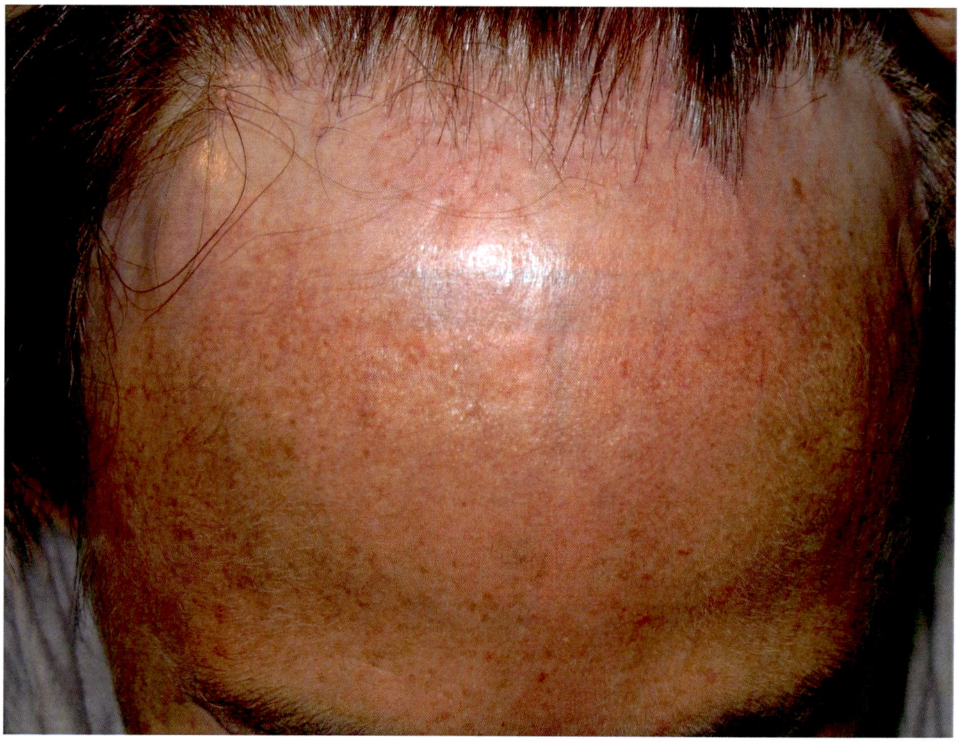

Fig. 22.1 Frontal fibrosing alopecia. Clinical examination reveals a symmetric, cicatricial band of frontal hairline recession. The frontoparietal area may be involved. The frontal hair-bearing margin shifts at a rate of about 0.3–1.7 mm per month [5]. Mild perifollicular scaling may be visible. Eyebrow involvement commonly is observed. Characteristically, eyebrow loss begins at the lateral end of the brow and may progress to total eyebrow loss at an advanced stage of the disease [5–7]. The coexistence of noninflammatory follicular papules of the face is common. The patient may perceive these small papules as roughness of the skin [14]

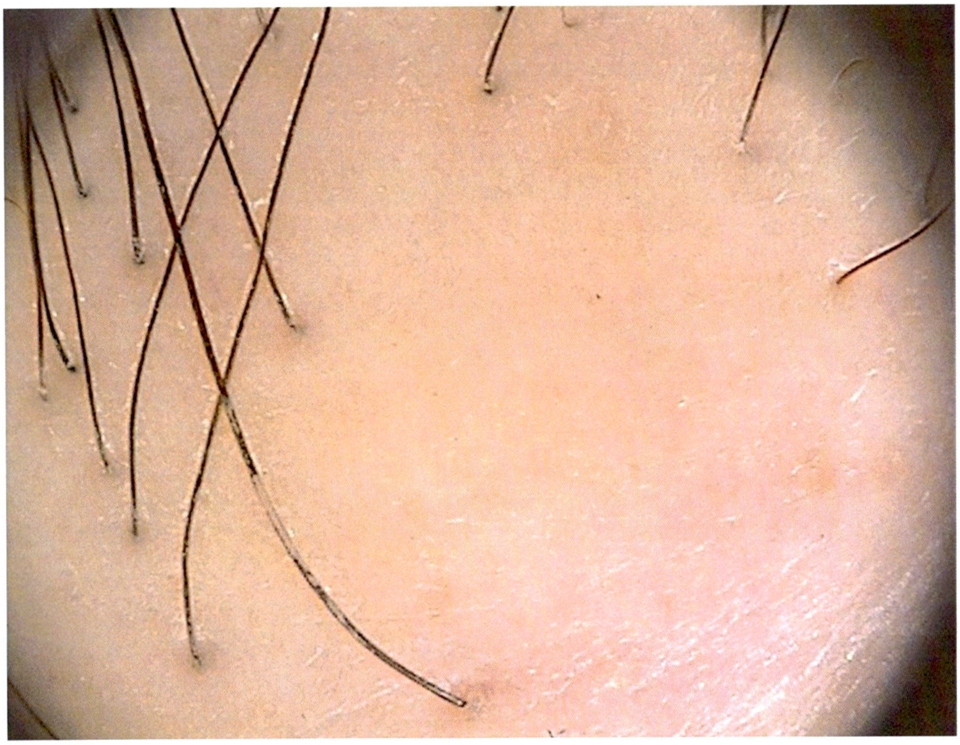

Fig. 22.2 Loss of follicular openings and ivory-colored background in frontal fibrosing alopecia. Recession of the frontal hair-bearing margin is associated with loss of follicular openings. The background color is usually ivory white or ivory beige, and rarely ivory pink. This differentiates FFA from classic lichen planopilaris and other types of cicatricial alopecia, in which the fibrotic areas are white or milky red. At the hair-bearing margin, a strong predominance of follicular openings with only one hair may be observed (×20)

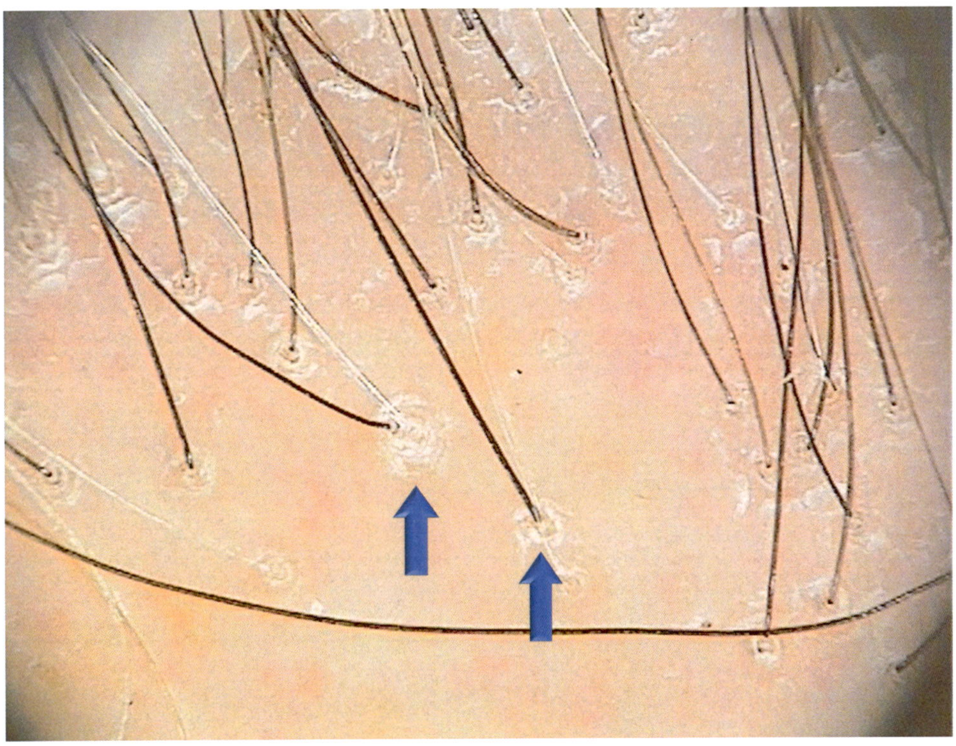

Fig. 22.3 Mild perifollicular scaling in frontal fibrosing alopecia. Dry trichoscopy reveals mild perifollicular scaling. Subtle tubular scaling may be observed in some cases (*arrows*). In contrast to classic lichen planopilaris and folliculitis decalvans, tubular scaling, which entangles the proximal end of the emerging hair shafts, is rare and significantly less severe. Follicular units with only one emerging hair may be observed at the hair-bearing margin (*top*). A lack of follicular openings and an ivory-white background with an erythematous tint are visible in the area of fibrosis (*bottom*) (×20)

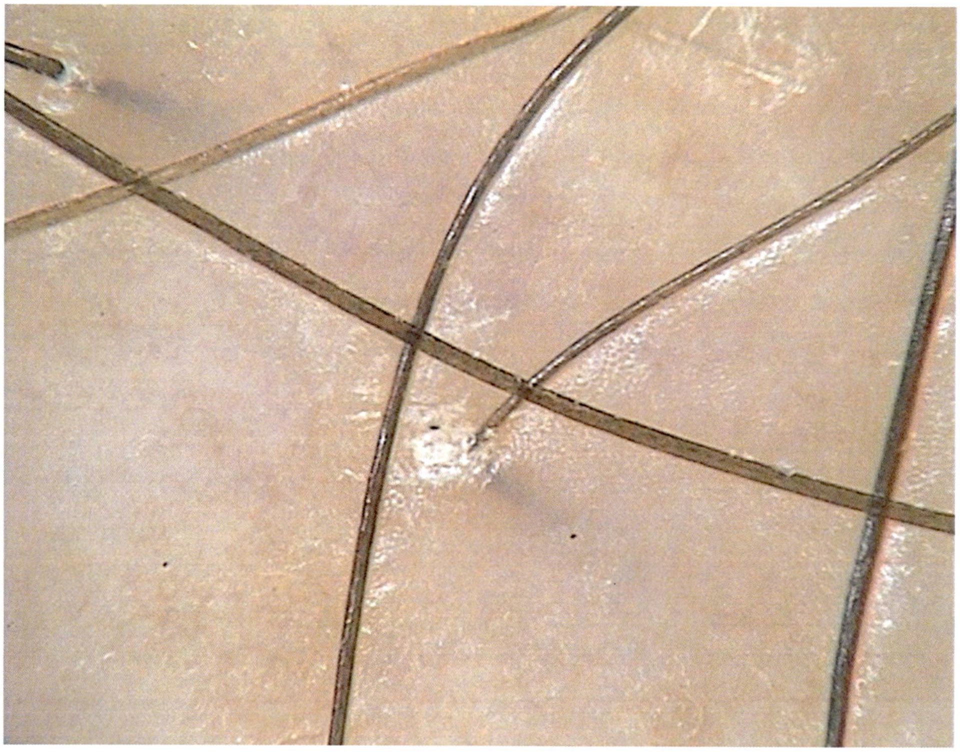

Fig. 22.4 **Mild perifollicular scaling in frontal fibrosing alopecia**. High magnification reveals a single hair shaft with mild perifollicular scaling. Characteristically, the skin surface surrounding the affected hair is almost ideally flat and homogenous in color. This differs from the starburst pattern hyperplasia observed in folliculitis decalvans and the multicolor background of early fibrosis in classic lichen planopilaris or discoid lupus erythematosus (×70)

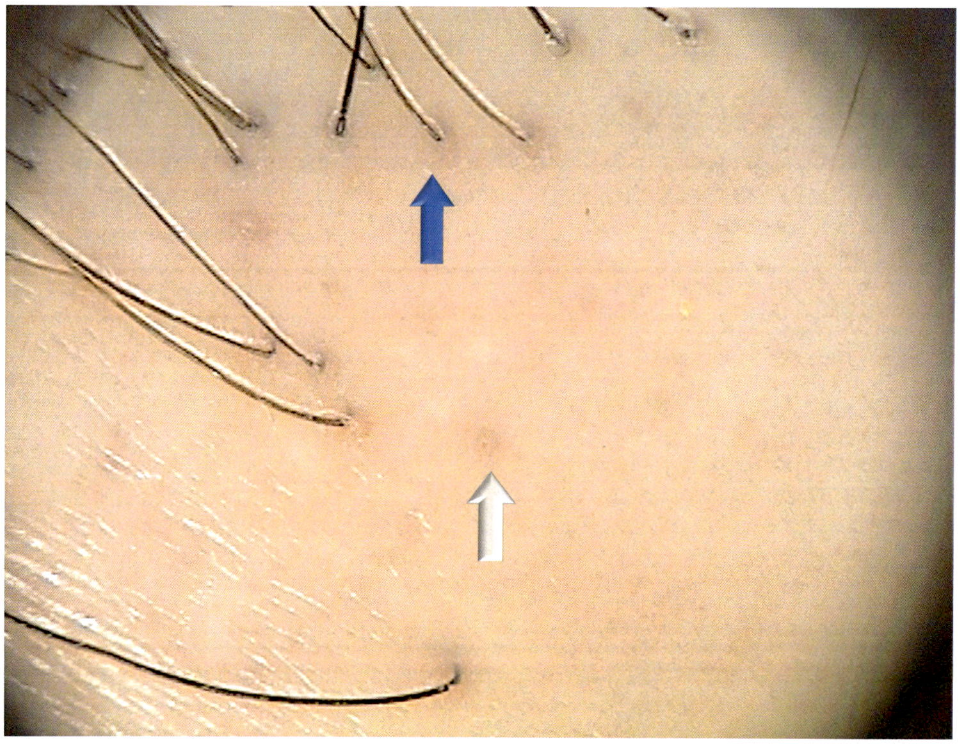

Fig. 22.5 **Brown and brown-violet perifollicular discoloration in frontal fibrosing alopecia**. Brown or brown-violet discoloration around hair follicles (*blue arrow*) may be present in patients with FFA. This finding is more common in patients with dark skin phototypes than in Caucasians. Empty hair follicle openings (*white arrow*) occasionally may be seen close to the hair-bearing margin. Very fine parallel folds of fibrotic skin may be observed at the *bottom left* of the image (×20)

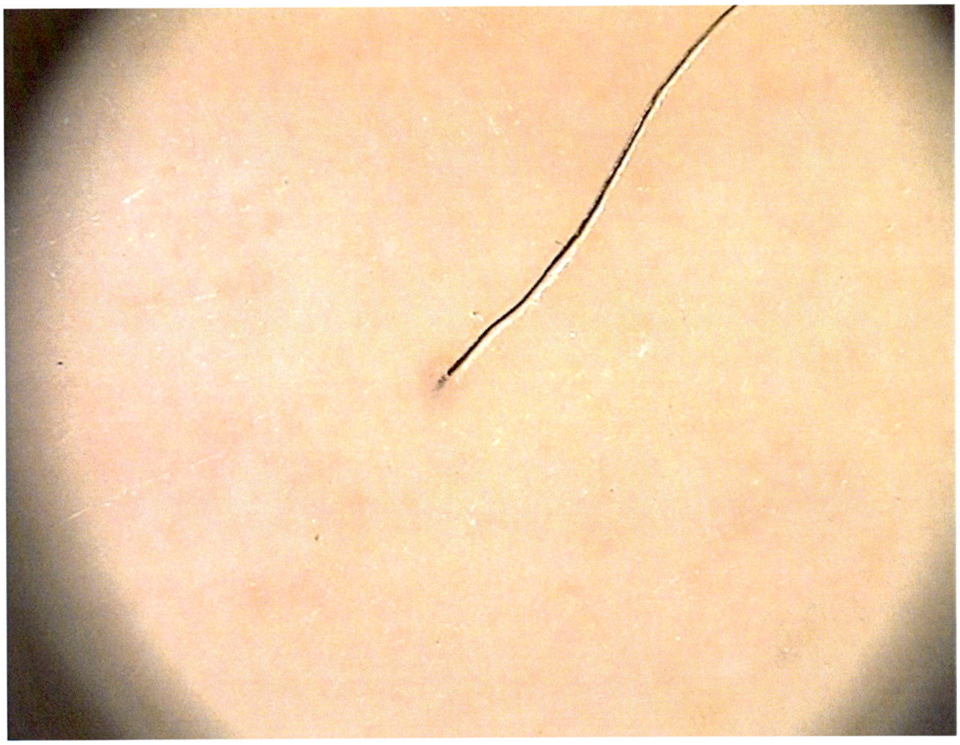

Fig. 22.6 Lonely hair in frontal fibrosing alopecia. "Lonely hairs" have been described as a clue to clinical (macroscopic) diagnosis of FFA [15]. These are isolated terminal hairs, often present in the middle of the forehead at the site of the original hairline. Lonely hairs are a few centimeters long and may be accompanied by perifollicular scaling. A similar phenomenon may be observed on trichoscopy of FFA. In this image, an isolated terminal shaft is visible. Subtle erythema and minimal scaling may be observed. The surrounding background is a homogenous ivory. An isolated hair on trichoscopy is not pathognomonic for FFA; a similar finding may be observed in classic lichen planopilaris and other types of primary cicatricial alopecia. It must be emphasized that there are no clear-cut trichoscopic criteria for diagnosing FFA. The diagnosis cannot be established without knowing the clinical details (×20)

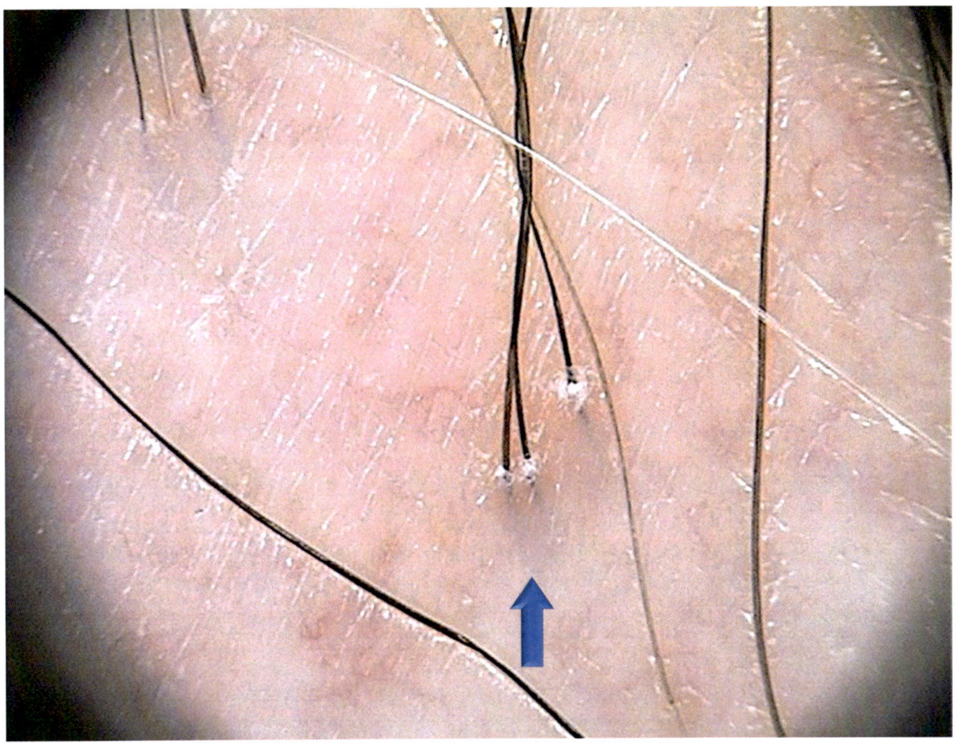

Fig. 22.7 Frontal fibrosing alopecia with skin atrophy due to topical corticosteroids. The ivory background is a characteristic, but not constant, finding in FFA. Shown here is a trichoscopic image from a 78-year-old woman with longstanding FFA and a history of chronic topical application of potent corticosteroids. The characteristic ivory color is not present. Also, unlike most trichoscopic results in FFA, in which avascular areas predominate, this image shows some thin arborizing vessels. Typical mild perifollicular scaling is visible. The hair follicle openings are surrounded by subtle brown-violet areas (*arrow*) (×20)

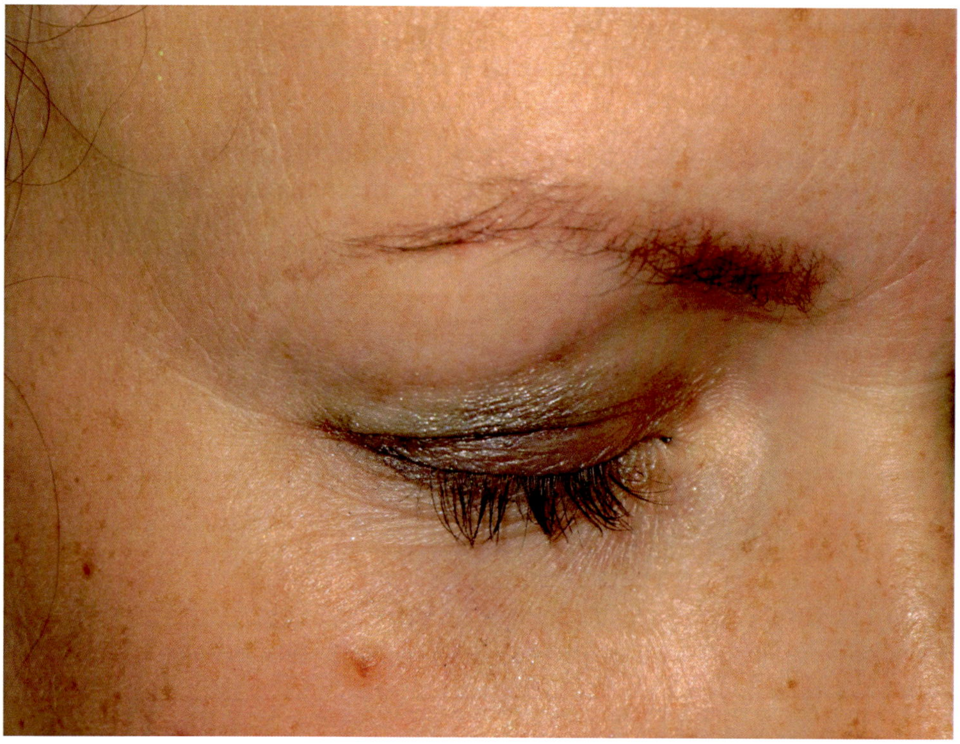

Fig. 22.8 Lateral loss of eyebrows in frontal fibrosing alopecia. Partial or complete loss of eyebrows is observed in 50–83 % of patients with FFA. Eyebrow loss begins symmetrically at the lateral third of the brows and may progress to total eyebrow loss. Loss of other body hairs has been observed in 27–77 % of patients with FFA [5–7]. Thus, a concept was created suggesting that FFA is a generalized, rather than localized, fibrotic process in the spectrum of lichen planopilaris [3]

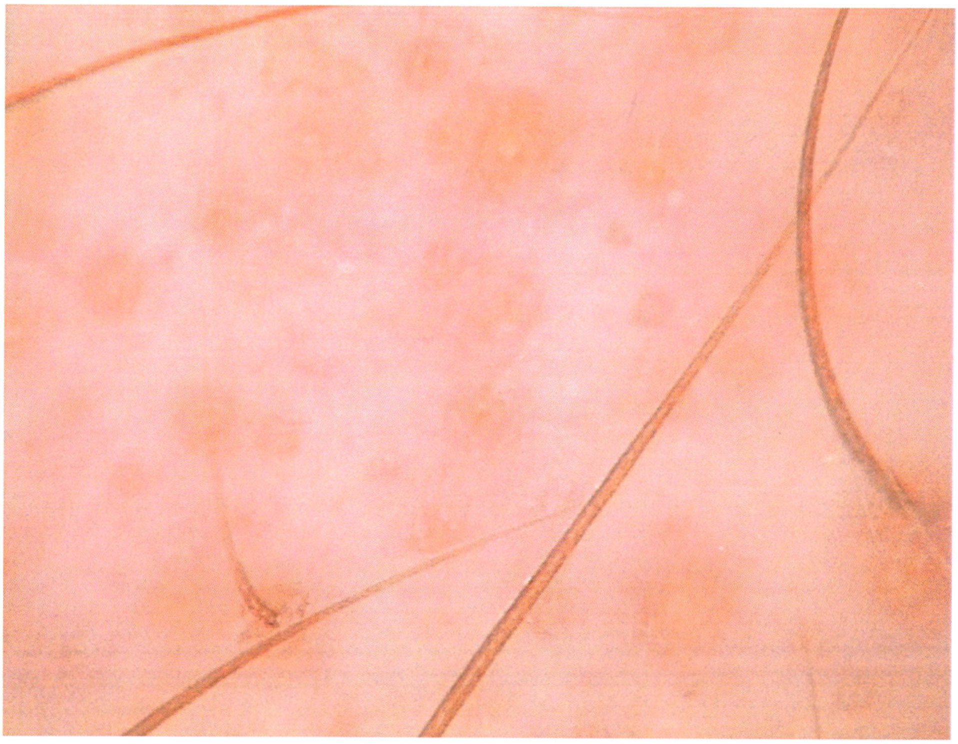

Fig. 22.9 Red dots in the eyebrow area in frontal fibrosing alopecia. In patients with FFA, trichoscopy of the eyebrow area shows features different from those of the scalp. Multiple empty follicles are visible; they appear as red dots in the early phase of the disease and change their color to more grayish over time. In this image, a new, regrowing eyebrow with perifollicular scaling also is visible (×70)

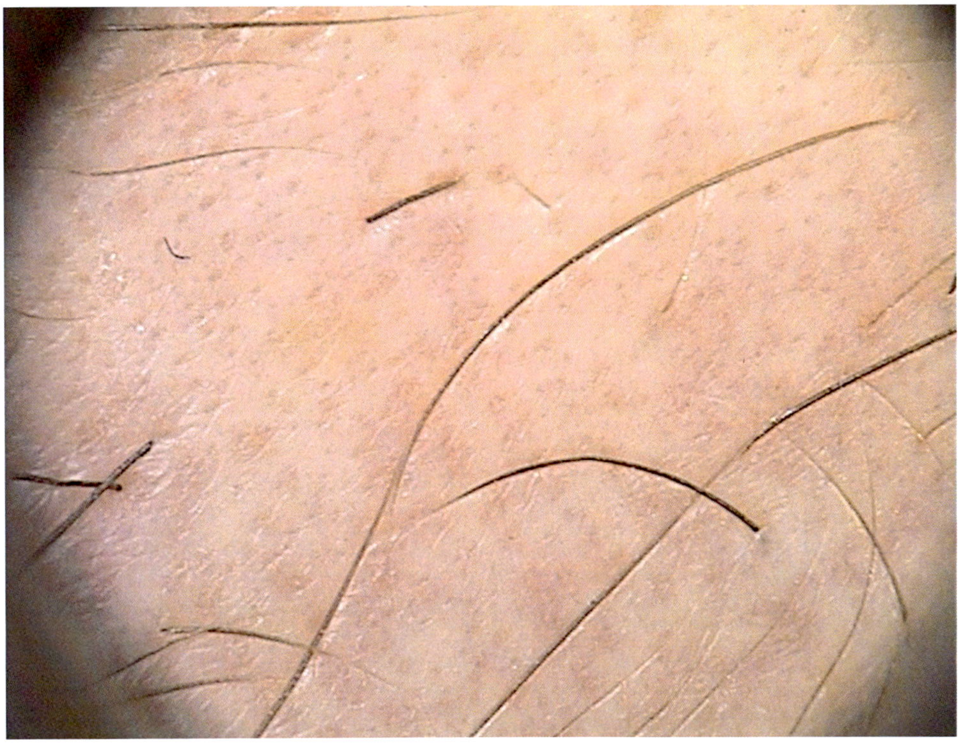

Fig. 22.10 Gray dots in the eyebrow area in frontal fibrosing alopecia. Shown is advanced eyebrow loss in a patient with advanced FFA. Several densely packed empty follicles are visible; they appear as gray or grayish dots. In FFA, trichoscopy of the eyebrow area rarely shows features of fibrosis with total loss of follicles. This may explain why it is possible to induce eyebrow regrowth in these patients [16] whereas hair regrowth in the fibrotic frontal scalp area is not possible (×20)

References

1. Olsen EA, Bergfeld WF, Cotsarelis G, Price VH, Shapiro J, Sinclair R, et al. Summary of North American Hair Research Society (NAHRS)-sponsored Workshop on Cicatricial Alopecia, Duke University Medical Center, February 10 and 11, 2001. J Am Acad Dermatol. 2003;48(1):103–10.
2. Samrao A, Chew AL, Price V. Frontal fibrosing alopecia: a clinical review of 36 patients. Br J Dermatol. 2010;163(6):1296–300.
3. Chew AL, Bashir SJ, Wain EM, Fenton DA, Stefanato CM. Expanding the spectrum of frontal fibrosing alopecia: a unifying concept. J Am Acad Dermatol. 2010;63(4):653–60.
4. Poblet E, Jimenez F, Pascual A, Pique E. Frontal fibrosing alopecia versus lichen planopilaris: a clinicopathological study. Int J Dermatol. 2006;45(4):375–80.
5. Tan KT, Messenger AG. Frontal fibrosing alopecia: clinical presentations and prognosis. Br J Dermatol. 2009;160(1):75–9.
6. Tosti A, Piraccini BM, Iorizzo M, Misciali C. Frontal fibrosing alopecia in postmenopausal women. J Am Acad Dermatol. 2005; 52(1):55–60.
7. Kossard S, Lee MS, Wilkinson B. Postmenopausal frontal fibrosing alopecia: a frontal variant of lichen planopilaris. J Am Acad Dermatol. 1997;36(1):59–66.
8. Rubegni P, Mandato F, Fimiani M. Frontal fibrosing alopecia: role of dermoscopy in differential diagnosis. Case Rep Dermatol. 2010; 2(1):40–5.
9. Inui S, Nakajima T, Shono F, Itami S. Dermoscopic findings in frontal fibrosing alopecia: report of four cases. Int J Dermatol. 2008;47(8):796–9.
10. Rudnicka L, Olszewska M, Rakowska A, Slowinska M. Trichoscopy update 2011. J Dermatol Case Rep. 2011;5(4):82–8.
11. Rakowska A, Slowinska M, Kowalska-Oledzka E, Olszewska M, Rudnicka L. Trichoscopy in cicatricial alopecia. J Drugs Dermatol. 2012;11:753–8.
12. Miteva M, Whiting D, Harries M, Bernardes A, Tosti A. Frontal fibrosing alopecia in black patients. Br J Dermatol. 2012; 167(1):208–10. doi:10.1111/j.1365-2133.2012.10809.x.
13. Duque-Estrada B, Tamler C, Sodre CT, Barcaui CB, Pereira FB. Dermoscopy patterns of cicatricial alopecia resulting from discoid lupus erythematosus and lichen planopilaris. An Bras Dermatol. 2010;85(2):179–83.
14. Donati A, Molina L, Doche I, Valente NS, Romiti R. Facial papules in frontal fibrosing alopecia: evidence of vellus follicle involvement. Arch Dermatol. 2011;147(12):1424–7.
15. Tosti A, Miteva M, Torres F. Lonely hair: a clue to the diagnosis of frontal fibrosing alopecia. Arch Dermatol. 2011;147(10):1240.
16. Donovan JC, Samrao A, Ruben BS, Price VH. Eyebrow regrowth in patients with frontal fibrosing alopecia treated with intralesional triamcinolone acetonide. Br J Dermatol. 2010;163(5):1142–4.

Discoid Lupus Erythematosus

23

Lidia Rudnicka, Malgorzata Olszewska,
and Adriana Rakowska

Abstract
The most characteristic trichoscopic features of active discoid lupus erythematosus are large yellow dots (keratotic plugs), thick arborizing vessels, scattered dark-brown discoloration, red dots, and blue-gray dots. Longstanding, inactive disease is characterized by the presence of structureless milky red or white areas and a lack of follicular openings. Thick arborizing vessels also may be present.

Keywords
Amicrobial pustulosis • Arborizing vessels • Blue-gray dots • Brown discoloration Cutaneous lupus erythematosus • Cicatricial alopecia • Cicatricial pemphigoid • Discoid lupus erythematosus • Eyebrow • Pink areas • Systemic lupus erythematosus • White areas • Whitish halo • Red dots • Yellow dots

Although discoid lupus erythematosus (DLE) has been classified as primary lymphocytic cicatricial alopecia [1], some authors emphasize that DLE cannot be considered a primary cicatricial alopecia because the hair follicle is not the primary target of a folliculocentric inflammatory attack [2].

DLE may occur at any age, but the onset is most frequent in persons between the ages of 20 and 40 years. Women are affected more frequently than men [3]. DLE lesions may develop in the course of systemic lupus erythematosus.

A lesion begins as a well-demarcated round or oval purplish macule or papule and enlarges into an alopecic patch with follicular plugging, erythema, and adherent scaling. The lesions may be hypo- or hyperpigmented. Symptoms may include itching, pain, burning, and tenderness. End-stage disease is characterized by fibrotic, atrophic, smooth white plaques lacking follicular ostia [3]. Longstanding DLE is clinically indistinguishable from other diseases in the spectrum of primary cicatricial alopecia [4–6].

The diagnosis is based on direct immunofluorescence, which shows IgG deposits at the dermoepidermal border, and histopathology.

The most characteristic trichoscopic features of active DLE are large yellow dots (keratotic plugs), thick arborizing vessels, scattered dark-brown discoloration, and blue-gray dots. Large yellow dots in DLE differ from the yellow dots observed in alopecia areata and androgenetic alopecia. The yellow dots in DLE have a mean diameter of 653 ± 125 μm (mean ± SD), whereas those in alopecia areata have a diameter of 212 ± 66 μm and those in androgenetic alopecia are 190 ± 71 μm [7, 8]. The large yellow dots in DLE are darker than those seen in other diseases and are usually dark yellow to yellow brown. Large yellow dots with radial, thin arborizing vessels emerging from the dot are considered highly characteristic of late, prefibrotic DLE lesions [7, 8]. This feature has been compared with a "red spider in a yellow dot" [7, 8].

L. Rudnicka (✉)
Faculty of Health Sciences, Medical University of Warsaw, Poland

Department of Dermatology, CSK MSW,
Woloska 137, Warsaw 02-502, Poland
e-mail: lidia.rudnicka@euderm.eu

M. Olszewska
Department of Dermatology, Medical University of Warsaw,
Warsaw, Poland

A. Rakowska
Department of Dermatology, CSK MSW, Warsaw, Poland

L. Rudnicka et al. (eds.), *Atlas of Trichoscopy*,
DOI 10.1007/978-1-4471-4486-1_23,

Thick arborizing vessels commonly are present at the periphery of the lesion. The average thickness of the widest vessel in a DLE lesion is 114 ± 28 μm (mean ± SD), which is significantly wider than that of arborizing vessels in the normal scalp or in seborrheic dermatitis (36 ± 17, $p < 0.05$) [7, 8]. The thick arborizing vessels observed in DLE are almost indistinguishable from those commonly seen in basal cell carcinoma.

Dark-brown discoloration of the skin, giving it a "dirty" appearance, is observed in active DLE lesions. This finding corresponds to pigment incontinence on histopathology [7, 8]. This finding does not seem to correspond to blue-gray dots forming a "speckled" pattern in DLE lesions, as described by Duque-Estrada et al. [9] in a DLE patient with a dark skin phototype.

Follicular red dots were described in DLE by Tosti et al. [10] as a characteristic feature of active DLE and a good prognostic factor for hair regrowth.

Longstanding inactive DLE lesions differ from active lesions. They are characterized by the presence of structureless milky red or white areas and a lack of follicular openings. Arborizing vessels also may be present.

Table 23.1 Trichoscopic features of discoid lupus erythematosus

Active (early) lesions
Thick arborizing vessels
Large yellow dots (follicular keratotic plugs)
Fine interfollicular scaling
Scattered brown discoloration
Red dots
Blue-gray dots (on dark or sun-exposed skin)
Inactive (end-stage) lesions
Loss of follicular openings
Pink areas
White areas
Arborizing vessels
Yellow dots containing thin spider vessels (in prefibrotic lesions)

Table 23.2 Trichoscopic differential diagnosis of discoid lupus erythematosus

Basal cell carcinoma
Seborrheic dermatitis
Psoriasis
Actinic keratosis
Pseudopelade of Brocq
Lichen planopilaris
Cicatricial pemphigoid

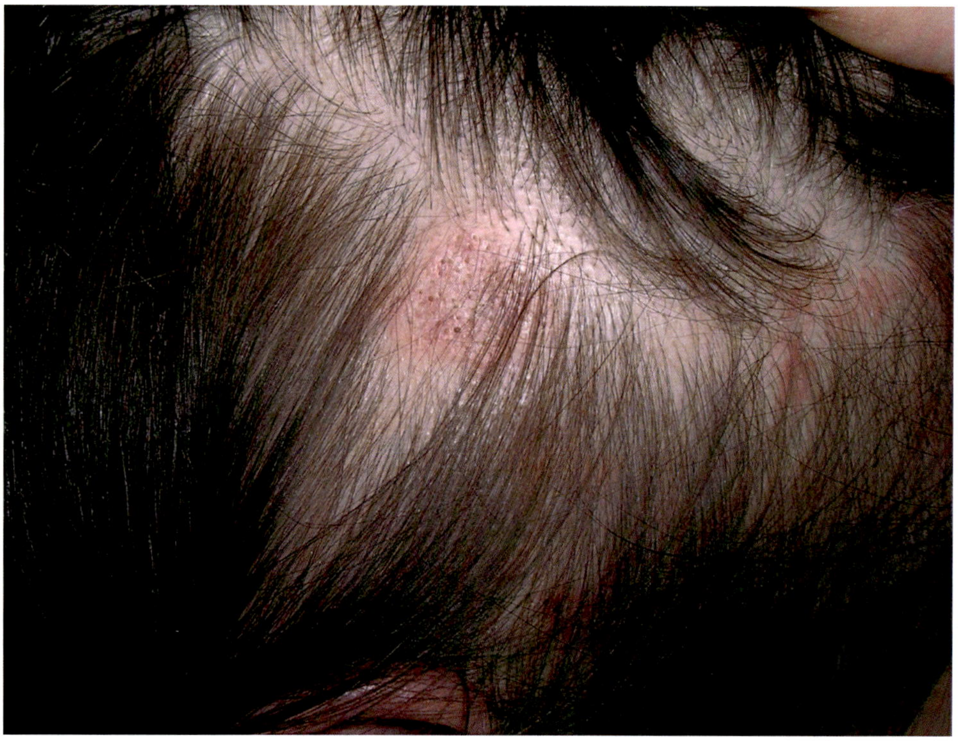

Fig. 23.1 Discoid lupus erythematosus. Shown is the typical rounded appearance of an early DLE lesion. Only minor hair loss may be observed

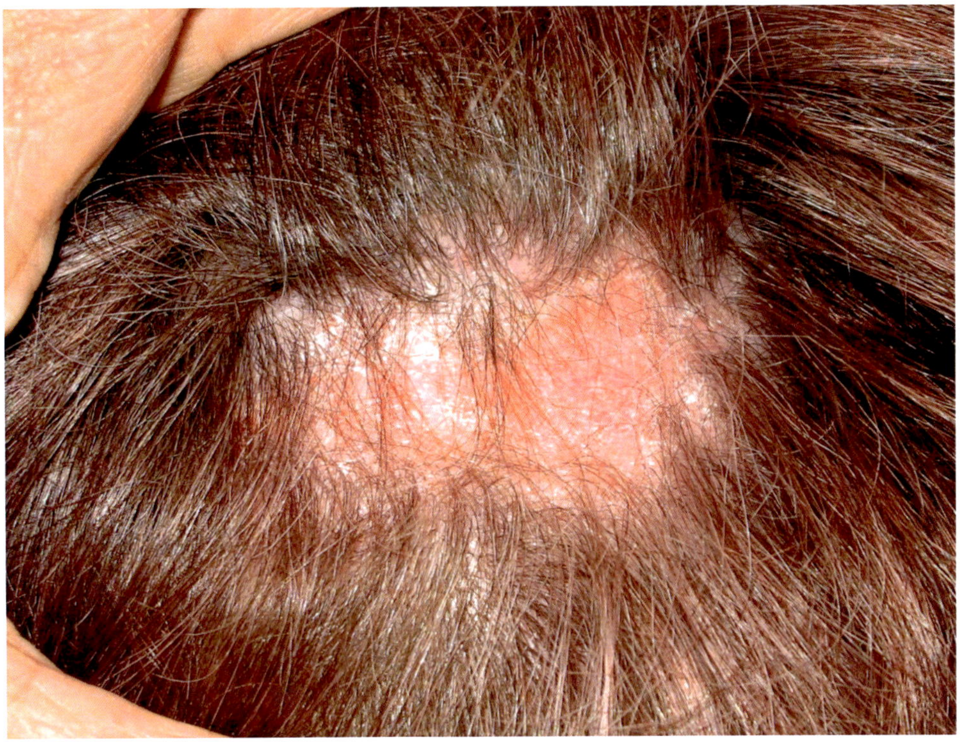

Fig. 23.2 Discoid lupus erythematosus. This image shows cicatricial alopecia in the course of longstanding DLE. The trichoscopic characteristics of DLE depend on disease duration and activity

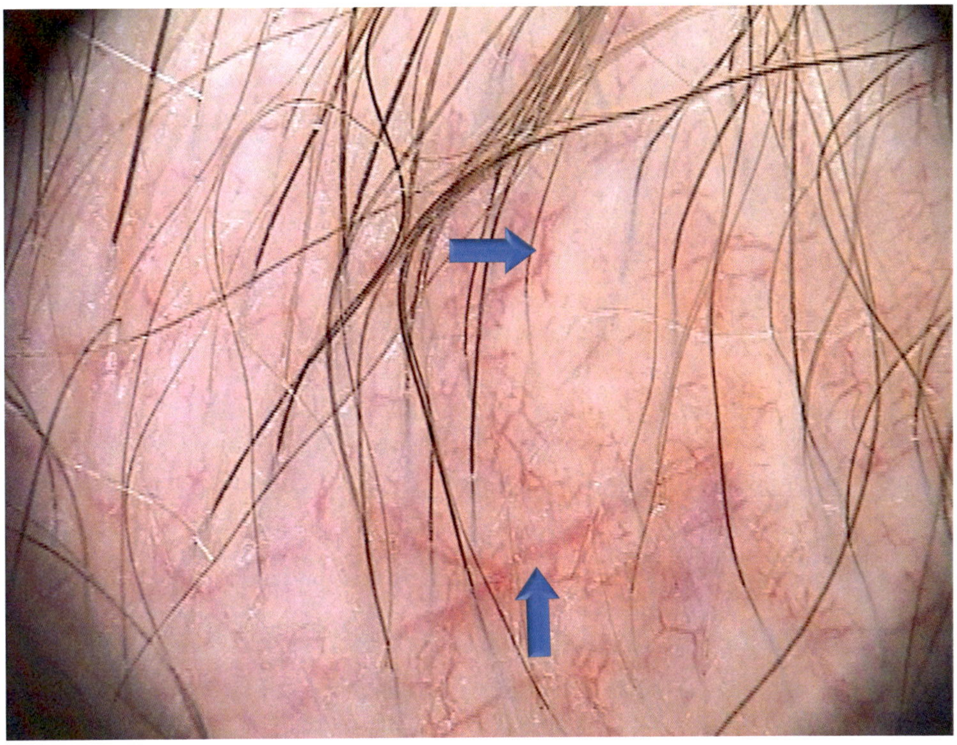

Fig. 23.3 Thick arborizing vessels in discoid lupus erythematosus. Thick arborizing vessels (*arrows*) may be observed on trichoscopy in two distinct clinical situations: DLE and basal cell carcinoma. Thus, DLE may be misdiagnosed as basal cell carcinoma when the diagnosis is based only on the presence of this type of vessel. Other diseases that manifest with thick arborizing vessels are rarely localized on the scalp (×20)

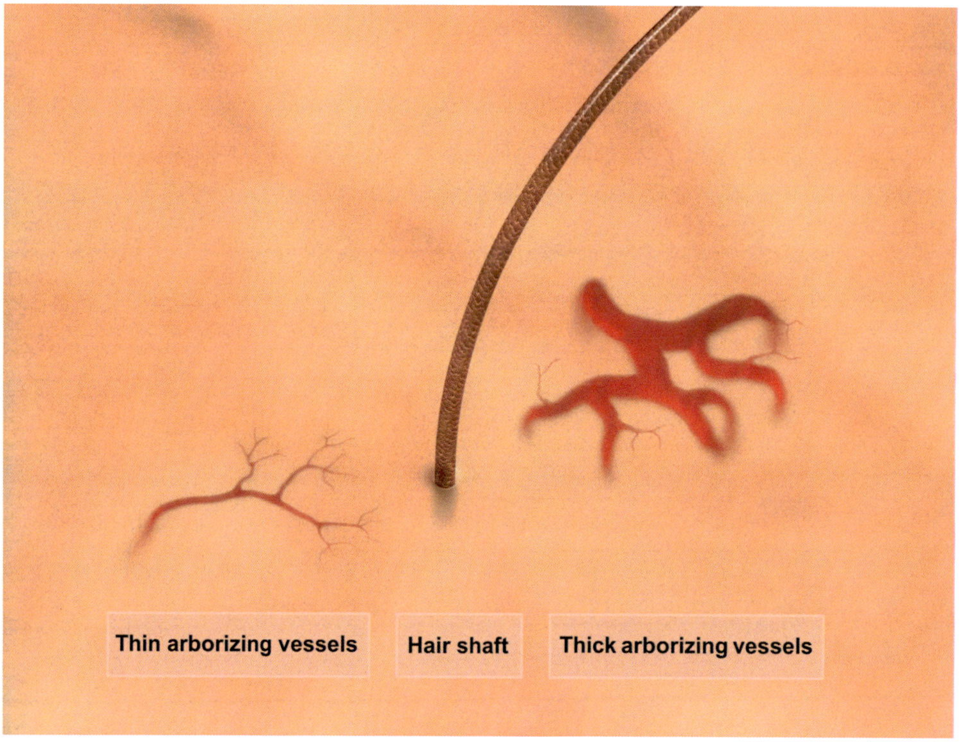

Fig. 23.4 Thick arborizing vessels in discoid lupus erythematosus; the "vessel-hair test." Thick arborizing vessels are observed in DLE and basal cell carcinoma and rarely in other diseases. They may be distinguished from thin arborizing vessels in healthy individuals by a test comparing blood vessel thickness with hair shaft thickness [8]. Most hair shafts are 55–100 μm thick. Normal, thin arborizing vessels usually are thinner than 50 μm, whereas most thick arborizing vessels are thicker than 100 μm. Thus, these blood vessels may be distinguished by comparing their thickness to that of an average hair shaft in the field of view. Normal, thin arborizing vessels are thinner than a hair shaft. About 80 % of thick arborizing vessels are thicker than a hair shaft. The thickest blood vessel in the field of view should be compared with an average hair shaft (*Graphic by* Dr. Wawrzyniec Podrzucki, courtesy of *Journal of Dermatological Case Reports*)

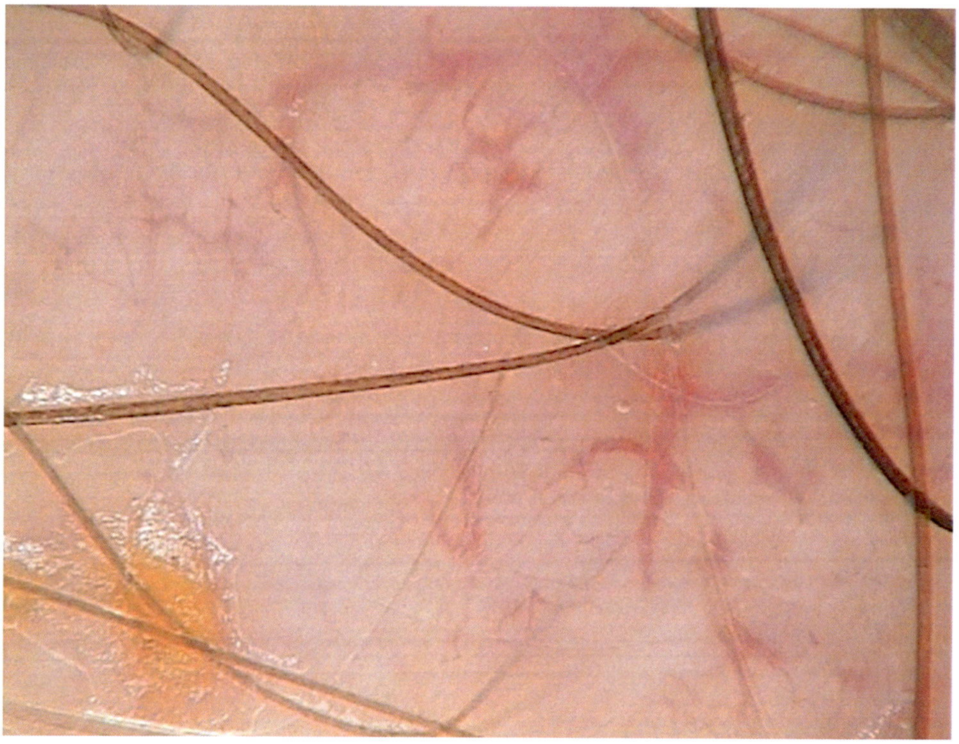

Fig. 23.5 Thick arborizing vessels in discoid lupus erythematosus. The thickest vessels in this image are thicker than an average hair shaft. Trichoscopy also shows a large yellow dot, another characteristic feature of DLE (×70)

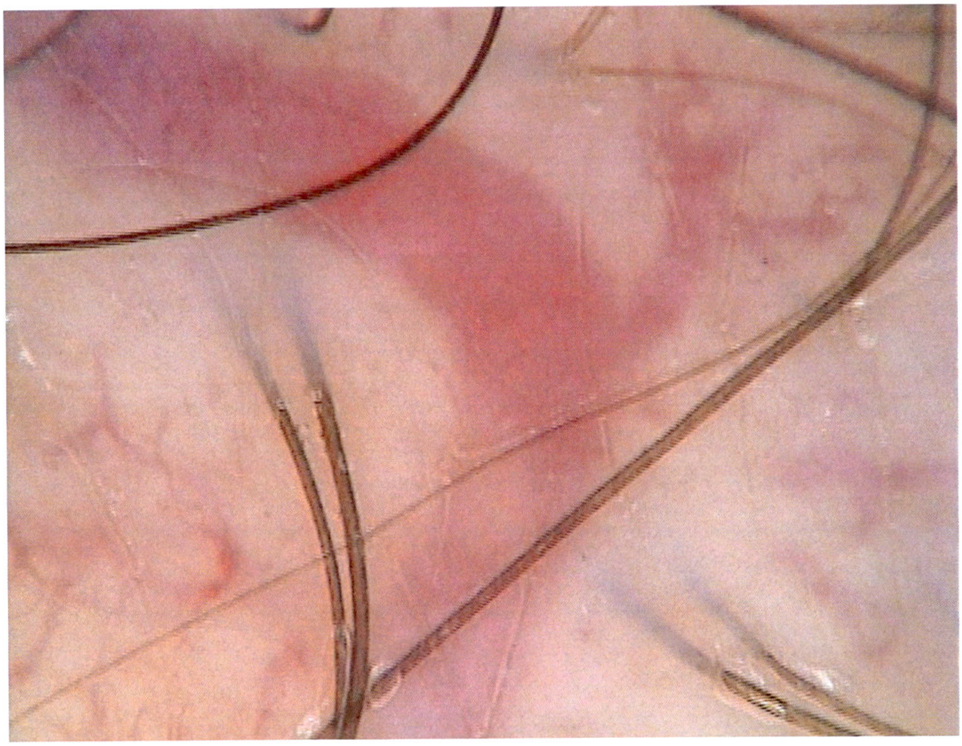

Fig. 23.6 Thick arborizing vessels in discoid lupus erythematosus. This giant blood vessel is significantly thicker than the average hair shaft in this image. The vessel is clearly visible through a thinned epidermis (×70)

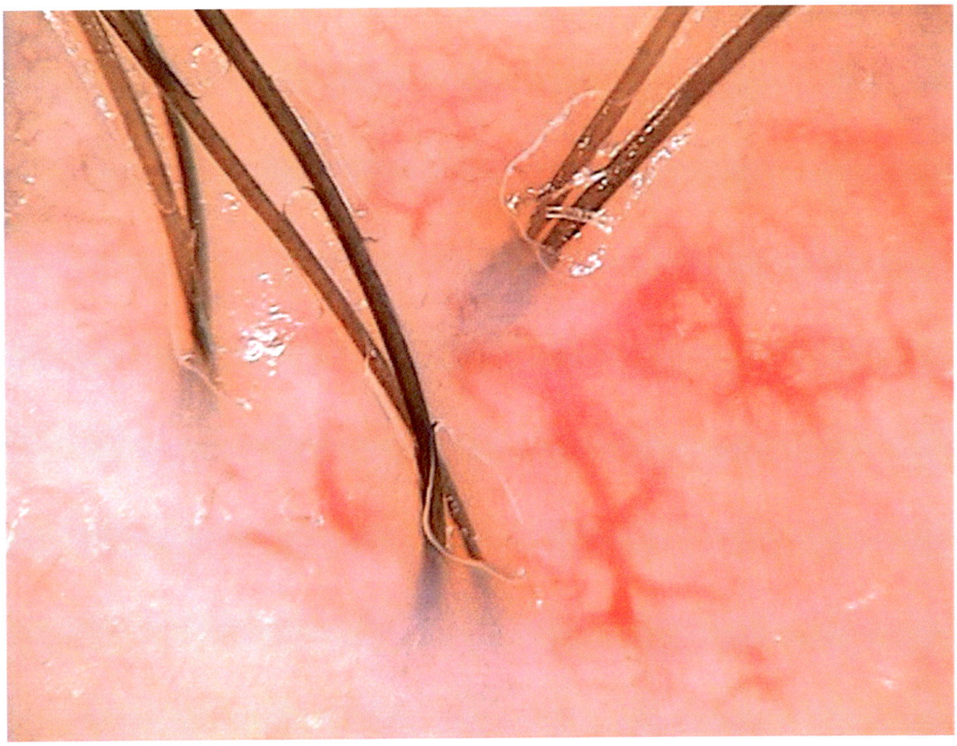

Fig. 23.7 Thick arborizing vessels in active discoid lupus erythematosus. Thick arborizing vessels appear most frequently at the periphery of active lesions. They may be replaced by cicatricial tissue during the process of fibrosis or may remain visible for many years despite a significant decrease in disease activity (×70)

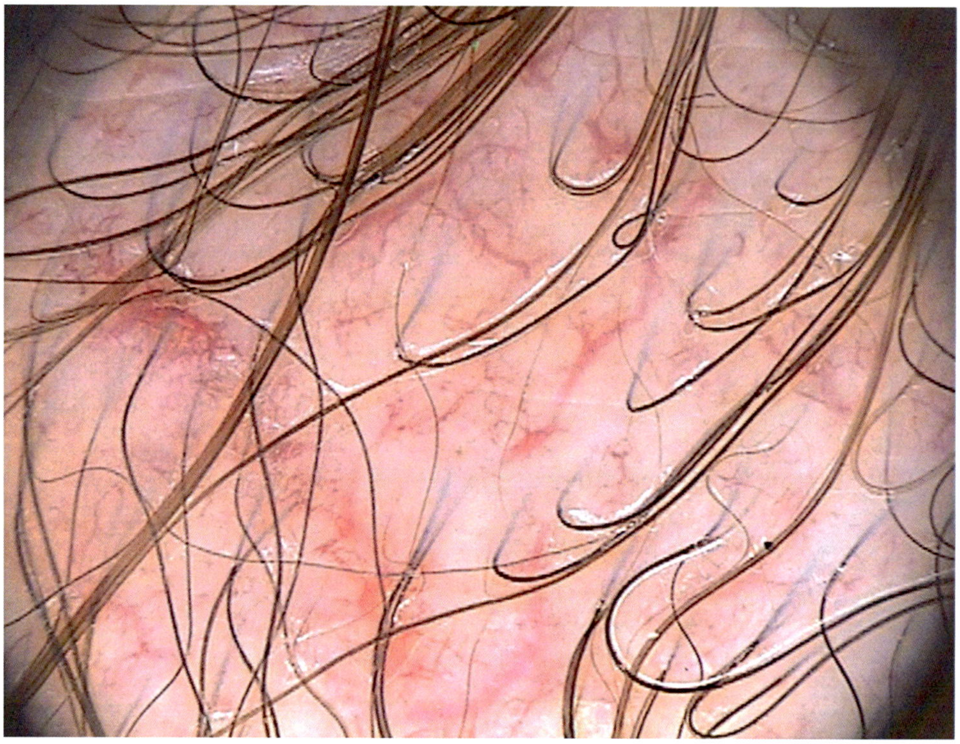

Fig. 23.8 **Thick arborizing vessels in inactive discoid lupus erythematosus**. This image of a nonactive DLE lesion (after successful treatment) shows thick arborizing vessels and root-like vessels. A dense network of thin vessels may result from corticosteroid treatment. Long fragments of hair shafts are visible below the skin surface, reflecting a notable thinning of the epidermis. Note the partial hair regrowth within this lesion (×20)

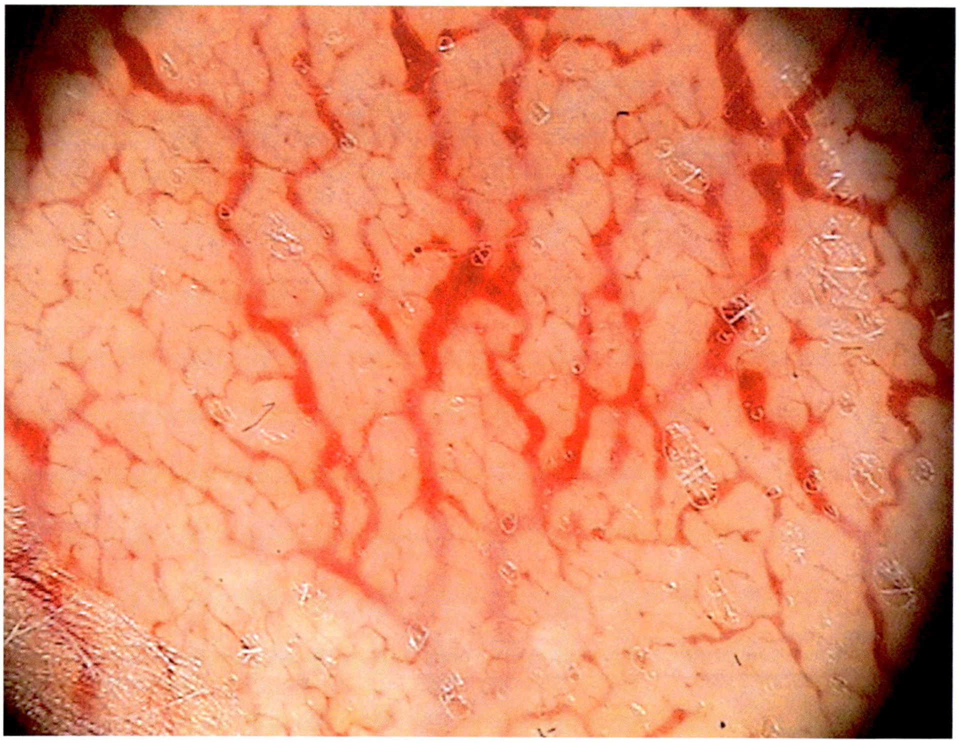

Fig. 23.9 **Thick arborizing vessels in discoid lupus erythematosus of the forehead**. Because of the absence of hairs and follicle openings in this image, the structure of the vessels may be analyzed in greater detail. One can clearly see that the large arborizing vessels belong to a large subepidermal network (×20)

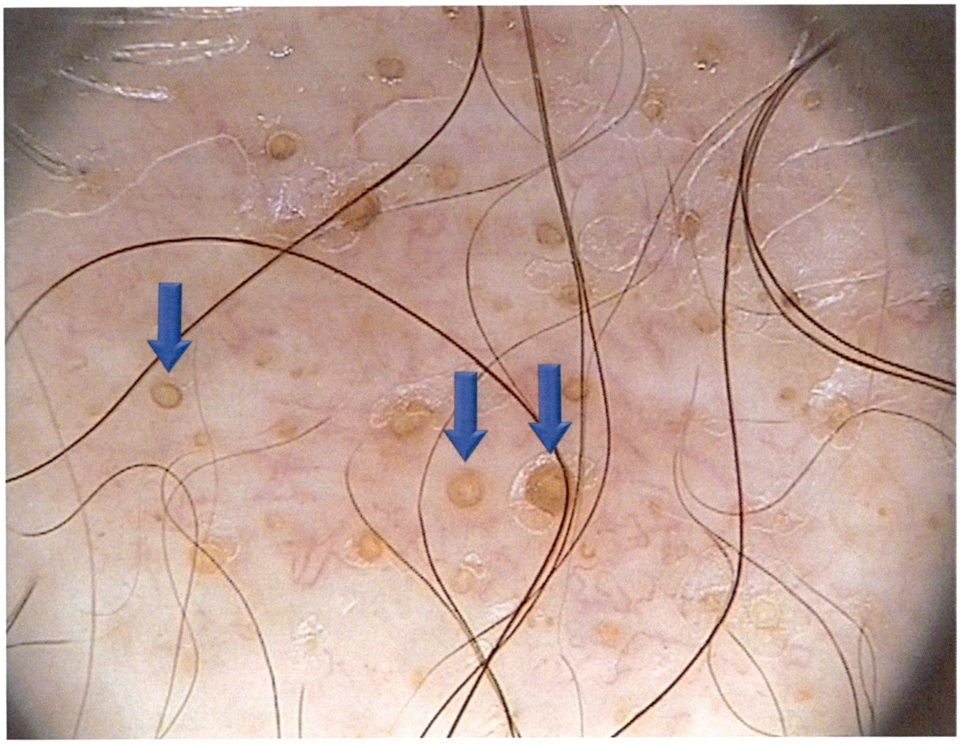

Fig. 23.10 Large yellow dots in discoid lupus erythematosus. Yellow dots in DLE (*arrows*) are bigger and darker than those seen in alopecia areata and androgenetic alopecia. They correspond to follicular hyperkeratotic plugs. Large yellow dots are a marker of active disease (×20)

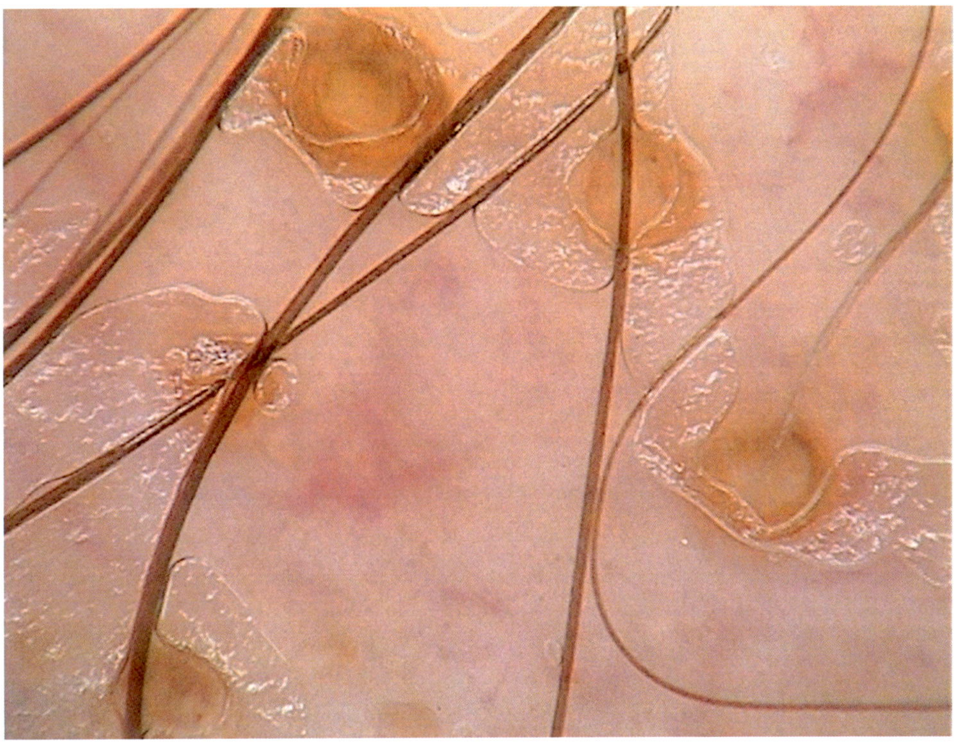

Fig. 23.11 Large yellow dots in discoid lupus erythematosus. High magnification shows that the yellow dots in DLE are sharply demarcated and have a double margin (×70)

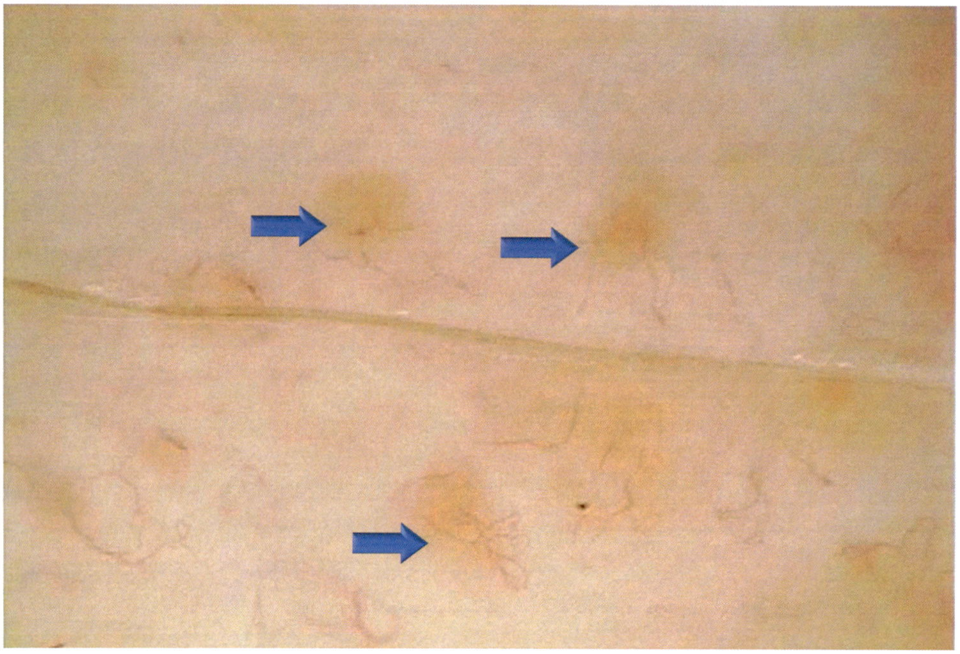

Fig. 23.12 Yellow dots containing thin spider vessels in inactive discoid lupus erythematosus. In inactive DLE, yellow dots become less prominent. They are flat and pale and have blurred borders. Occasionally, long thin arborizing vessels are superimposed over these dots (*arrows*). This feature is called "red spider in a yellow dot" and is characteristic of late, inactive DLE lesions (×70)

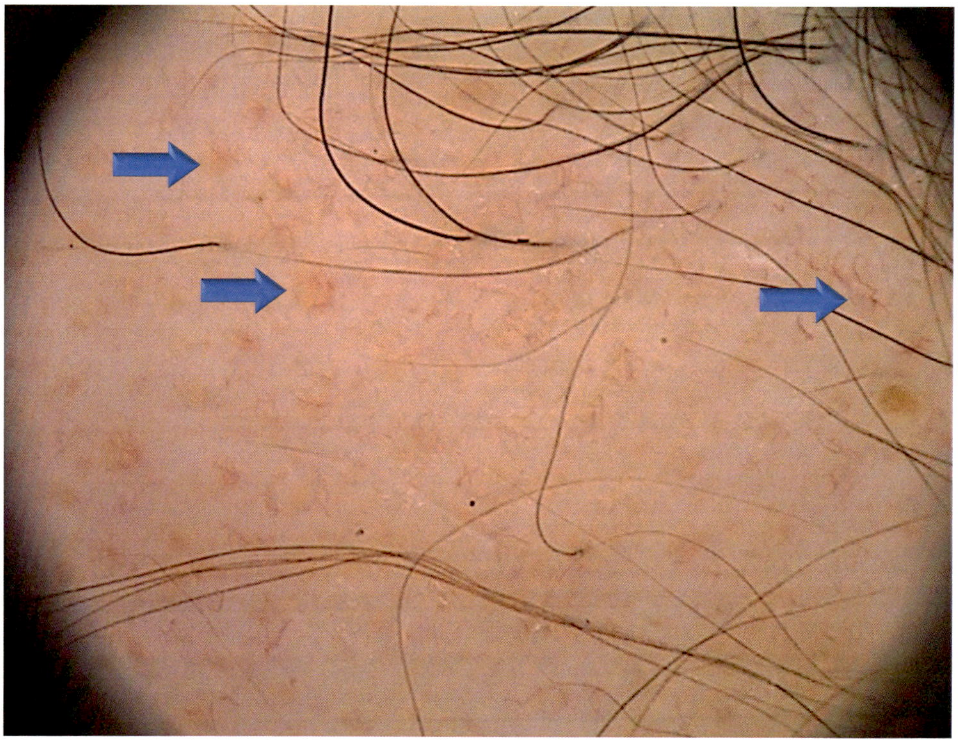

Fig. 23.13 Yellow dots containing thin spider vessels in inactive discoid lupus erythematosus. On low-magnification trichoscopy, the red spiders in yellow dots are barely visible. The *arrows* point to yellow dots showing the characteristic superimposed thin red vessels (×20)

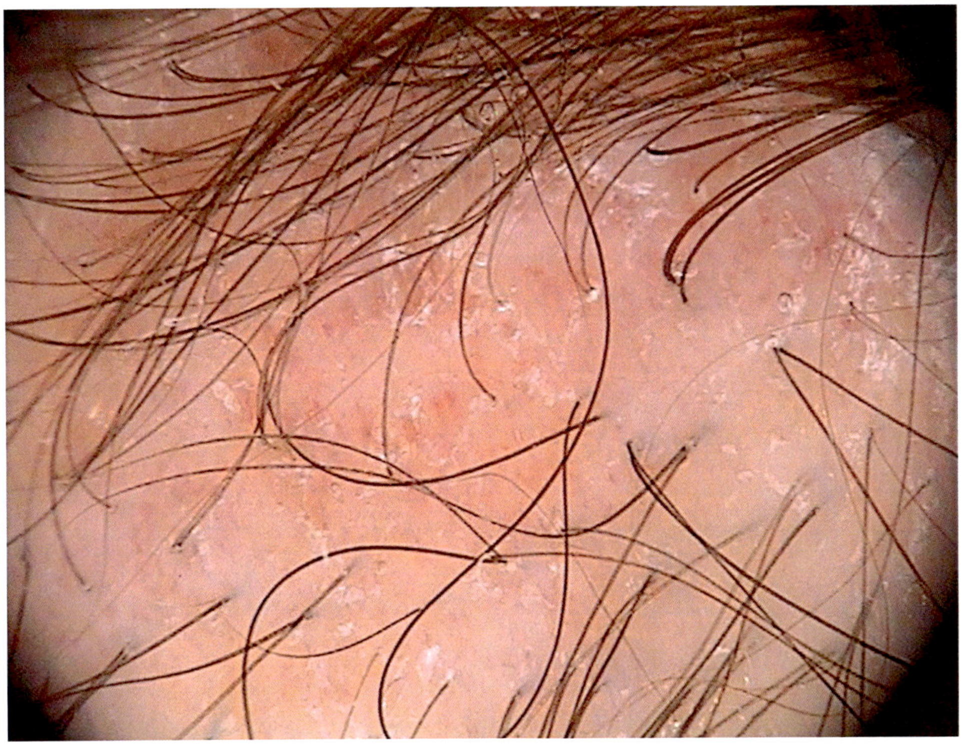

Fig. 23.14 Fine scaling in discoid lupus erythematosus. Scaling is a frequent finding in active DLE lesions. Scales are fine and firmly adhere to the epidermis. Scaling usually directly precedes or coexists with fibrosis. In this image, the fine scaling is associated with a disseminated decrease in the number of follicular openings and with pink coloration, which corresponds to fibrosis of recent onset (×20)

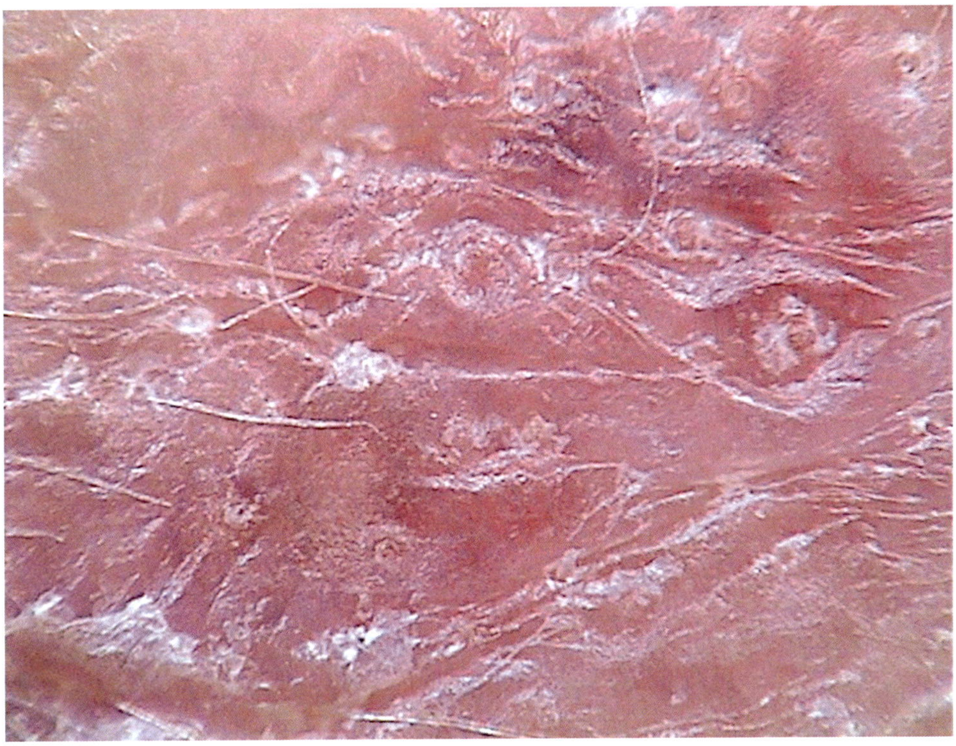

Fig. 23.15 Fine scaling associated with fibrosis in discoid lupus erythematosus. In the course of DLE, a newly formed scar covered by fine scaling with follicular accentuation is a common finding [11]. Characteristic circular flakes are superimposed over fibrosing follicular openings (×70)

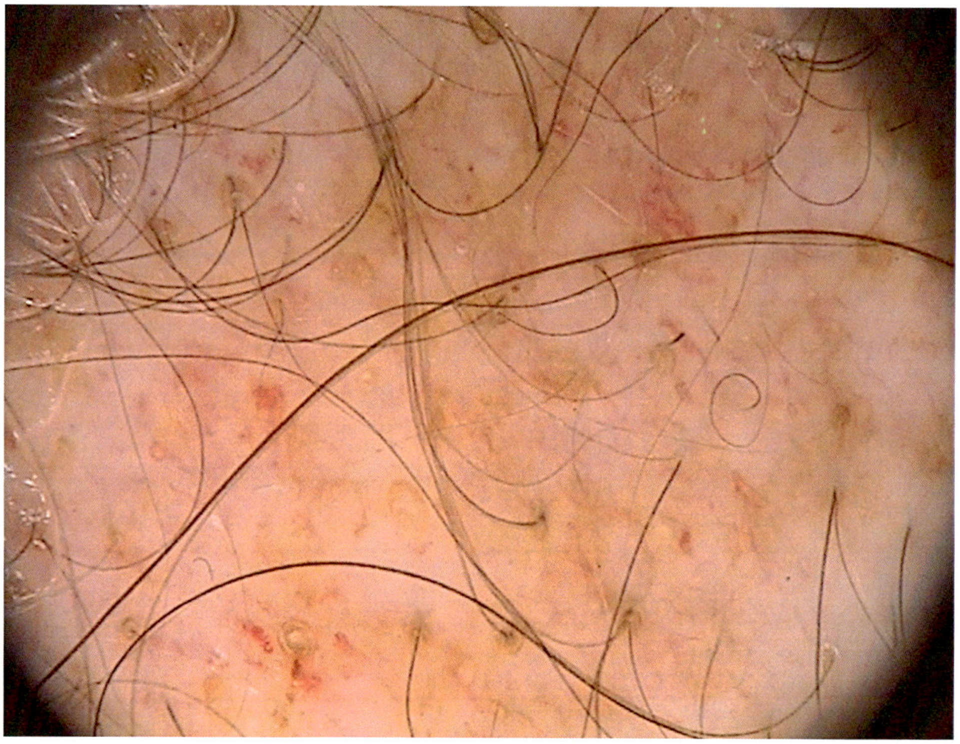

Fig. 23.16 Scattered brown skin discoloration in active discoid lupus erythematosus. Scattered brown skin discoloration is observed in active lesions of DLE. This feature corresponds to the pigment incontinence seen on histopathology. Other DLE features visible in this picture are thick arborizing vessels, a linear helical vessel, and a large yellow dot (×20)

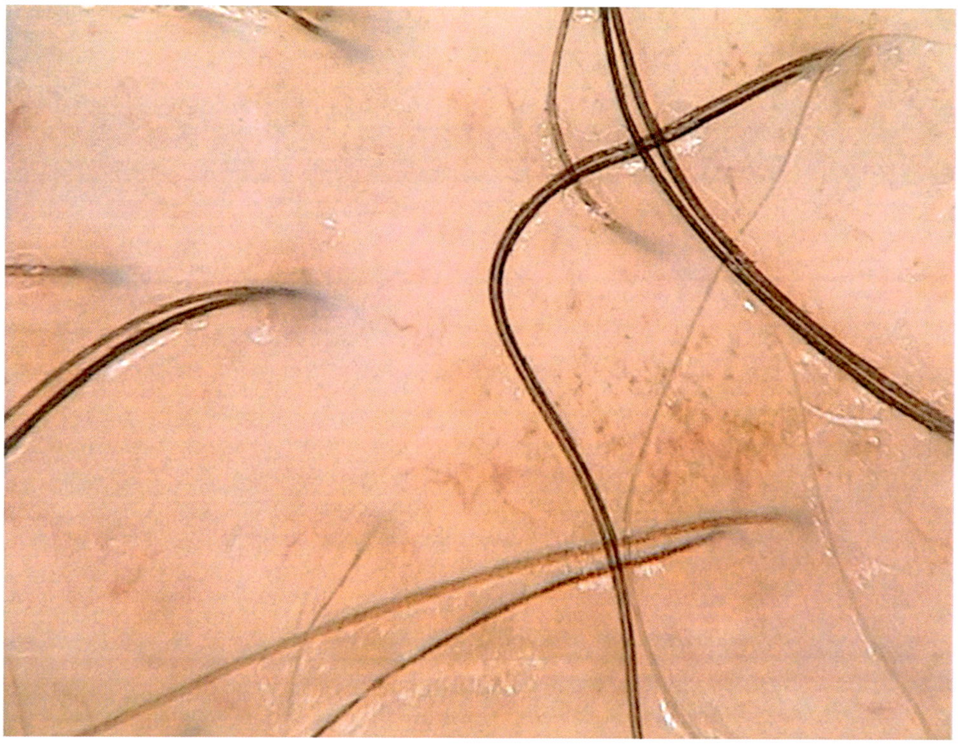

Fig. 23.17 Scattered brown skin discoloration in active discoid lupus erythematosus. High magnification reveals disseminated brown granules, giving the skin a "dirty" appearance. This distribution of brown skin pigmentation must be differentiated from a similar finding in actinic keratosis and from a brow dye used for hair coloring (×70)

Fig. 23.18 Red dots in discoid lupus erythematosus. Red dots are observed in 5–38 % of patients with DLE [7, 10]. The dots appear as erythematous, polycyclic, concentric structures with a diameter ranging from 0.16 to 0.47 mm and are regularly distributed in and around the follicular ostia. The color of the dots may range from light to dark red. Red dots correspond to widened infundibula with dense perivascular lymphocytic infiltrates, dilated vessels, and extravasated erythrocytes [10]. Hair regrowth is possible in areas with red dots (×70)

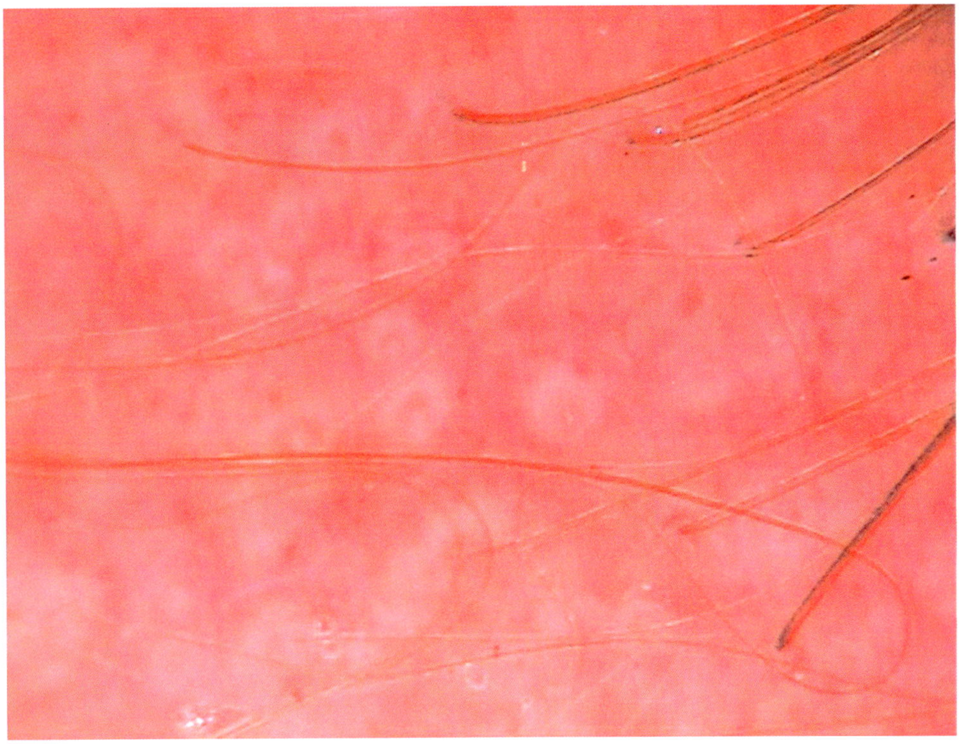

Fig. 23.19 Cicatricial alopecia in the course of discoid lupus erythematosus. White and milky red areas lacking follicular openings correspond to fibrosis. At the hair-bearing margin, hairs are thinner than normal, with only one hair per follicular unit. Faint thick blood vessels are visible close to the hair-bearing margin. In the midpart of the lesion, (*bottom left*) no blood vessels are visible, indicating longstanding fibrosis (×70)

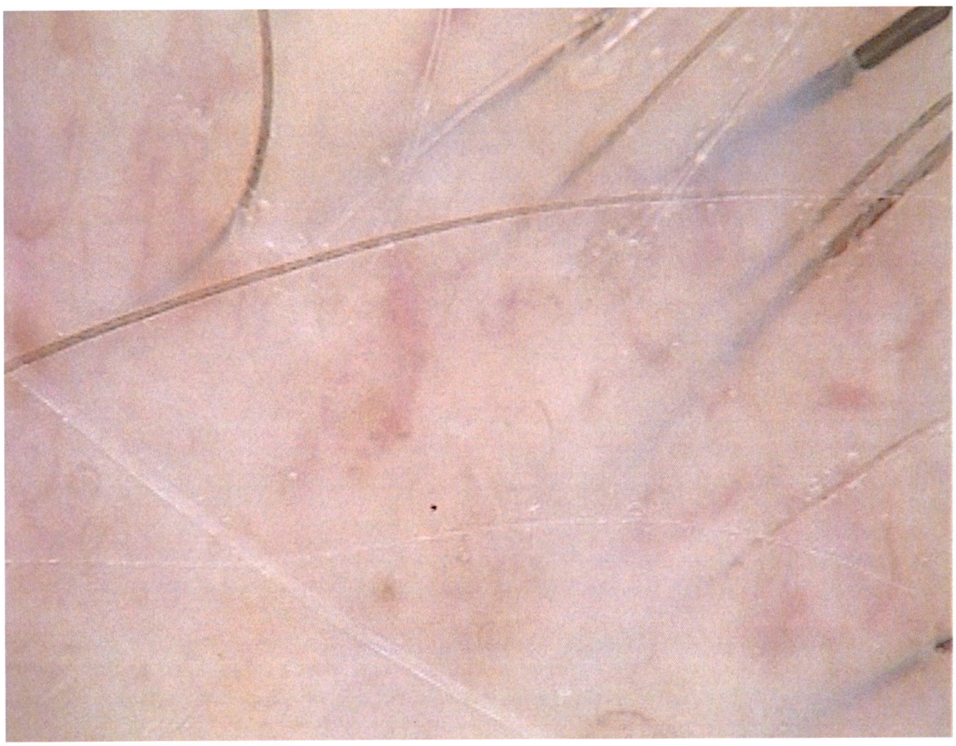

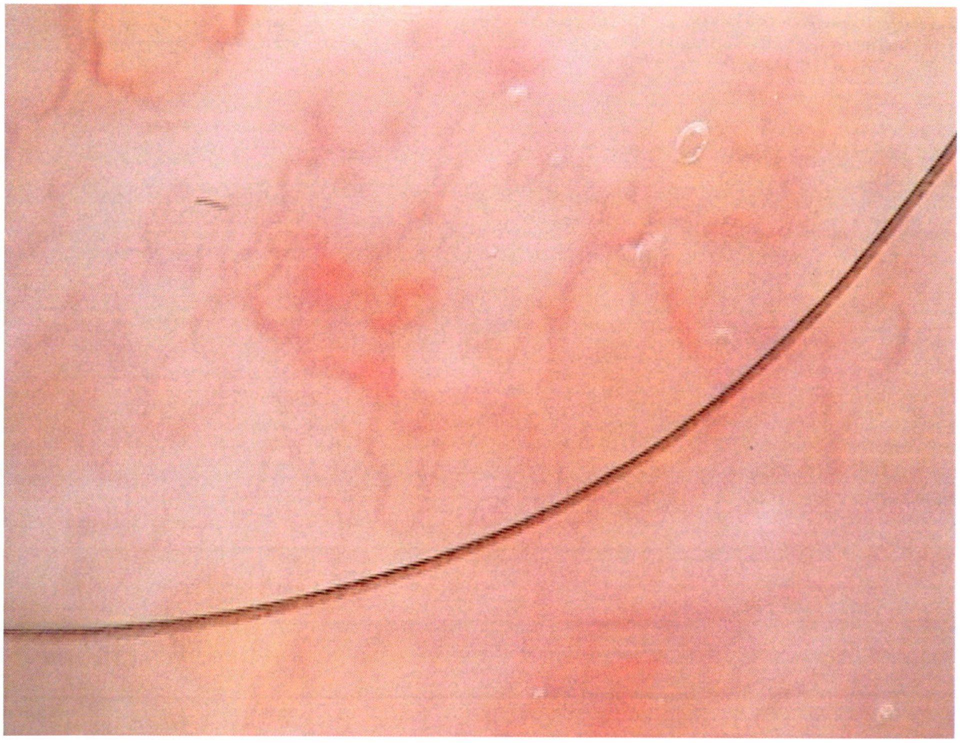

Fig. 23.20 Cicatricial alopecia in the course of discoid lupus erythematosus. Shown is end-stage fibrosis in the course of DLE. Note the lack of follicular openings. The diagnosis may be suspected based on the presence of several thick arborizing vessels. Note also that in DLE, the areas of fibrosis are not ivory white, as in most other types of cicatricial alopecia. The milky red (*pink*) color results from the vascular network, which is visible through the thinned epidermis (×70)

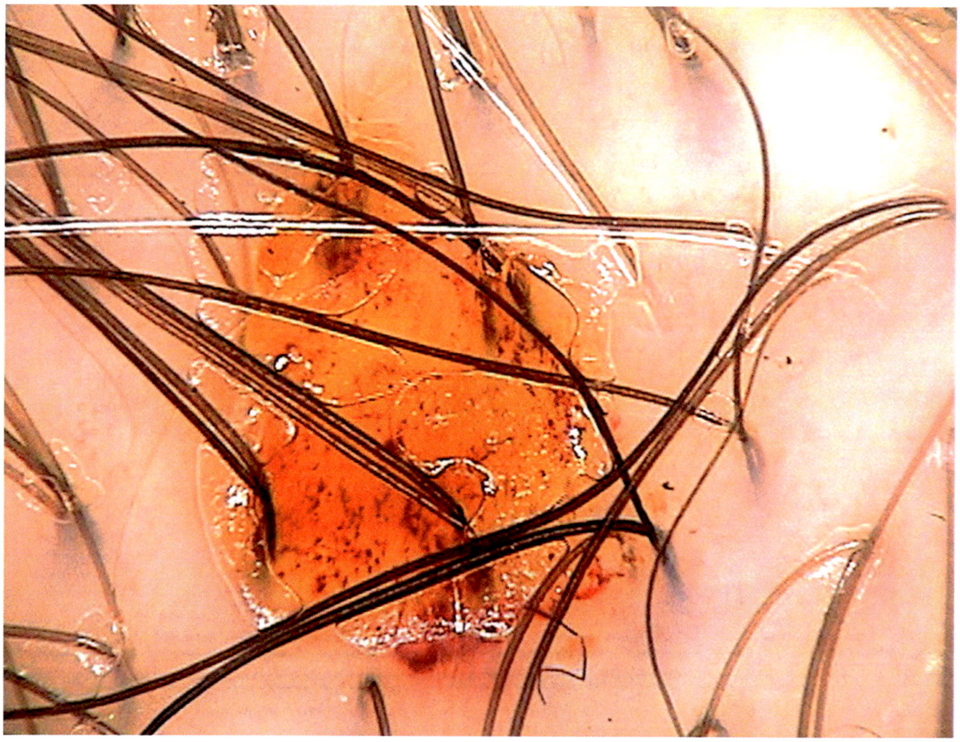

Fig. 23.21 Amicrobial pustulosis associated with discoid lupus erythematosus. Amicrobial pustulosis associated with autoimmune disease is a clinical entity characterized by the recurrent acute onset of pustular lesions, predominantly involving the skin of the scalp, ears, and genital area, and the skin folds. This condition may develop during the course of various autoimmune diseases. Shown here is an amicrobial pustule in a patient with DLE in the course of systemic lupus erythematosus. These pustules are large, bulging, and yellow, and have a glossy surface. They contain several short linear blood vessels and small extravasations (×70)

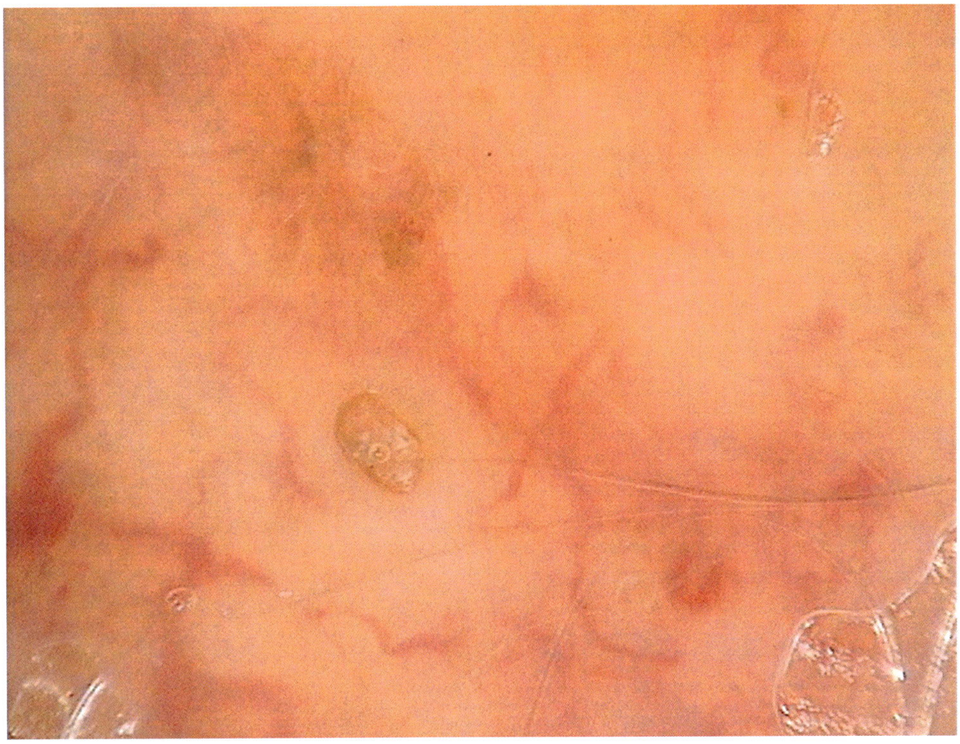

Fig. 23.22 Trichoscopic pattern of discoid lupus erythematosus. The simultaneous presence of large yellow dots, thick arborizing vessels, and scattered brown skin discoloration is a characteristic pattern of DLE (×70)

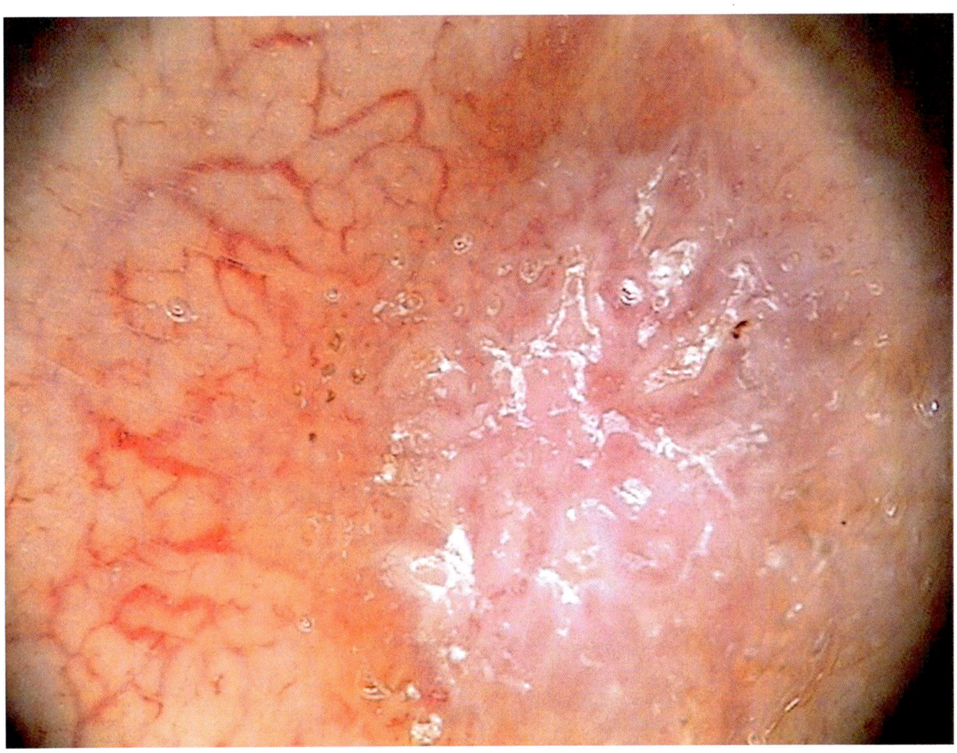

Fig. 23.23 A discoid lupus erythematosus lesion. This DLE lesion shows the evolution (*from left to right*) of the most characteristic features of the disease: thick arborizing vessels, large yellow dots, scattered brown skin discoloration, fine scaling, and white areas of fibrosis (×20)

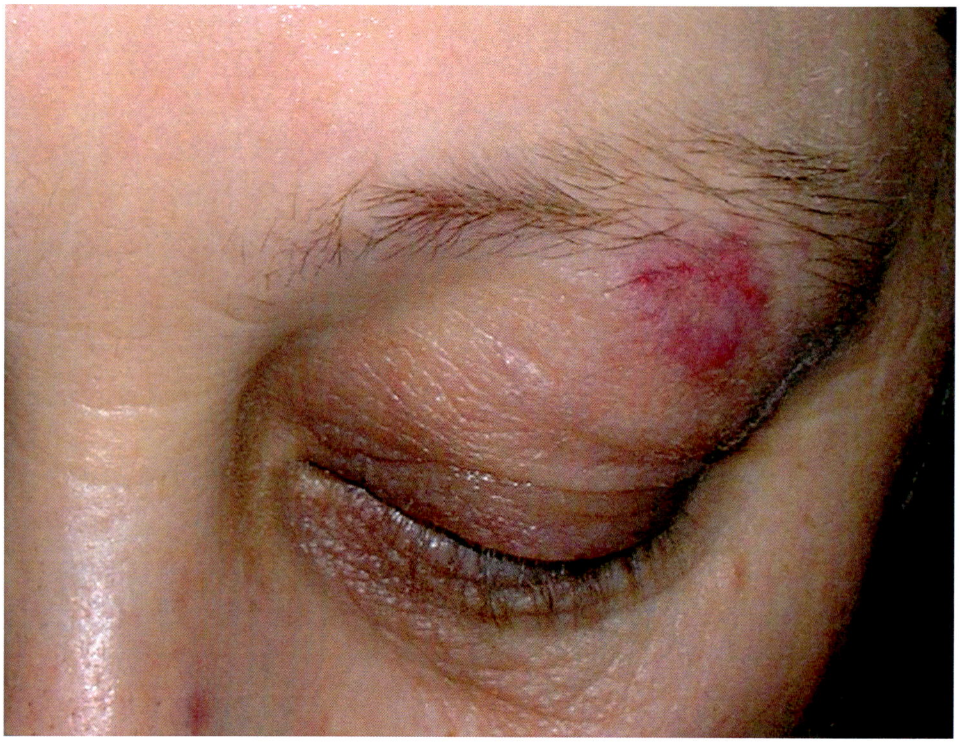

Fig. 23.24 A discoid lupus erythematosus lesion in the eyebrow area. Shown is a characteristic DLE lesion in the eyebrow area. Interestingly, in some diseases, such as DLE, trichoscopy of the eyebrow area reveals predominant trichoscopic features that are different from those of the scalp

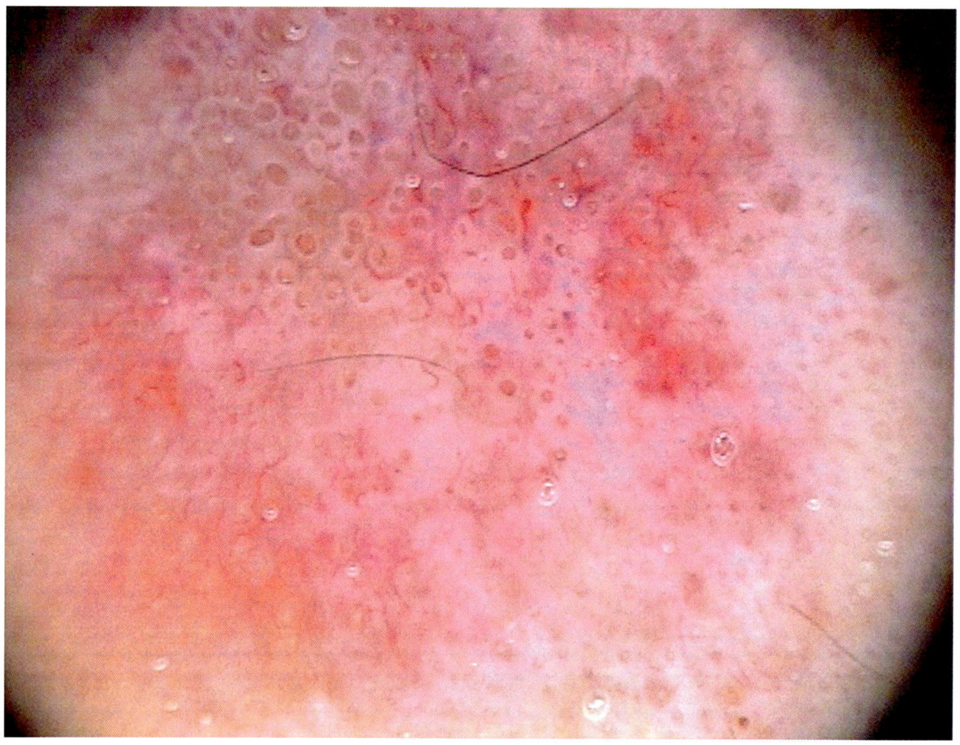

Fig. 23.25 Follicular red dots in the eyebrow area in discoid lupus erythematosus. Trichoscopy shows multiple red dots, which are densely packed and surrounded by a whitish halo. Arborizing vessels are thin. The diffuse redness reflects an active inflammatory process. Blurred milky white areas reveal fibrosis of recent onset (×20)

References

1. Olsen E, Stenn K, Bergfeld W, Cotsarelis G, Price V, Shapiro J, et al. Update on cicatricial alopecia. J Investig Dermatol Symp Proc. 2003;8(1):18–9.
2. Price V, Mirmirani P, editors. Cicatricial alopecia: an approach to diagnosis and management. New York: Springer; 2011.
3. Walling HW, Sontheimer RD. Cutaneous lupus erythematosus: issues in diagnosis and treatment. Am J Clin Dermatol. 2009;10(6): 365–81.
4. Hordinsky M. Cicatricial alopecia: discoid lupus erythematosus. Dermatol Ther. 2008;21(4):245–8.
5. Fabbri P, Amato L, Chiarini C, Moretti S, Massi D. Scarring alopecia in discoid lupus erythematosus: a clinical, histopathologic and immunopathologic study. Lupus. 2004;13(6):455–62.
6. Stefanato CM. Histopathology of alopecia: a clinicopathological approach to diagnosis. Histopathology. 2010;56(1):24–38.
7. Rakowska A, Slowinska M, Kowalska-Oledzka E, Olszewska M, Rudnicka L. Trichoscopy in cicatricial alopecia. J Drugs Dermatol. 2012;11(6):753–8.
8. Rudnicka L, Olszewska M, Rakowska A, Slowinska M. Trichoscopy update 2011. J Dermatol Case Rep. 2011;5(4):82–8.
9. Duque-Estrada B, Tamler C, Sodre CT, Barcaui CB, Pereira FB. Dermoscopy patterns of cicatricial alopecia resulting from discoid lupus erythematosus and lichen planopilaris. An Bras Dermatol. 2010;85(2):179–83.
10. Tosti A, Torres F, Misciali C, Vincenzi C, Starace M, Miteva M, et al. Follicular red dots: a novel dermoscopic pattern observed in scalp discoid lupus erythematosus. Arch Dermatol. 2009;145(12): 1406–9.
11. Lopez-Tintos BO, Garcia-Hidalgo L, Orozco-Topete R. Dermoscopy in active discoid lupus. Arch Dermatol. 2009;145(3):358.

24 Folliculitis Decalvans

Adriana Rakowska, Catherine Stefanato, Joanna Czuwara, Malgorzata Olszewska, and Lidia Rudnicka

Abstract

Trichoscopy of active folliculitis decalvans shows tufted hairs surrounded by perifollicular hyperplasia, which may be arranged in a starburst pattern (starburst sign). Other common trichoscopic features of active disease include yellowish tubular scaling and follicular pustules with emerging hair shafts in their midpart. In longstanding lesions, white and milky red areas lacking follicular openings predominate.

Keywords

Blood vessels • Drug-induced • Follicular pustule • Folliculitis decalvans • Hair transplants • Lichen planopilaris • Milky red areas • Pemphigus • Starburst sign • Tinea capitis • Tubular scaling • Tufted folliculitis • Yellow discharge • White areas • White dots

Folliculitis decalvans is a neutrophilic primary cicatricial alopecia [1]. The term *decalvans* is derived from the Latin *decalvare*, which means "remove hair."

The disease predominantly involves the vertex and occipital area of the scalp. Rarely, the beard and other extracranial hairs are affected. The hallmark of folliculitis decalvans is the presence of multiple hairs emerging from one single dilated follicular opening [2–5]. These follicular tufts usually consist of 5 to 20 or more hairs [2]. The tufts form by the clustering of adjacent follicular units due to fibrosis and retention of telogen hairs within the involved follicles [6, 7].

In the active phase, the disease is characterized by recurrent follicular pustules. Additional findings are erythema, dark yellow-gray scales, follicular hyperkeratosis, erosions, and hemorrhagic crusts, most prominent around the follicles. Symptoms include scalp pain, itching, and burning sensations [2–4]. In the course of the disease, small to extensive irregularly shaped patches of cicatricial alopecia develop. With progression, the bare patches coalesce to form large areas of cicatricial alopecia [2–5].

Mild to moderate growth of *Staphylococcus aureus* in bacterial culture is observed in about 20–75 % of patients [8].

It has been debated whether tufted folliculitis is an entity of its own or a variant of folliculitis decalvans. Many authors indicate that the clinical features and histopathology of the two conditions are indistinguishable. However, Price and Mirmirani [9] point out that in tufted folliculitis, usually only one or more small areas are affected, hair loss is minimal, and the prognosis is better compared with folliculitis decalvans.

Trichoscopy of tufted folliculitis and folliculitis decalvans shows similar features. The most frequent finding is tufted hairs. At the base, these hair tufts are surrounded by a band of yellowish scales and perifollicular epidermal hyperplasia, which may be arranged in a starburst pattern (starburst sign)

A. Rakowska • J. Czuwara
Department of Dermatology, CSK MSW, Warsaw, Poland

C. Stefanato
Department of Dermatopathology,
St. John's Institute of Dermatology, St. Thomas' Hospital,
London, UK

M. Olszewska
Department of Dermatology,
Medical University of Warsaw, Warsaw, Poland

L. Rudnicka (✉)
Faculty of Health Sciences, Medical University of Warsaw, Poland

Department of Dermatology, CSK MSW, Woloska 137,
Warsaw 02-502, Poland
e-mail: lidia.rudnicka@euderm.eu

L. Rudnicka et al. (eds.), *Atlas of Trichoscopy*,
DOI 10.1007/978-1-4471-4486-1_24, © Springer-Verlag London 2012

[10]. Other trichoscopic features of active folliculitis decalvans include yellowish tubular scaling, follicular pustules, and yellow discharge [10–12]. In longstanding lesions, white and milky red areas lacking follicular openings predominate in trichoscopic images [10, 12]. White dots were observed in a patient described by Baroni and Romano [13] and in one patient in our recent study [10]. There seems to be no specific vascular pattern. Elongated loops and lace-like and coiled vessels have been observed [12–14]. In the early phase of pustule formation, a perifollicular concentration of blood vessels may be present [12–14].

Table 24.1 Characteristic trichoscopic features of folliculitis decalvans

Active disease
Tufts of five or more hairs in one follicular unit
Yellow follicular pustules
Yellowish tubular scaling with collar formation
Yellow discharge
Starburst sign
Folds of epidermal hyperplasia
Vessels: elongated loops, coiled vessels, concentric perifollicular arrangement
Late-stage, inactive disease
Folds of epidermal hyperplasia
Milky red areas lacking follicular openings
White areas lacking follicular openings

Table 24.2 Diseases with the presence of tufted hairs

- Tufted folliculitis (by definition)
- Folliculitis decalvans (very frequent)
- Lichen planopilaris (frequent)
- Discoid lupus erythematosus (rare)
- Central centrifugal cicatricial alopecia (rare)
- Acne keloidalis (rare)
- Dissecting cellulitis (rare)
- Tinea capitis (very rare)
- Folliculitis keloidalis nuchae[a]
- Dissecting cellulitis[a]
- Pemphigus[a]
- Associated with anticancer drugs that target epidermal growth factor receptor[a]
- Associated with immunosuppressive therapy[a]
- Hair transplants[a]

[a]Case reports

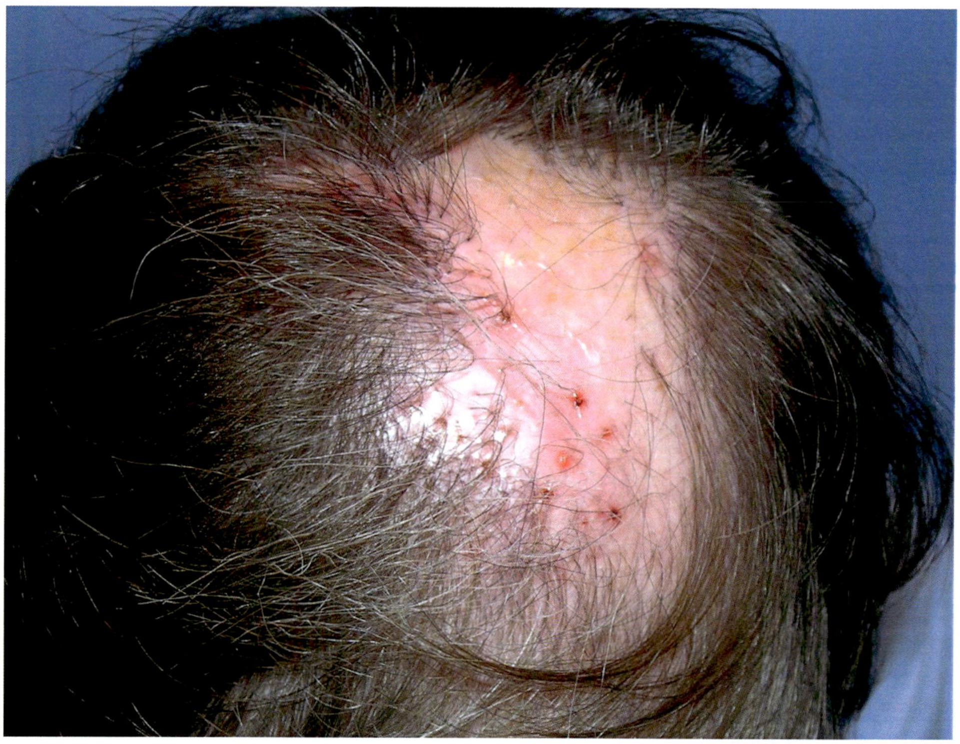

Fig. 24.1 Folliculitis decalvans. Folliculitis decalvans predominantly involves the vertex and occipital area of the scalp. The most characteristic clinical feature is the presence of multiple hairs emerging from one dilated follicular opening. These follicular tufts usually consist of 5–20 hairs. The active phase of disease is characterized by development of recurrent follicular pustules, erythema, yellow-gray scales, follicular hyperkeratosis, erosions, and hemorrhagic crusts, which are most prominent around the hair follicle openings. Scalp pain, itching, and burning sensations may be present. During the course of the disease, small to extensive irregularly shaped patches of cicatricial alopecia develop. With disease progression, the bare patches coalesce to form large areas of cicatricial alopecia [2–5]

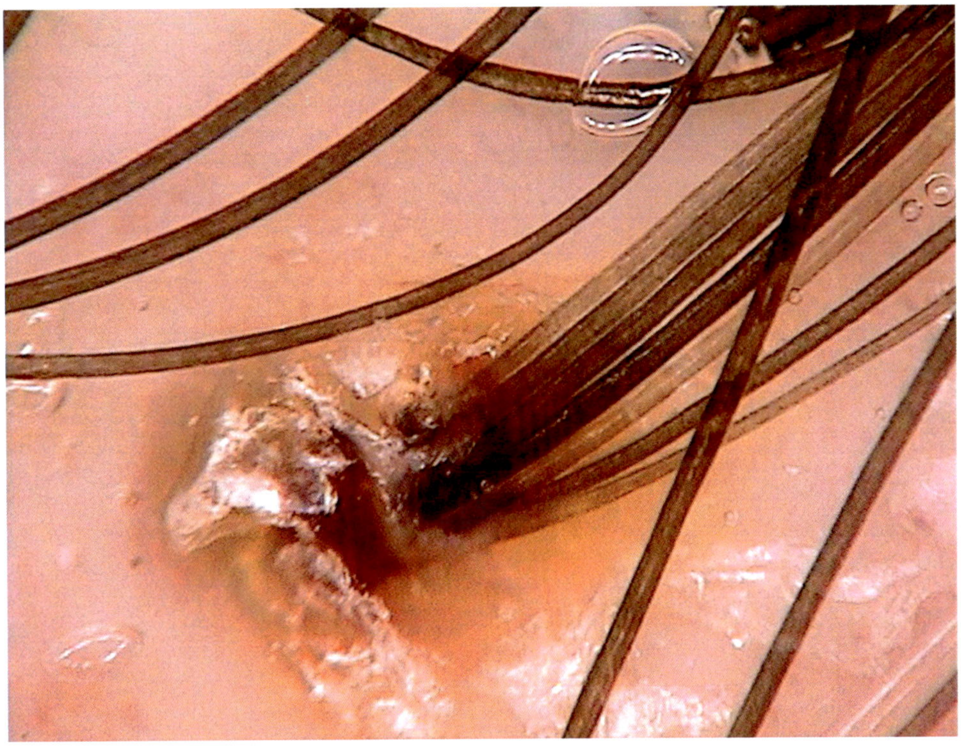

Fig. 24.2 Tufted hairs in folliculitis decalvans. In folliculitis decalvans, several hairs (five or more) emerge from one dilated follicular opening. This image shows a follicular opening with seven hairs. Prominent perifollicular scaling is visible (×70)

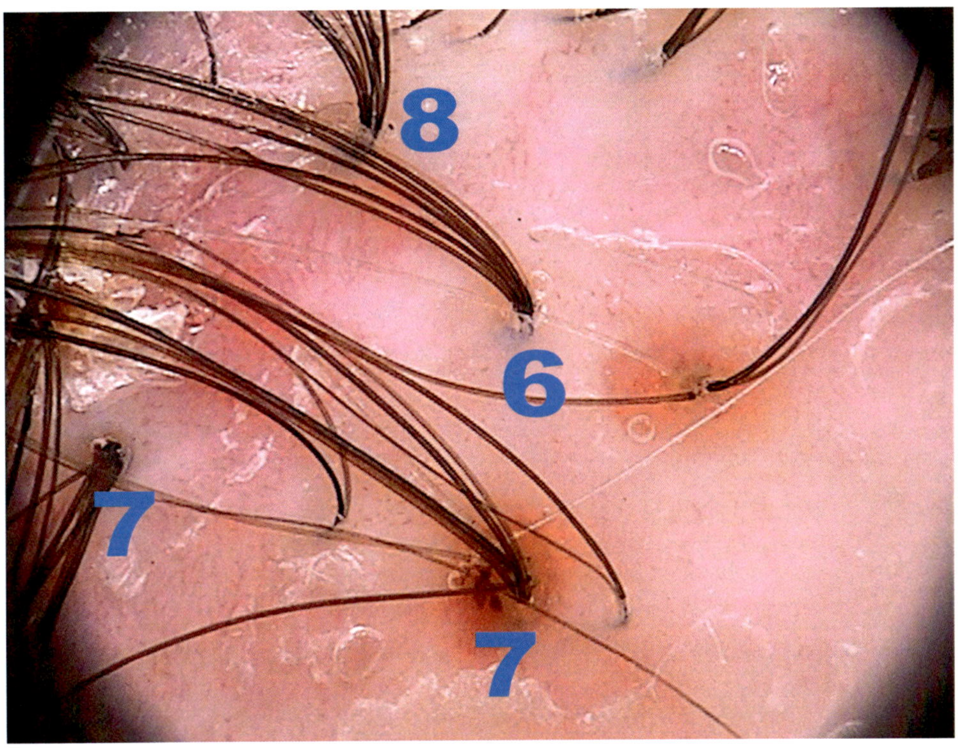

Fig. 24.3 Tufted hairs in folliculitis decalvans. Hair tufts with six to eight hairs emerging from each follicular unit. The numbers correspond to the number of hair shafts emerging from each follicular unit. The presence and size of the follicular pustules (yellow-red areas surrounding the follicular openings) does not correspond to the size of the tuft (×20)

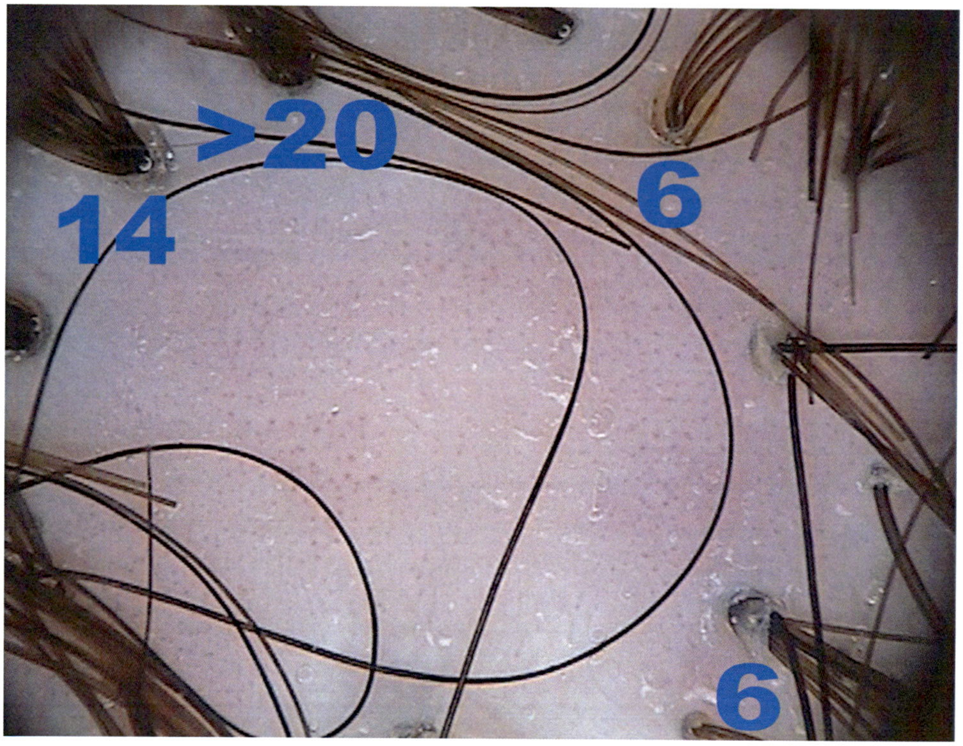

Fig. 24.4 Tufted hairs in folliculitis decalvans. Shown are hair tufts of various sizes at the hair-bearing margin in a patient with long-lasting folliculitis decalvans. The numbers indicate the number of hairs per one follicular unit. The midpart of the image shows an area of cicatricial alopecia, characterized by a lack of follicular openings. Pinpoint vessels are visible in this area (×20)

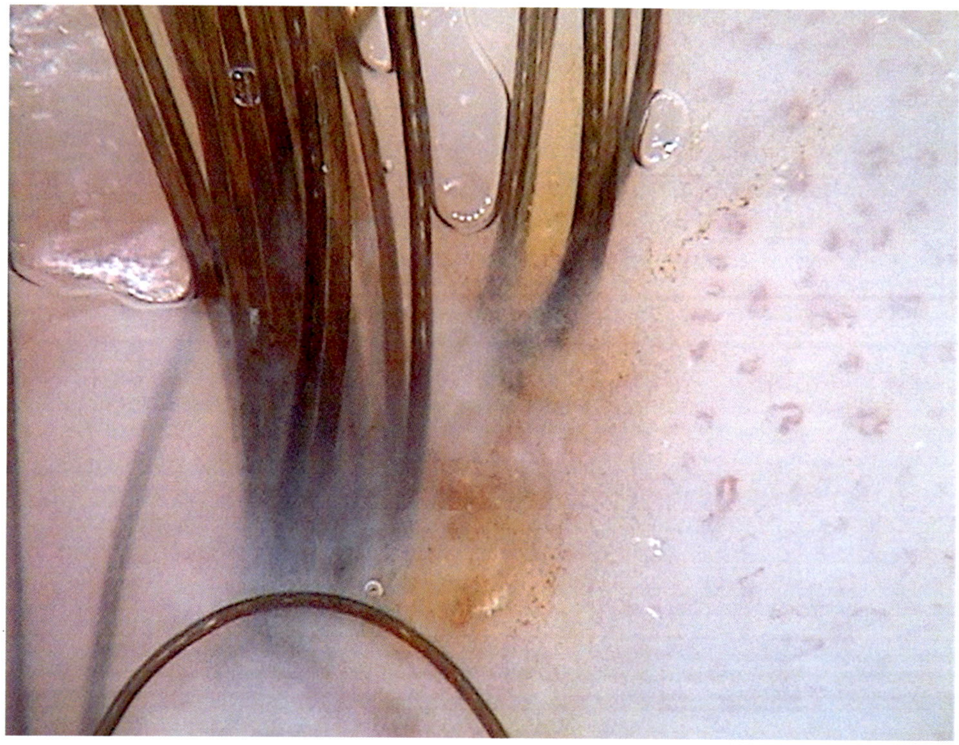

Fig. 24.5 A hair tuft containing approximately 13 hairs. Hair tufts in folliculitis decalvans occasionally may contain more than 100 hairs. A minor purulent area is visible; multiple coiled vessels and elongated loops indicate an active inflammatory process (×70)

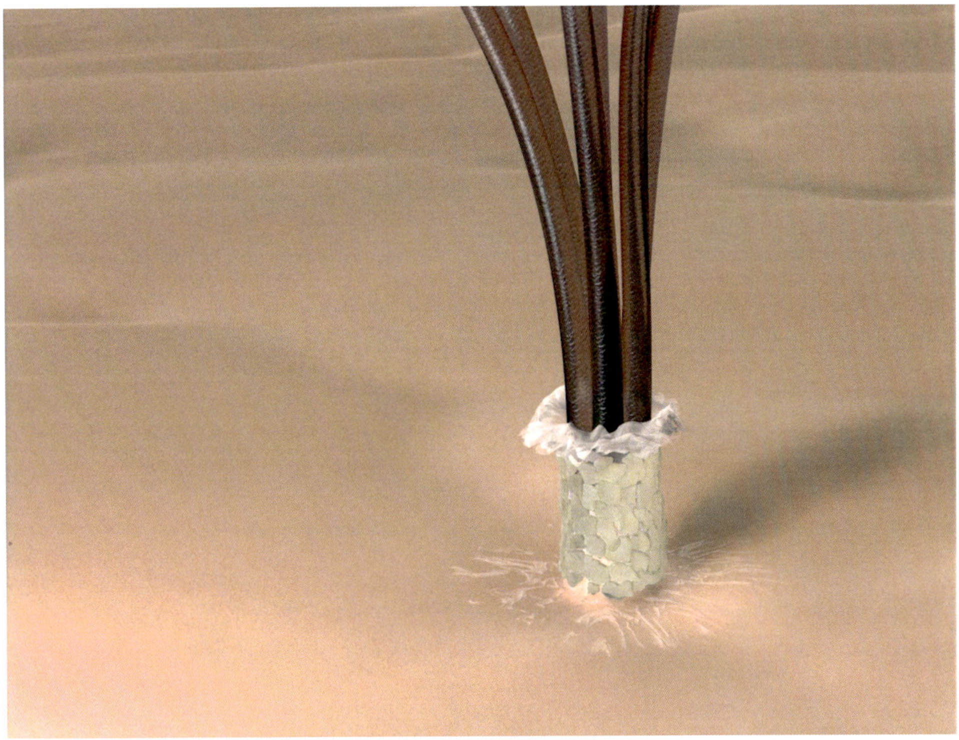

Fig. 24.6 Yellowish tubular scaling with collar formation in folliculitis decalvans. A characteristic feature of folliculitis decalvans, present in over 60 % of patients [10], is tubular scaling, which entangles a hair shaft or a tuft of hairs. This type of tubular scaling is similar to that observed in lichen planopilaris. In folliculitis decalvans, more frequently than in lichen planopilaris, the scales roll away from the hair shaft at the distal end of the "tube" and form collar-like structures. Another feature that differentiates the tubular scaling observed on trichoscopy of folliculitis decalvans from that seen in lichen planopilaris is the yellowish color of the scales. This feature results from the purulent contents of the scaly structures and is a frequent, but not constant, finding in folliculitis decalvans

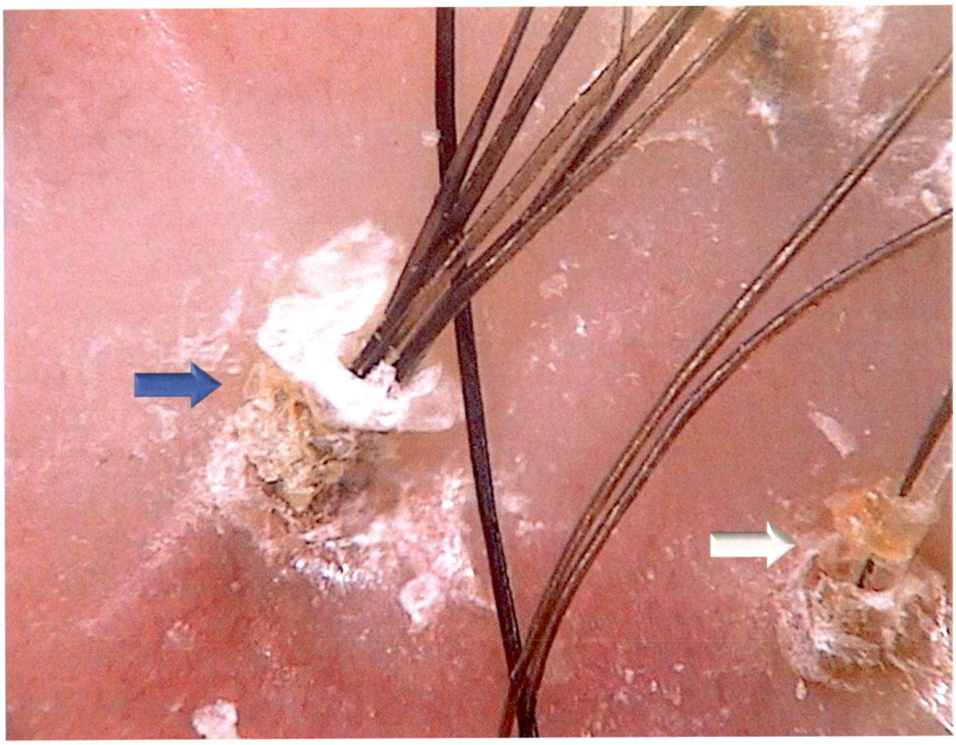

Fig. 24.7 Yellowish tubular scaling with collar formation in folliculitis decalvans. The *blue arrow* points to characteristic tubular scaling with yellowish scales surrounding a tuft of five hairs. The scales roll away from the hairs and form a collar-like structure. The *white arrow* points to tubular scaling around two hairs emerging from a follicular unit. In this case, the scales are also yellowish but the collar-like structure is absent (×70) (*Courtesy of Journal of Dermatological Case Reports*)

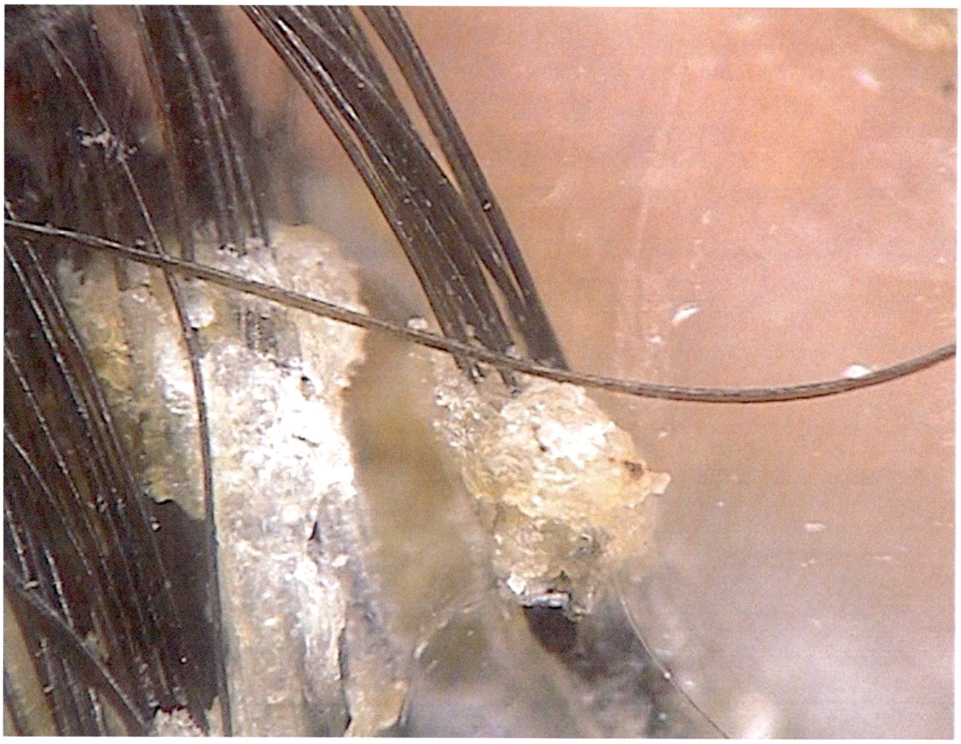

Fig. 24.8 Hair casts in folliculitis decalvans. Occasionally, the yellowish, scaly, tubular structures detach from the scalp surface and remain attached to the hair shafts as they grow. This image shows a hair cast (*right*) attached to a tuft of hairs. Hair casts are less common in folliculitis decalvans than in lichen planopilaris. They differ in their yellowish color and entangled whole tufts of hairs (×70)

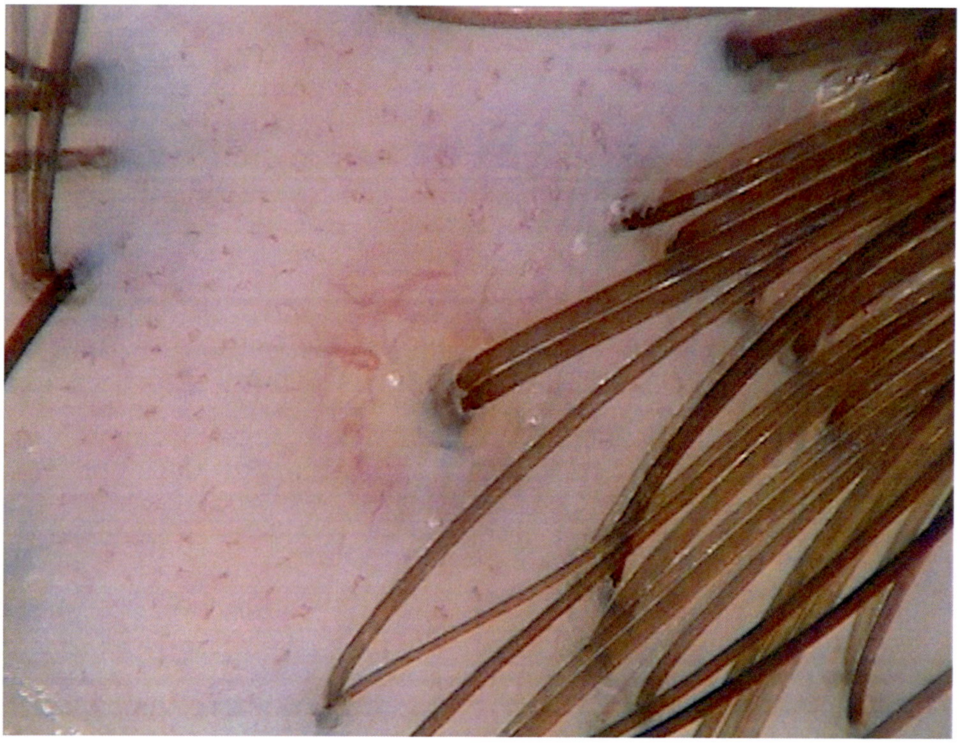

Fig. 24.9 Development of a follicular pustule in folliculitis decalvans: stage 1. In the first stage, formation of a follicular pustule is visible as yellowish discoloration of the perifollicular area, with a slightly bulging appearance. Elongated looped blood vessels are arranged concentrically around the emerging hair shaft (×20)

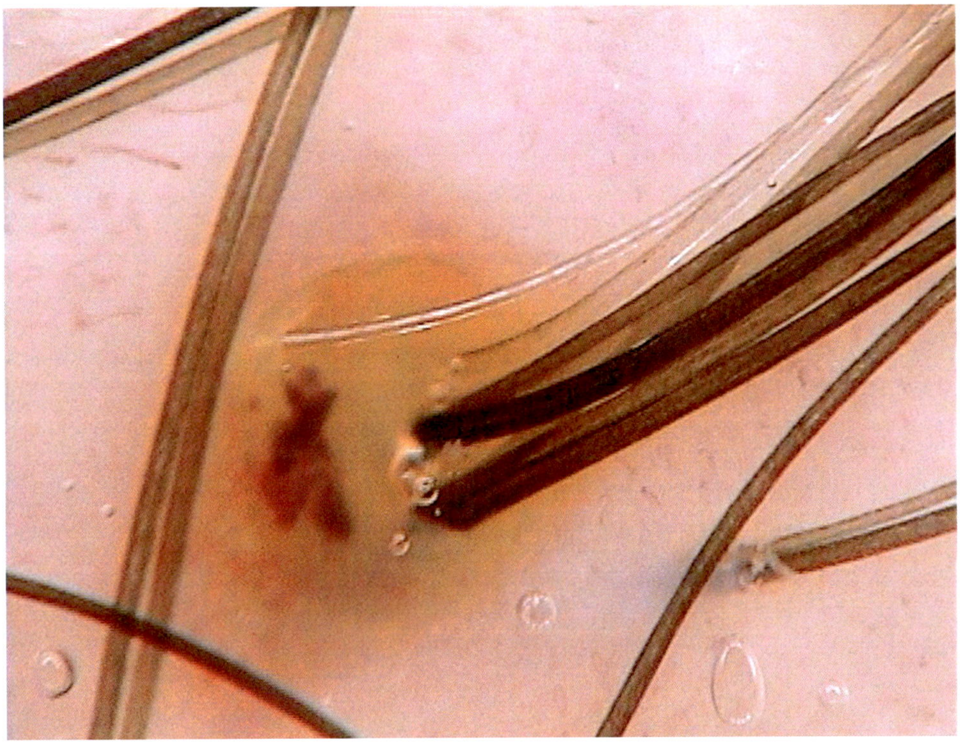

Fig. 24.10 Formation of a follicular pustule in folliculitis decalvans: stage 2. In the second stage, there is yellow perifollicular discoloration with visible bulging of the perifollicular area. The concentric blood vessels are no longer visible. A reddish halo may be present. At this stage, blood extravasations usually are visible within the pustule (×70)

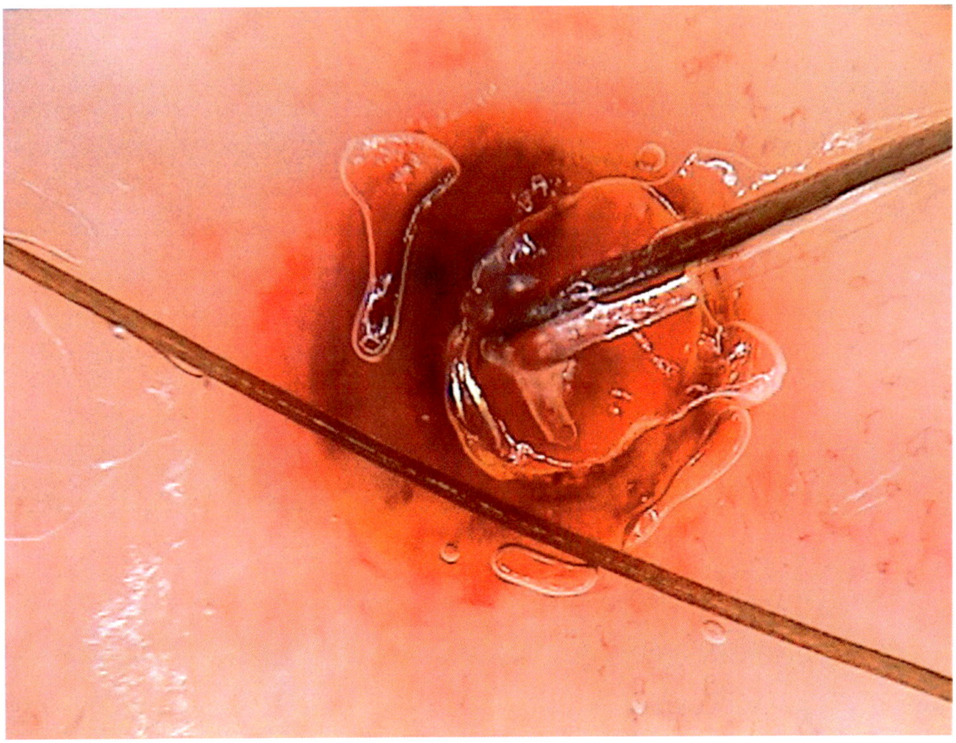

Fig. 24.11 Formation of a follicular pustule in folliculitis decalvans: stage 3. In the third stage, a dark red area surrounding the follicular units may be observed as residue of the pustule. Prominent blood extravasation is present. Rarely, in the last stage of development, the follicular pustule or its purulent discharge dries without blood extravasation (×70)

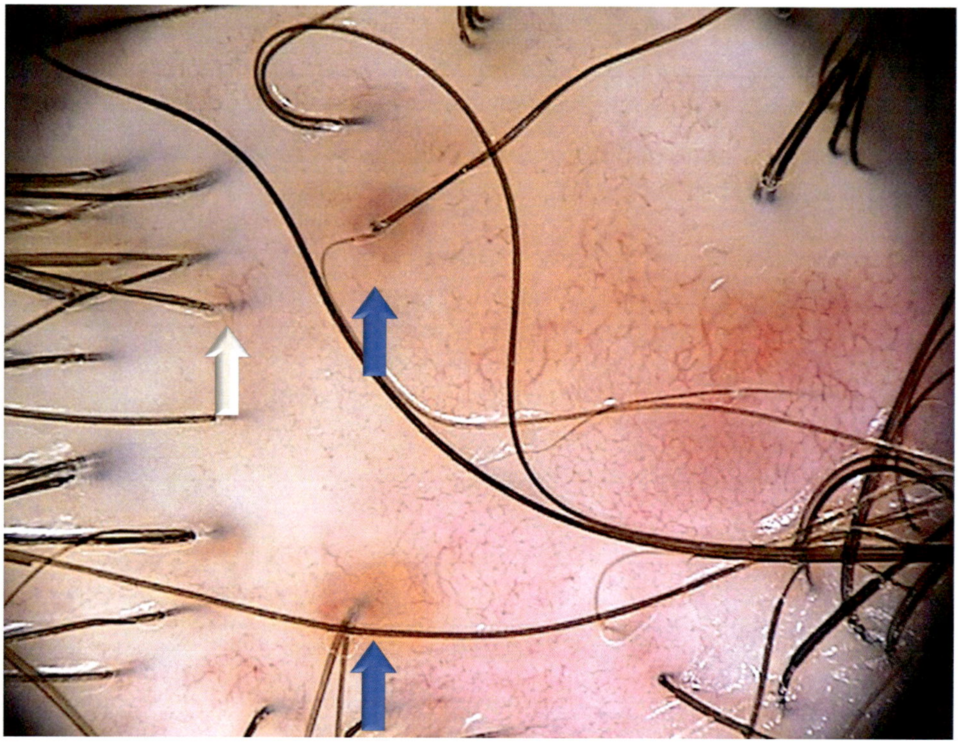

Fig. 24.12 Follicular pustules in folliculitis decalvans. A few pustules (*blue arrows*), visible as yellow sharply demarcated areas around the follicular units, may be recognized. They are located at the hair-bearing margin, next to an area of fibrosis, characterized by the absence of follicular openings (dots). Concentration of elongated blood vessels around the follicular units (*white arrow*) may indicate a possible pre-pustule stage, and we hypothesize that this feature is a marker of disease activity in folliculitis decalvans (×20)

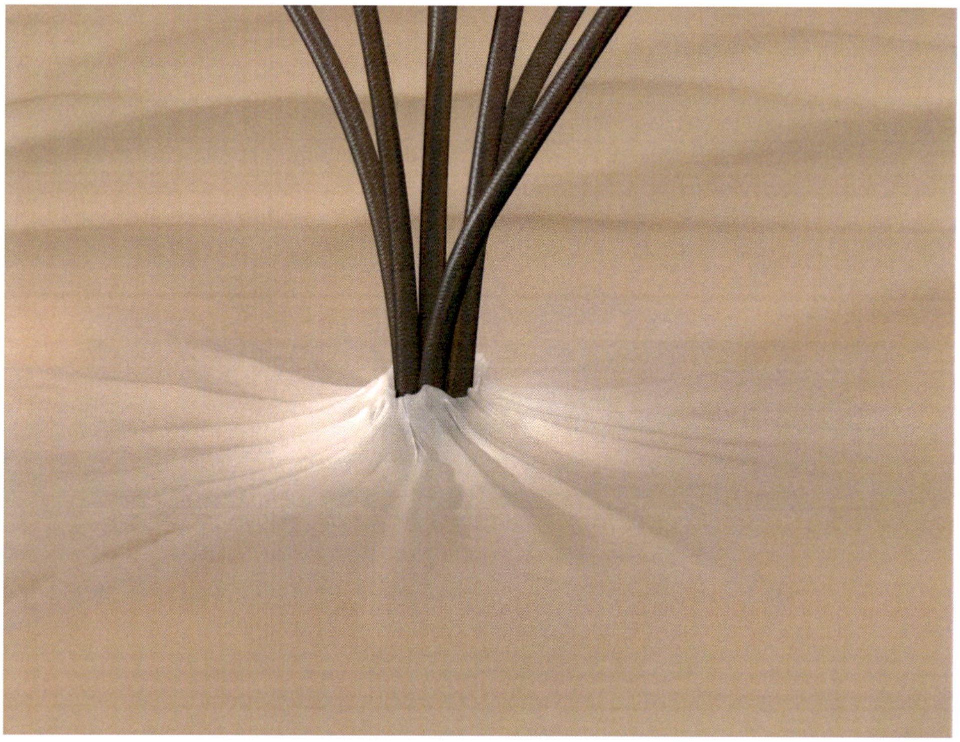

Fig. 24.13 Starburst pattern hyperplasia in folliculitis decalvans (starburst sign). Epidermal hyperplasia observed on histopathology of folliculitis decalvans may be arranged in a starburst pattern around the hair follicle openings. This is a characteristic feature of folliculitis decalvans, present in 66 % of patients [10]. Very rarely (in less than 5 % of patients), delicate starburst hyperplasia–like structures may be observed in patients with lichen planopilaris. The starburst sign frequently is associated with follicular units containing hair tufts. This characteristic feature seems more evident and more frequent in patients with large hair tufts during the course of folliculitis decalvans. This finding corresponds to a combination of epidermal hyperplasia and hyperkeratosis with the underlying pandermal fibrosis observed on histopathology. Dermal fibrosis with a loss of elastic fibers may be responsible for the radiating, undulatory appearance that characterizes the finding

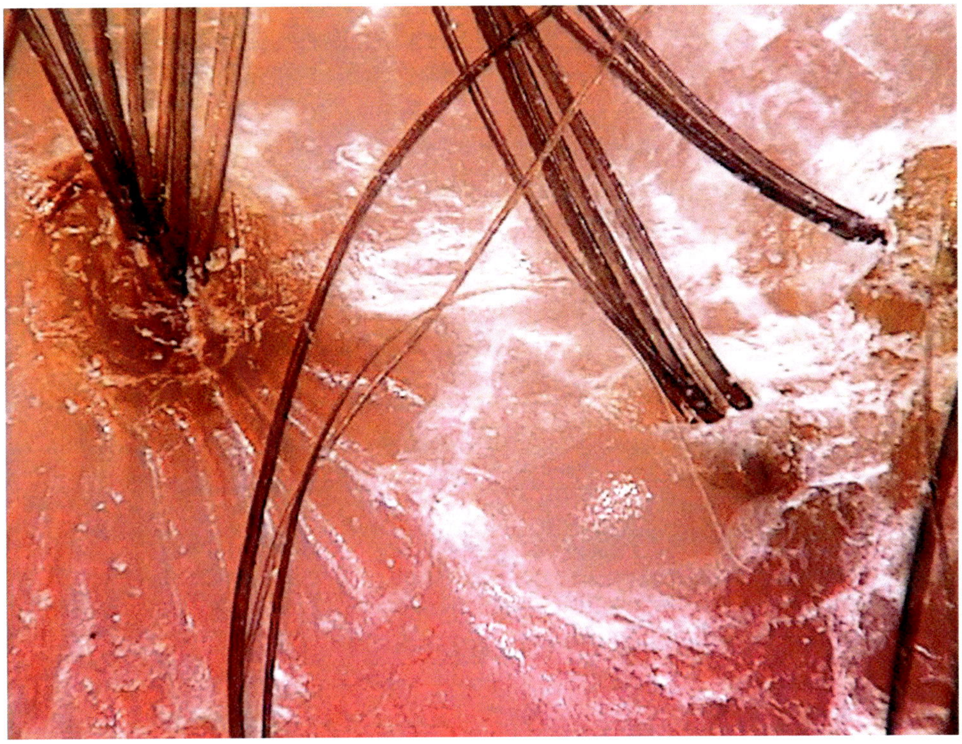

Fig. 24.14 Starburst pattern hyperplasia in folliculitis decalvans (starburst sign). Starburst hyperplasia surrounds a tuft containing eight hairs (*left*). There is prominent perifollicular hyperkeratosis and scaling, a frequent finding in folliculitis decalvans. The right part of the image shows irregular epidermal hyperplasia adjacent to another follicular unit (×70) (*Courtesy of Journal of Dermatological Case Reports*)

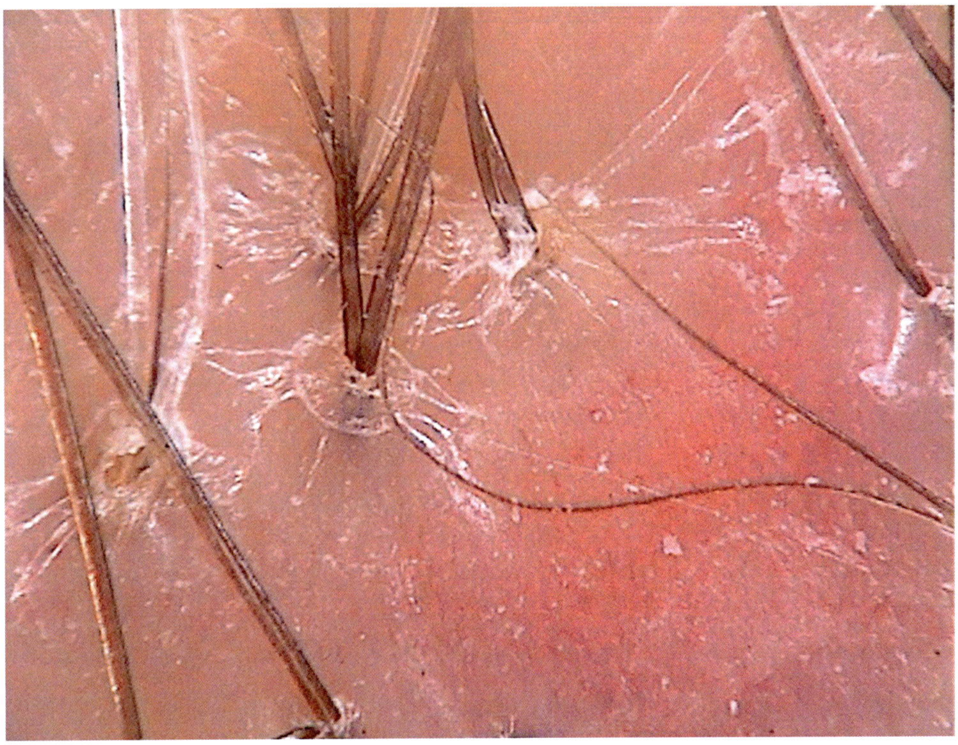

Fig. 24.15 Starburst pattern hyperplasia in folliculitis decalvans (starburst sign). Several small areas of starburst pattern hyperplasia surround follicular units with two to six hairs each in a patient with folliculitis decalvans. The milky red area lacking follicular openings indicates fibrosis of recent onset (×70)

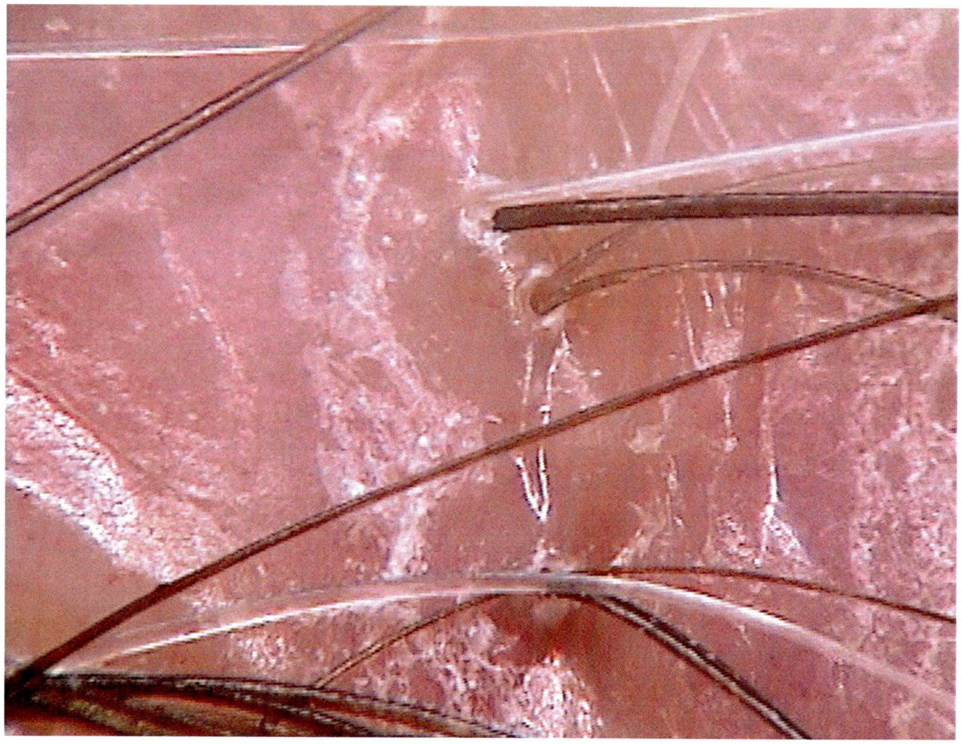

Fig. 24.16 Epidermal hyperplasia in folliculitis decalvans. Shown is epidermal hyperplasia with the partial formation of elements of a starburst sign. Note that in this case, fibrosis and starburst sign formation are associated with follicular units of two to three hairs. Only one hair tuft is visible at the *bottom left* (×70)

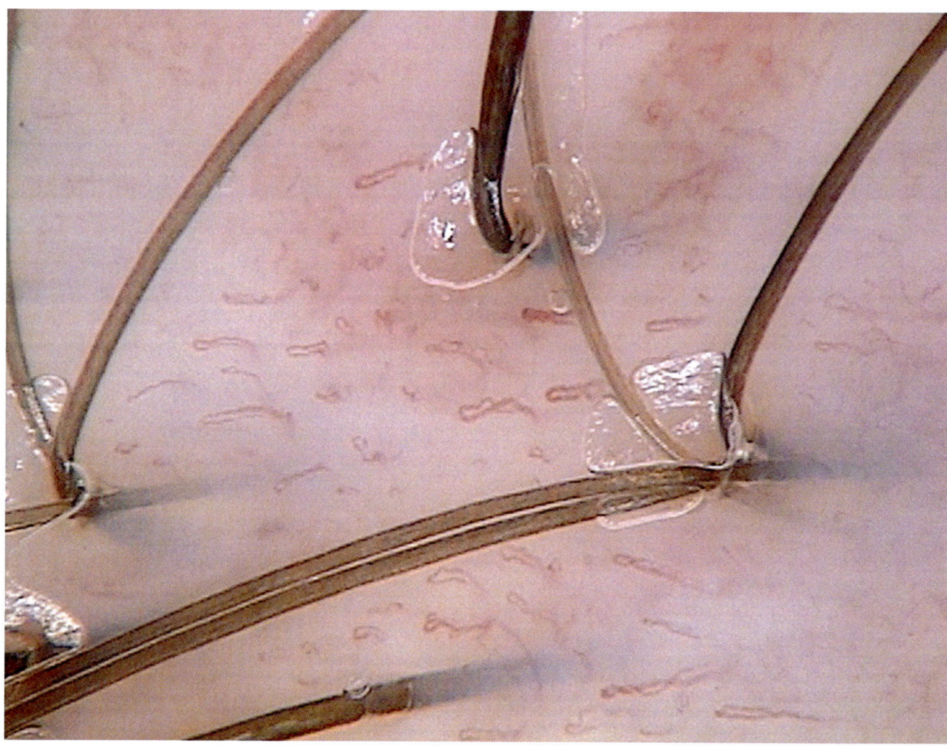

Fig. 24.17 Vascular pattern of folliculitis decalvans. Several vascular abnormalities are observed on trichoscopy of folliculitis decalvans. This image shows several elongated looped and lace-like vessels, which are oriented in one direction. Other abnormalities include coiled vessels and a perifollicular concentration of elongated vessels. These vessels may be distributed concentrically, as shown in Fig. 24.9 (×70)

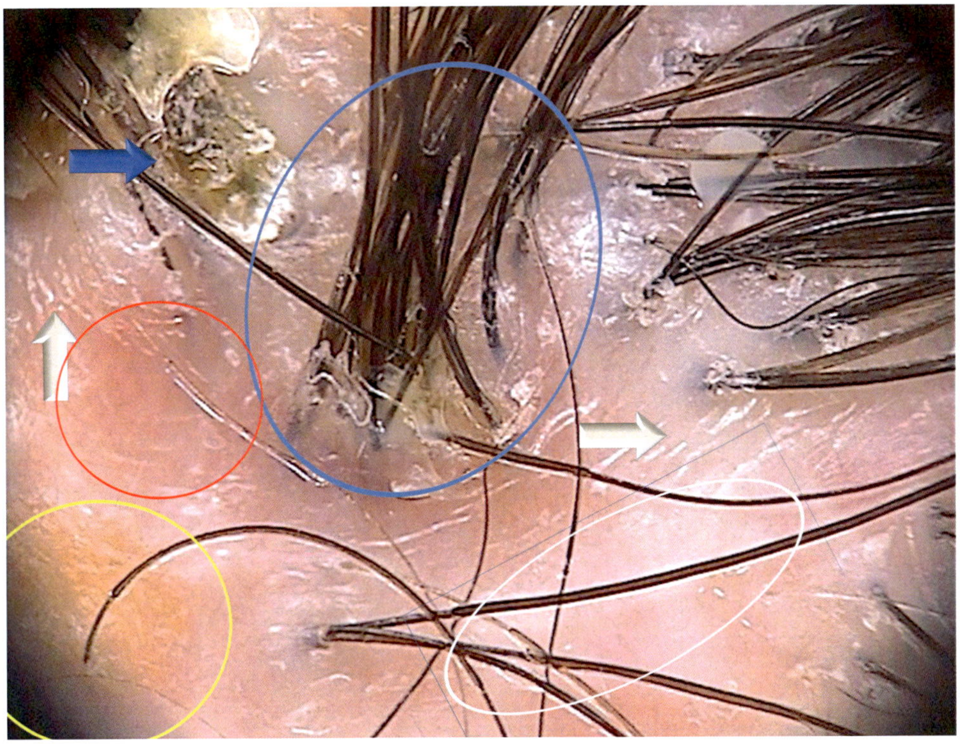

Fig. 24.18 Folliculitis decalvans. The characteristic pattern of folliculitis decalvans includes tufts of five or more hairs in one follicular unit (*blue ring*), yellow follicular pustules (*yellow ring*), yellowish tubular scaling with collar formation (*blue arrow*), milky red areas lacking follicular openings (*red ring*), white areas lacking follicular openings (*white ring*), and folds of epidermal hyperplasia (*white arrows*). This image shows the coexistence of various stages of disease progression, from active inflammatory lesions to features of end-stage fibrosis (×20)

References

1. Somani N, Bergfeld WF. Cicatricial alopecia: classification and histopathology. Dermatol Ther. 2008;21(4):221–37.
2. Otberg N, Kang H, Alzolibani AA, Shapiro J. Folliculitis decalvans. Dermatol Ther. 2008;21(4):238–44.
3. Mirmirani P, Willey A, Headington JT, Stenn K, McCalmont TH, Price VH. Primary cicatricial alopecia: histopathologic findings do not distinguish clinical variants. J Am Acad Dermatol. 2005;52(4):637–43.
4. Wu WY, Otberg N, McElwee KJ, Shapiro J. Diagnosis and management of primary cicatricial alopecia: part II. Skinmed. 2008;7(2):78–83.
5. Stefanato CM. Histopathology of alopecia: a clinicopathological approach to diagnosis. Histopathology. 2010;56(1):24–38.
6. Elston DM. Tufted folliculitis. J Cutan Pathol. 2011;38(7):595–6.
7. Baroni A, Ruocco E, Aiello FS, Faccenda F, Lo Schiavo A, Satriano RA, et al. Tinea capitis mimicking tufted hair folliculitis. Clin Exp Dermatol. 2009;34(8):e699–701.
8. Chandrawansa PH, Giam YC. Folliculitis decalvans-a retrospective study in a tertiary referred centre, over five years. Singapore Med J. 2003;44(2):84–7.
9. Price V, Mirmirani P, editors. Cicatricial alopecia: an approach to diagnosis and management. New York: Springer; 2011.
10. Rakowska A, Slowinska M, Kowalska-Oledzka E, Olszewska M, Rudnicka L. Trichoscopy in cicatricial alopecia. J Drugs Dermatol. 2012;11:753–8.
11. Trueb RM. Systematic approach to hair loss in women. J Dtsch Dermatol Ges. 2010;8(4):284–97, 298.
12. Rudnicka L, Olszewska M, Rakowska A, Slowinska M. Trichoscopy update 2011. J Dermatol Case Rep. 2011;5(4):82–8.
13. Baroni A, Romano F. Tufted hair folliculitis in a patient affected by pachydermoperiostosis: case report and videodermoscopic features. Skinmed. 2011;9(3):186–8.
14. Rudnicka L, Olszewska M, Rakowska A, Slowinska M. Trichoscopy. How it may help the clinician. Dermatol Clin. 2013 (in press). doi:10.1016/j.det.2012.08.011.

Dissecting Cellulitis

25

Adriana Rakowska, Malgorzata Olszewska, Joanna Czuwara, Elzbieta Kowalska-Oledzka, and Lidia Rudnicka

Abstract

In dissecting cellulitis, trichoscopy shows yellow structureless areas and yellow (soap bubble) dots with a "three-dimensional" structure imposed over dystrophic hair shafts. Black dots occasionally are present. Pinpoint-like vessels with a whitish halo may be present. Fibrotic lesions are characterized by confluent ivory-white or white areas lacking follicular openings.

Keywords

Acne keloidalis nuchae • Black dots • Dissecting cellulitis • Dissecting folliculitis Folliculitis decalvans • Mycosis fungoides • Perifolliculitis capitis abscedens et suffodiens • Soap bubble dots • Tinea capitis • Tufts • Vessels • Yellow areas

Dissecting cellulitis (dissecting folliculitis, perifolliculitis capitis abscedens et suffodiens) is a chronic, progressive, inflammatory disease that occurs most commonly in young adults with dark skin phototypes. Men are affected more commonly than women [1]. The disease usually starts with occlusion of follicular openings on the scalp vertex or occiput. Later, perifollicular pustules, nodules, and abscesses with interconnecting sinus tracts develop. Nodules are firm or fluctuant and contain purulent material. Tufted hairs may be present [2–5]. Lesions expand peripherally. Bacterial culture of the purulent discharge is sterile, but secondary bacterial infection may occur [2]. The disease course is chronic, relapsing, and progressive. Occasionally, the disease may be associated with musculoskeletal symptoms [6, 7].

Together with acne conglobata, hidradenitis suppurativa, and pilonidal cysts, the disease forms a syndrome called the "follicular occlusion tetrad" (or "follicular occlusion triad" when only two of these diseases coexist with dissecting cellulitis) [7, 8].

In dissecting cellulitis, trichoscopy shows yellow structureless areas and yellow dots with a "three-dimensional (3D)" structure imposed over dystrophic hair shafts. Black dots occasionally are present. Pinpoint-like vessels with a whitish halo have been described in patients with dissecting folliculitis, but they are not uncommon in other scalp diseases [9]. End-stage fibrotic lesions are characterized by confluent ivory-white or white areas lacking follicular openings. At this stage of the disease, the trichoscopic findings are indistinguishable from those of scarring alopecia of other origins [9, 10].

A. Rakowska • J. Czuwara • E. Kowalska-Oledzka
Department of Dermatology, CSK MSW, Warsaw, Poland

M. Olszewska
Department of Dermatology,
Medical University of Warsaw, Warsaw, Poland

L. Rudnicka (✉)
Faculty of Health Sciences, Medical University of Warsaw, Poland

Department of Dermatology, CSK MSW,
Woloska 137, Warsaw 02-502, Poland
e-mail: lidia.rudnicka@euderm.eu

L. Rudnicka et al. (eds.), *Atlas of Trichoscopy*,
DOI 10.1007/978-1-4471-4486-1_25, © Springer-Verlag London 2012

Table 25.1 Trichoscopic features of active dissecting cellulitis

- Yellow structureless areas
- Yellow 3D (soap bubble) dots with or without hair shafts
- Black dots
- Pinpoint-like vessels with a whitish halo
- Cutaneous clefts with emerging hairs
- Hair tufts

Table 25.2 Trichoscopic differential diagnosis of active dissecting folliculitis

- Acne keloidalis nuchae
- Folliculitis decalvans
- Folliculotropic mycosis fungoides
- Alopecia mucinosa
- Tinea capitis
- Tinea capitis favosa

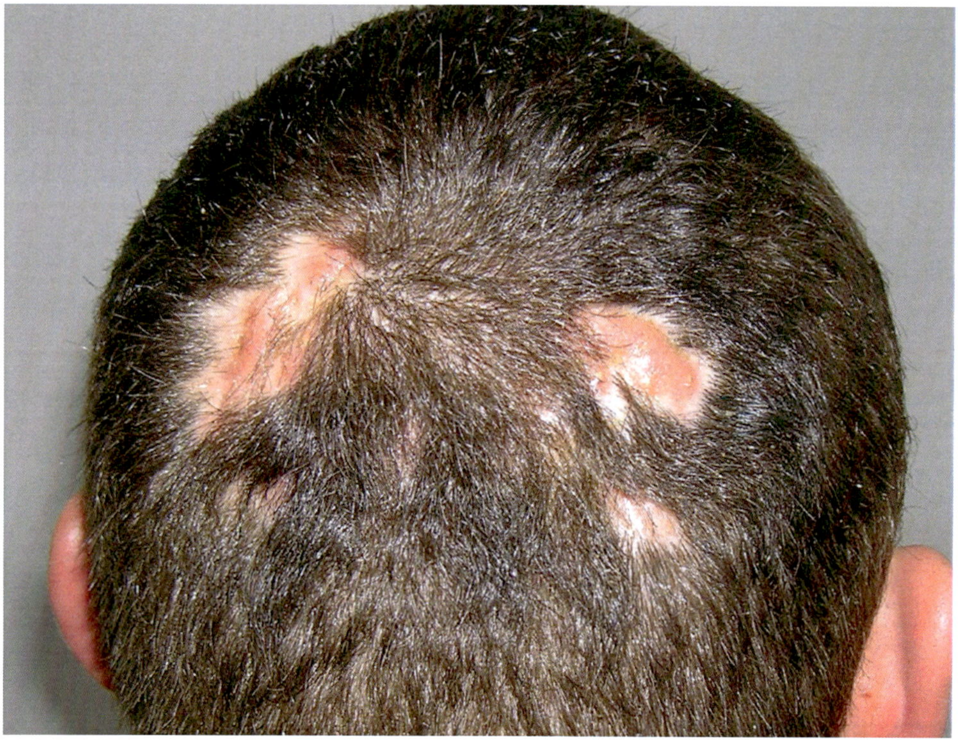

Fig. 25.1 Dissecting cellulitis. Dissecting cellulitis (perifolliculitis capitis abscedens et suffodiens, dissecting folliculitis) is characterized clinically by the formation of pustules, nodules, abscesses, and sinuses that evolve into scarring alopecia. The disease usually begins at the vertex or occipital area. The initial lesion is a pustule that rapidly transforms into a painful bulbous, firm, or fluctuant nodule. Nodules range from a few millimeters to several centimeters in diameter. The pressure of a fluctuant nodule releases a purulent discharge from the nodule itself or from an interconnected nodule. Lesions at different stages may persist for many years. In an active phase of the disease, a nonscarring alopecia develops over the nodules. Cervical or occipital lymphadenopathy may be present. The advanced stage of the disease is characterized by cicatricial alopecia with either atrophic or hypertrophic scarring. Dissecting cellulitis may coexist with acne conglobata, hidradenitis suppurativa, and pilonidal cysts. The concomitant occurrence of three of four of these diseases is called the "follicular occlusion triad" or "follicular occlusion tetrad," depending on the number of coexisting components of the syndrome. In dissecting cellulitis, usually no systemic symptoms are evident, but occasionally the disease may be associated with musculoskeletal symptoms [1, 6–8]

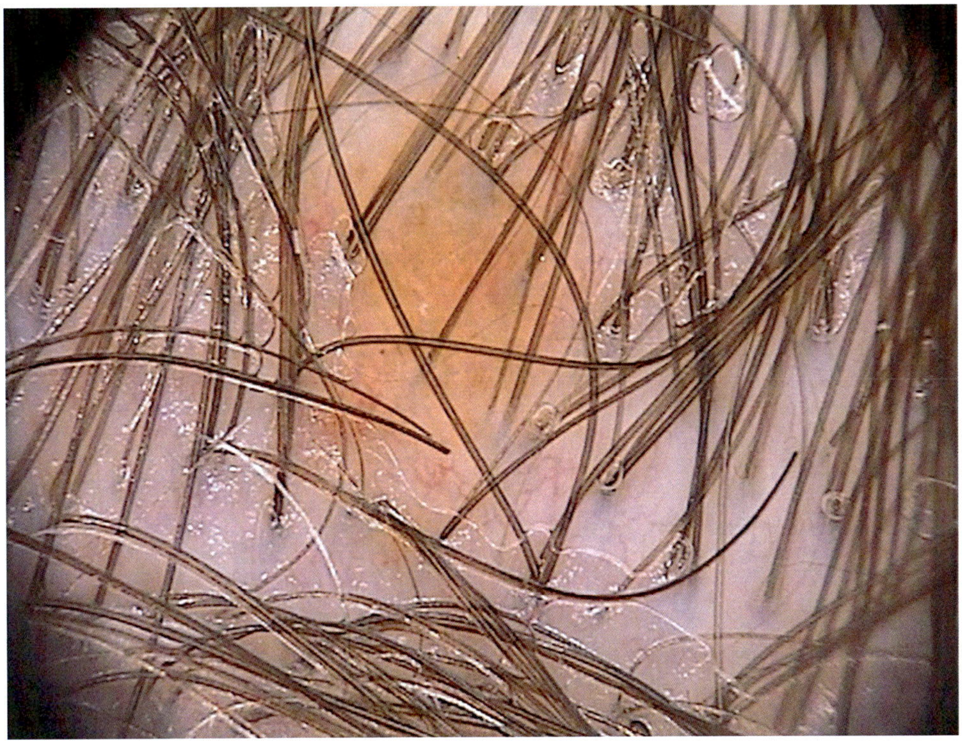

Fig. 25.2 Perifollicular pustules in dissecting cellulitis. Large perifollicular pustules are the earliest trichoscopic finding in dissecting cellulitis. These pustules are indistinguishable from amicrobial or microbial pustules in the course of other diseases (×20)

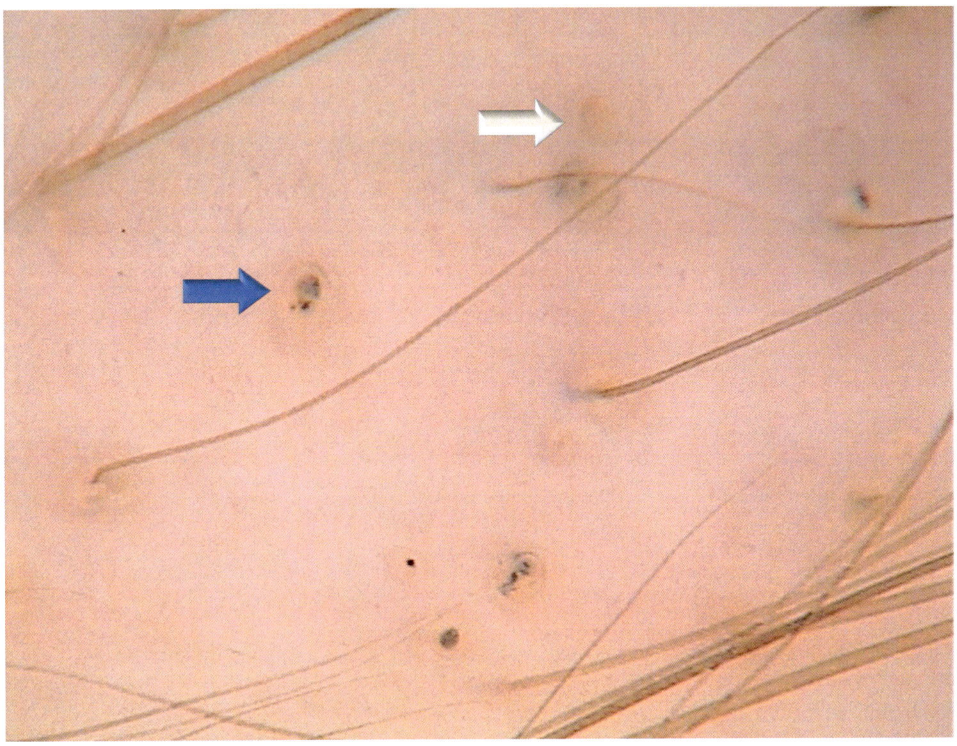

Fig. 25.3 Yellow 3D (soap bubble) dots in dissecting cellulitis. The characteristic yellow dots with a 3D structure have been observed in 100 % of patients with dissecting cellulitis. The term *soap bubble dots* has been suggested for this finding (Dr. Sami Abdennader; personal communication). These structures usually contain a centrally located black dot (*blue arrow*), but soap bubble dots without a black element also are visible in this image (*white arrow*) (×70)

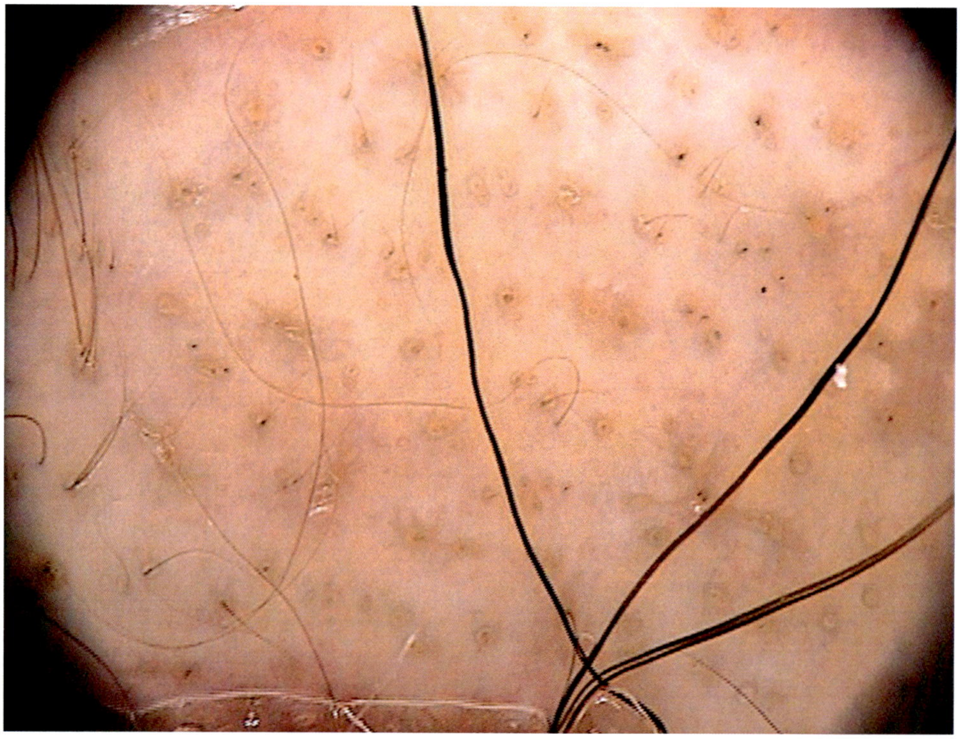

Fig. 25.4 Yellow 3D (soap bubble) dots in dissecting cellulitis. Multiple yellow 3D dots with and without black dots in their center predominate in this image. Thin hairs emerge from some of these follicular openings. Yellow structureless areas are visible. These areas correspond to dense neutrophilic dermal infiltrates on histopathology. Acquired dystrophy of terminal hairs is an additional, nonspecific finding (×20)

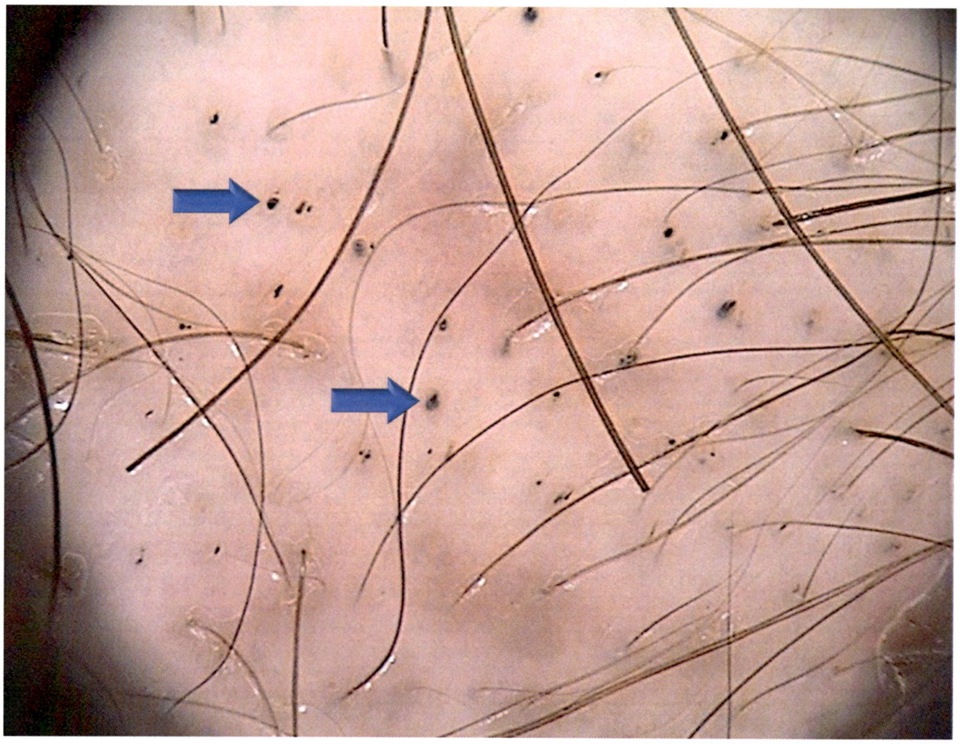

Fig. 25.5 Black dots in dissecting cellulitis. Black dots (*arrows*) are a nonspecific finding in dissecting cellulitis. The image also shows multiple upright regrowing hairs. Irregular violaceous areas, corresponding to pigment incontinence, also may be observed in lichen planopilaris and discoid lupus erythematosus (×20)

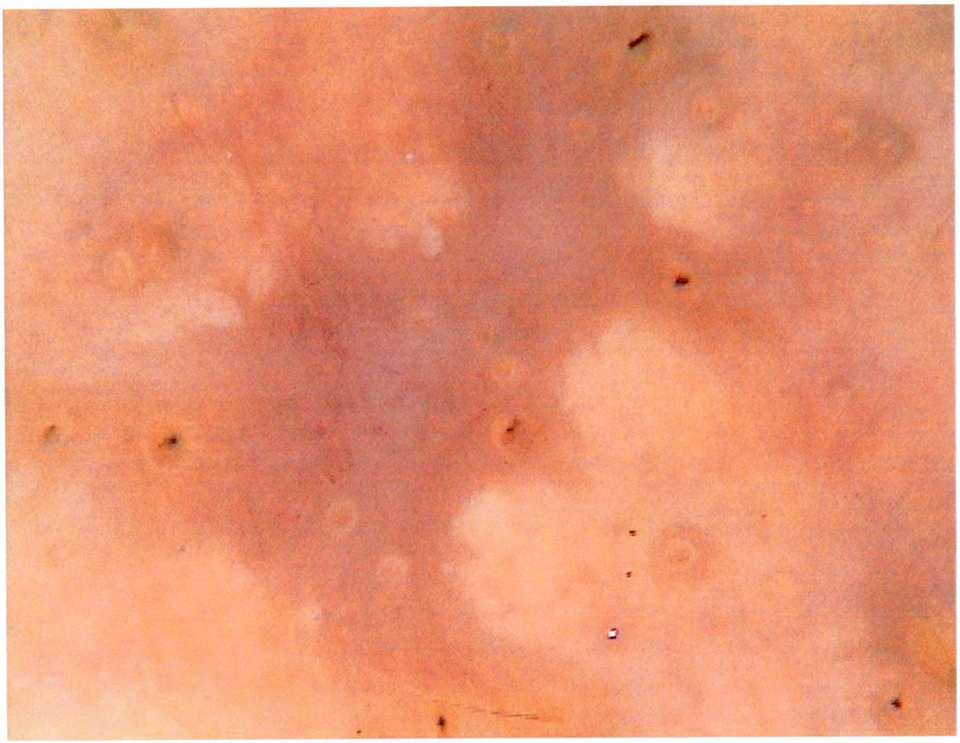

Fig. 25.6 Yellow structureless areas in dissecting cellulitis. Perifollicular yellow structureless areas appear highly characteristic of dissecting cellulitis. In a study including 84 patients with primary cicatricial alopecia, this feature was observed only in those with dissecting cellulitis [9]. Note the yellow dot in the midpart of the yellow area. Yellow 3D dots imposed over black dots also are visible in this image. A few pinpoint vessels with a whitish halo are present (×70)

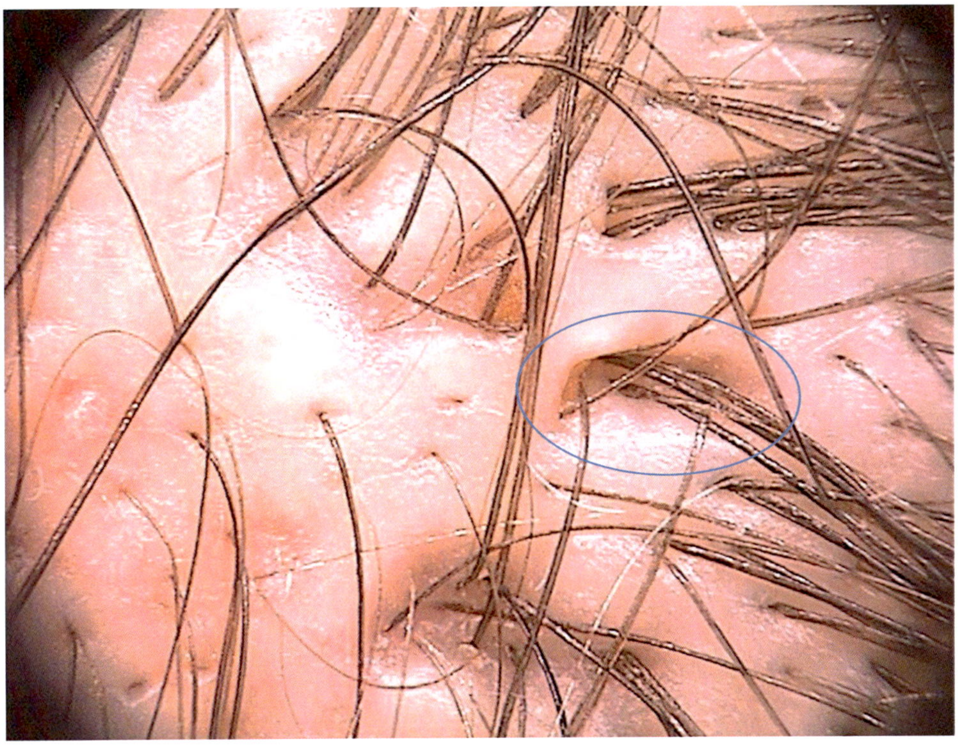

Fig. 25.7 Cutaneous clefts with emerging hairs in dissecting cellulitis. Cutaneous clefts (*blue ring*) containing hair shafts appear to be highly characteristic of dissecting cellulitis. Frequently, small hair tufts (five to eight hairs) emerge from these clefts. Other trichoscopic features of dissecting cellulitis in this image include empty hair follicle openings and a whitish area of developing fibrosis (×20)

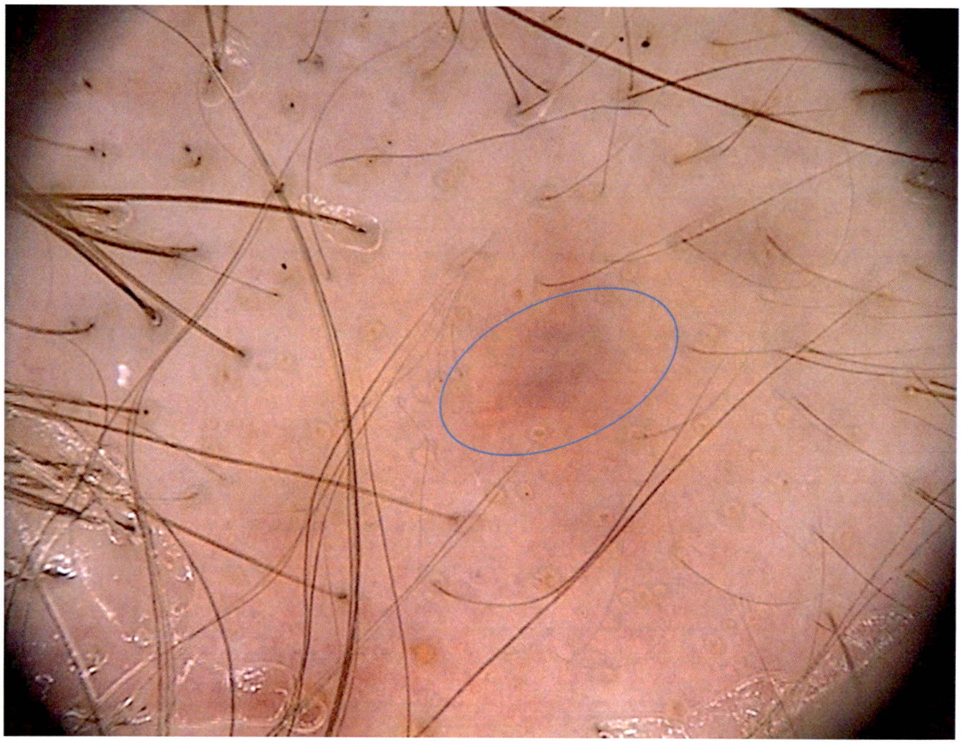

Fig. 25.8 Violaceous areas in dissecting cellulitis. Violaceous areas (*blue ring*) are visible in the late, prefibrotic stages of dissecting cellulitis. On the periphery of this area, multiple 3D dots are visible. The presence of multiple upright regrowing hairs indicates hair regrowth after successful therapy (×20)

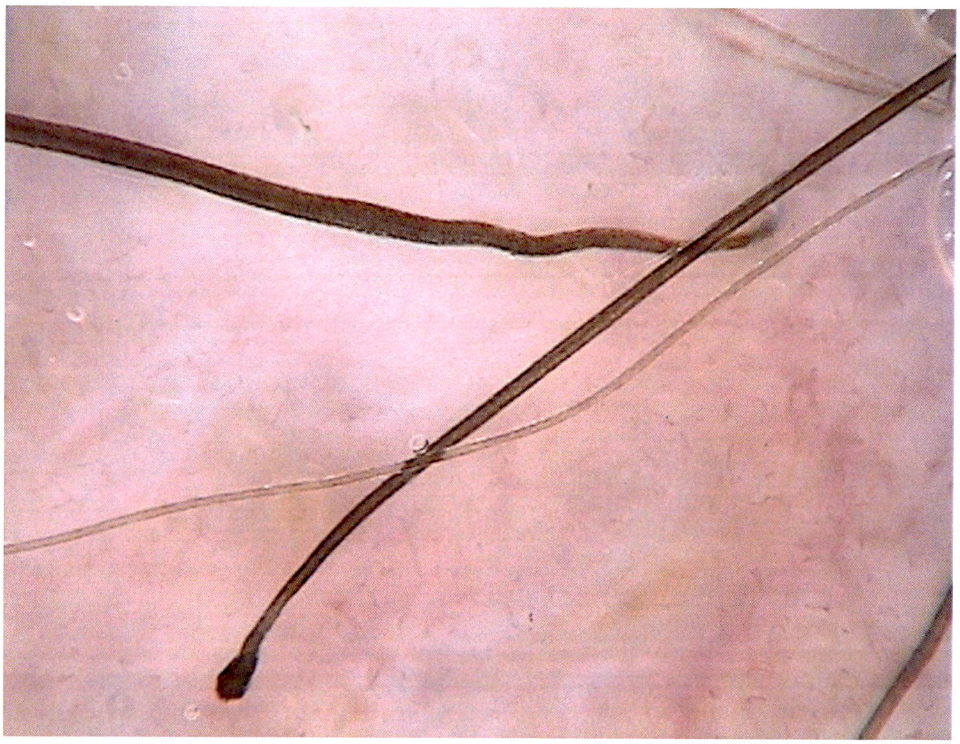

Fig. 25.9 White areas of fibrosis in dissecting cellulitis. The white background indicates a late disease phase with ongoing fibrosis. An irregularly shaped single hair shaft resulting from fibrotic changes in the perifollicular area is visible. This is a frequent finding in all types of cicatricial alopecia. An unusual finding is the anagen bulb, just after being pulled from a nearby follicle with minimal force of the dermoscope lens. A few pinpoint vessels with a whitish halo are present at the periphery of the area of fibrosis (×70)

References

1. Price V, Mirmirani P, editors. Cicatricial alopecia: an approach to diagnosis and management. New York: Springer; 2011.
2. Lugovic Mihic L, Tomas D, Situm M, Krolo I, Sebetic K, Sjerobabski-Masnec I. Perifolliculitis capitis abscedens et suffodiens in a caucasian: diagnostic and therapeutic challenge. Acta Dermatovenerol Croat. 2011;19(2):98–102.
3. Branisteanu DE, Molodoi A, Ciobanu D, Badescu A, Stoica LE, Branisteanu D, et al. The importance of histopathologic aspects in the diagnosis of dissecting cellulitis of the scalp. Rom J Morphol Embryol. 2009;50(4):719–24.
4. Wu WY, Otberg N, McElwee KJ, Shapiro J. Diagnosis and management of primary cicatricial alopecia: part II. Skinmed. 2008;7(2):78–83.
5. Tchernev G. Folliculitis et perifolliculitis capitis abscedens et suffodiens controlled with a combination therapy: systemic antibiosis (metronidazole plus clindamycin), dermatosurgical approach, and high-dose isotretinoin. Indian J Dermatol. 2011;56(3):318–20.
6. Scheinfeld NS. A case of dissecting cellulitis and a review of the literature. Dermatol Online J. 2003;9(1):8.
7. Thein M, Hogarth MB, Acland K. Seronegative arthritis associated with the follicular occlusion triad. Clin Exp Dermatol. 2004;29(5):550–2.
8. Deschamps ME, Payet S, Tournadre A, Soubrier M, Souteyrand P, D'Incan M. Efficacy of infliximab in the treatment of follicular occlusion triad [in French]. Ann Dermatol Venereol. 2010;137(8–9):546–50.
9. Rakowska A, Slowinska M, Kowalska-Oledzka E, Olszewska M, Rudnicka L. Trichoscopy in cicatricial alopecia. J Drugs Dermatol. 2012;11:753–8.
10. Rudnicka L, Olszewska M, Rakowska A, Slowinska M. Trichoscopy update 2011. J Dermatol Case Rep. 2011;5(4):82–8.

Pseudopelade of Brocq

26

Malgorzata Olszewska, Adriana Rakowska, and Lidia Rudnicka

Abstract
The trichoscopic features of classic pseudopelade of Brocq are nonspecific and include loss of follicular openings, porcelain-white areas, and, occasionally, dystrophic hairs at the periphery of the lesion. The trichoscopic features characteristic of other primary cicatricial alopecias are not present. Thus, pseudopelade of Brocq is a diagnosis of exclusion.

Keywords
Cicatricial alopecia • Pseudopelade of Brocq

Pseudopelade of Brocq is a lymphocytic primary scarring alopecia. Females are affected more often than males. The peak age of onset is between 30 and 50 years. The typical patient is a middle-aged woman with skin phototype II [1–3].

The disease was first described in the French literature in 1905 [4], and the term *pseudopelade* was derived from the French word *pelade*, meaning "alopecia areata." Accordingly, *pseudopelade* refers to the resemblance of the disease to alopecia areata. Pseudopelade of Brocq is characterized clinically by asymptomatic, noninflamed white or porcelain-white, small oval/round, reticulate, or large, irregular patches located in the central scalp area [1, 2]. The distribution of alopecic patches in pseudopelade of Brocq may imitate "footprints in the snow" [2]. The small patches of alopecia may coalesce to form larger patches. The course is slowly progressive, and no inflammatory lesions are observed throughout the disease course.

Clinically, the disease differs from alopecia areata by the irregular, nonsymmetric shape of the patches and by the smooth cicatricial lesion surface lacking follicular openings.

Most authors emphasize that pseudopelade of Brocq is a distinct entity. The term *pseudopelade of Brocq* should not be used to describe end-stage, nonspecific cicatricial alopecia resulting from any inflammatory disease when the clinical features are no longer distinguishable [2, 5, 6].

The trichoscopic features of classic pseudopelade of Brocq are nonspecific and include loss of follicular openings and, occasionally, solitary dystrophic hairs at the periphery of the lesion. The background most frequently appears in various shades of white (porcelain, gray, beige, erythematous) and may differ depending on the thickness of the epidermis, disease duration, or sun exposure. Trichoscopy of the eyebrows is normal. Unlike other authors, we have not observed white dots in pseudopelade of Brocq. The trichoscopic features characteristic of other primary cicatricial alopecias, such as tubular perifollicular scaling in lichen planopilaris, starburst pattern hyperplasia in folliculitis decalvans, and large arborizing vessels in discoid lupus erythematosus, are not present [7]. Thus, both clinically and trichoscopically, pseudopelade of Brocq is a diagnosis of exclusion.

M. Olszewska
Department of Dermatology,
Medical University of Warsaw, Warsaw, Poland

A. Rakowska
Department of Dermatology, CSK MSW, Warsaw, Poland

L. Rudnicka (✉)
Faculty of Health Sciences, Medical University of Warsaw, Poland

Department of Dermatology, CSK MSW, Woloska 137,
Warsaw 02-502, Poland
e-mail: lidia.rudnicka@euderm.eu

L. Rudnicka et al. (eds.), *Atlas of Trichoscopy*,
DOI 10.1007/978-1-4471-4486-1_26, © Springer-Verlag London 2012

Table 26.1 Trichoscopic features of pseudopelade of Brocq

- No follicular openings
- Smooth white areas
- Occasionally, dystrophic hairs at the periphery of the lesion
- No features indicative of other types of cicatricial alopecia

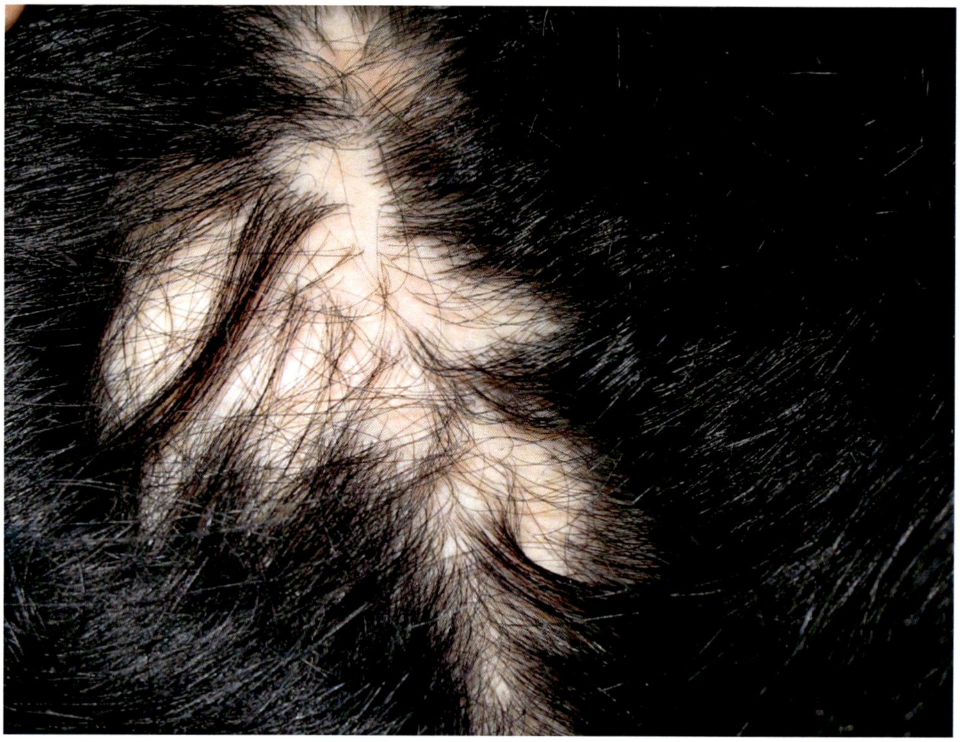

Fig. 26.1 Pseudopelade of Brocq. Pseudopelade of Brocq is characterized clinically by white or porcelain-white, oval/round, or reticulate irregular patches [1, 2]. The small patches of alopecia may merge and form larger areas lacking hair. No clinical features of inflammation are observed. The course of disease is slowly progressive

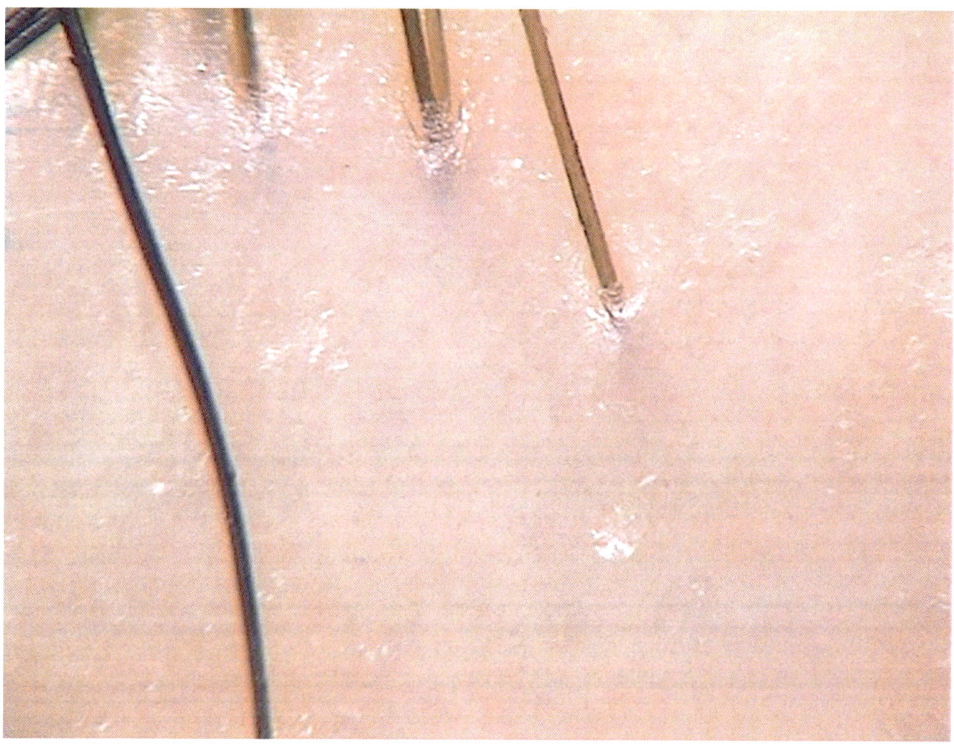

Fig. 26.2 Pseudopelade of Brocq. The hair-bearing margin of a hairless area in a patient with pseudopelade of Brocq shows no features of inflammation and no perifollicular scaling. No follicular openings are present. The skin color usually is porcelain white but may have a subtle erythematous tint, as in this image (dry trichoscopy, ×70)

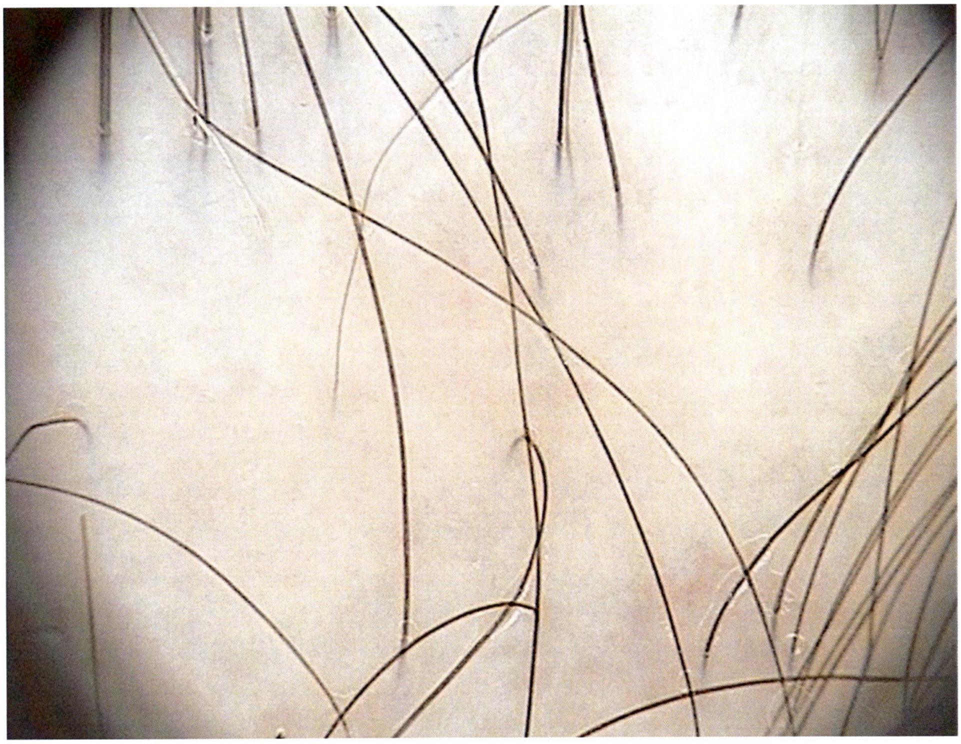

Fig. 26.3 Pseudopelade of Brocq. This image shows a typical small pseudopelade of Brocq lesion in an early phase of the disease. The hairless area is about 1 cm in diameter. Single hairs emerging from the central part of the lesion are still present. The background most frequently appears in various shades of white (porcelain, gray, beige, erythematous) and may differ depending on various factors, such as the use of potent topical corticosteroids, the thickness of the epidermis, the disease duration, or sun exposure (×20)

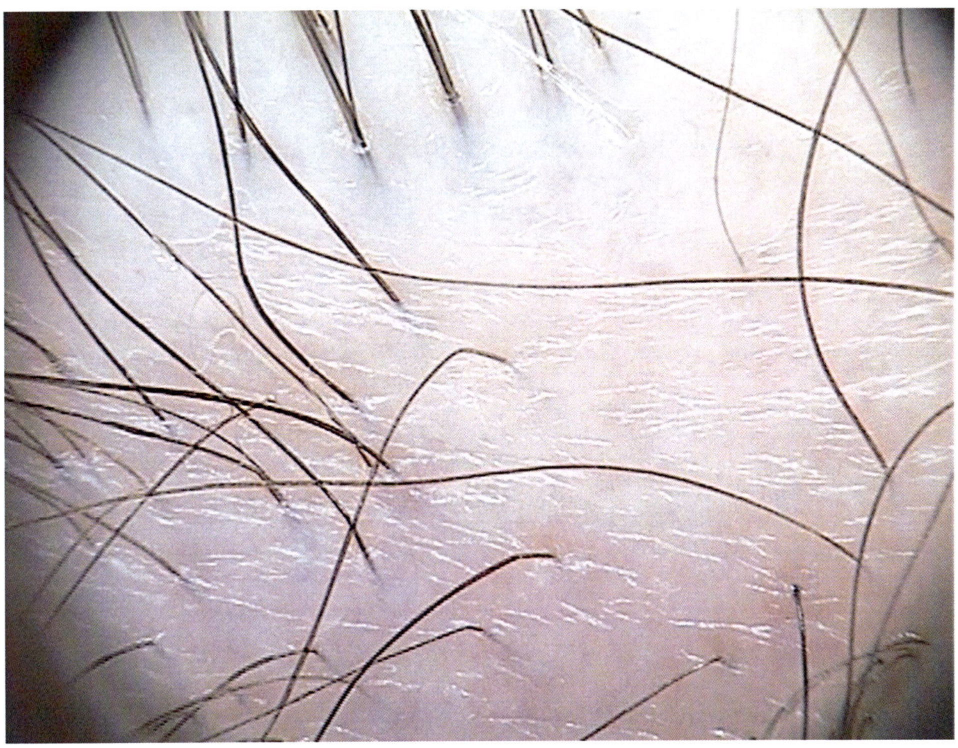

Fig. 26.4 Pseudopelade of Brocq. As in the previous image, a characteristic small hairless patch is surrounded on at least three sides by a hair-bearing margin with most follicular units containing only one hair. These small patches merge into bigger lesions during the course of the disease. Fine parallel folds indicate cicatricial alopecia (dry trichoscopy, ×20)

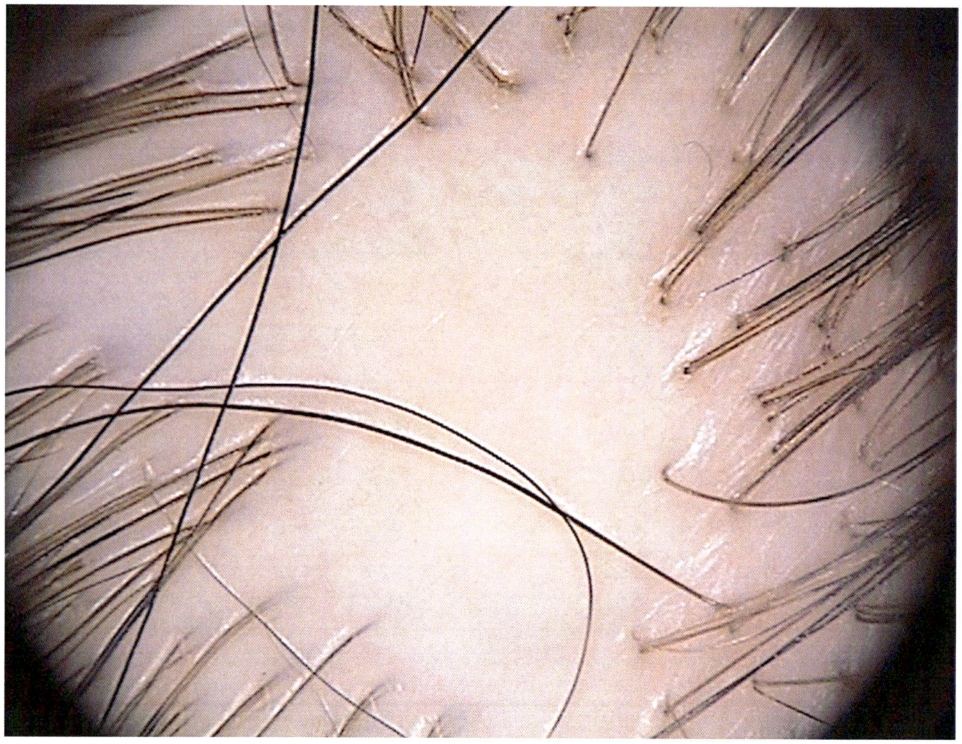

Fig. 26.5 Pseudopelade of Brocq. Shown is a small smooth patch lacking follicular openings and fine parallel folds at the periphery, indicating cicatricial alopecia. This type of image rarely is seen in the course of other types of primary cicatricial alopecia. The background color has a subtle erythematous tone (×20)

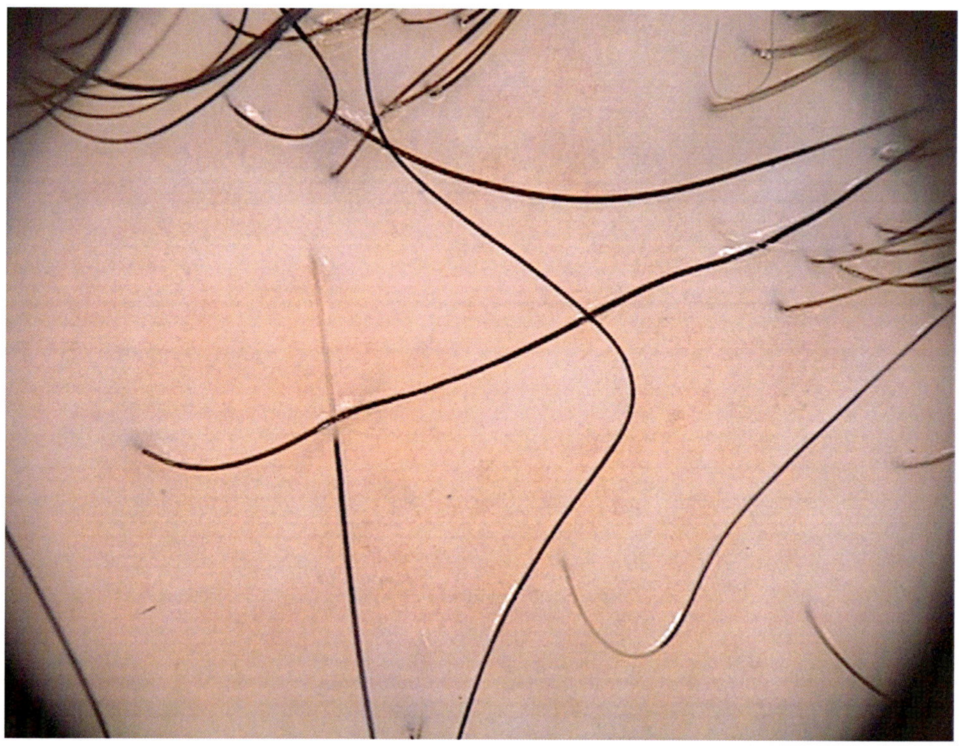

Fig. 26.6 Pseudopelade of Brocq. Shown is a very smooth surface lacking follicular openings. In the midpart of the lesion, a dystrophic hair of irregular shape and thickness is visible. Irregularly shaped hair shafts and pili torti commonly are observed in cicatricial alopecia, independent of the cause. A subtle pigment network is visible (×20)

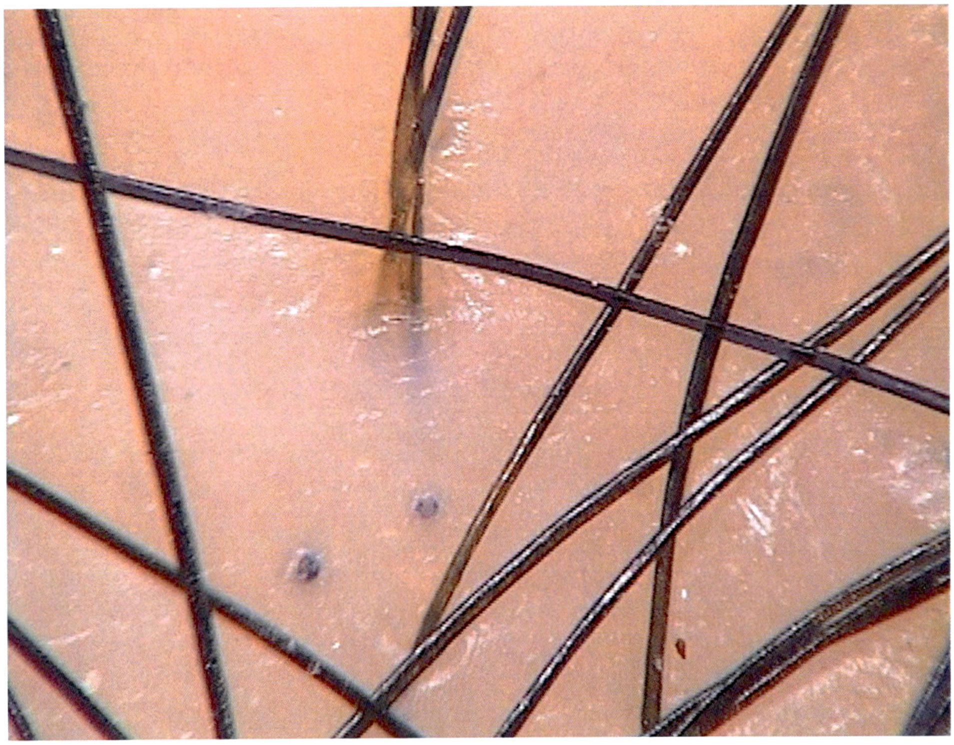

Fig. 26.7 Hair-bearing margins of a patch of pseudopelade of Brocq. Two black dots seen in this area correspond to hair residues. On trichoscopy, pseudopelade of Brocq may be suspected based on the presence of small smooth hairless areas lacking follicular openings when no features indicating other types of cicatricial alopecia (such as tubular perifollicular scaling in lichen planopilaris, starburst pattern hyperplasia in folliculitis decalvans, or large arborizing vessels in discoid lupus erythematosus) are present. The main trichoscopic differential diagnoses are late-stage cicatricial alopecia of other origin and longstanding alopecia areata (×70)

References

1. Alzolibani AA, Kang H, Otberg N, Shapiro J. Pseudopelade of Brocq. Dermatol Ther. 2008;21(4):257–63.
2. Price V, Mirmirani P, editors. Cicatricial alopecia: an approach to diagnosis and management. New York: Springer; 2011.
3. Kluger N, Assouly P. Pseudopelade of Brocq [in French]. Ann Dermatol Venereol. 2011;138(5):430–3; quiz 429, 434.
4. Brocq L, Lenglet E, Ayrignac J. Recherches sur l'alopecie atrophiante, variete pseudo-pelade. Ann Dermatol Syphil (France). 1905;6: 1–32.
5. Trueb RM. Systematic approach to hair loss in women. J Dtsch Dermatol Ges. 2010;8(4):284–97, 298.
6. Yu M, Bell RH, Ross EK, Lo BK, Isaac-Renton M, Martinka M, et al. Lichen planopilaris and pseudopelade of Brocq involve distinct disease associated gene expression patterns by microarray. J Dermatol Sci. 2010;57(1):27–36.
7. Rudnicka L, Olszewska M, Rakowska A, Slowinska M. Trichoscopy update 2011. J Dermatol Case Rep. 2011;5(4):82–8.

Part IX

Hair Transplantation

Hair Transplantation

27

Malgorzata Olszewska, Adriana Rakowska, and Lidia Rudnicka

Abstract

In most patients, trichoscopy performed after hair transplantation shows no significant abnormalities. However, trichoscopy may be a useful tool for early differential diagnosis of surgical complications. Posttransplant folliculitis appears as yellowish, well-demarcated areas surrounding emerging hair shafts. In secondary lichen planopilaris, trichoscopy shows typical features of the disease, such as perifollicular scaling and areas lacking follicular openings. Performed before hair transplantation, trichoscopy may be useful in detecting features of prodromal lichen planopilaris and predicting possible risk for this complication.

Keywords

Arborizing vessels • Folliculitis • Folliculitis decalvans • Frontal fibrosing alopecia • Hair transplantation • Hair restoration • Lichen planopilaris • Perifollicular inflammation Perifollicular scaling • Pili torti

Hair transplantation is a surgical method for restoring hair in female and male patients with androgenetic alopecia. Occasionally, this method is used in patients with inactive scarring alopecia.

The first hair transplantation for male androgenetic alopecia was performed in 1952 by Orentreich. In 1984, the minigrafting technique was initiated, and in 1995 follicular unit transplantation was introduced [1]. Today, the technique of follicular unit transplantation is a standard procedure [2, 3].

There currently are no reports on trichoscopy in hair transplant patients. Our experience shows that in most patients, trichoscopy performed after hair transplantation shows no significant abnormalities. Minor indications of a prior hair transplantation include accentuation of hair follicle openings and a tendency for transplanted thick terminal hairs to grow in slightly different directions compared with local thin hairs ("signpost sign"). Minimal posttransplant perifollicular fibrosis may induce hair shaft structure abnormalities, such as hair twisting and curling. Pili torti may be observed after successful hair transplantation. Large arborizing vessels occasionally are seen at grafting sites.

Trichoscopy also may be applied in the differential diagnosis of surgical complications. According to Salanitri et al. [4], who analyzed a large series of 533 hair transplantations in 425 patients, the rate of surgical complications is 4.7 %. Folliculitis that resolves without sequelae is one of the most common complications [4]. These lesions may be observed on trichoscopy as yellowish, relatively well-demarcated areas surrounding emerging hair shafts.

Lichen planopilaris developing after hair transplantation has been reported; Chiang et al. [5] described seven such cases. Both types of the disease affecting the scalp—classic lichen planopilaris and frontal fibrosing alopecia—have been observed. The authors suggest that this disease may be induced by surgical trauma in the form of Koebner phenom-

M. Olszewska
Department of Dermatology,
Medical University of Warsaw, Warsaw, Poland

A. Rakowska
Department of Dermatology, CSK MSW, Warsaw, Poland

L. Rudnicka (✉)
Faculty of Health Sciences, Medical University of Warsaw, Poland

Department of Dermatology, CSK MSW, Woloska 137,
Warsaw 02-502, Poland
e-mail: lidia.rudnicka@euderm.eu

L. Rudnicka et al. (eds.), *Atlas of Trichoscopy*,
DOI 10.1007/978-1-4471-4486-1_27, © Springer-Verlag London 2012

enon. In these patients, trichoscopy shows typical features of the respective disease (classic lichen planopilaris and/or frontal fibrosing alopecia). Other cases of lichen planopilaris after hair restoration surgery were described by Kossard and Shiell [6] and Crisóstomo et al. [7]. Trichoscopy was not performed in these cases.

Our experience shows that patients who develop lichen planopilaris after hair transplantation tend to have more pronounced perifollicular erythema compared with other patients with the disease. This most probably corresponds to pronounced lichenoid inflammation concentrated around the infundibulum of the involved hair follicles, as observed by Kossard et al. [6].

The coexistence of trichoscopic features of lichen planopilaris with those of folliculitis decalvans occasionally may be observed. Thus far, only one case of true folliculitis decalvans after hair transplantation has been reported. In that case, folliculitis decalvans developed 20 years after hair restoration surgery with punch grafts [8].

In conclusion, in most patients who have undergone follicular unit transplantation, trichoscopy shows no abnormalities. Trichoscopy may be useful in the early differential diagnosis of surgical complications and for detecting features of prodromal lichen planopilaris before surgery.

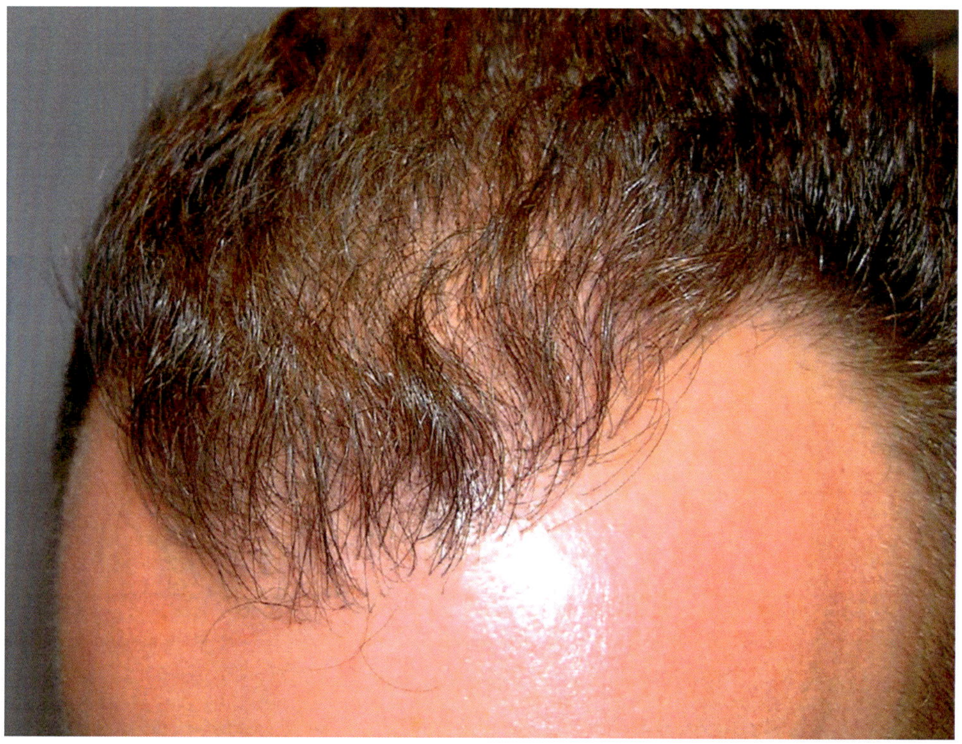

Fig. 27.1 A patient with androgenetic alopecia after follicular unit hair transplantation. In such cases, trichoscopy usually shows no abnormalities. Current data indicate that trichoscopy may be rather useful in the early differential diagnosis of surgical complications. In our opinion, trichoscopy also should be performed before hair transplantation. This would allow one to (1) verify the clinical diagnosis, (2) exclude unknown causes of hair loss coexisting with androgenetic alopecia, and (3) exclude features of prodromal lichen planopilaris and predict possible risk for this complication

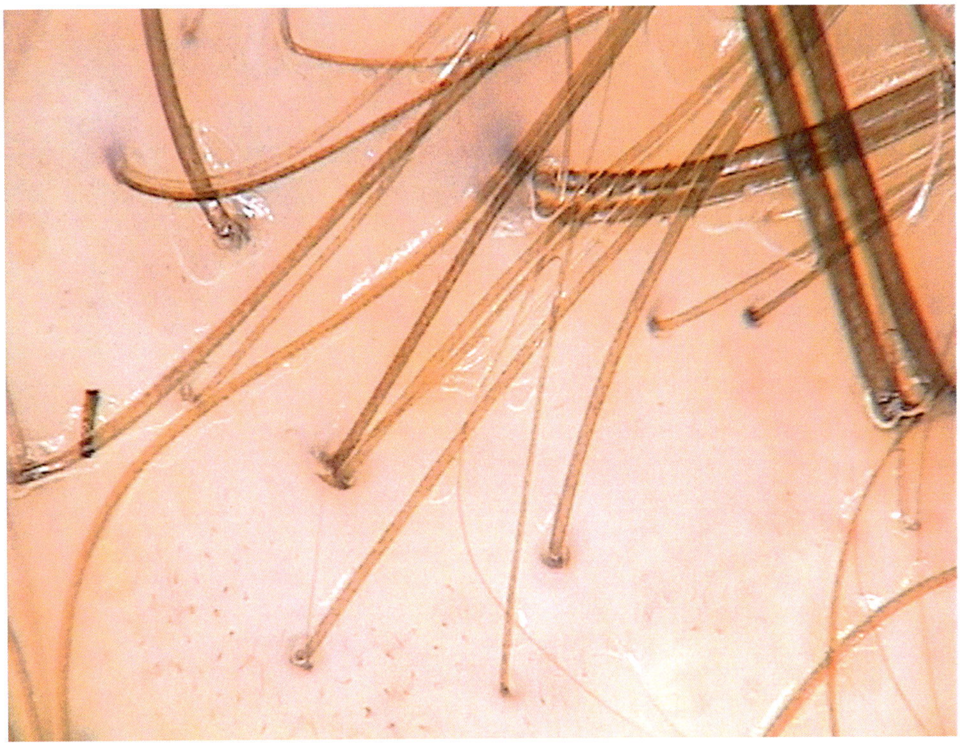

Fig. 27.2 Normal trichoscopy of the recipient area after hair transplantation. Transplanted follicular units consist of thick terminal hairs growing in different directions. Accentuation of the follicular opening is visible. Trichoscopic features of androgenetic alopecia are present despite clinically successful surgery. Hair shaft thickness heterogeneity, thin hairs, and yellow dots are visible in this image (×70)

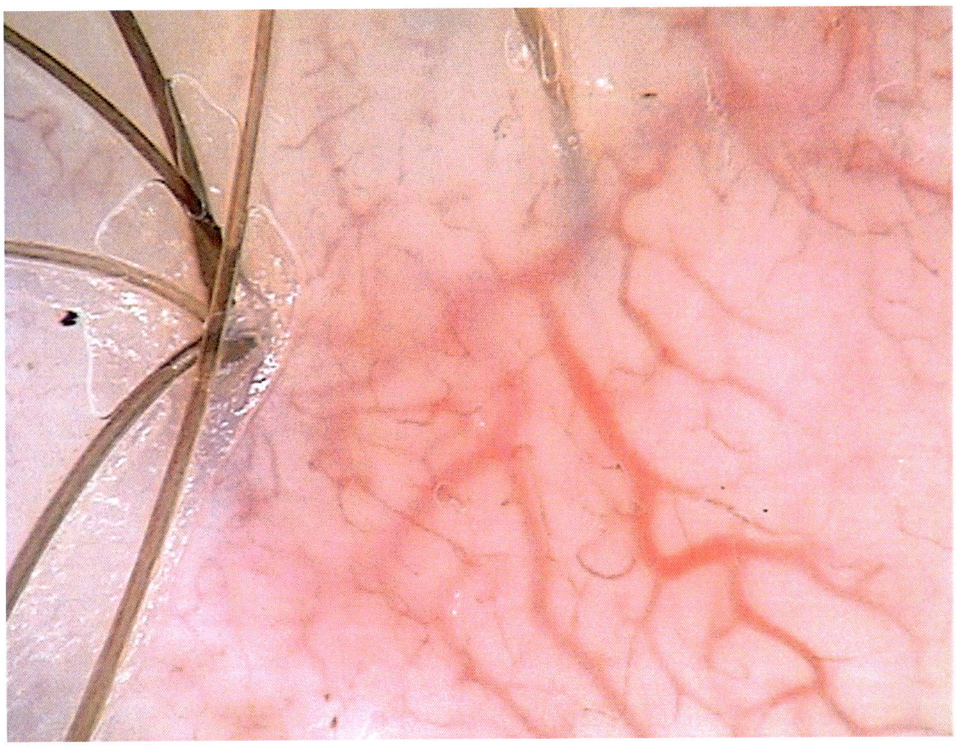

Fig. 27.3 Recipient area after hair transplantation. A follicular unit with four hairs was transplanted into this area. Each hair in this unit is growing in a different direction. This distinguishes transplanted follicular units from natural ones, in which all the hairs in one follicular unit grow in the same direction. We call this characteristic feature of transplanted follicular units the *signpost sign*. Large arborizing vessels result from the formation of an atrophic scar. Note that such scars are a few millimeters in diameter and may not be visible macroscopically (×70)

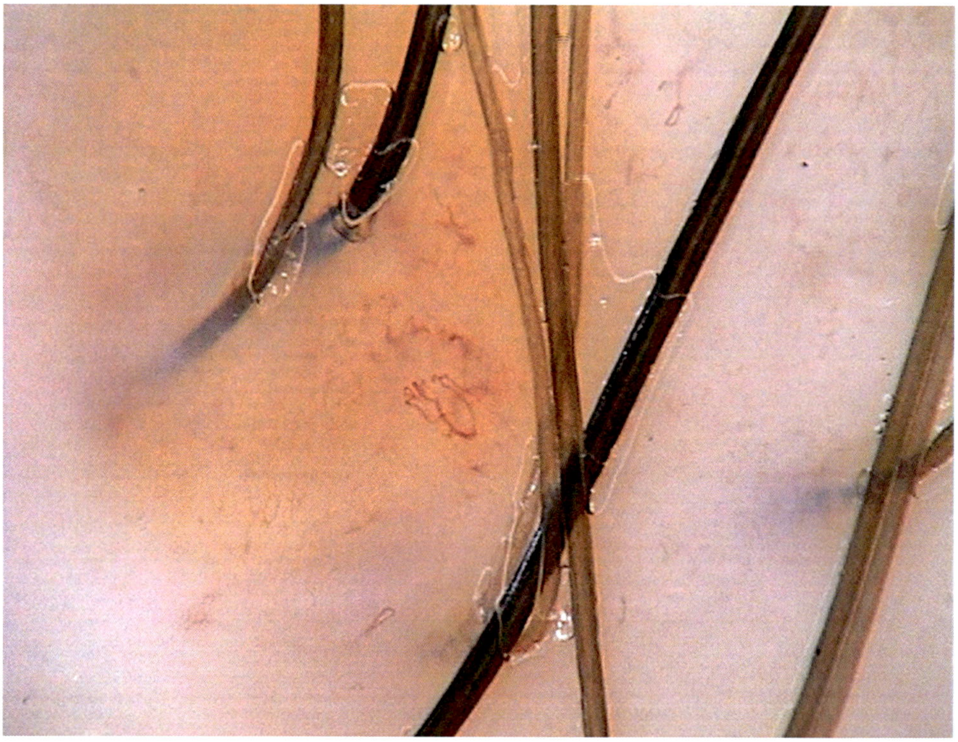

Fig. 27.4 Folliculitis after hair transplantation. Folliculitis developing after follicular unit transplantation presents as pustules that appear as relatively well-demarcated yellowish areas surrounding the grafted follicular unit. The whitish area adjacent to the transplanted follicular unit indicates early fibrosis. These pustules closely resemble the follicular pustules observed in folliculitis decalvans (×70)

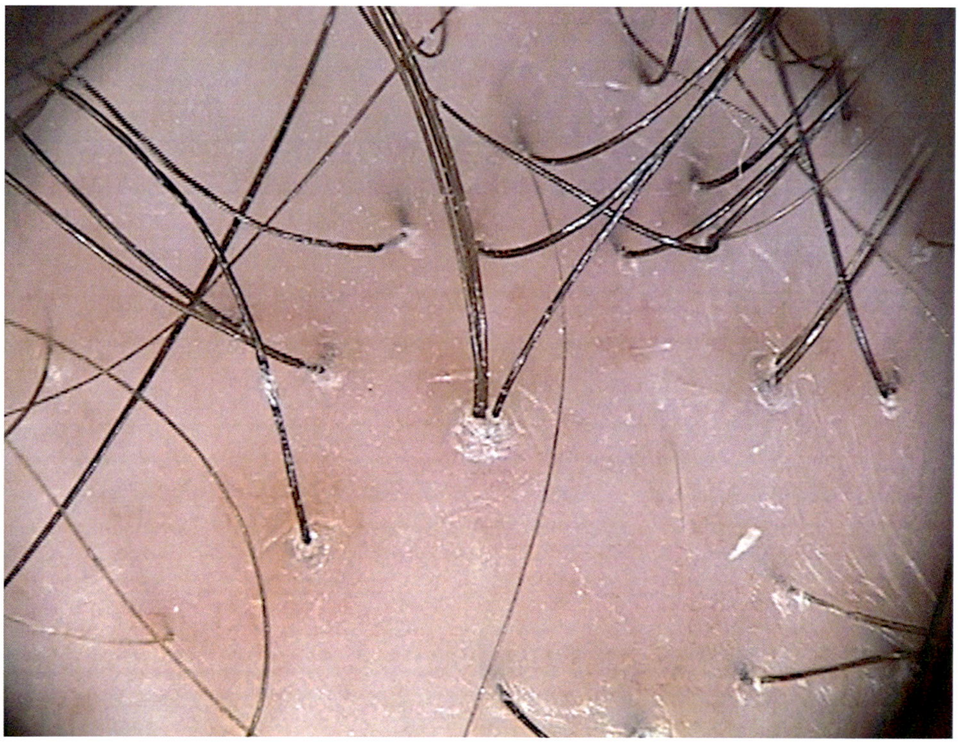

Fig. 27.5 Lichen planopilaris after hair transplantation. A 30-year-old male patient with androgenetic alopecia developed cicatricial alopecia a few months after follicular unit transplantation. Trichoscopy shows features of lichen planopilaris: areas lacking follicular openings, perifollicular scaling, and the whitish red background color of early fibrosis. Perifollicular erythema is more common in patients with lichen planopilaris associated with transplantation than in other patients with this disease (×20)

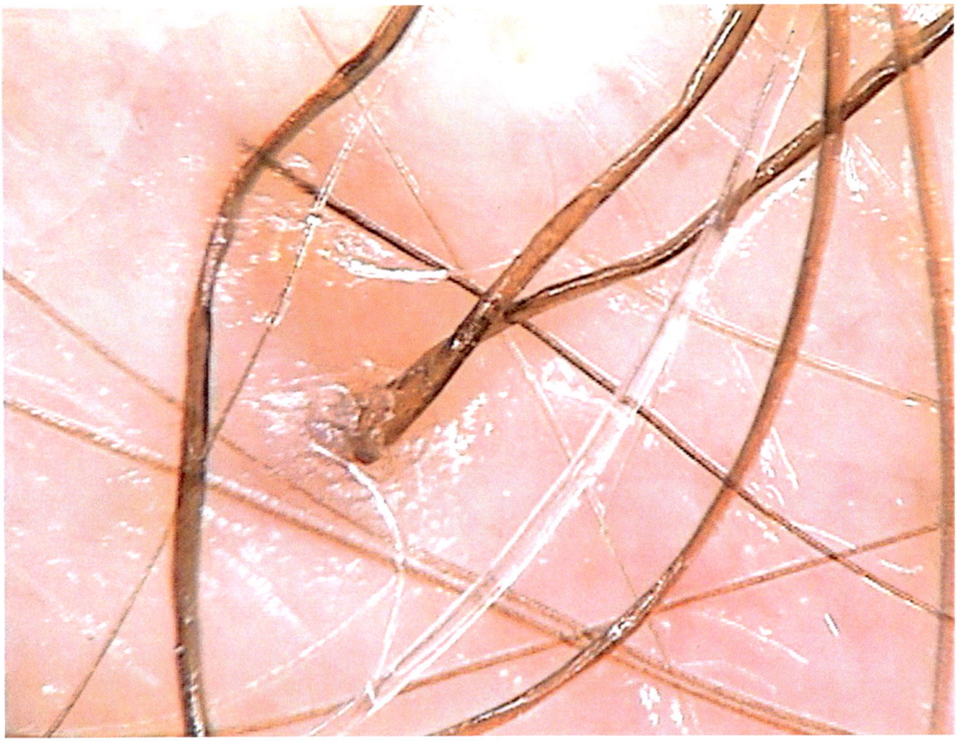

Fig. 27.6 Pili torti after hair transplantation. Inflammation or scarring surrounding the transplanted follicular unit may result in hair shaft twisting and curling. This image shows pili torti and other hair shaft abnormalities in a 42-year-old woman who developed chronic perifollicular inflammation after a follicular unit transplantation (×70)

References

1. Bernstein RM, Rassman WR. The logic of follicular unit transplantation. Dermatol Clin. 1999;17(2):277–95, viii; discussion 296.
2. Rose PT. The latest innovations in hair transplantation. Facial Plast Surg. 2011;27(4):366–77.
3. Sadick NS, White MP. Basic hair transplantation: 2007. Dermatol Ther. 2007;20(6):436–47.
4. Salanitri S, Goncalves AJ, Helene Jr A, Lopes FH. Surgical complications in hair transplantation: a series of 533 procedures. Aesthet Surg J. 2009;29(1):72–6.
5. Chiang YZ, Tosti A, Chaudhry IH, Lyne L, Farjo B, Farjo N, et al. Lichen planopilaris following hair transplantation and face-lift surgery. Br J Dermatol. 2012;166(3):666–70.
6. Kossard S, Shiell RC. Frontal fibrosing alopecia developing after hair transplantation for androgenetic alopecia. Int J Dermatol. 2005; 44(4):321–3.
7. Crisóstomo MR, Crisóstomo MC, Crisóstomo MG, Gondim VJ, Benevides AN. Hair loss due to lichen planopilaris after hair transplantation: a report of two cases and a literature review. An Bras Dermatol. 2011;86(2):359–62.
8. Otberg N, Wu WY, Kang H, Martinka M, Alzolibani AA, Restrepo I, et al. Folliculitis decalvans developing 20 years after hair restoration surgery in punch grafts: case report. Dermatol Surg. 2009;35(11): 1852–6.

Part X

Infections and Inflammatory Scalp Diseases

Parasitic Scalp Infections

28

Francesco Lacarrubba, Franco Dinotta, and Giuseppe Micali

Abstract

Videodermatoscopy represents a useful noninvasive diagnostic tool for pediculosis and scabies. It is quick and easy to perform and well-accepted by patients, as it does not cause physical or psychological discomfort. Moreover, videodermatoscopic examination may be useful in assessing the activity of different topical treatments and may enhance patient compliance with therapy, showing the presence, persistence, or resolution of the infestation on a monitor.

Keywords

Crab louse • Head louse • Lice • Nits • Parasitic infections • Pediculosis capitis • *Phthirus pubis* • Scabies • *Sarcoptes scabiei*

Pediculosis capitis is a parasitosis caused by *Pediculus humanus* var *capitis* (head louse), a blood-sucking insect and obligate parasite of humans that predominantly affects children aged 4–14 years. The diagnostic clue of pediculosis capitis is represented by identification of lice and/or nits, which may be seen at close-up observation; however, searching for lice is time consuming, and sometimes nits may be overlooked or misdiagnosed as scales of seborrheic dermatitis, debris of hairspray or gel, or hair casts. Dermatoscopy, and particularly videodermatoscopy, may be used as a diagnostic tool, rapidly confirming the diagnosis in some puzzling cases in which parasites and nits may not be easily identified [1]. Videodermatoscopy at low magnification (×10–50) unequivocally shows the presence of lice (Fig. 28.1) and viable nits fixed to the hair shaft (Fig. 28.2). It allows rapid differentiation among scales of different origins or pseudo-nits (Fig. 28.3), as well as more detailed identification of full-versus-empty, nonviable nits (Fig. 28.4), the latter appearing as translucent structures with a plane and fissured free ending, thus providing useful information about therapeutic response [1]. Videodermatoscopy does not require hair pulling, so a large scalp area may be investigated with minimal discomfort for the patient. Moreover, videodermatoscopic examination may enhance patient compliance with therapy by showing the presence, persistence, or resolution of the infestation on a monitor. Finally, videodermatoscopy also allows "in vivo" evaluation of the movements and physiology of lice and nits and may be useful in assessing the pediculocidal activity of different topical products [2, 3].

The diagnostic effectiveness of videodermatoscopy may be extended to phthiriasis pubis due to *Phthirus pubis* (crab louse); both lice and nits may rarely be found on the margin of the scalp (Fig. 28.5), especially in children, who lack pubic hair.

Scabies is a parasitic infestation caused by *Sarcoptes scabiei* var *hominis*. Scalp involvement generally is limited to newborn and immunocompromised patients. Scalp localization is rare in adult immunocompetent patients but may be responsible for some cases of persistent infestation, representing the reservoir of the mite, as this site generally is spared from standard therapies. Videodermatoscopy is a useful noninvasive technique for diagnosing scabies [1, 4, 5]; it easily may be used for routine observation of the scalp, especially in cases that are persistent or resistant to therapy [6]. Videodermatoscopy allows detailed inspection of the

F. Lacarrubba • F. Dinotta
Dermatology Clinic, University of Catania, Catania, Italy

G. Micali, M.D. (✉)
Dermatology Clinic, University of Catania,
A.O.U. Policlinico-Vittorio Emanuele, Via Santa Sofia 78,
Catania 95123, Italy
e-mail: cldermct@nti.it

L. Rudnicka et al. (eds.), *Atlas of Trichoscopy*,
DOI 10.1007/978-1-4471-4486-1_28, © Springer-Verlag London 2012

scalp with rapid and clear detection of the diagnostic features of scabies, such as burrows and mites at magnifications ranging from ×40 to ×200 (Figs. 28.6 and 28.7) and eggs or feces at higher magnifications (up to×600). False negative results are rare, and there is no chance of false positive results, as the images obtained are unequivocal. In most cases, it is possible to detect mites moving inside the burrows. Videodermatoscopy is quick and easy to perform and is well-accepted by patients, as it does not cause physical or psychological discomfort. Moreover, it may be useful for nontraumatic screening of family members and for post-therapeutic follow-up [3, 7].

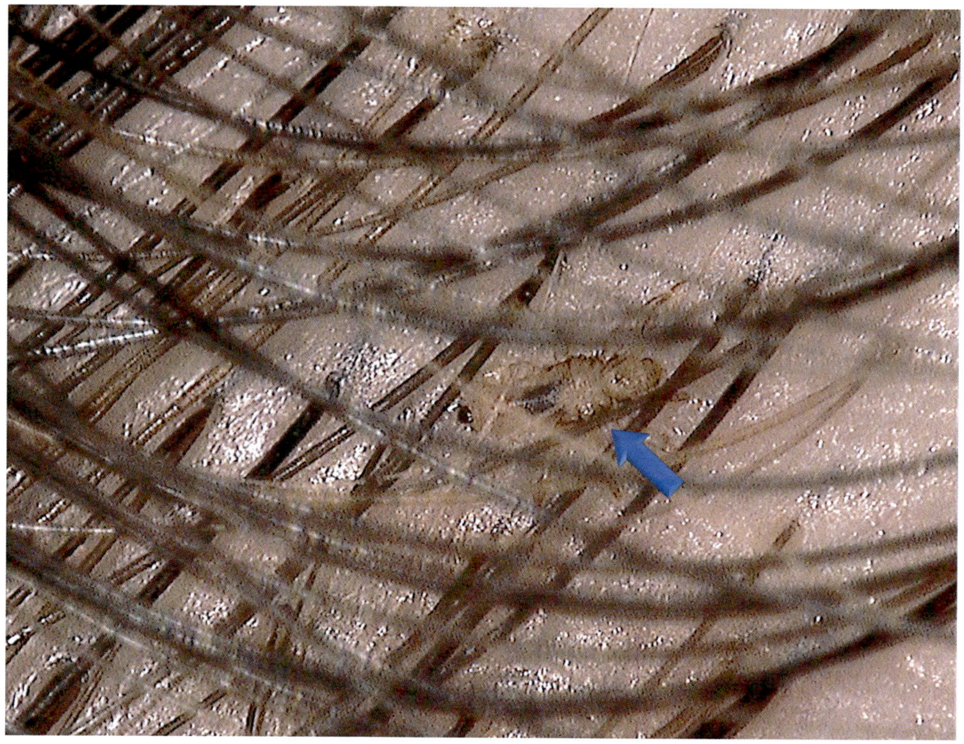

Fig. 28.1 Head lice. Shown is the scalp of a patient with infestation of *Pediculus capitis* (*arrow*), a blood-sucking insect and obligate parasite of humans. *P. capitis* is 1–3 mm long, is dorsoventrally flattened, and has three pairs of legs (×50)

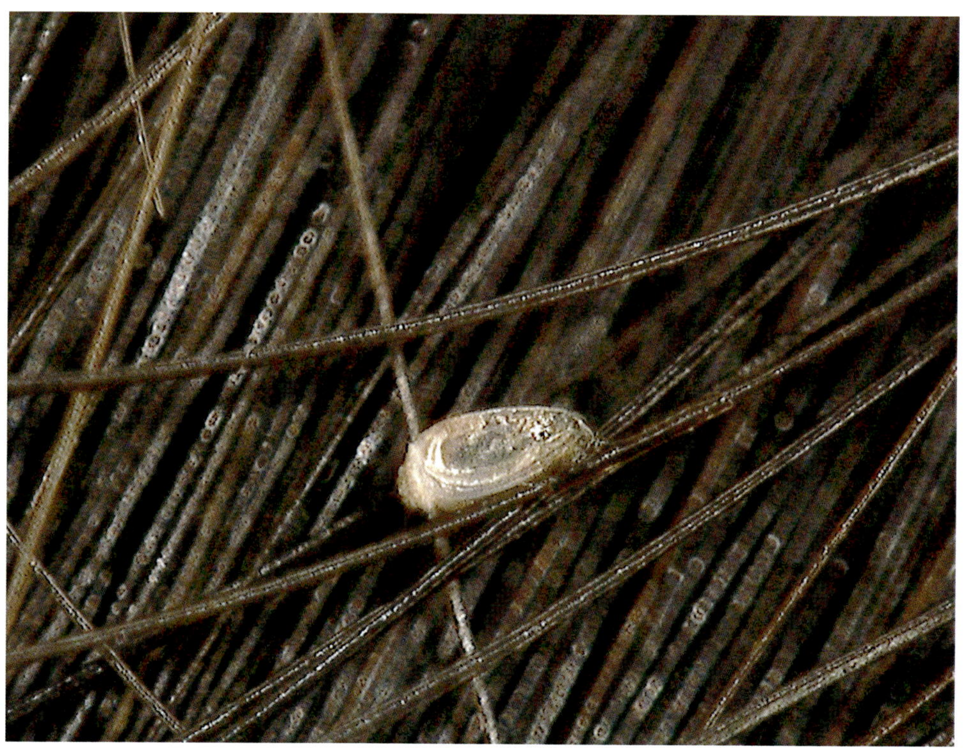

Fig. 28.2 Head lice. A full, viable nit of *P. capitis* fixed to the hair shaft, appearing as an opaque structure with a convex free ending (×50)

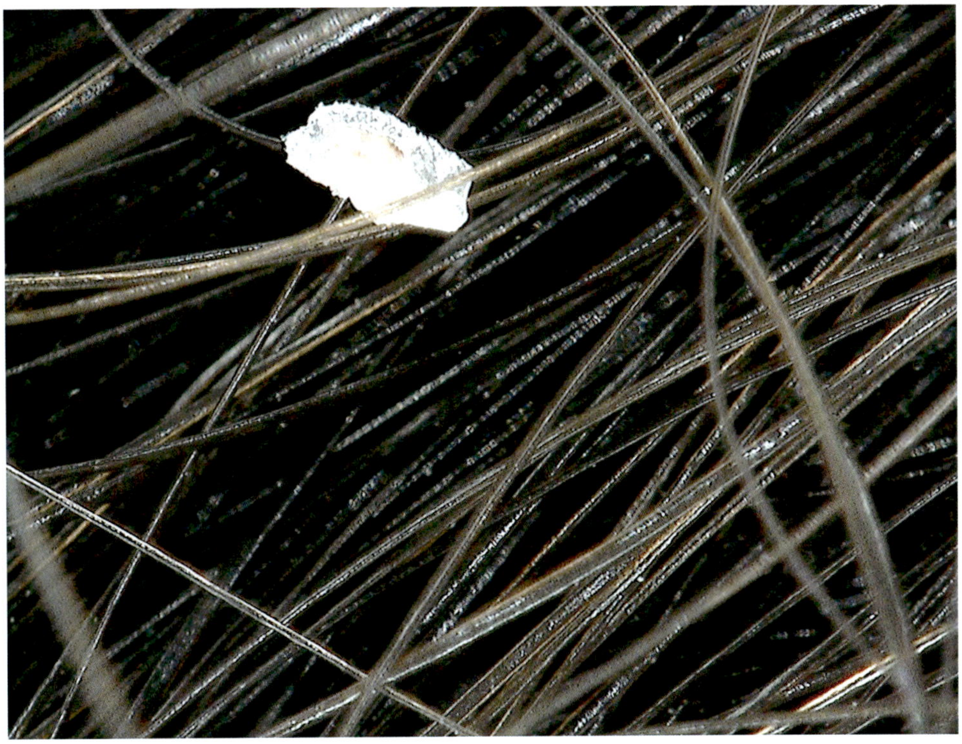

Fig. 28.3 Pseudo-nit. Shown is a scale of seborrheic dermatitis. Pseudo-nits also include debris of hairspray or gel and hair casts, and sometimes are misdiagnosed as nits on simple naked-eye observation (×50)

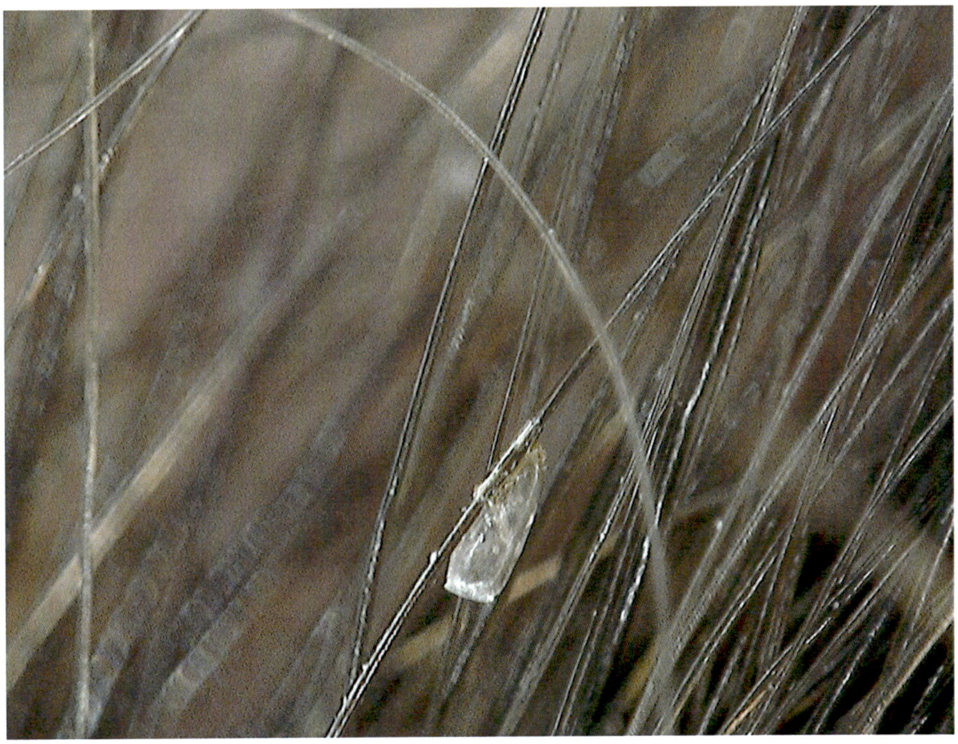

Fig. 28.4 Head lice. Shown is an empty, nonviable nit of *P. capitis* fixed to a hair shaft, appearing as a translucent structure with a plane and fissured free ending (×50)

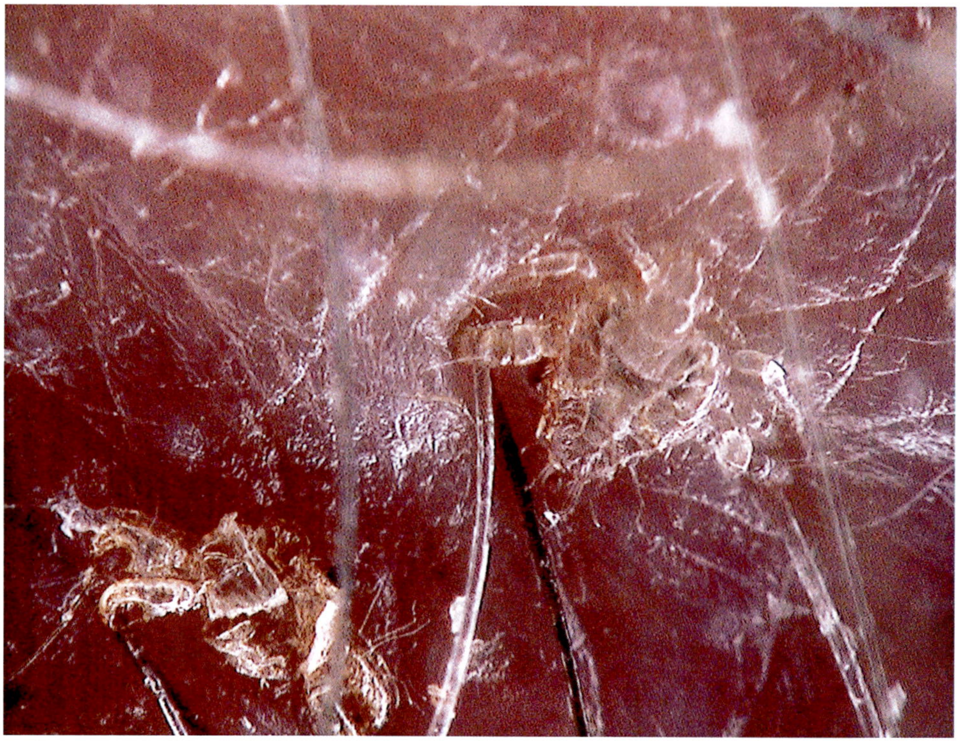

Fig. 28.5 Crab lice. Margin of the scalp showing the presence of two samples of *Phthirus pubis*. Rarely, the louse and nits may be found in this body area, especially in children, who lack pubic hair (×50)

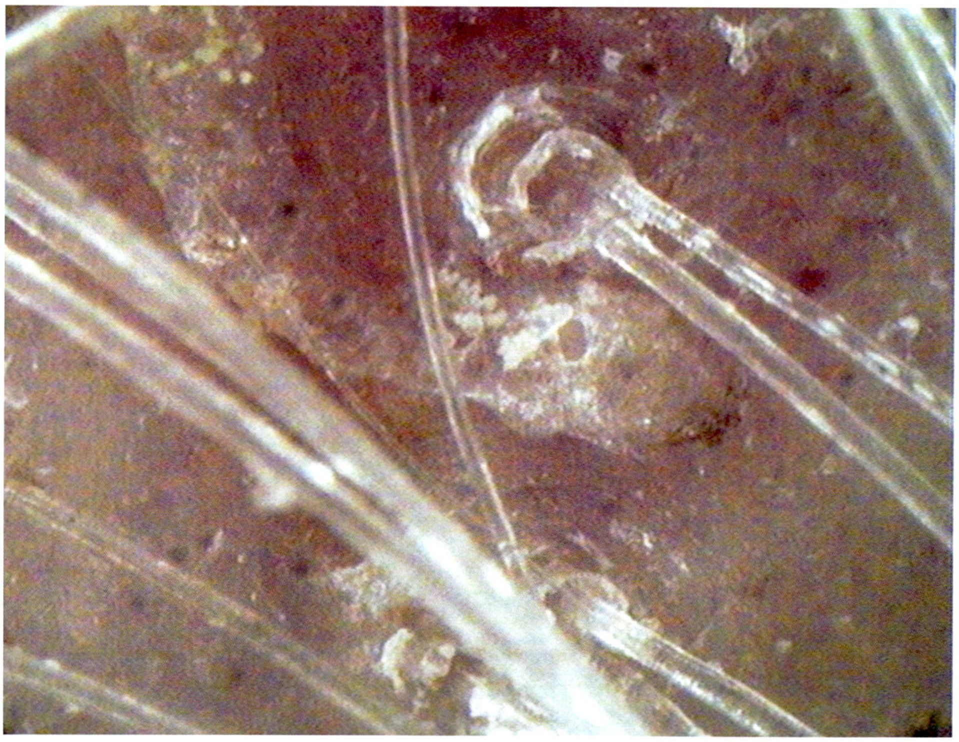

Fig. 28.6 Scabies. Burrow on the scalp with the presence of the roundish body of *Sarcoptes scabiei* at the extremity. Scalp involvement of scabies is rare in adult immunocompetent patients but may be responsible for some cases of persistent infestation, representing the reservoir of the mite (×200)

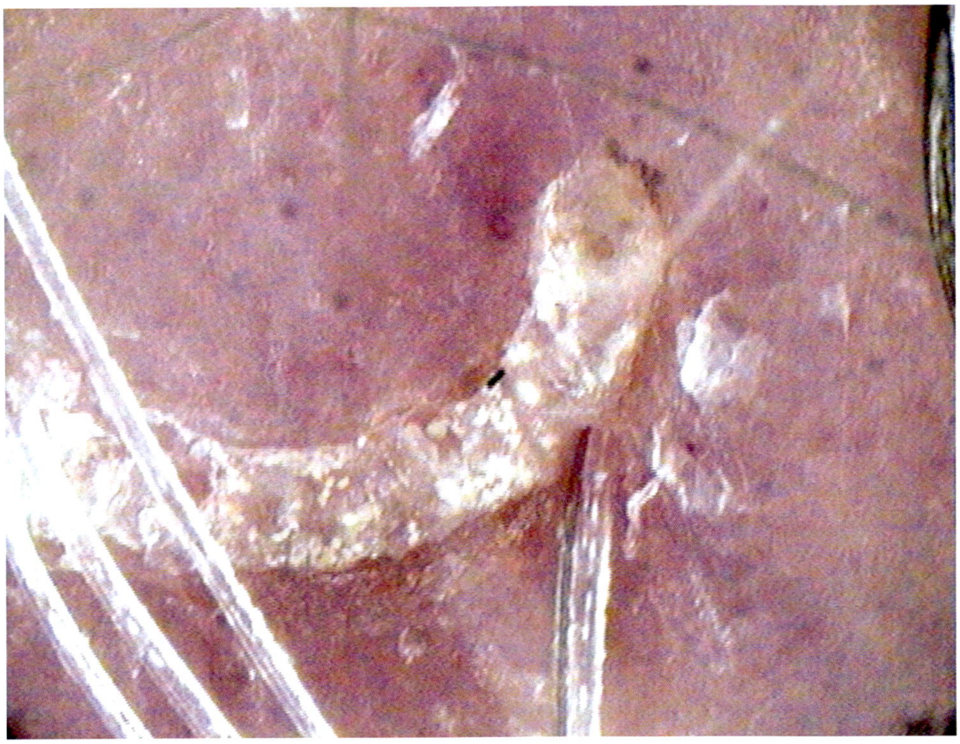

Fig. 28.7 **Scabies**. Shown is a burrow on the scalp containing the roundish body of *Sarcoptes scabiei* with a darkened head part (×200)

References

1. Micali G, Lacarrubba F, Massimino D, Schwartz RA. Dermatoscopy: alternative uses in daily clinical practice. J Am Acad Dermatol. 2011;64:1135–46.
2. Lacarrubba F, Nardone B, Milani M, Botta G, Micali G. Head lice: ex vivo videodermatoscopy evaluation of the pediculocidal activity of two different topical products. G Ital Dermatol Venereol. 2006;141:233–5.
3. Micali G, Tedeschi A, West DP, Dinotta F, Lacarrubba F. The use of videodermatoscopy to monitor treatment of scabies and pediculosis. J Dermatol Treat. 2011;22:133–7.
4. Micali G, Lacarrubba F, Lo Guzzo G. Scraping versus videodermatoscopy for the diagnosis of scabies: a comparative study. Acta Derm Venereol. 2000;79:396.
5. Lacarrubba F, Musumeci ML, Caltabiano R, Impallomeni R, West DP, Micali G. High-magnification videodermatoscopy: a new noninvasive diagnostic tool for scabies in children. Pediatr Dermatol. 2001;18:439–41.
6. Lacarrubba F, Micali G. Videodermatoscopy enhances the diagnostic capability in a case of scabies of the scalp. G Ital Dermatol Venereol. 2008;143:351–2.
7. Micali G, Lacarrubba F, Tedeschi A. Videodermatoscopy enhances the ability to monitor efficacy of scabies treatment and allows optimal timing of drug application. J Eur Acad Dermatol. 2004;18:153–4.

Tinea Capitis

29

Lidia Rudnicka, Jacek C. Szepietowski, Monika Slowinska, Malgorzata Lukomska, Malgorzata Maj, and Ana Maria Costa Pinheiro

Abstract

Typical trichoscopic features of tinea capitis are comma hairs and corkscrew hairs. Other commonly observed abnormalities are interrupted, Morse code hairs; block hairs; i-hairs; and zigzag hairs. Tinea capitis favosa does not affect the hair structure significantly. The most characteristic trichoscopic feature of tinea capitis favosa is the presence of large amorphous yellow areas and large wax-colored perifollicular areas. Ultraviolet-enhanced trichoscopy, which uses the effect of Wood's light, increases the diagnostic potential of trichoscopy.

Keywords

Black dots • Cicatricial alopecia • Comma hairs • Corkscrew hairs • Favus • i-Hairs • Tinea capitis • Tinea capitis favosa • Morse code hairs • Tufted folliculitis • Ultraviolet-enhanced trichoscopy • Wood's light • Zigzag hairs

Tinea capitis is a fungal infection of the scalp and hair [1]. Children are most commonly affected. *Microsporum* and *Trichophyton* are the genera most commonly associated with tinea capitis [2].

According to a morphologic classification, three types of *in vivo* hair invasion are distinguished: ectothrix, endothrix, and favus. In ectothrix, fungal hyphae and arthroconidia cover the outside of the hair up to the zone of keratinization and may damage the hair cuticle. In endothrix, the hair shaft is filled with fungal hyphae and arthroconidia. All elements of the hair shaft may be weakened. In favus (endothrix favosa), caused most frequently by *Trichophyton schoenleinii*, hair invasion is associated with formation of characteristic air spaces within the infected hair shaft [3–6].

A clinical classification also distinguishes three types of tinea capitis: noninflammatory, inflammatory, and favus. Noninflammatory (epidemic) tinea capitis most frequently is caused by anthropophilic fungi and predominantly affects children. Foci of short hairs broken at different lengths and black dots are characteristic clinical features. Minimal scaling may be present. Noninflammatory tinea capitis due to *Microsporum canis* may be associated with subtle erythema. Inflammatory tinea capitis usually is caused by zoophilic or geophilic fungi. Pustules, abscesses, or kerions with or without pustules may be observed. Favus (tinea capitis favosa) presents clinically as crusts and amorphous material containing hair residues, dermatophyte hyphae, and keratin debris. Yellowish white scutula are specific for favus but not always present. Clinically, the hair shafts appear normal. In the late phase of the disease, tinea capitis favosa causes cicatricial hair loss [7–13].

L. Rudnicka (✉)
Faculty of Health Sciences, Medical University of Warsaw, Poland

Department of Dermatology, CSK MSW, Woloska 137, Warsaw 02-502, Poland
e-mail: lidia.rudnicka@euderm.eu

J.C. Szepietowski
Department of Dermatology, Venereology, and Allergology, Medical University (University Hospital), Wroclaw, Poland

M. Slowinska • M. Lukomska • M. Maj
Department of Dermatology, CSK MSW, Warsaw, Poland

A.M.C. Pinheiro
Department of Internal Medicine, Hospital Universitario de Brasilia, Brasilia, Brazil

L. Rudnicka et al. (eds.), *Atlas of Trichoscopy*,
DOI 10.1007/978-1-4471-4486-1_29, © Springer-Verlag London 2012

The diagnosis of tinea capitis is based on microscopic examination of infected hairs and mycologic culture, which allows precise identification of the fungal pathogen.

Examination of the scalp with Wood's light (340–450 nm; peak, 365 nm) may be helpful in diagnosing some forms of tinea capitis. The characteristic bright green fluorescence may be observed in tinea capitis due infection with *Microsporum audouinii*, *M. canis*, *Microsporum distortum*, *Microsporum ferrugineum*, and *Microsporum gypseum*. *T. schoenleinii* fluoresces a faint blue color. *Trichophyton tonsurans* and *Trichophyton verrucosum* do not produce fluorescence on Wood's light examination [14, 15].

The usefulness of trichoscopy as a supplementary method for the differential diagnosis of tinea capitis was first documented in 2008 by Slowinska et al. [16], who described characteristic comma hairs in a patient with tinea capitis due to *M. canis*. Sandoval et al. [17] documented that comma hairs are associated with both the ectothrix and endothrix types of fungal invasion. In their patients, comma hairs were associated with *M. canis* and *T. tonsurans* infection. Hughes et al. [18] described the presence of comma hairs in black patients with tinea capitis due to *Trichophyton violaceum*, *Trichophyton soudanense*, and *Microsporum langeronii*. In patients with *T. soudanense* infection, the hairs were coiled more intensely than typical comma hairs. The authors called this type of abnormality *corkscrew hairs*. All authors have described the presence of broken hairs on trichoscopy of tinea capitis, which is a common but nonspecific finding [16, 18].

Cases of tinea capitis with clinical and trichoscopic features of tufted folliculitis have been described [11, 19].

Ultraviolet (UV)-enhanced trichoscopy, first described in 2011 by Rudnicka et al. [20], is a new method that may help identify tinea capitis. This method is based on trichoscopy, but regular light is replaced by UV light at a wavelength overlapping or partly overlapping Wood's light [20].

Table 29.1 Trichoscopic features of tinea capitis

- Comma hairs (highly characteristic)
- Corkscrew hairs (highly characteristic)
- Interrupted (Morse code) hairs
- Block hairs
- i-Hairs
- Zigzag hairs
- Black dots
- Elongated blood vessels
- Yellow amorphous areas (favus)
- Wax-colored perifollicular areas (favus)

Box 29.1

UV-enhanced trichoscopy combines features of trichoscopy with Wood's light.

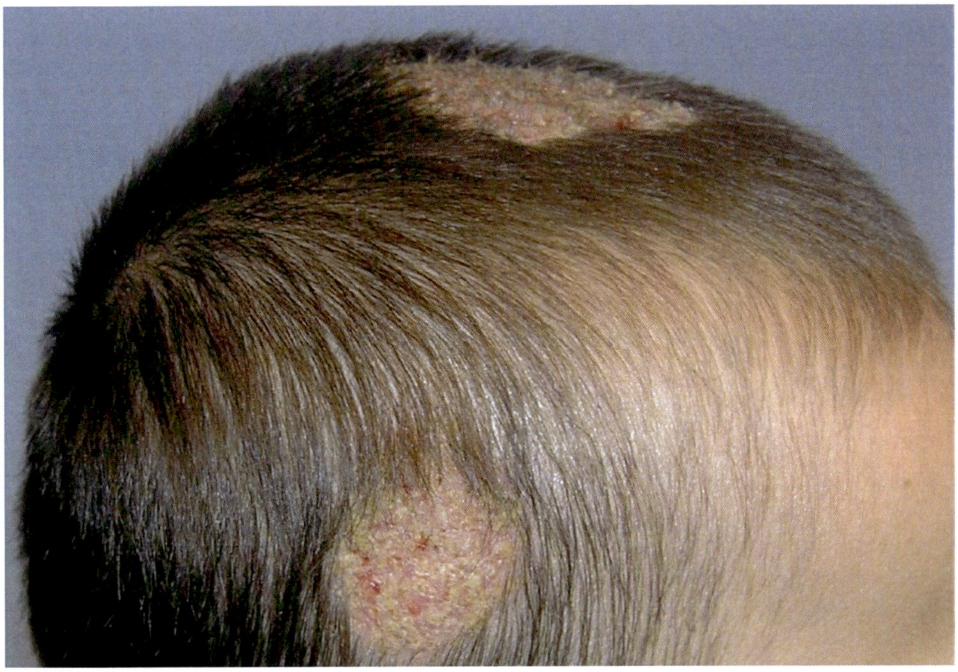

Fig. 29.1 **Tinea capitis**. The clinical presentation of tinea capitis varies depending on the type of fungal infection. The following types of tinea capitis may be distinguished: noninflammatory tinea capitis, inflammatory tinea capitis, and tinea capitis favosa (favus). In noninflammatory tinea capitis, hairs broken at different lengths and black dots may be observed. The term *black dots* refers to the clinical appearance of the abnormality and is not necessarily equivalent to the "black dots" observed on trichoscopy. Minimal scaling and subtle erythema may be present. Inflammatory tinea capitis is characterized by the presence of pustules, abscesses, or kerions (edematous nodules) with or without pustules. In favus (tinea capitis favosa), crusts and a yellowish amorphous discharge are the most frequent clinical findings. The typical scutula and "mousy" smell are not always present. Cicatricial alopecia may develop secondary to tinea capitis favosa. Tinea capitis may mimic folliculitis decalvans: and several other inflammatory scalp diseases

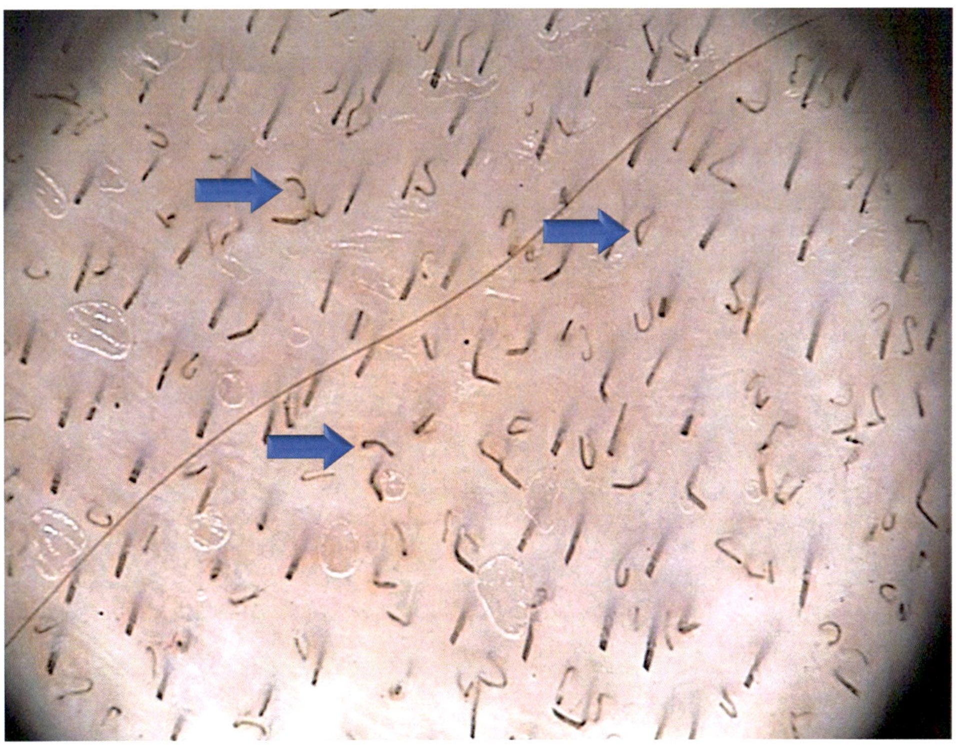

Fig. 29.2 **Comma hairs in tinea capitis**. Focal alopecia with multiple comma hairs (*arrows*) is a characteristic feature of tinea capitis. It has been documented that comma hairs may be associated with both the ectothrix and endothrix types of fungal invasion. Comma hairs have been detected in tinea capitis due to *M. canis*, *M. langeronii*, *T. tonsurans*, *T. violaceum*, and *T. soudanense* [16–18] (×20)

Fig. 29.3 Comma hairs in tinea capitis. Bending of infected hair shafts and formation of comma hairs probably are a result of partial damage to hair shafts filled with hyphae or damage to the hair cuticle [16]. Comma hairs bend and form curved shapes resembling commas. Comma hairs are homogeneous in thickness and evenly pigmented. The *arrow* points to the most characteristic comma hair, but other hairs in this image exhibit a tendency to bend and form comma-like shapes (×70)

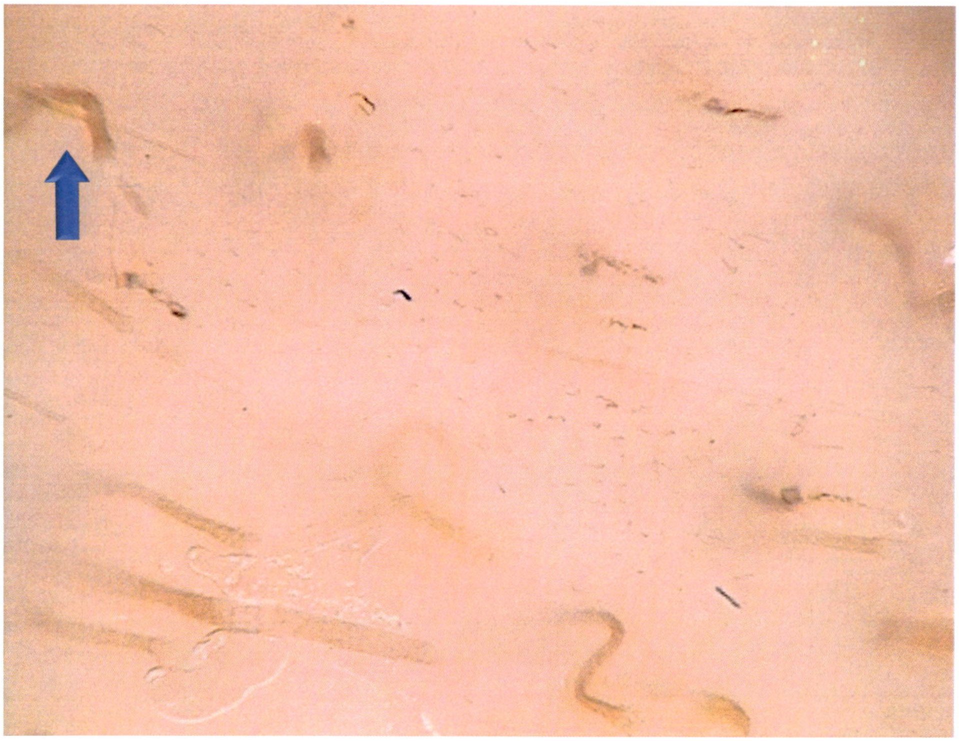

Fig. 29.4 Corkscrew hairs in tinea capitis. Corkscrew hairs observed on trichoscopy of tinea capitis differ from comma hairs by the presence of multiple twists and an intensely coiled shape. These hairs were first described in an African American child with *T. soudanense* infection, but experience has shown that most dermatophytes (of the genera *Trichophyton* and *Microsporum*) may induce formation of corkscrew hairs. This image shows corkscrew hairs (*arrow*) in a Brazilian child with *T. tonsurans* infection (×20)

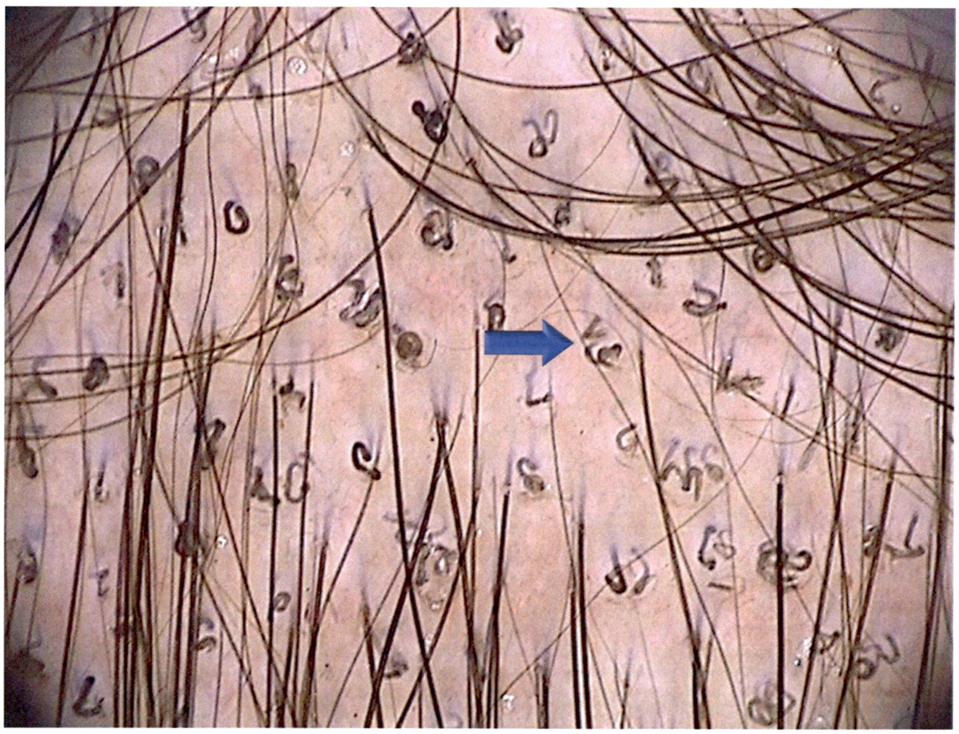

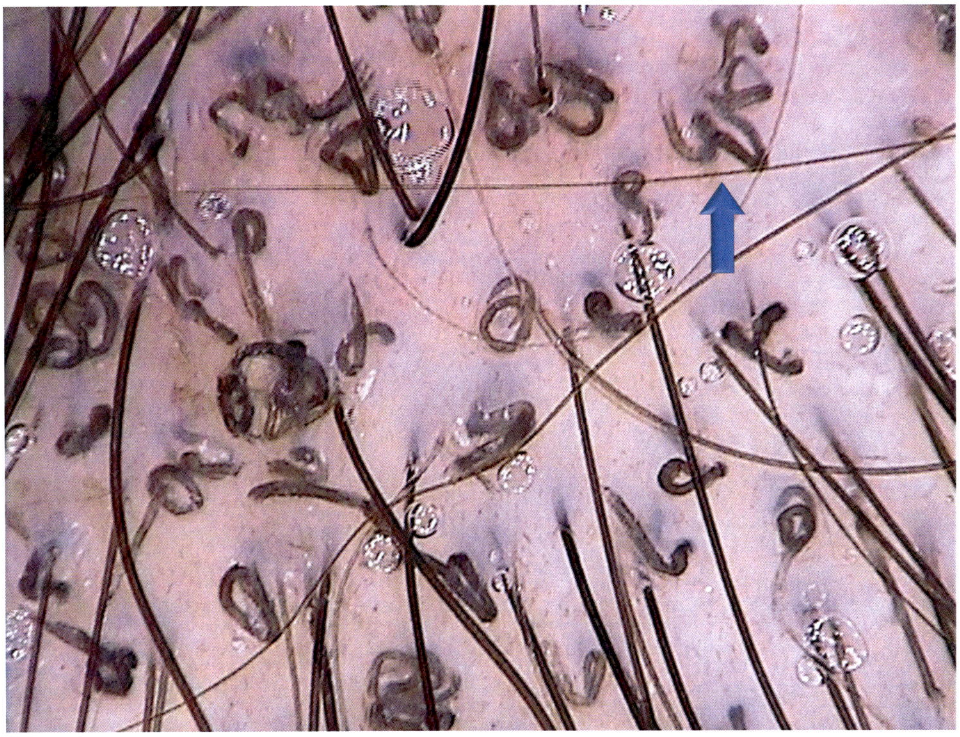

Fig. 29.5 Corkscrew hairs in tinea capitis. The *arrow* points to the most characteristic spiral corkscrew hair, but most hairs in this image have multiple twists and fulfill the definition of corkscrew hairs. The term *corkscrew hairs* in trichoscopy of tinea capitis must be distinguished from the historical meaning of this term. Historically, corkscrew hairs were defined as normal terminal body hairs that curl spontaneously in patients with hypovitaminosis C (scurvy) [21]. These two types of corkscrew hairs share the same name, but their clinical appearance and etiopathogenesis are different (×70)

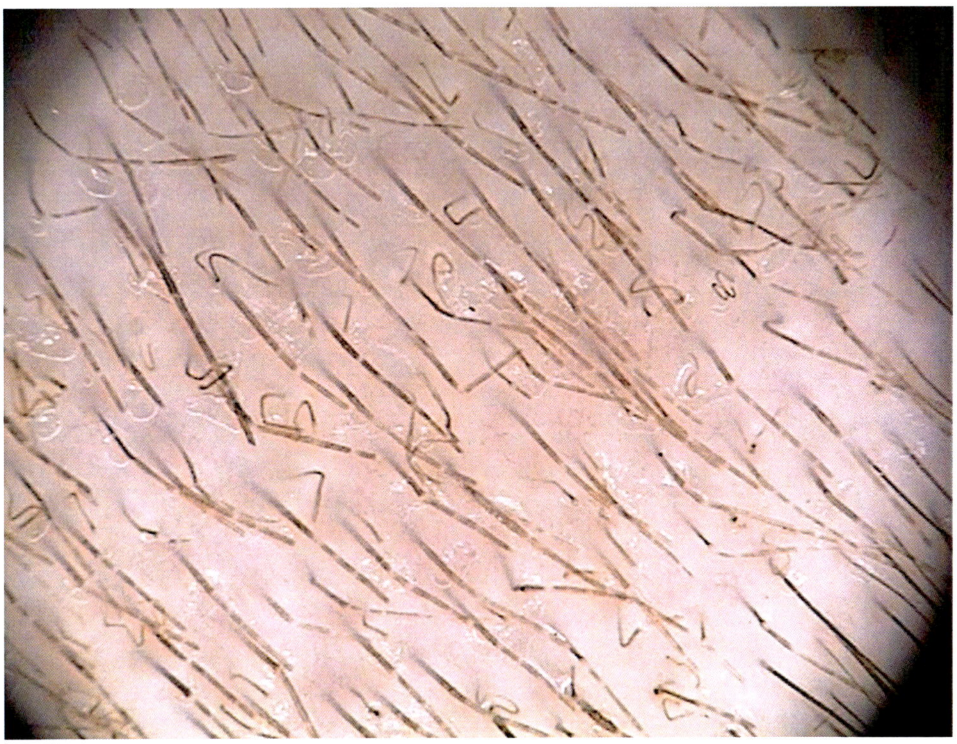

Fig. 29.6 Morse code hairs in tinea capitis. Morse code (or interrupted) hairs are characterized by the presence of multiple transverse bands (gaps) relatively regularly distributed throughout the hair shaft. This trichoscopic image shows trichoscopy in a child with tinea capitis due to *M. canis* (×20)

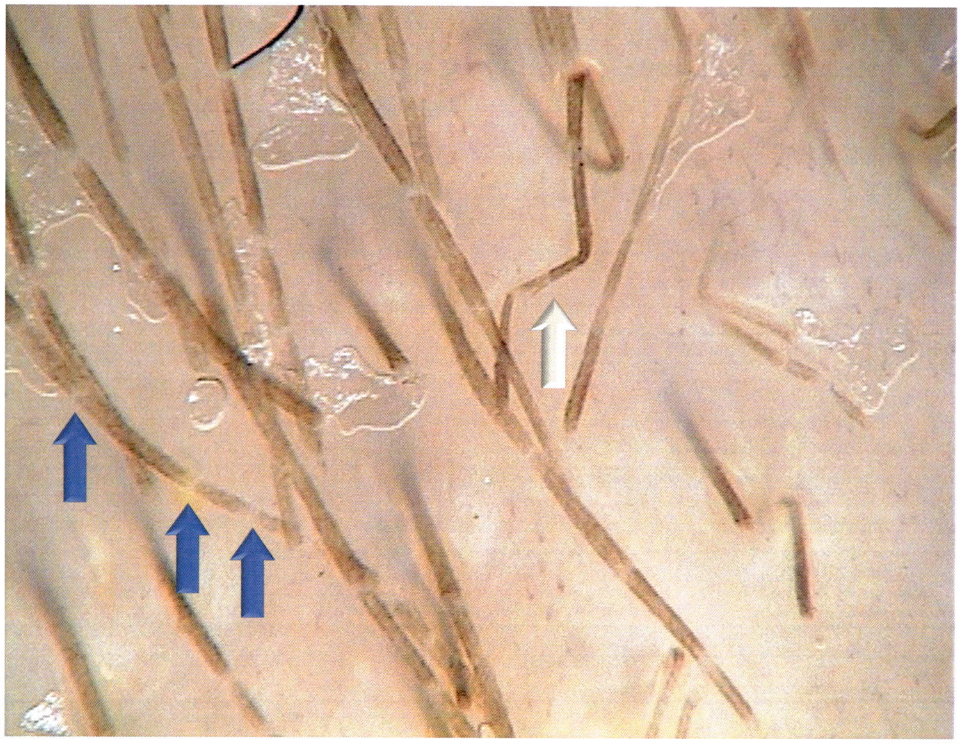

Fig. 29.7 **Morse code hairs and zigzag hairs in tinea capitis**. A high-magnification view of Morse code hairs shows that these hairs have a tendency to bend at points of the transverse bands or gaps (*blue arrows*) and to form zigzag shapes (*white arrow*). Zigzag hairs are sharply bent at multiple points and may fracture easily at the bending sites. The mechanism leading to formation of Morse code and then zigzag hairs in tinea capitis remains unclear. Zigzag hairs are indicative of tinea capitis but also may be seen in other hair and scalp diseases, such as trichorrhexis nodosa, monilethrix, and alopecia areata (×70)

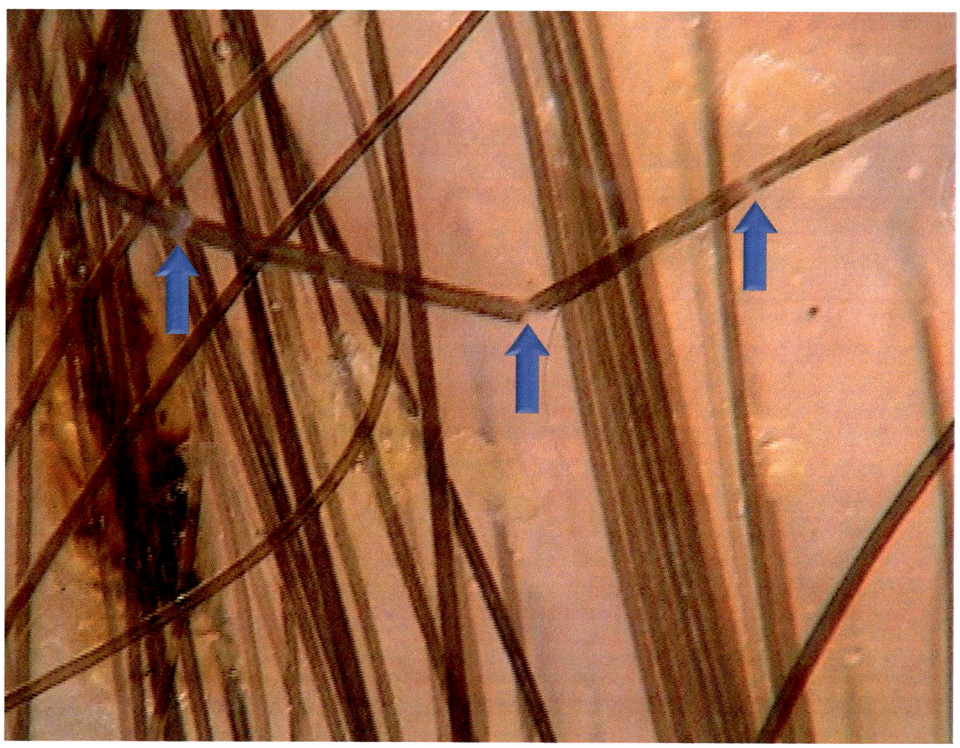

Fig. 29.8 **Morse code hairs and formation of a zigzag hair in tinea capitis**. Transverse bands (gaps) in a Morse code hair are indicated by the *arrows*. These bands may be difficult to distinguish from trichorrhexis nodosa on trichoscopy with immersion fluid. Thus, dry trichoscopy may be performed to aid the differential diagnosis. On dry trichoscopy, tinea capitis bands appear transparent, whereas trichorrhexis nodosa appears white (see Chap. 10 for details). Zigzag hairs resulting from trichorrhexis nodosa may be observed in the early phase of acute alopecia areata (×70)

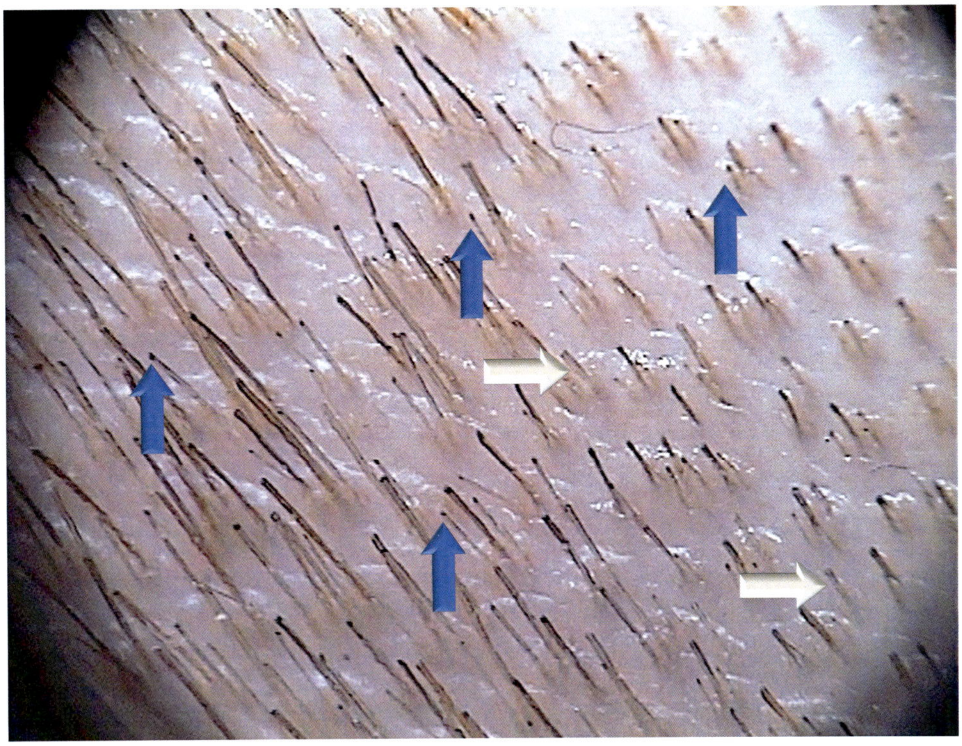

Fig. 29.9 "i-Hairs" in tinea capitis. i-Hairs are short broken hairs with an accentuated distal end (*blue arrows*). There may be a thin hypopigmented band (gap) directly beneath the dark distal end, making these hairs look even more like the letter *i*. Short rectangular hairs with no distal accentuation (*white arrows*) are "block hairs." Shown here is a trichoscopic image of tinea capitis due to *M. canis* (×20)

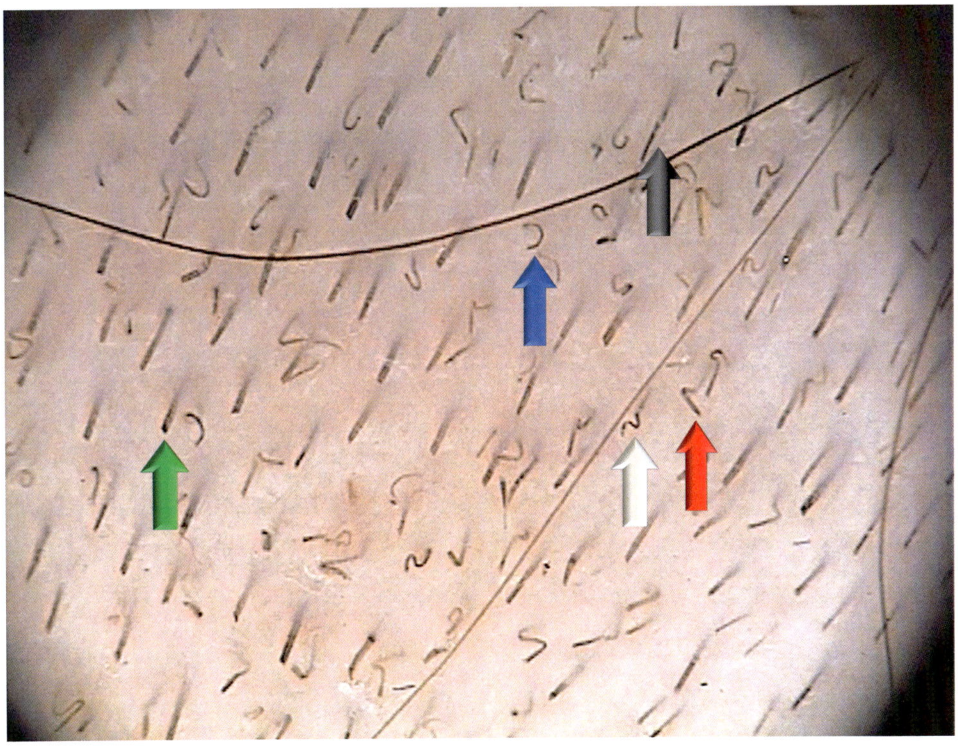

Fig. 29.10 Trichoscopic features of tinea capitis. The typical trichoscopic pattern in tinea capitis includes comma hairs (*blue arrow*), corkscrew hairs (*white arrow*), i-hairs (*green arrow*), interrupted Morse code hairs (*gray arrow*), and zigzag hairs (*red arrow*). At this point, there are no data allowing trichoscopic patterns to be classified according to the type of fungus causing the disease (×20)

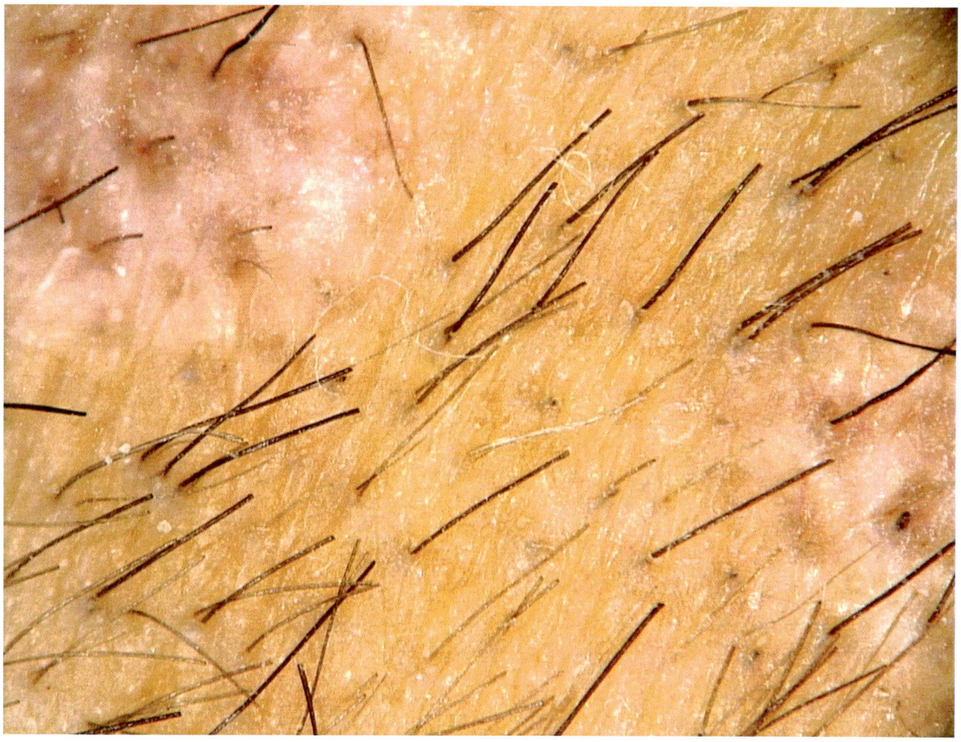

Fig. 29.11 Yellow amorphous areas in tinea capitis favosa (favus). Tinea capitis favosa, caused most frequently by *T. schoenleinii*, shows trichoscopic results that vary greatly among patients with different stages of the disease as well as in different scalp areas of the same patient. Our experience shows that irrespective of typical scutula, large amorphous yellow areas are the most common finding. They are best visible on dry dermoscopy and must be differentiated from similar findings in seborrheic dermatitis and dissecting cellulitis. The hair shafts may be normal, slightly curved, or absent. An early phase of hair loss is visible in the *upper left corner* of the image. Other trichoscopic features of tinea capitis favosa may include yellow scales; big yellow dots lacking hair shafts; large yellowish, wax-colored perifollicular areas; black dots; elongated blood vessels; and, at late stages of the disease, large areas lacking hair (dry trichoscopy, ×20)

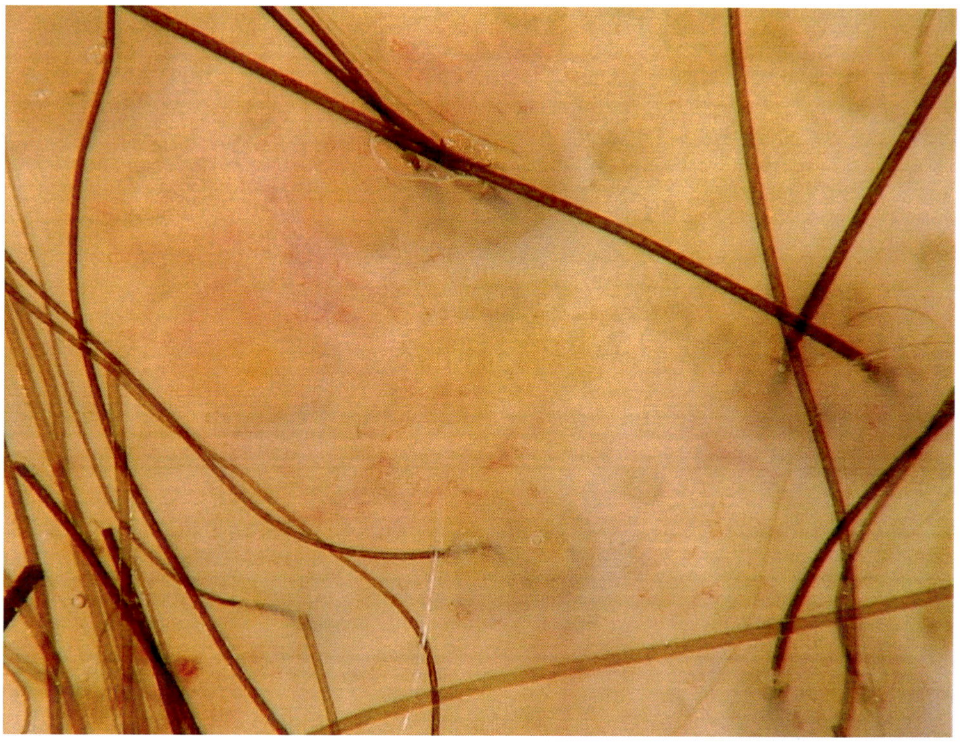

Fig. 29.12 Wax-colored perifollicular areas in tinea capitis favosa (favus). Visible are areas lacking hair shafts; large yellowish, wax-colored perifollicular areas; big yellow dots with a double margin; and yellow amorphous areas. The hair shaft structure rarely is affected in tinea capitis favosa. This image was taken with immersion fluid. Note that the yellowish amorphous area in the midpart of the image presents slightly different features compared with those of the dry trichoscopic image in Fig. 29.11 (×70)

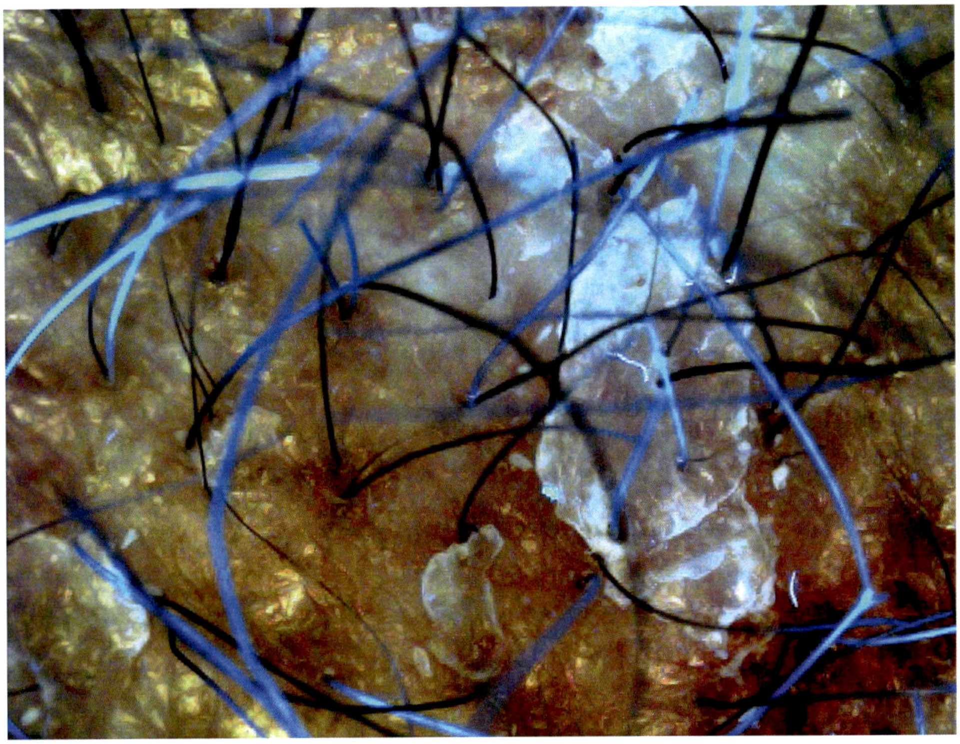

Fig. 29.13 Ultraviolet-enhanced trichoscopy. UV-enhanced trichoscopy is a method that combines trichoscopy with the effect of a Wood's lamp examination. UV light, at a wavelength overlapping or partly overlapping the Wood's light (340–450 nm), induces different types of fluorescence, depending on the type of infection [20]. In this method, the following colors may be expected: dull blue (*T. schoenleinii*); blue green (*M. audouinii*, *M. canis*, *M. ferrugineum*, *M. distortum*); yellow (*M. gypseum*); and orange (*Malassezia furfur*) (Kong UV camera [Bomtech Electronics Co., Seoul, Korea]; ×80)

References

1. Patel GA, Schwartz RA. Tinea capitis: still an unsolved problem? Mycoses. 2011;54(3):183–8.
2. Grimalt R. A practical guide to scalp disorders. J Investig Dermatol Symp Proc. 2007;12(2):10–4.
3. Mebazaa A, Oumari KE, Ghariani N, Mili AF, Belajouza C, Nouira R, et al. Tinea capitis in adults in Tunisia. Int J Dermatol. 2010;49(5):513–6.
4. Ilkit M. Favus of the scalp: an overview and update. Mycopathologia. 2010;170(3):143–54.
5. Sarabi K, Khachemoune A. Tinea capitis: a review. Dermatol Nurs. 2007;19(6):525–9; quiz 30.
6. Niczyporuk W, Krajewska-Kulak E, Lukaszuk C. Tinea capitis favosa in Poland. Mycoses. 2004;47(5–6):257–60.
7. Elewski BE. Tinea capitis: a current perspective. J Am Acad Dermatol. 2000;42(1 Pt 1):1–20; quiz 1–4.
8. Gupta AK, Summerbell RC. Tinea capitis. Med Mycol. 2000; 38(4):255–87.
9. Jankowska-Konsur A, Dylag M, Szepietowski JC. Tinea capitis in southwest Poland. Mycoses. 2009;52(2):193–4.
10. Raszeja-Kotelba B, Adamski Z, Pawlowicz A. A case of tinea favosa capitis caused by Trichophyton schoenleinii. Przegl Dermatol. 1993;80:518–24.
11. Baroni A, Ruocco E, Aiello FS, Faccenda F, Lo Schiavo A, Satriano RA, et al. Tinea capitis mimicking tufted hair folliculitis. Clin Exp Dermatol. 2009;34(8):e699–701.
12. Mirmirani P, Willey A, Chamlin S, Frieden IJ, Price VH. Tinea capitis mimicking cicatricial alopecia: what host and dermatophyte factors lead to this unusual clinical presentation? J Am Acad Dermatol. 2009;60(3):490–5.
13. Szepietowski J. Dermatomycoses and onychomycosis. A practical guide. Krakow: Medycyna Praktyczna; 2001.
14. Asawanonda P, Taylor CR. Wood's Light in dermatology. Int J Dermatol. 1999;38(11):801–7.
15. Wigger-Alberti W, Elsner P. Fluorescence with Wood's light. Current applications in dermatologic diagnosis, therapy follow-up and prevention [in German]. Hautarzt. 1997;48(8):523–7.
16. Slowinska M, Rudnicka L, Schwartz RA, Kowalska-Oledzka E, Rakowska A, Sicinska J, et al. Comma hairs: a dermatoscopic marker for tinea capitis: a rapid diagnostic method. J Am Acad Dermatol. 2008;59(5 Suppl):S77–9.
17. Sandoval AB, Ortiz JA, Rodriguez JM, Vargas AG, Quintero DG. Dermoscopic pattern in tinea capitis [in Spanish]. Rev Iberoam Micol. 2010;27(3):151–2.
18. Hughes R, Chiaverini C, Bahadoran P, Lacour JP. Corkscrew hair: a new dermoscopic sign for diagnosis of tinea capitis in black children. Arch Dermatol. 2011;147(3):355–6.
19. Tangjaturonrusamee C, Piraccini BM, Vincenzi C, Starace M, Tosti A. Tinea capitis mimicking folliculitis decalvans. Mycoses. 2011;54(1):87–8.
20. Rudnicka L, Olszewska M, Rakowska A, Slowinska M. Trichoscopy update 2011. J Dermatol Case Rep. 2011;5(4):82–8.
21. Nguyen RT, Cowley DM, Muir JB. Scurvy: a cutaneous clinical diagnosis. Australas J Dermatol. 2003;44(1):48–51.

30 Seborrheic Dermatitis

Lidia Rudnicka, Justyna Sicinska, Adriana Rakowska, and Olga Warszawik-Hendzel

Abstract
The most characteristic trichoscopic findings of seborrheic dermatitis include the presence of multiple thin arborizing vessels and yellowish scaling. Thin arborizing vessels also may be present in healthy individuals, but they are less abundant in healthy persons than in individuals with seborrheic dermatitis. Yellowish scaling is characteristic, but not specific, for this condition. Thus, in most cases, seborrheic dermatitis is a trichoscopic diagnosis of exclusion. In this chapter, we also discuss differential diagnoses of seborrheic dermatitis, including ichthyosis vulgaris and contact dermatitis of the scalp.

Keywords
Arborizing vessels • Contact dermatitis • Ichthyosis vulgaris • Multicomponent vascular pattern • Psoriasis • Scaling • Sebopsoriasis • Seborrheic dermatitis

Seborrheic dermatitis is a common chronic relapsing inflammatory skin condition with a predilection for areas rich in sebaceous glands. The scalp, central face, and anterior chest are affected most frequently. The disorder is characterized by scaling and poorly defined erythematous patches, with large variations in extent and morphologic characteristics [1–3]. Young adults are affected most commonly, and men are affected more often than women. The estimated prevalence is 2.3–11 % [4, 5].

The etiopathogenesis of the disease is not fully understood. The role of *Malassezia spp* in the pathogenesis of seborrheic dermatitis has long been suggested and debated in the literature. It has been hypothesized that seborrheic dermatitis develops as an altered cutaneous response to *Malassezia spp* or their toxins, or to the free fatty acids produced by *Malassezia spp* lipases [6, 7].

Clinical variants of seborrheic dermatitis include pityriasis capitis (dandruff), blepharitis (scaling and erythema of the eyelid margin), flexural seborrheic dermatis (involving body folds, especially the retroauricular area), and erythroderma [1–3]. In infants, seborrheic dermatitis may present clinically as scalp seborrheic dermatitis (cradle cap) or Leiner's disease. Drug-induced seborrheic dermatitis–like skin lesions are most commonly associated with anticancer drugs [1]. Some authors have linked *Malassezia* (*Pityrosporum*) folliculitis to seborrheic dermatitis [1].

HIV-related seborrheic dermatitis, another clinical variant of the disease, is often diffuse and severe [1]. In a recent study including an 18-year-old male cohort, the occurrence of scalp seborrheic dermatitis was associated with white skin and a higher body fat content [8].

The clinical differential diagnosis includes psoriasis, atopic dermatitis, tinea capitis, discoid lupus erythematosus, pemphigus foliaceus, pemphigus erythematosus, contact dermatitis, and other inflammatory diseases of the scalp.

The trichoscopic features of scalp seborrheic dermatitis have been studied extensively in recent years [9–12]. The most frequent trichoscopic finding is the presence of multiple thin arborizing vessels. Featureless areas with no particular vascular pattern also may be found. Scaling typically is

L. Rudnicka (✉)
Faculty of Health Sciences, Medical University of Warsaw, Poland

Department of Dermatology, CSK MSW, Woloska 137, Warsaw 02-502, Poland
e-mail: lidia.rudnicka@euderm.eu

J. Sicinska • A. Rakowska • O. Warszawik-Hendzel
Department of Dermatology, CSK MSW, Warsaw, Poland

L. Rudnicka et al. (eds.), *Atlas of Trichoscopy*,
DOI 10.1007/978-1-4471-4486-1_30, © Springer-Verlag London 2012

yellowish, which differentiates seborrheic dermatitis from psoriasis. Globular lines and rings, which are most characteristic of psoriasis, are absent in seborrheic dermatitis [9–12]. The hair shafts appear normal on trichoscopy.

A recent atomic force microscopic study of hair shafts in patients with seborrheic dermatitis showed that the cuticle is significantly thicker in these patients than in control hairs [13].

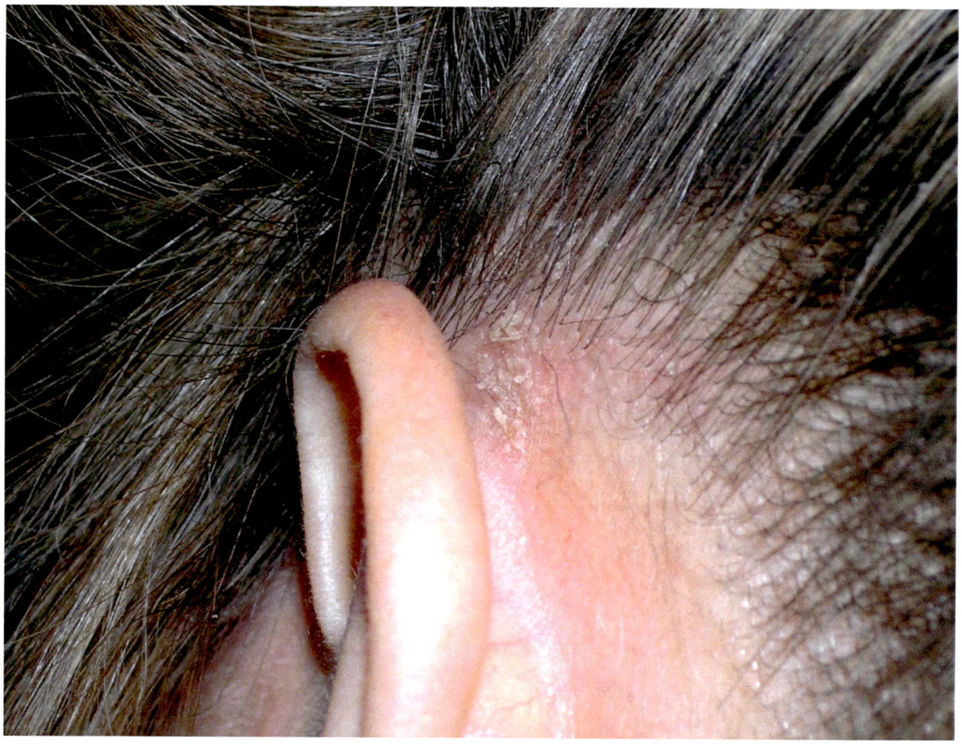

Fig. 30.1 Seborrheic dermatitis. Seborrheic dermatitis is a chronic relapsing inflammatory skin disease located predominantly in areas rich in sebaceous glands. The scalp almost always is affected. Other common sites are the face, chest, and retroauricular area. Blepharoconjunctivitis may occur in isolation, or it may be associated with skin lesions. Clinically, the disorder is characterized by poorly defined erythematous patches covered by white to yellowish scales. The lesional skin surface may appear slightly moist [1]. Lesions in the retroauricular area, as in this patient, require differential diagnosis with psoriasis and discoid lupus erythematosus

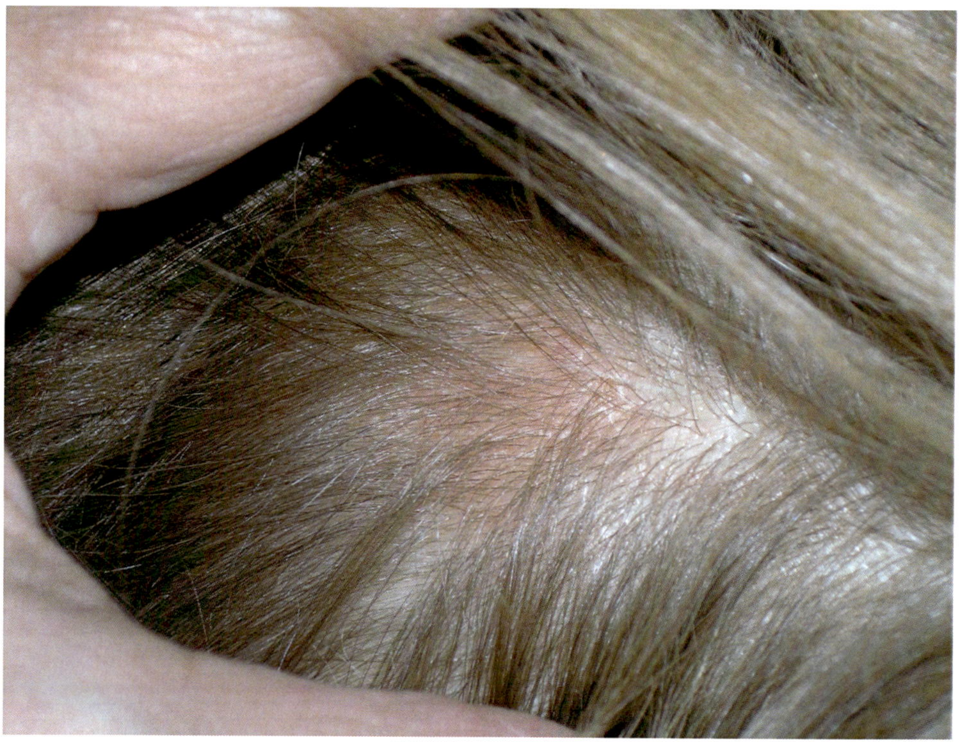

Fig. 30.2 A typical, not well-defined, erythematous patch covered by scales in seborrheic dermatitis. Scaling may be very mild, as in this patient, to severe. Clinical variants of seborrheic dermatitis include pityriasis capitis (dandruff with no erythematous lesions), blepharitis (scaling and erythema of the eyelid margin), flexural seborrheic dermatitis (involving body folds, especially the retroauricular area), erythroderma [1], and pityriasis amiantacea (pseudo–tinea amiantacea) [14]. The existence of sebopsoriasis (i.e., the coexistence of seborrheic dermatitis and psoriasis) is a matter of controversy [15]. In infants, seborrheic dermatitis may present clinically as scalp seborrheic dermatitis, Leiner's disease, or pityriasis amiantacea [1]

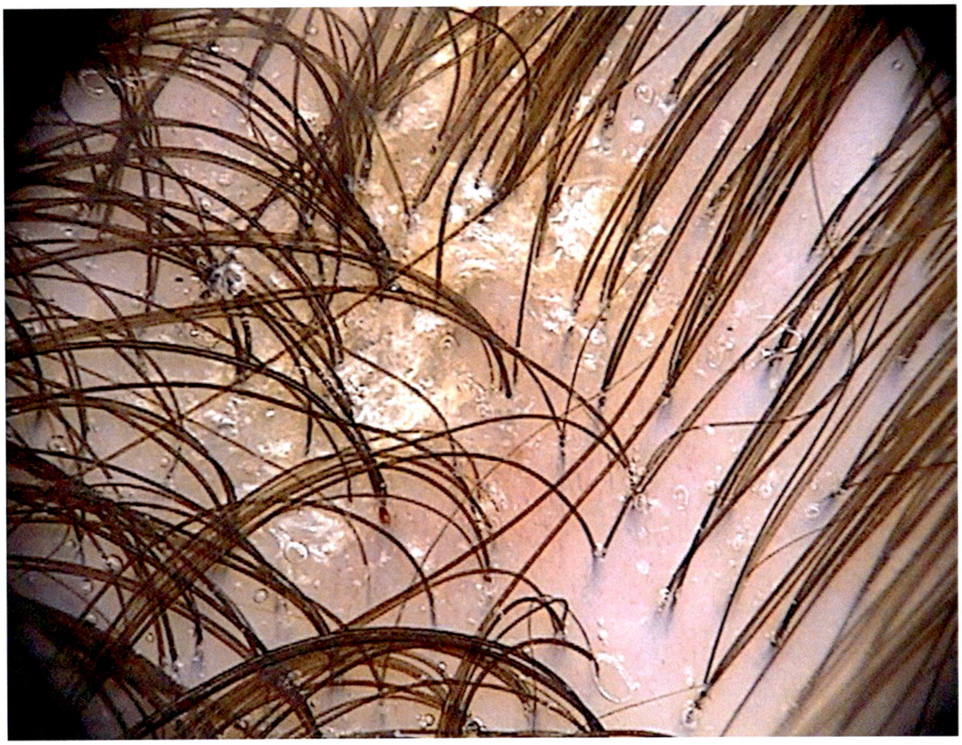

Fig. 30.3 Yellow scaling in seborrheic dermatitis. Dry trichoscopy typically reveals yellowish scales in a diffuse distribution. The background color may be slightly erythematous. The hair structure and density are normal (dry trichoscopy, ×20)

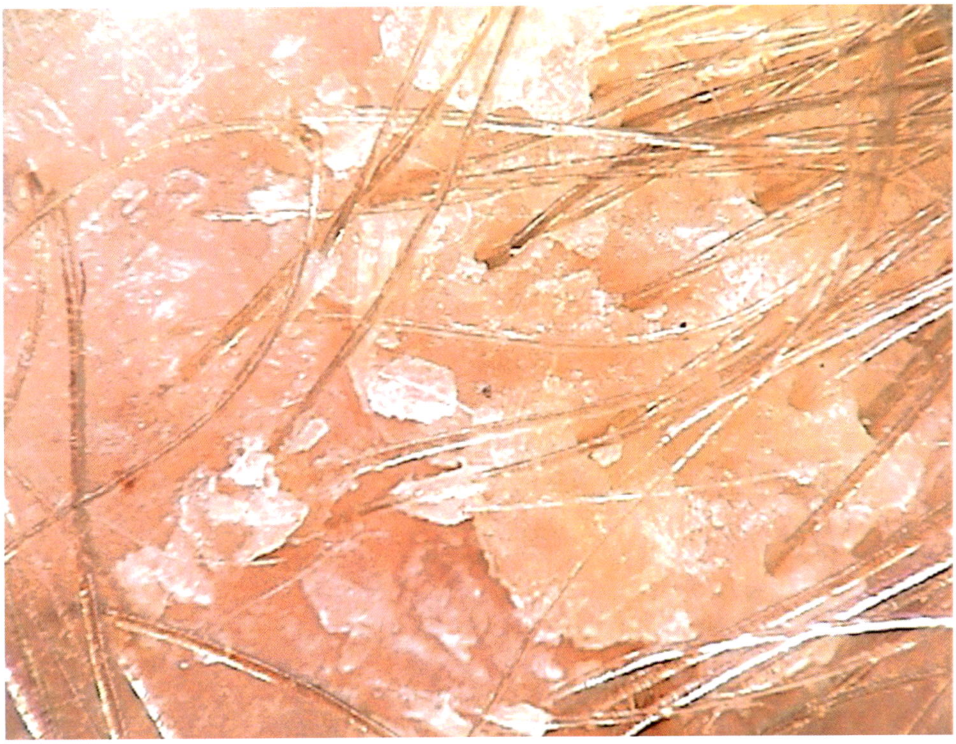

Fig. 30.4 Yellow scaling in seborrheic dermatitis. Higher magnification shows yellowish scales distributed among follicular units. Single scales and clusters of scales are visible in this image. Scaling in psoriasis may be differentiated by the more common presence of white or silver-white scales. Lichen planopilaris may be differentiated by a tendency toward perifollicular or tubular scaling (×70)

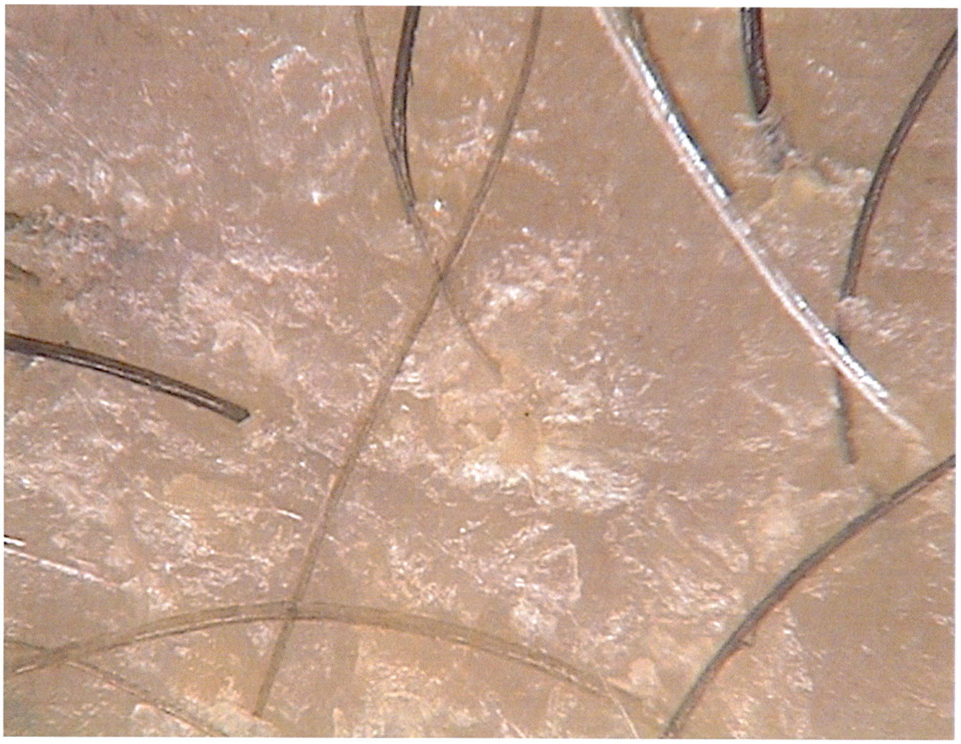

Fig. 30.5 Yellow scaling in seborrheic dermatitis. In this image obtained with dry trichoscopy, the lesional skin surface appears slightly moist. Moderate yellow scaling is present. Hair shaft density is decreased, and follicular units with only one hair predominate, which may indicate coexisting hair loss unrelated to seborrheic dermatitis (×70)

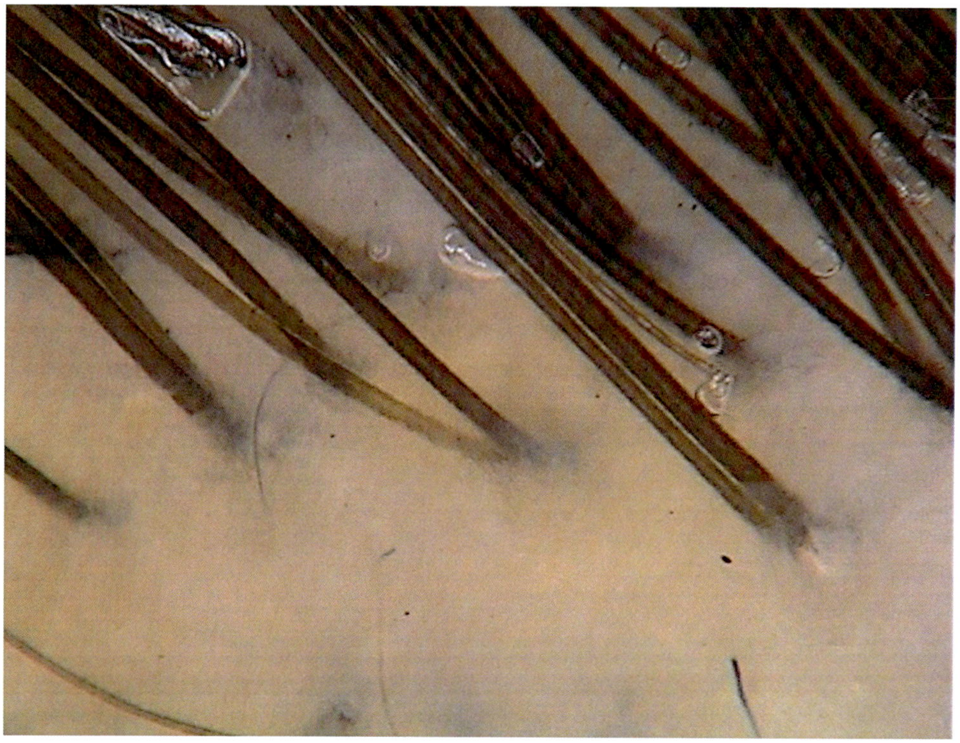

Fig. 30.6 Yellow areas in seborrheic dermatitis. On trichoscopy performed with immersion fluid, yellow scaling is visible as yellowish areas or a yellowish background color, which requires wide differential diagnosis (e.g., dissecting cellulitis, tinea favosa, purulent discharge). In such cases, the vascular pattern may not be visible because it is covered by a thick layer of scales (×70)

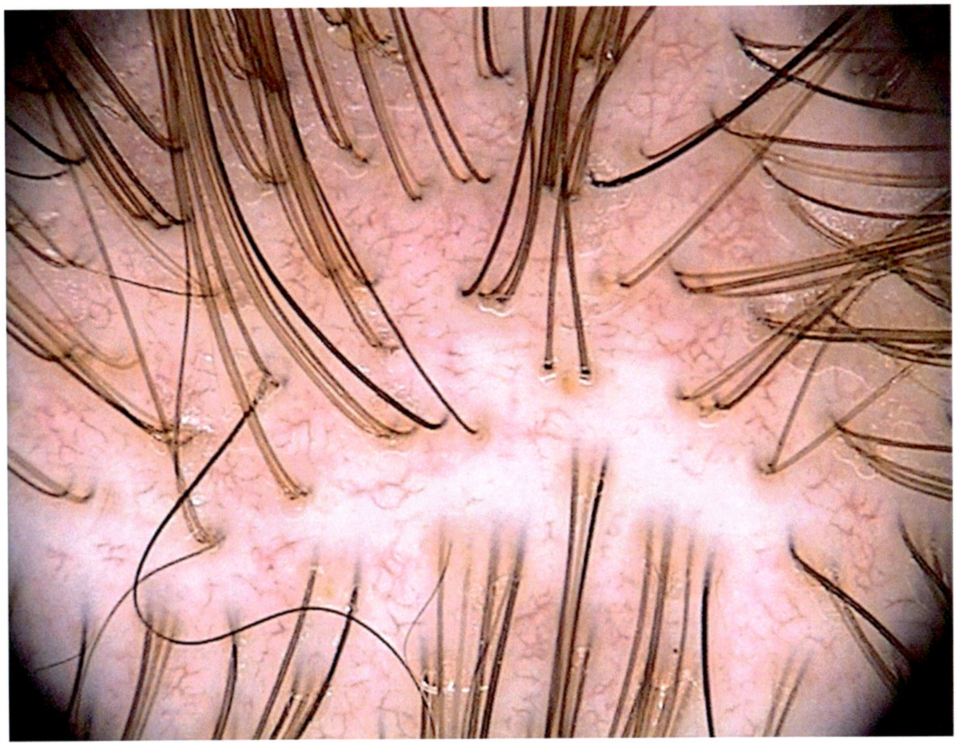

Fig. 30.7 Thin arborizing vessels in seborrheic dermatitis. Thin arborizing vessels may be present in healthy individuals but are observed more commonly in patients with seborrheic dermatitis, and in significantly increased numbers. In a recent study, Kim et al. [9] observed arborizing vessels in 49 % of patients with seborrheic dermatitis and in only 9 % of those with psoriasis. The corresponding number in healthy persons is estimated at 20–80 %, with the highest density of arborizing vessels observed in the occipital area [16]. Thus, the presence of thin arborizing vessels alone has no diagnostic significance. However, in seborrheic dermatitis, the number of arborizing vessels appears to be increased compared with healthy controls. The cut-off number (for seborrheic dermatitis vs normal) remains to be established (×20)

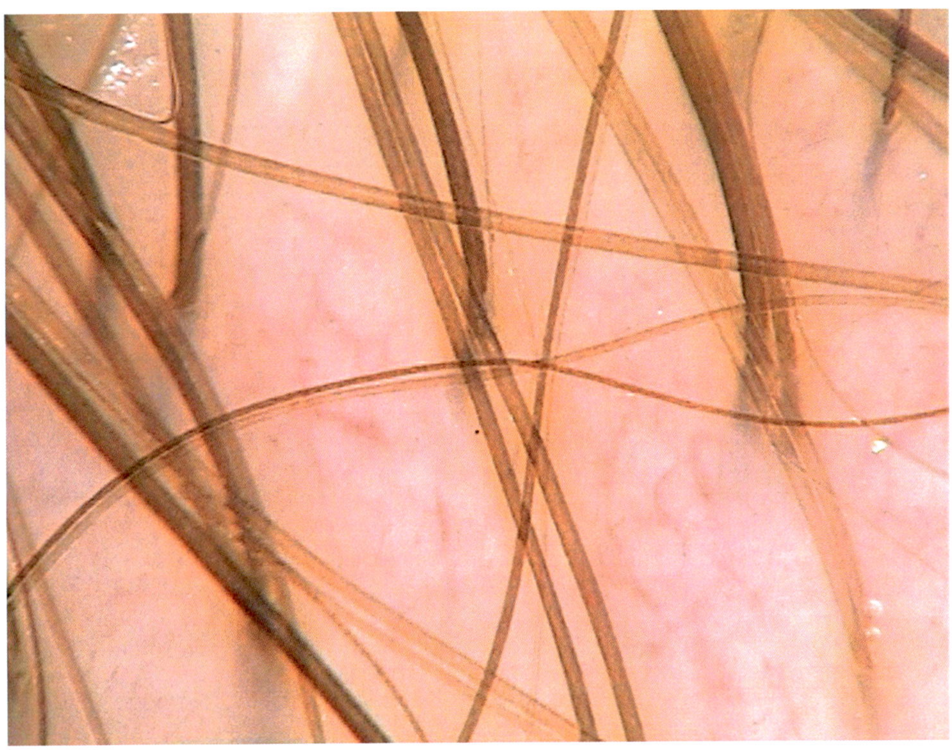

Fig. 30.8 Thin arborizing vessels in seborrheic dermatitis. Thin arborizing vessels in seborrheic dermatitis and in healthy individuals must be distinguished from thick arborizing vessels in discoid lupus erythematosus and basal cell carcinoma. A simple method to distinguish these vessels is to compare their thickness with the thickness of an average hair shaft in the area. Thin arborizing vessels are thinner than a hair, whereas thick arborizing vessels are thicker. See Fig. 23.4 for details about this method of evaluation (×70)

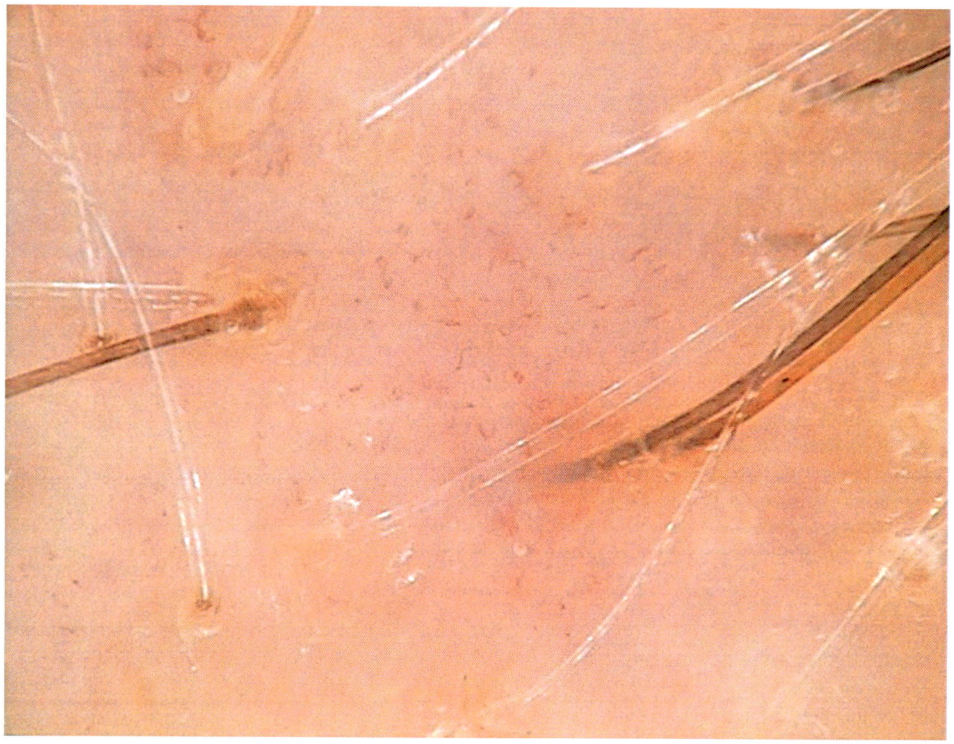

Fig. 30.9 Multicomponent vascular pattern in seborrheic dermatitis. Areas with multiple dotted, comma, linear, and very small arborizing vessels are highly characteristic of seborrheic dermatitis. This multicomponent vascular pattern may be found in most patients with seborrheic dermatitis and differs from the regular, homogeneous pattern seen in psoriasis. Small areas of yellowish scaling are visible in this image (×70)

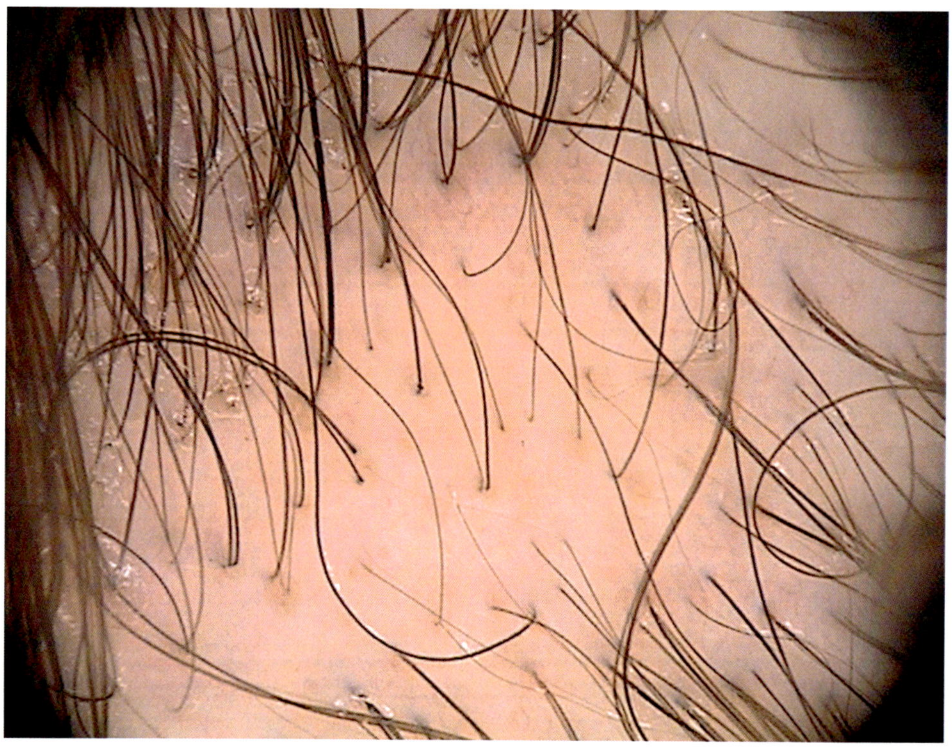

Fig. 30.10 Featureless areas in seborrheic dermatitis. Featureless areas devoid of any particular vascular patterns are observed frequently in seborrheic dermatitis [9]. These areas are practically indistinguishable from a healthy scalp. This trichoscopic image shows the frontal area of a 36-year-old woman with seborrheic dermatitis and female androgenetic alopecia. A slightly yellowish tint in the background color may provide a weak indication of seborrheic dermatitis (×20)

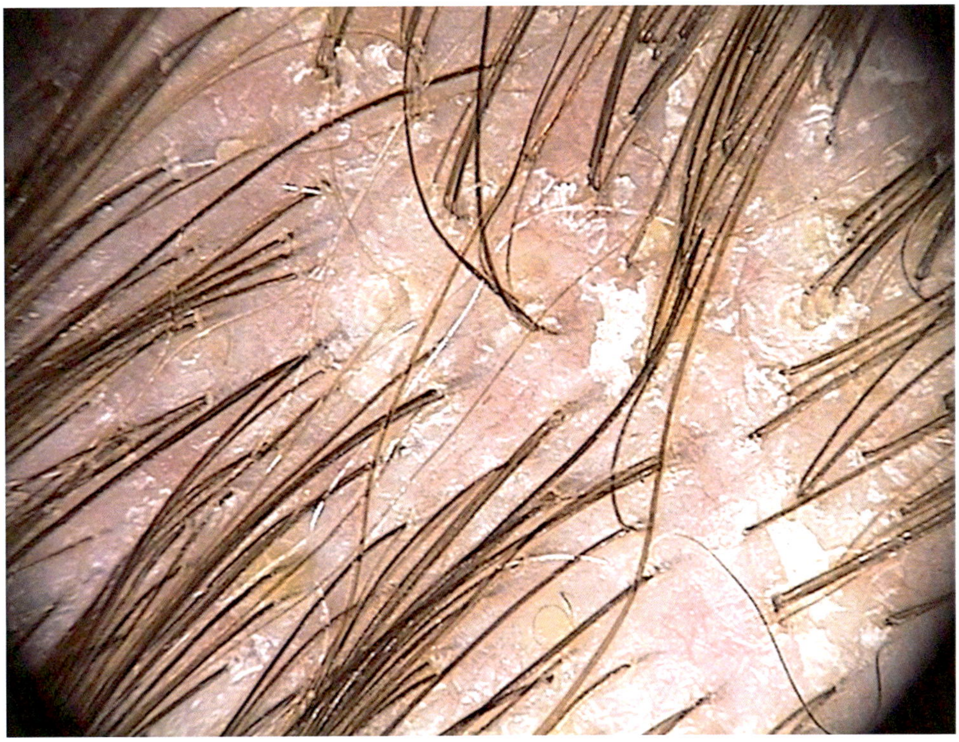

Fig. 30.11 Scaling in ichthyosis vulgaris. Scaling on trichoscopy is most commonly associated with seborrheic dermatitis, psoriasis, discoid lupus erythematosus, or folliculitis decalvans (see Chap. 24 for details). Contact dermatitis and ichthyosis also must be considered in the differential diagnosis. Trichoscopy of contact dermatitis of the scalp was investigated by Tosti et al. [17], who found no statistically significant abnormalities in scaling or blood vessel structure associated with contact dermatitis. This image shows white diffuse scaling in a patient with ichthyosis vulgaris. Small areas of yellowish scales, contaminated with sebum, are visible. Dirty gray to brown scales also may be observed in this condition (dry trichoscopy, ×20)

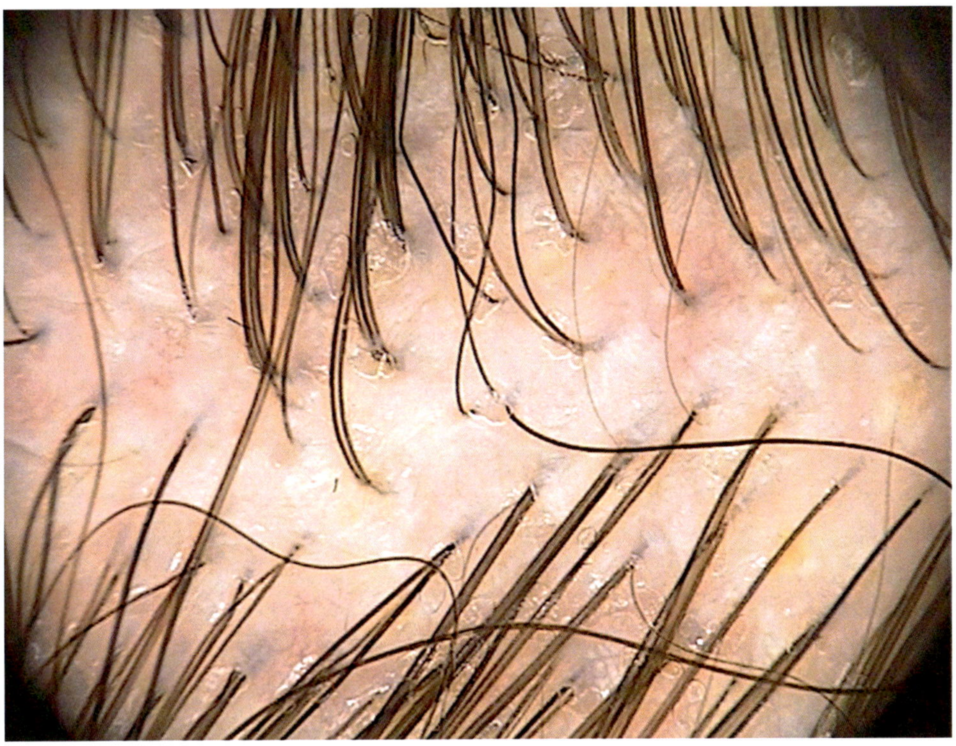

Fig. 30.12 Scaling in ichthyosis vulgaris. Scaling in ichthyosis vulgaris, observed on trichoscopy with immersion fluid, may be difficult to distinguish from seborrheic dermatitis. In this 28-year-old patient with acquired ichthyosis vulgaris, scaling presents as irregular, semitransparent white areas with small islands of yellowish, sebum-contaminated zones. Acquired ichthyosis, usually appearing for the first time in adulthood, is considered a marker of systemic disease. This condition may be associated with various systemic diseases, including malignancies (especially lymphoproliferative disorders), sarcoidosis, leprosy, thyroid diseases, hyperparathyroidism, nutritional disorders, chronic renal failure, and HIV infection [18] (×20)

References

1. Naldi L, Rebora A. Clinical practice. Seborrheic dermatitis. N Engl J Med. 2009;360(4):387–96.
2. Schwartz RA, Janusz CA, Janniger CK. Seborrheic dermatitis: an overview. Am Fam Physician. 2006;74(1):125–30.
3. Olsen EA, Callender V, McMichael A, Sperling L, Anstrom KJ, Shapiro J, et al. Central hair loss in African American women: incidence and potential risk factors. J Am Acad Dermatol. 2011;64(2):245–52.
4. Breunig Jde A, de Almeida Jr HL, Duquia RP, Souza PR, Staub HL. Scalp seborrheic dermatitis: prevalence and associated factors in male adolescents. Int J Dermatol. 2012;51(1):46–9.
5. Palamaras I, Kyriakis K, Stavrianeas N. Seborrheic dermatitis: lifetime detection rates. J Eur Acad Dermatol Venereol. 2012;26(4):524–6.
6. Hay RJ. Malassezia, dandruff and seborrhoeic dermatitis: an overview. Br J Dermatol. 2011;165 Suppl 2:2–8.
7. Kim GK. Seborrheic dermatitis and Malassezia species: how are they related? J Clin Aesthet Dermatol. 2009;2(11):14–7.
8. de Avelar Breunig J, de Almeida Jr HL, Duquia RP, Souza PR, Staub HL. Scalp seborrheic dermatitis: prevalence and associated factors in male adolescents. Int J Dermatol. 2012;51(1):46–9.
9. Kim GW, Jung HJ, Ko HC, Kim MB, Lee WJ, Lee SJ, et al. Dermoscopy can be useful in differentiating scalp psoriasis from seborrhoeic dermatitis. Br J Dermatol. 2011;164(3):652–6.
10. Ross EK, Vincenzi C, Tosti A. Videodermoscopy in the evaluation of hair and scalp disorders. J Am Acad Dermatol. 2006;55(5):799–806.
11. Rosina P, Zamperetti MR, Giovannini A, Girolomoni G. Videocapillaroscopy in the differential diagnosis between psoriasis and seborrheic dermatitis of the scalp. Dermatology. 2007;214(1):21–4.
12. Rudnicka L, Olszewska M, Rakowska A, Slowinska M. Trichoscopy update 2011. J Dermatol Case Rep. 2011;5(4):82–8.
13. Kim KS, Shin MK, Ahn JJ, Haw CR, Park HK. A comparative study of hair shafts in scalp psoriasis and seborrheic dermatitis using atomic force microscopy. Skin Res Technol. 2012. doi:10.1111/j.1600-0846.2011.00608.x.
14. Abdel-Hamid IA, Agha SA, Moustafa YM, El-Labban AM. Pityriasis amiantacea: a clinical and etiopathologic study of 85 patients. Int J Dermatol. 2003;42(4):260–4.
15. Wozel G, Klein E, Mrowietz U, Reich K, Sebastian M, Streit V. Scalp psoriasis. J Dtsch Dermatol Ges. 2011;9(1):70–4.
16. Rakowska A. Trichoscopy (hair and scalp videodermoscopy) in the healthy female. Method standardization and norms for measurable parameters. J Dermatol Case Rep. 2009;3(1):14–9.
17. Tosti A, Donati A, Vincenzi C, Fabbrocini G. Videodermoscopy does not enhance diagnosis of scalp contact dermatitis due to topical minoxidil. Int J Trichol. 2009;1(2):134–7.
18. Okulicz JF, Schwartz RA. Hereditary and acquired ichthyosis vulgaris. Int J Dermatol. 2003;42(2):95–8.

Psoriasis

31

Lidia Rudnicka, Adriana Rakowska,
Malgorzata Olszewska, Justyna Sicinska,
Malgorzata Maj, Magdalena Majsterek,
Monika Slowinska, and Olga Warszawik-Hendzel

Abstract

The trichoscopic diagnosis of scalp psoriasis is based on the evaluation of microvascular alterations. At low magnifications, red globular rings and red globular lines may be observed. High magnification reveals that the "globules" are coiled (glomerular) capillaries arranged into rings or lines. Other types of capillaries (linear looped, lace-like, comma vessels) may be present. A consistent finding is the presence of regularly distributed clusters of multiple vessels. White or white-silver scaling is a very frequent, nonspecific finding.

Keywords

Blood extravasations • Bowen's disease • Clear cell acanthoma • Erythematous background Extravasations • Glomerular vessels • Homogeneous vascular pattern • Pityriasis amiantacea Pseudo–tinea amiantacea • Psoriasis • Sebopsoriasis • Red globular lines • Red dots Red globular rings • Red globules • VSCAPSI • White scaling

Psoriasis is a chronic inflammatory cutaneous disorder with multisystem involvement. The scalp is the most common site of disease manifestation. The frequency of scalp involvement in patients with psoriasis ranges from 50–80 % [1, 2]. The scalp may be the site of the first or only manifestation of the disease. Scalp psoriasis is characterized by sharply bordered erythematous lesions covered to varying degrees by silver or white scales. The lesions often spread over the anterior hairline into the forehead and may also affect the retroauricular region [1–3].

L. Rudnicka (✉)
Faculty of Health Sciences, Medical University of Warsaw, Poland

Department of Dermatology, CSK MSW, Woloska 137, Warsaw 02-502, Poland
e-mail: lidia.rudnicka@euderm.eu

A. Rakowska • J. Sicinska • M. Maj • M. Majsterek • M. Slowinska
O. Warszawik-Hendzel
Department of Dermatology, CSK MSW, Warsaw, Poland

M. Olszewska
Department of Dermatology, Medical University of Warsaw, Warsaw, Poland

Defining scalp psoriasis severity may be challenging. Most scoring systems include evaluation of the surface size covered by psoriatic plaques, lesion thickness, scaling intensity, facial involvement, or pruritus. The most popular system, especially in clinical trials, is the Psoriasis Scalp Severity Index (PSSI). The PSSI is a score based on the addition of partial scores for erythema, induration, and desquamation multiplied by a score for the extent of scalp area involved. The scores range from 0 to 72, with higher scores indicating more severe disease. A less time-consuming system, and one probably more adequate for clinical practice, is the European Score, an algorithm developed by Ortonne et al. in 2009 [2]. This algorithm classifies scalp psoriasis as mild, moderate, or severe [2].

Occasionally, psoriasis may be associated with either increased hair density [4] or psoriatic alopecia. Psoriatic alopecia is very rarely cicatricial [5]. In most patients with psoriasis hair loss is noncicatricial and reversible [6].

In patients with scalp psoriasis, a common comorbidity is seborrheic dermatitis. An overlap between psoriasis and seborrheic dermatitis is often called *sebopsoriasis* [1]. This coexistence makes differential diagnosis even more

L. Rudnicka et al. (eds.), *Atlas of Trichoscopy*,
DOI 10.1007/978-1-4471-4486-1_31, © Springer-Verlag London 2012

complex. However, the existence and diagnostic criteria for sebopsoriasis remain controversial.

The diagnosis of scalp psoriasis usually is based on clinical evaluation. Histopathology may be performed in uncertain cases. Trichogram results are nonspecific [1, 7].

Trichoscopy of scalp psoriasis has been studied extensively [4, 8–12]. Similar to dermoscopy of plaque psoriasis on glabrous skin, the evaluation of microvascular alterations seems to have the highest diagnostic value. The images produced at low magnification (i.e., from a handheld dermoscope) are somewhat different from those obtained with high-magnification trichoscopy (>×50) produced by digital videodermoscopes. At low magnification, rings or lines consisting of red globules may be observed as the most characteristic finding. High magnification reveals that the "globules" are coiled (glomerular) capillaries [13–16].

Another type of vascular abnormality commonly observed in psoriasis is the presence of clusters of multiple vessels homogeneously distributed in the field of view. These vessels may be linear, looped, lace-like, or comma shaped [13–16]. The vessel caliber tends to be slightly larger than that of capillaries in normal skin. Vascular abnormalities in scalp psoriasis usually coexist with white or white-silver scaling.

Clinically and trichoscopically, the most relevant differential diagnosis is seborrheic dermatitis [10, 12].

It must be emphasized that the diagnosis of psoriasis is based principally on clinical features. Dermoscopy (on glabrous skin) and trichoscopy (on hair-bearing skin) have only accessory value. The vascular patterns observed in psoriasis also may be observed in skin tumors such as Bowen's disease or clear cell acanthoma [17].

Table 31.1 Trichoscopic features of scalp psoriasis

Low magnification
White interfollicular scaling
Red dots and globules
Red globular rings (dots and globules in circular arrangement)
Red globular lines (dots and globules in linear arrangement)
Erythematous background
High magnification
Glomerular (coiled) vessels arranged in lines or rings
Clusters of multiple vessels arranged in a homogenous pattern (linear, looped, comma-like, lace-like)
Blood extravasations

Table 31.2 Trichoscopic differential diagnosis of scalp psoriasis and seborrheic dermatitis

Feature	Psoriasis	Seborrheic dermatitis
Scaling	Diffuse, interfollicular, white	Diffuse, interfollicular, yellowish
Most commonly observed vessels	Glomerular (coiled)	Thin arborizing
Arrangement of blood vessels	Clusters of multiple, homogeneously distributed vessels arranged in rings or lines	Not regularly arranged
Extravasations	Common (round shaped)	Uncommon (linear excoriations)

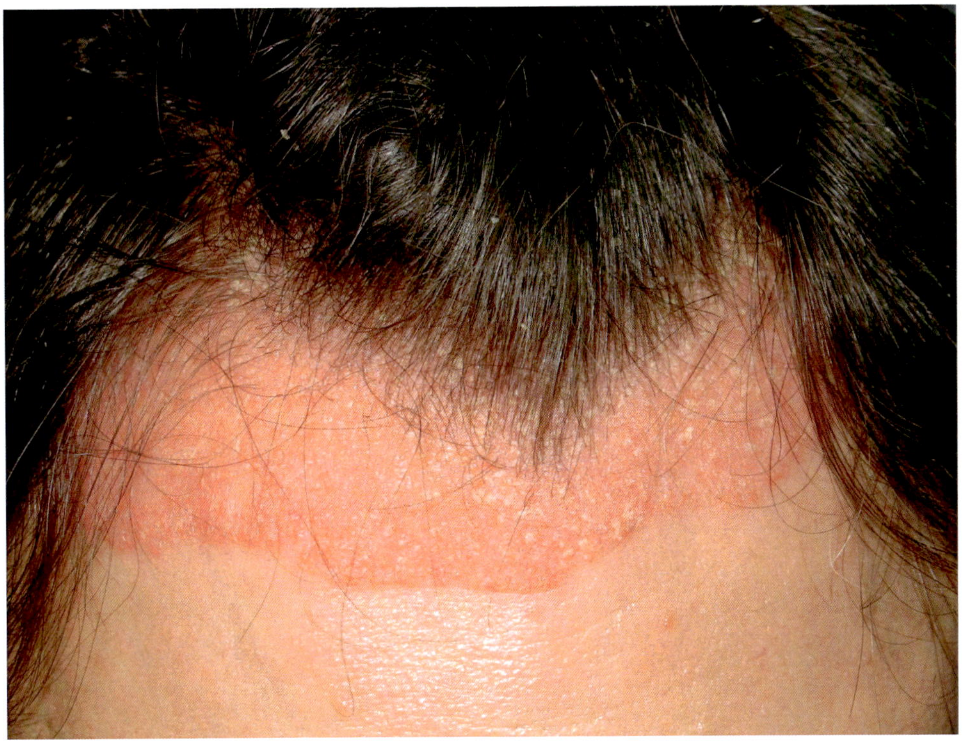

Fig. 31.1 Scalp psoriasis. Scalp psoriasis is characterized by sharply bordered erythematous lesions covered to varying degrees by silver or white scales. The lesions often spread onto the forehead and into the postauricular region [1–3]. In this patient, scalp psoriasis was classified as severe according to the European Score [2]. The European Score classifies scalp psoriasis as mild, moderate, or severe. Mild scalp psoriasis affects less than 50 % of the scalp (mild erythema, mild scaling, minimal thickness, or mild pruritus). Moderate scalp psoriasis also affects less than 50 % of the scalp (moderate erythema, moderate scaling, moderate thickness, or mild to moderate pruritus). Severe scalp psoriasis affects more than 50 % of the scalp (severe erythema, severe scaling, very thick infiltration, moderate to severe pruritus, or evidence of hair loss with scarring or forehead involvement) [2]

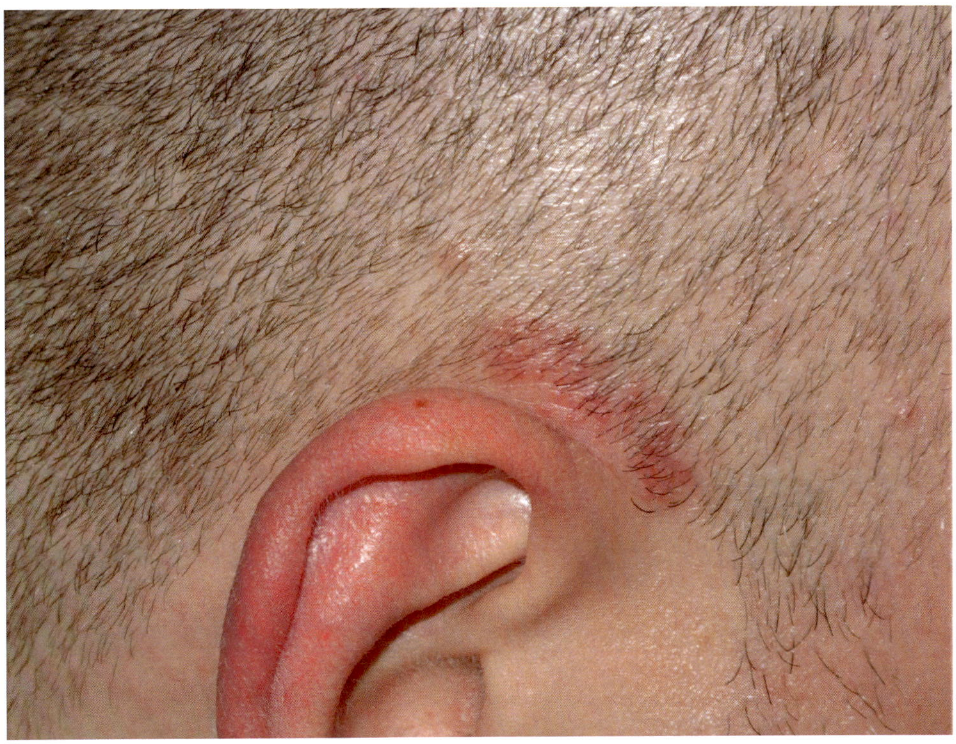

Fig. 31.2 Scalp psoriasis. The scalp is the most common site of disease manifestation in psoriasis. The frequency of scalp involvement in patients with psoriasis ranges from 50 to 80 %. Commonly, the scalp is the only site of clinical manifestation of the disease [1, 2]. In this patient, a small sharply demarcated erythematous plaque is the only manifestation of psoriasis. Trichoscopy is most useful in cases such as this one, in which the clinical differential diagnosis is difficult and includes seborrheic dermatitis, discoid lupus erythematosus, lichen planus, tinea capitis, pemphigus erythematosus, and other inflammatory scalp diseases

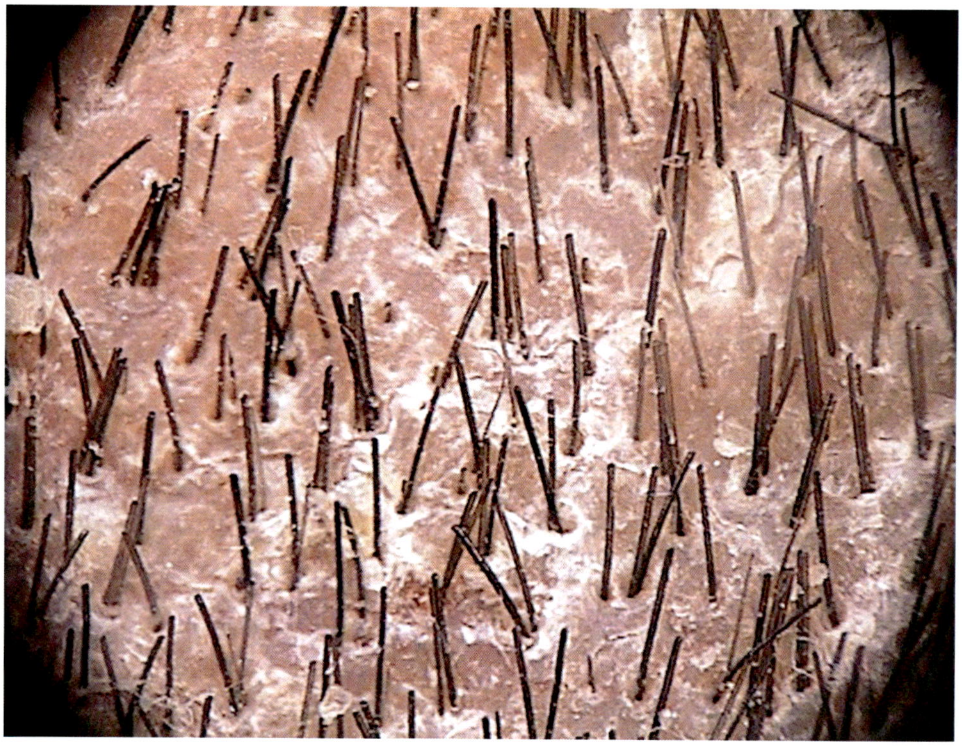

Fig. 31.3 White scaling in scalp psoriasis. Scaling in scalp psoriasis is diffuse and interfollicular. There is no perifollicular scaling, and hair casts are very rare. Scaling appears as a widespread scaly area firmly adhering to the scalp surface. Unlike in seborrheic dermatitis, discernment of single scales often is not possible. The scaling is almost always white, which also distinguishes psoriasis from seborrheic dermatitis. This image of the frontal scalp area of a 43-year-old man with psoriasis shows increased hair density with a high percentage of follicular units with three to four hairs (dry trichoscopy, ×20)

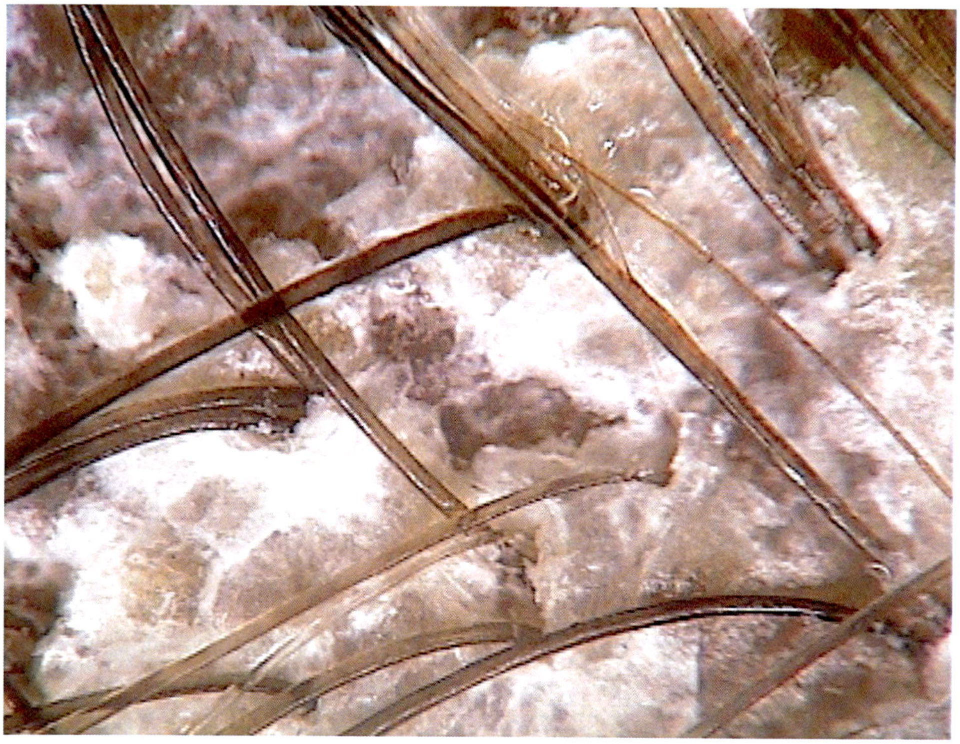

Fig. 31.4 White scaling in scalp psoriasis. White fluffy, diffuse scaling is a characteristic, but not specific, finding in psoriasis. In such cases, visualization of characteristic blood vessel abnormalities is possible only after removing the scales with a keratolytic agent. Our experience shows that the characteristic blood vessel structure and arrangement may be seen even after 2–3 weeks of treatment with keratolytic agents (e.g., salicylic acid) combined with potent corticosteroids for 2 weeks. In a study performed on nonscaly, glabrous skin lesions in patients with plaque psoriasis, 15 days of topical therapy with betamethasone dipropionate induced the thinning of abnormal blood vessels by about 10–20 % [18] (dry trichoscopy, ×70)

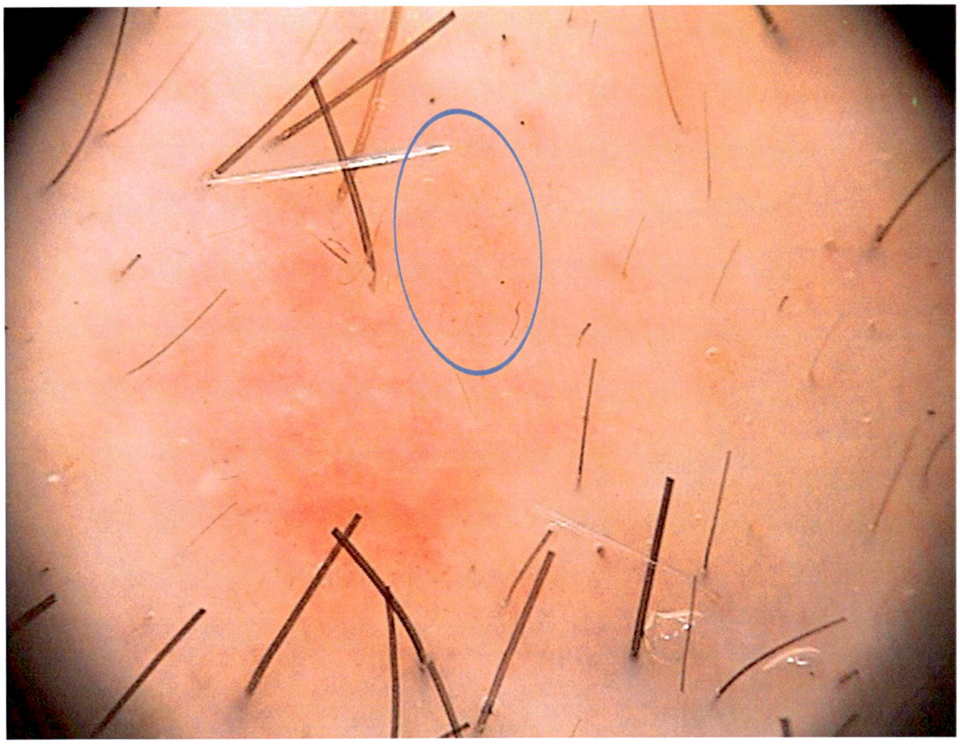

Fig. 31.5 Red dots and globules in psoriasis. This low-magnification image of a small psoriatic plaque shows an erythematous area with clusters of multiple regularly distributed red dots and globules (*blue ring*). Red dots and globules observed at low magnification (e.g., with a handheld dermoscope) correspond to twisted glomerular blood vessels, which may be observed in detail at a higher magnification. These blood vessels tend to align into a linear pattern ("red globular lines") or into rings ("red globular rings") (×20)

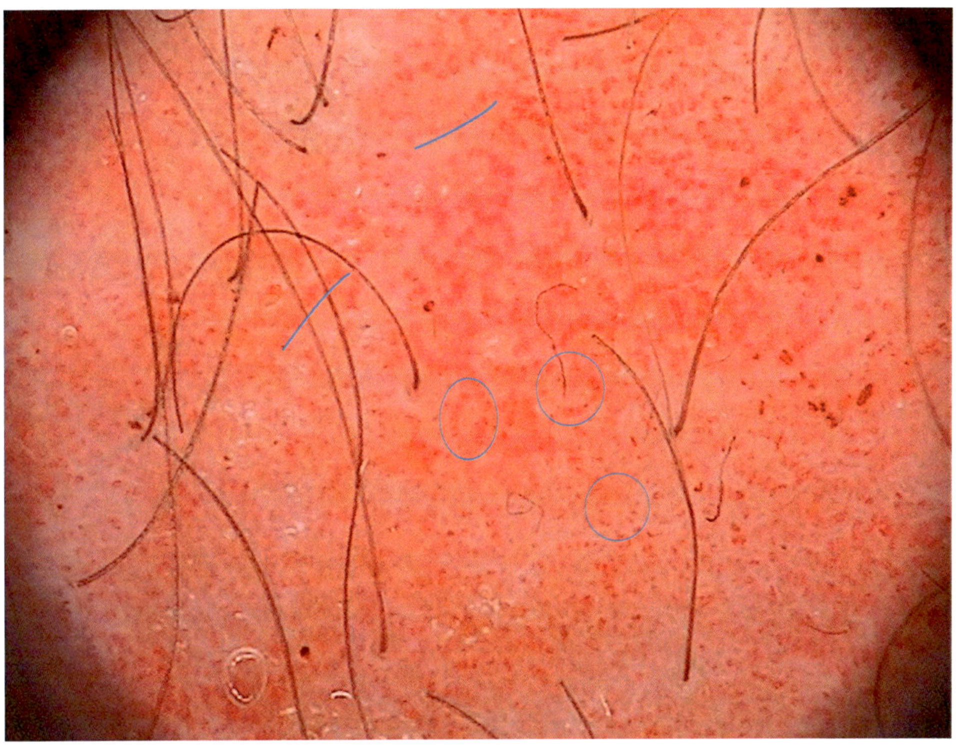

Fig. 31.6 Red globular rings in psoriasis. In this patient with highly active, severe psoriasis, red dots and globules are arranged in rings and lines. These circular structures are called *red globular rings* (marked by *blue rings*) [15]. The linearly arranged vessels are called *red globular lines* (vessels aligning along the *blue lines*). Red globular rings are more commonly visible on glabrous skin than on the scalp (×20)

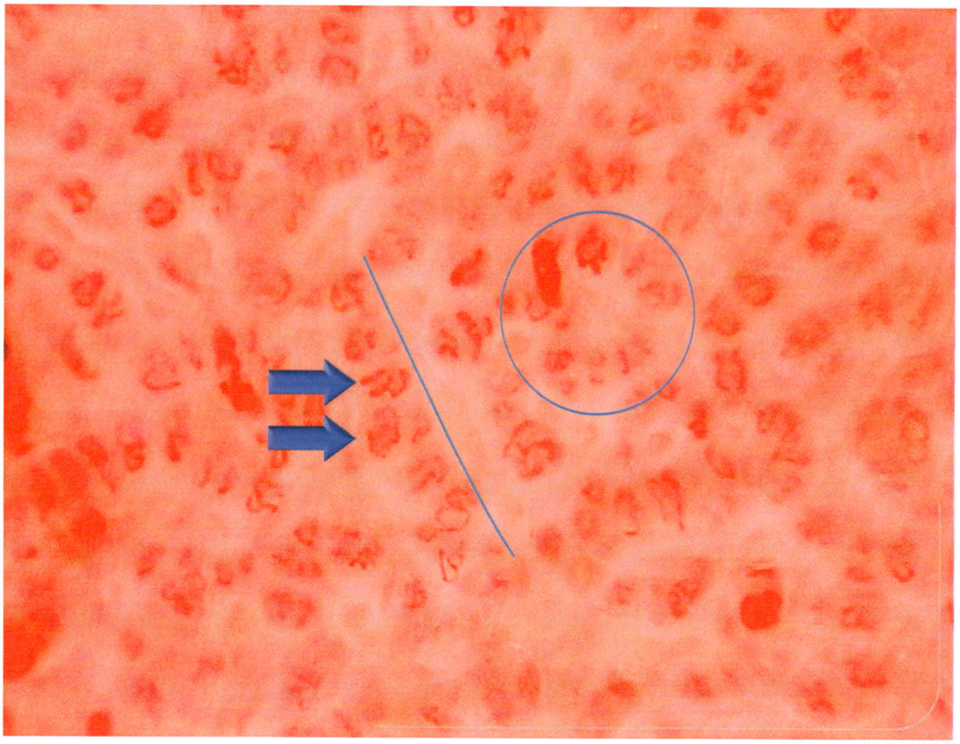

Fig. 31.7 Glomerular vessels in psoriasis. High magnification of the area presented in the previous image reveals the detailed glomerular nature of the blood vessels (*arrows*). The name *glomerular vessels* has been suggested because their appearance calls to mind the first report of the glomerular apparatus in the kidney [19]. Other names for these vessels are *coiled vessels* and *linear coiled vessels* [17]. The arrangement of these vessels in psoriasis may be linear (*blue line*) or circular (*blue circle*) (×70)

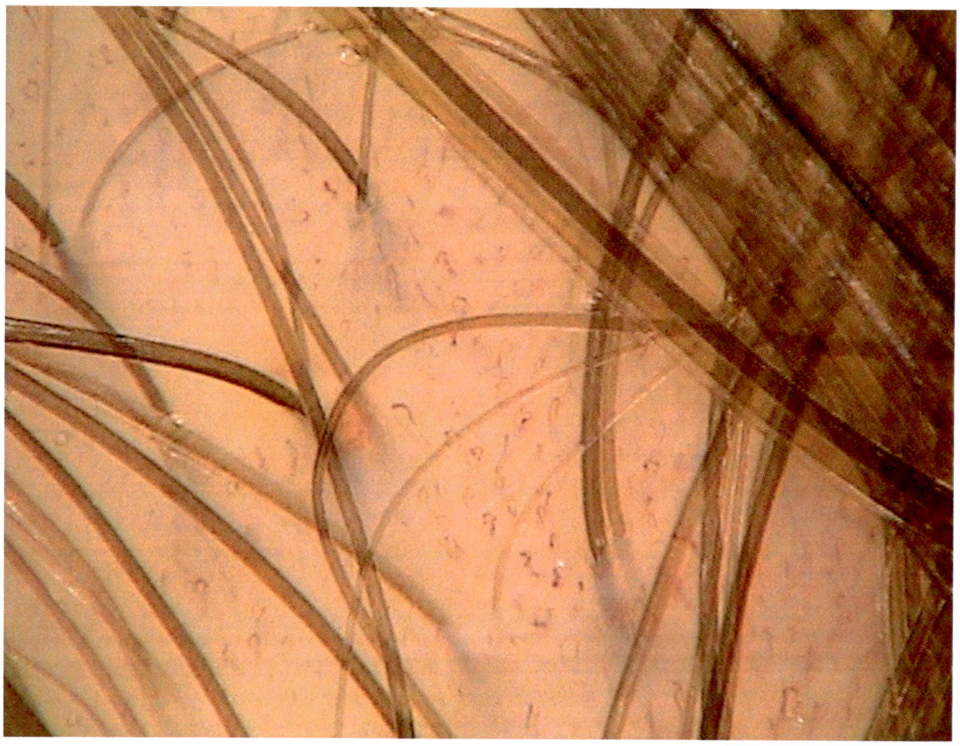

Fig. 31.8 Clusters of multiple vessels in psoriasis. In less severe cases of scalp psoriasis, vessels are arranged homogeneously in clusters, each containing multiple vessels. These clusters may contain several types of small vessels (lace-like, linear, looped, glomerular, small arborizing, linear, comma-like). A consistent characteristic feature is the regular homogeneous distribution of these vessels between pilosebaceous units. The tendency of vessels to align into a linear pattern is visible. Unlike diseases primarily affecting the perifollicular area (e.g., lichen planopilaris), blood vessels do not concentrate around the emerging hair shafts in psoriasis (×70)

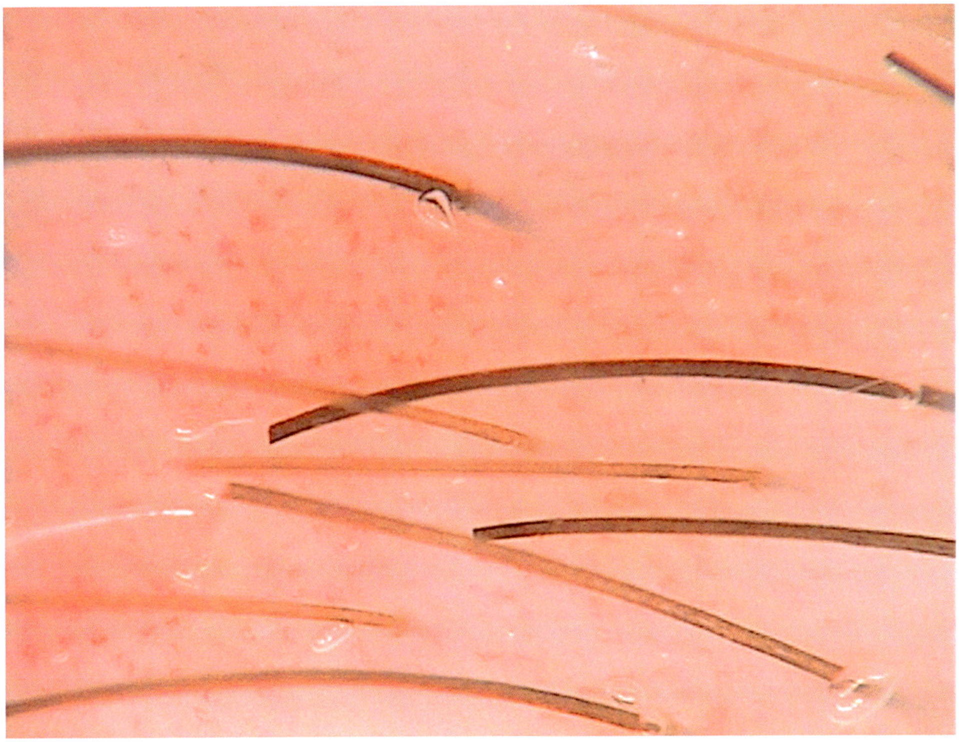

Fig. 31.9 Clusters of multiple vessels in psoriasis. Shown is a cluster of glomerular, looped, and lace-like vessels on an erythematous background. In this image, the blood vessels tend to merge with the erythematous background and their structure is not clearly defined. This phenomenon is most common in treated, fading, psoriatic lesions. Theoretically, it is possible to use trichoscopy for disease monitoring in psoriasis. For this purpose, the Videodermoscopy Scalp Psoriasis Severity Index (VSCAPSI) was developed [9]. This scoring system takes into account the clinical evaluation and videodermoscopic results (vascular pattern, erythema, desquamation). The complex VSCAPSI score is probably more useful in clinical trials than in daily practice. Our experience also shows that the most accurate results are obtained when the same videodermoscope is used for evaluation in the same patient. Each machine produces a slightly different shade of red, which may influence the evaluation of "erythema" (for details about this scoring system, see Chap. 40) (×70)

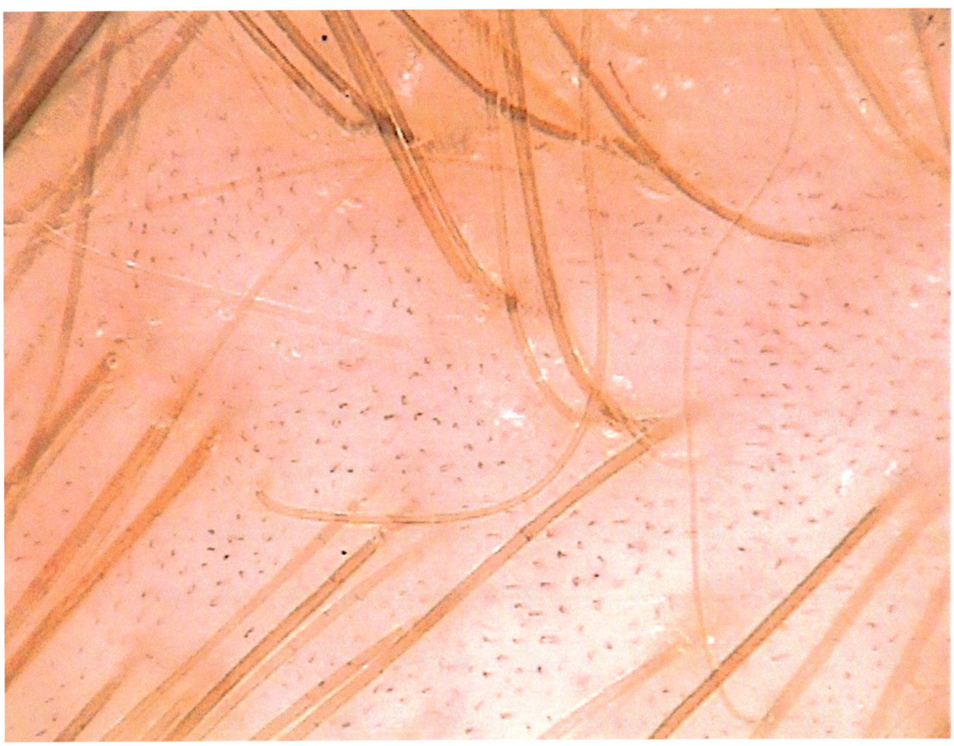

Fig. 31.10 Homogeneously distributed vessels in psoriasis. In this psoriatic scalp lesion, several types of vessels are visible (dotted, comma-like, looped, lace-like, linear). No glomerular vessels are present. The vessels are arranged in a homogeneous distribution; some are arranged linearly. The regular, homogeneous distribution of blood vessels between follicular units is a consistent finding in psoriasis. In such cases, the difference between healthy skin and psoriasis is quantitative rather than qualitative (×40)

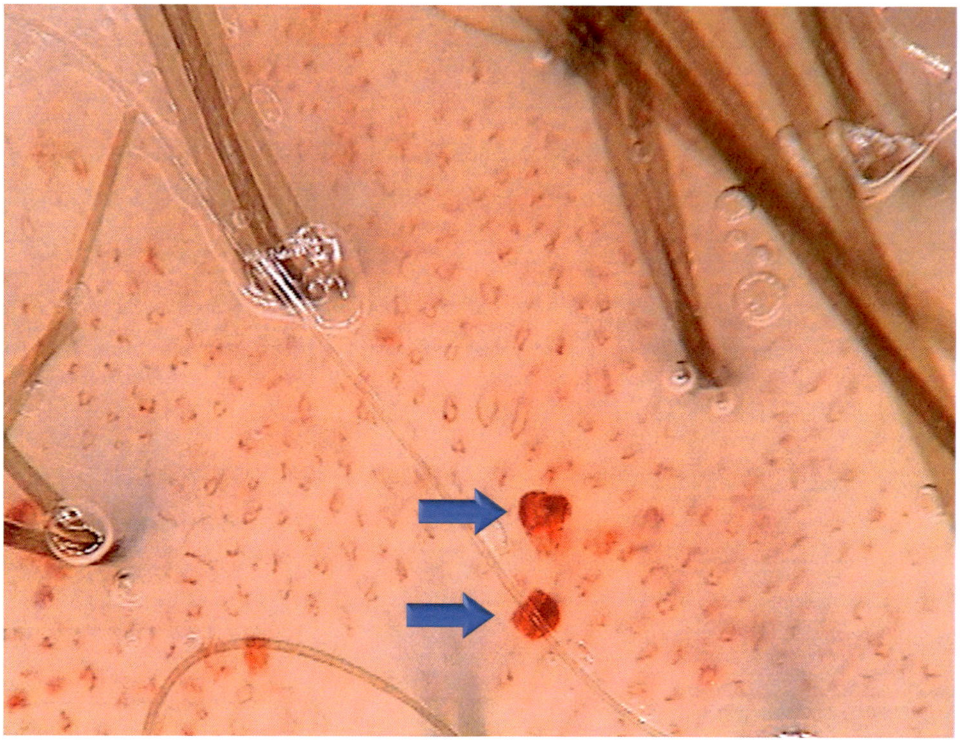

Fig. 31.11 Blood extravasations in psoriasis. Blood extravasations (*arrows*) are common in the active phase of scalp psoriasis. They usually are circular or oval in shape, which distinguishes them from artificial extravasations resulting from mechanical trauma (e.g., scratching). Other features of psoriasis in this image are lace-like, looped, and comma-like vessels in a homogeneous distribution (×70)

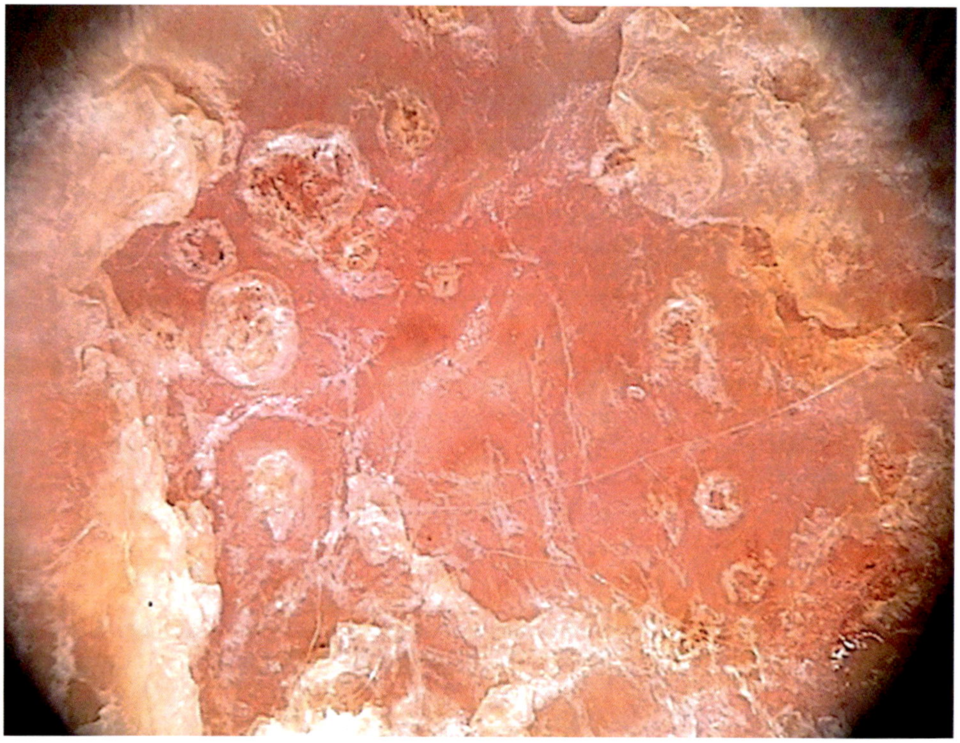

Fig. 31.12 Pustular psoriasis. The scalp rarely is involved in generalized pustular (von Zumbusch) psoriasis, and this disease usually can be diagnosed based on clinical appearance. Trichoscopy is not specific. In the early phase, small pustules surrounded by erythema are visible. When the pustules rupture, they release a yellow discharge. Dried discharge appears as circular yellow areas of crust on erythematous skin. This image shows pustular psoriasis on glabrous skin (×20)

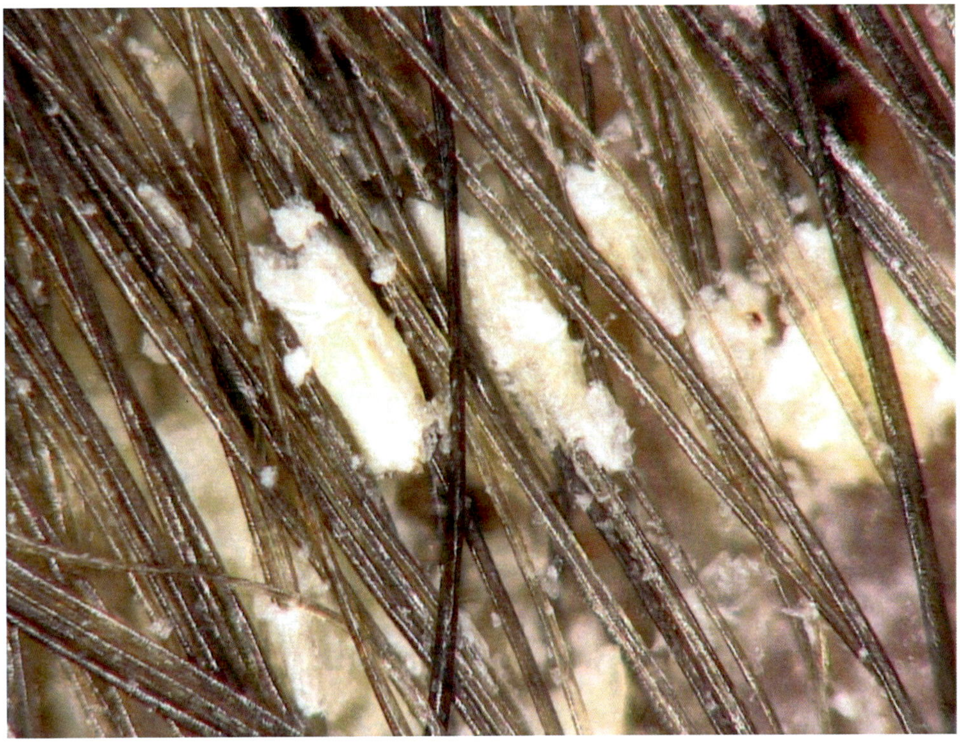

Fig. 31.13 Pityriasis (pseudo-tinea) amiantacea. Pityriasis amiantacea (formerly pseudo-tinea amiantacea) is a distinct clinical symptom characterized by thick, white, adherent scales that firmly adhere to hairs and bind them into hair tufts. Pityriasis amiantacea is a reaction pattern of the scalp to various inflammatory scalp diseases. Psoriasis is the most common cause of the condition. Other causes are seborrheic dermatitis, lichen planus, lichen simplex chronicus, and fungal or bacterial infections [20]. Trichoscopy shows fluffy white agglomerates of scales. In contrast to hair casts, which entangle the hair shafts or hair tufts as they emerge from the follicular opening, these scale agglomerates adhere to the hair shafts from the side and glue them together into tufts of various sizes (×70)

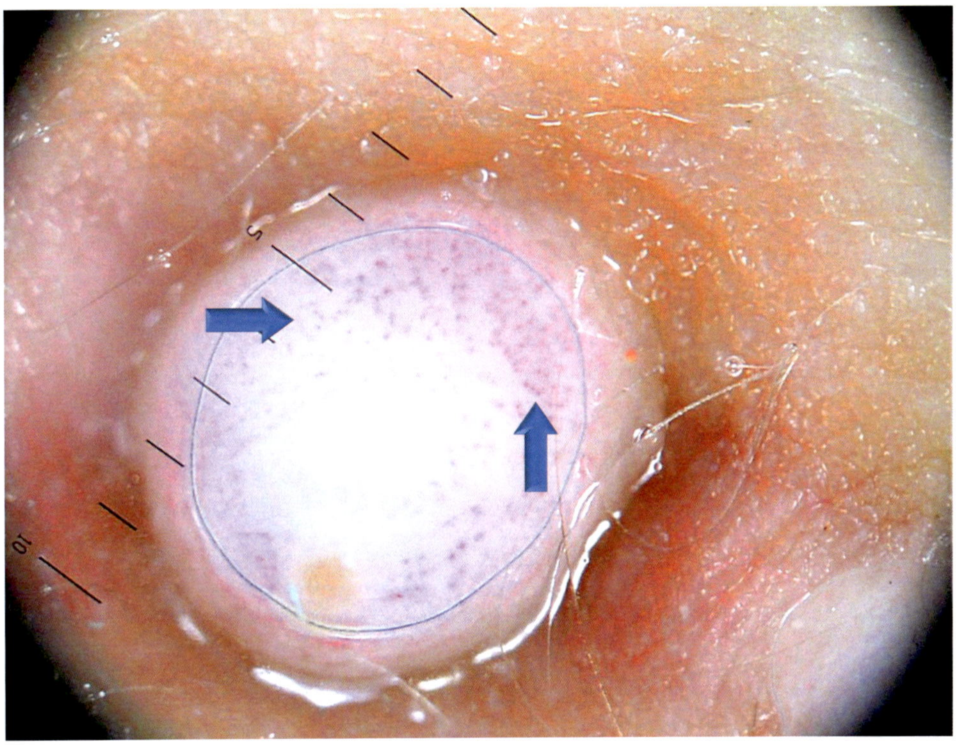

Fig. 31.14 Psoriasis-like vascular pattern in clear cell acanthoma. Red globular rings and lines (*arrows*) are not specific for psoriasis. A similar pattern has been described in clear cell acanthoma (*ring*). There is ongoing discussion as to whether the arrangement of these vessels is identical to that seen in psoriasis [21–23]. The differential diagnosis must take into account the clinical appearance of the lesion (×20)

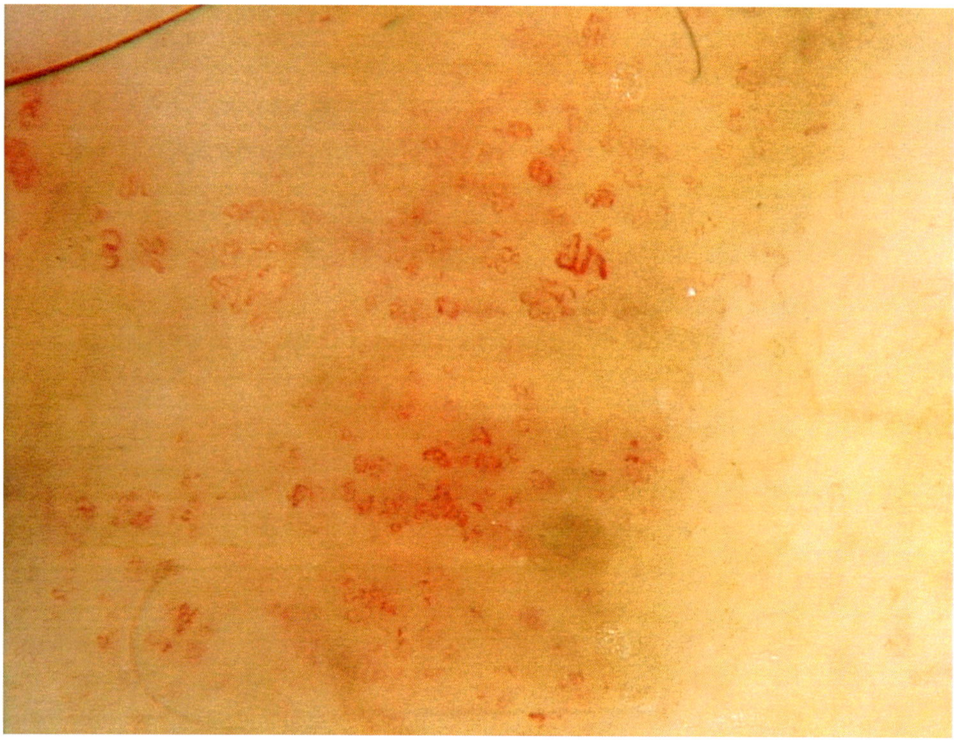

Fig. 31.15 Psoriasis-like vascular pattern in Bowen's disease. Dermoscopy of Bowen's disease is characterized by the presence of glomerular (coiled) vessels, which may be indistinguishable from vessels observed in psoriasis. Usually, they are organized slightly less regularly than those in psoriasis. Glomerular vessels are observed in most patients with nonpigmented Bowen's disease and in 80 % of those with pigmented (image) Bowen's disease [19]. An additional feature, which makes the differential diagnosis of Bowen's disease and psoriasis more complex, is the scaly surface that may be present in both diseases. The presence of glomerular vessels also has been described in squamous cell carcinoma and other cutaneous conditions. Thus, trichoscopy may be used as an accessory tool only, for differential diagnosis or for the confirmation of clinically suspected psoriasis (×50)

References

1. Wozel G, Klein E, Mrowietz U, Reich K, Sebastian M, Streit V. Scalp psoriasis. J Dtsch Dermatol Ges. 2011;9(1):70–4.
2. Ortonne J, Chimenti S, Luger T, Puig L, Reid F, Trueb RM. Scalp psoriasis: European consensus on grading and treatment algorithm. J Eur Acad Dermatol Venereol. 2009;23(12):1435–44.
3. Chan CS, Van Voorhees AS, Lebwohl MG, Korman NJ, Young M, Bebo Jr BF, et al. Treatment of severe scalp psoriasis: from the Medical Board of the National Psoriasis Foundation. J Am Acad Dermatol. 2009;60(6):962–71.
4. Sawan S, Descamps V. Scalp psoriasis: a paradigm of "switch-on" mechanism to anagen hair growth? Arch Dermatol. 2008;144(8): 1064–6.
5. Bardazzi F, Fanti PA, Orlandi C, Chieregato C, Misciali C. Psoriatic scarring alopecia: observations in four patients. Int J Dermatol. 1999;38(10):765–8.
6. Runne U, Kroneisen-Wiersma P. Psoriatic alopecia: acute and chronic hair loss in 47 patients with scalp psoriasis. Dermatology. 1992;185(2):82–7.
7. Stanimirovic A, Skerlev M, Stipic T, Beck T, Basta-Juzbasic A, Ivankovic D. Has psoriasis its own characteristic trichogram? J Dermatol Sci. 1998;17(2):156–9.
8. Ross EK, Vincenzi C, Tosti A. Videodermoscopy in the evaluation of hair and scalp disorders. J Am Acad Dermatol. 2006;55(5):799–806.
9. Rossi A, Mandel VD, Garelli V, Mari E, Fortuna MC, Carlesimo M, et al. Videodermoscopy scalp psoriasis severity index (VSCAPSI): a useful tool for evaluation of scalp psoriasis. Eur J Dermatol. 2011;21(4):546–51.
10. Rosina P, Zamperetti MR, Giovannini A, Girolomoni G. Videocapillaroscopy in the differential diagnosis between psoriasis and seborrheic dermatitis of the scalp. Dermatology. 2007;214(1): 21–4.
11. Slowinska M, Kardynal A, Warszawik O, Czuwara J, Rudnicka L. Alopecia areata developing paralell to improvement of psoriasis during ustekinumab therapy. J Dermatol Case Rep. 2010;4(1): 15–7.
12. Kim GW, Jung HJ, Ko HC, Kim MB, Lee WJ, Lee SJ, et al. Dermoscopy can be useful in differentiating scalp psoriasis from seborrhoeic dermatitis. Br J Dermatol. 2011;164(3):652–6.
13. Micali G, Lacarrubba F, Massimino D, Schwartz RA. Dermatoscopy: alternative uses in daily clinical practice. J Am Acad Dermatol. 2011;64(6):1135–46.
14. Lacarrubba F, Nasca MR, Micali G. Videodermatoscopy enhances diagnostic capability in psoriatic balanitis. J Am Acad Dermatol. 2009;61(6):1084–6.
15. Vazquez-Lopez F, Zaballos P, Fueyo-Casado A, Sanchez-Martin J. A dermoscopy subpattern of plaque-type psoriasis: red globular rings. Arch Dermatol. 2007;143(12):1612.
16. Zalaudek I, Argenziano G, Di Stefani A, Ferrara G, Marghoob AA, Hofmann-Wellenhof R, et al. Dermoscopy in general dermatology. Dermatology. 2006;212(1):7–18.
17. Zalaudek I, Kreusch J, Giacomel J, Ferrara G, Catricala C, Argenziano G. How to diagnose nonpigmented skin tumors: a review of vascular structures seen with dermoscopy: part II.

Nonmelanocytic skin tumors. J Am Acad Dermatol. 2010;63(3): 377–86; quiz 387–8.
18. Rosina P, Giovannini A, Gisondi P, Girolomoni G. Microcirculatory modifications of psoriatic lesions during topical therapy. Skin Res Technol. 2009;15(2):135–8.
19. Zalaudek I, Argenziano G. Glomerular vessels in Bowen's disease. Br J Dermatol. 2004;151(3):720.
20. Abdel-Hamid IA, Agha SA, Moustafa YM, El-Labban AM. Pityriasis amiantacea: a clinical and etiopathologic study of 85 patients. Int J Dermatol. 2003;42(4):260–4.
21. Bugatti L, Filosa G, Broganelli P, Tomasini C. Psoriasis-like dermoscopic pattern of clear cell acanthoma. J Eur Acad Dermatol Venereol. 2003;17(4):452–5.
22. Blum A, Metzler G, Bauer J, Rassner G, Garbe C. The dermatoscopic pattern of clear-cell acanthoma resembles psoriasis vulgaris. Dermatology. 2001;203(1):50–2.
23. Zalaudek I, Hofmann-Wellenhof R, Argenziano G. Dermoscopy of clear-cell acanthoma differs from dermoscopy of psoriasis. Dermatology. 2003;207(4):428; author reply 429.

Autoimmune Bullous Diseases

32

Marta Kurzeja, Malgorzata Olszewska,
and Lidia Rudnicka

Abstract

Trichoscopy of scalp lesions in pemphigus vulgaris and pemphigus foliaceous shows red, sharply demarcated, polygonal hemorrhagic areas; elongated serpentine blood vessels; dotted vessels with a whitish halo; large yellow dots with a whitish halo ("fried-egg sign"); and white lamellar structures. In pemphigoid, large yellow dots may be observed as well. Blisters and scarring features commonly are present. In dermatitis herpetiformis (Duhring's disease), trichoscopy is characterized by clusters of dotted blood vessels.

Keywords

Cicatricial alopecia • Cutaneous T-cell lymphoma • Dermatitis herpetiformis • Duhring's disease • Herpes zoster • Pemphigoid • Pemphigus foliaceus • Pemphigus vulgaris • Psoriasis Zoster

Scalp lesions in the course of autoimmune bullous diseases may be a diagnostic challenge if they are the first or only manifestation of disease. This chapter focuses on trichoscopy of the three most common autoimmune bullous diseases involving the scalp: pemphigus, pemphigoid, and dermatitis herpetiformis.

The pemphigus group includes autoimmune bullous diseases characterized immunologically by the presence of circulating and in vivo bound antibodies against desmogleins 1 and 3. In pemphigus vulgaris, bullae and erosions of the skin and mucous membranes are observed, whereas in pemphigus foliaceus, only skin lesions are present [1].

There is a discrepancy in the data regarding the incidence of scalp lesions and the type of hair loss in pemphigus. The estimated incidence of scalp involvement in pemphigus ranges from 5 to 50 % [2–6]. In some cases, scalp lesions, typically erosions, are the first manifestation of the disease [6, 7]. Case reports of very longstanding and treatment-resistant isolated pemphigus scalp lesions have been described [8, 9]. Wilson et al. [10] and Ioannides et al. [11] attributed the frequent scalp involvement in pemphigus to the high concentration of pemphigus antigens in the hair follicles. Whether pemphigus is associated with a certain type of hair loss remains controversial. Some authors indicate that pemphigus may be associated with telogen effluvium.

Pemphigoid is an autoimmune subepidermal bullous disease with various clinical and immunologic variants. Mucous membrane pemphigoid is associated with skin lesions (including those of the scalp) in 7 to 30 % cases [12]. Bullae, erosions, and scarring are typical clinical manifestations of scalp involvement.

Brunsting-Perry type pemphigoid is an immunologically heterogenous disease [13–15]. In Brunsting-Perry type pemphigoid, blisters and scarring are localized on the head,

M. Kurzeja
Department of Dermatology, CSK MSW, Warsaw, Poland

M. Olszewska (✉)
Department of Dermatology, Medical University of Warsaw, Koszykowa 82A, Warsaw 02-008, Poland
e-mail: malgorzata.olszewska@wum.edu.pl

L. Rudnicka
Faculty of Health Sciences, Medical University of Warsaw, Poland

Department of Dermatology, CSK MSW, Woloska 137, Warsaw 02-502, Poland

L. Rudnicka et al. (eds.), *Atlas of Trichoscopy*,
DOI 10.1007/978-1-4471-4486-1_32,

forehead, neck, and upper trunk, typically in elderly men [15]. Scarring alopecia may be seen in such cases.

In epidermolysis bullosa acquisita, antibody formation against collagen VII is observed. Bullae are located in the area of mechanical trauma and heal with scars and milia. Scalp involvement very rarely is observed [16].

Dermatitis herpetiformis is an autoimmune bullous disease associated with gluten-sensitive enteropathy [17]. A typical clinical manifestation is the presence of pruritic, symmetrically distributed vesicles on the skin. The scalp is a typical location of the disease: scalp lesions are observed in about 30 % of patients with dermatitis herpetiformis [16]. Very rarely, this location is the site of the first manifestation of the disease [18].

Trichoscopy of scalp lesions in most autoimmune bullous diseases has not been fully elucidated yet. In pemphigus, trichoscopy shows red, sharply demarcated, polygonal hemorrhagic areas; elongated serpentine blood vessels; dotted vessels with a whitish halo; large yellow dots with a whitish halo ("fried-egg sign"); and white lamellar structures [19]. There are no significant differences in the results of scalp lesion trichoscopy between pemphigus vulgaris and pemphigus foliaceus. In pemphigoid, large yellow dots may be observed as well. Blisters and features of scarring may be observed. In dermatitis herpetiformis, trichoscopy is characterized by clusters of multiple blood vessels that are regularly distributed and form linear and circular structures.

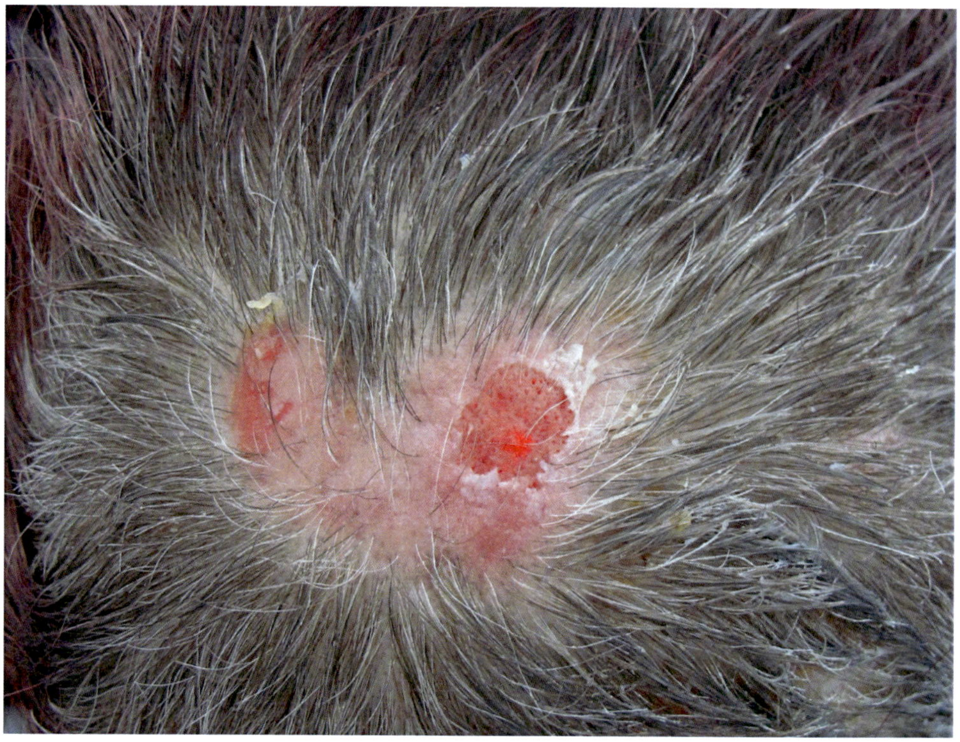

Fig. 32.1 Scalp lesions in pemphigus vulgaris. This image shows sharply demarcated erosions and detached epidermis in a 43-year-old patient with pemphigus vulgaris of recent onset. A hemorrhagic area is visible within the erosion. The estimated incidence of scalp involvement in pemphigus ranges from 5 to 50 % [2–6]. In some cases of pemphigus vulgaris and pemphigus foliaceus, scalp lesions are the first manifestation of the disease [6, 7]. In these cases, the diagnosis is most challenging. Case reports of very long-lasting and treatment-resistant isolated pemphigus scalp lesions have been described [8, 9]. Some authors indicate that scalp involvement in the course of pemphigus predicts more severe, long-lasting disease [7]

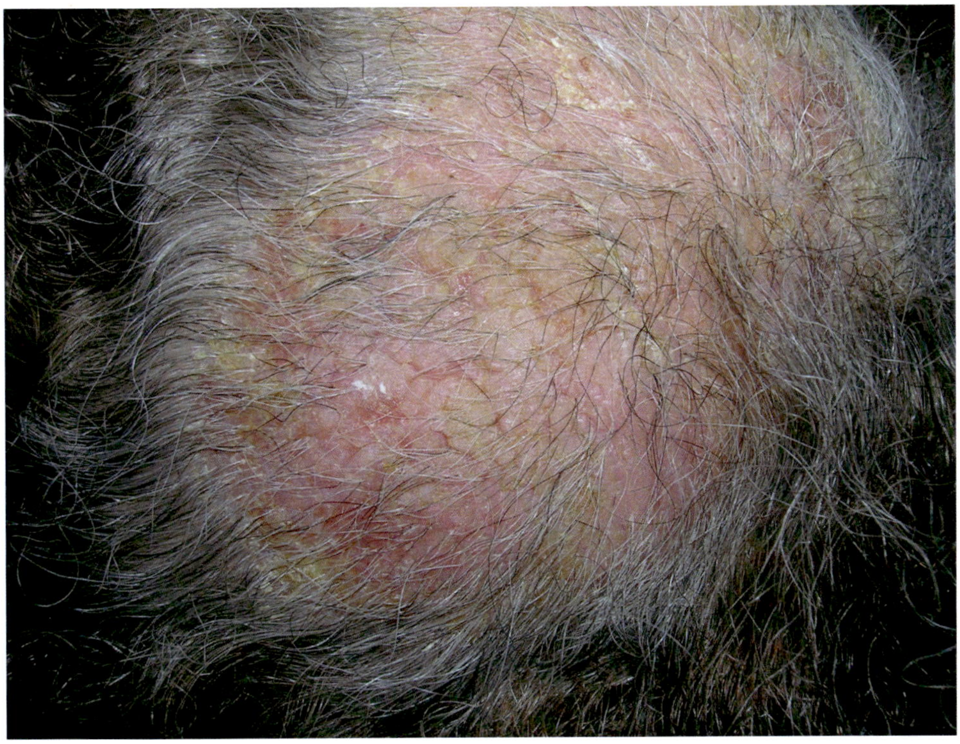

Fig. 32.2 Scalp lesions in pemphigus foliaceus. Shown is hair loss in a 57-year-old patient with long-lasting, therapy-resistant pemphigus vulgaris and a transition to pemphigus foliaceus during the course of the disease. Whether pemphigus is associated with a certain type of hair loss remains controversial. Some authors indicate that pemphigus may be associated with telogen effluvium. Stanley's group [20] described mice with a disruption of the desmoglein 3 gene, in which synchronous telogen hair loss was observed. The authors suggested that desmoglein 3 may play an important role in anchoring telogen hairs in the hair follicle. Schaerer and Trueb [21] showed that pemphigus antibodies bind to the outer root sheaths in pemphigus patients with or without skin lesions. These findings and subsequent reflectance confocal microscopic studies indicate that hair shafts may detach from the hair follicle as a result of acantholysis [22], which would result in anagen hair loss [6, 16, 23, 24]. Saijyo and Tagami [25], Petroni - Rosi et al. [26], and Jappe et al. [27] described tufted hair folliculitis in patients with pemphigus

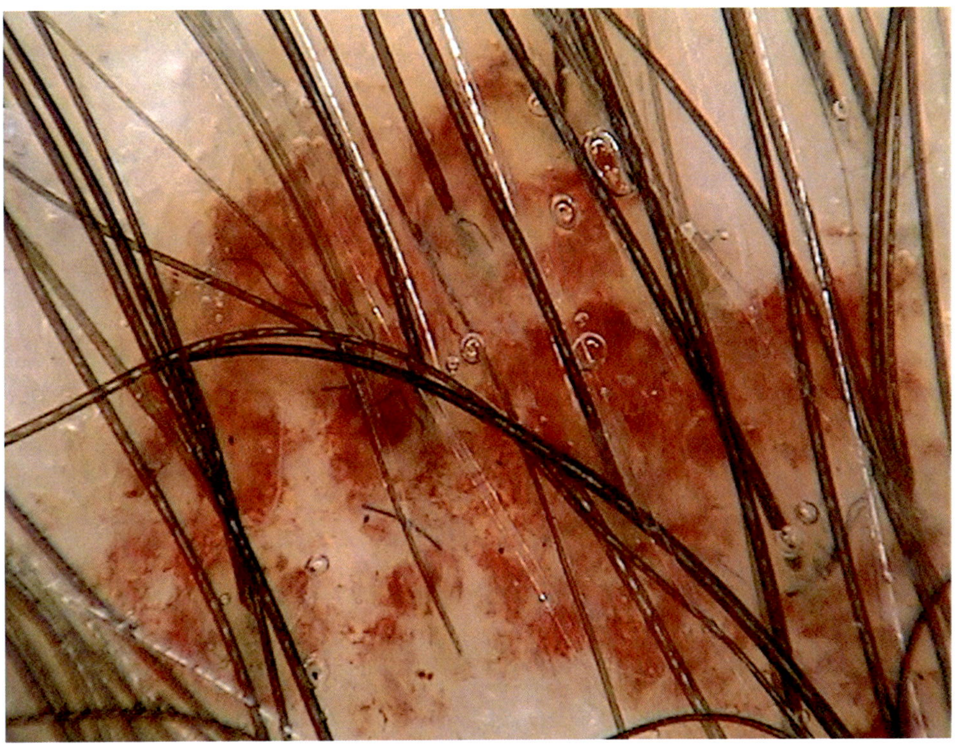

Fig. 32.3 Hemorrhagic areas in pemphigus vulgaris. Red, sharply demarcated, polygonal hemorrhagic areas usually develop within pemphigus vulgaris erosions of recent onset. This finding is more common in pemphigus vulgaris than pemphigus foliaceus [28](×70)

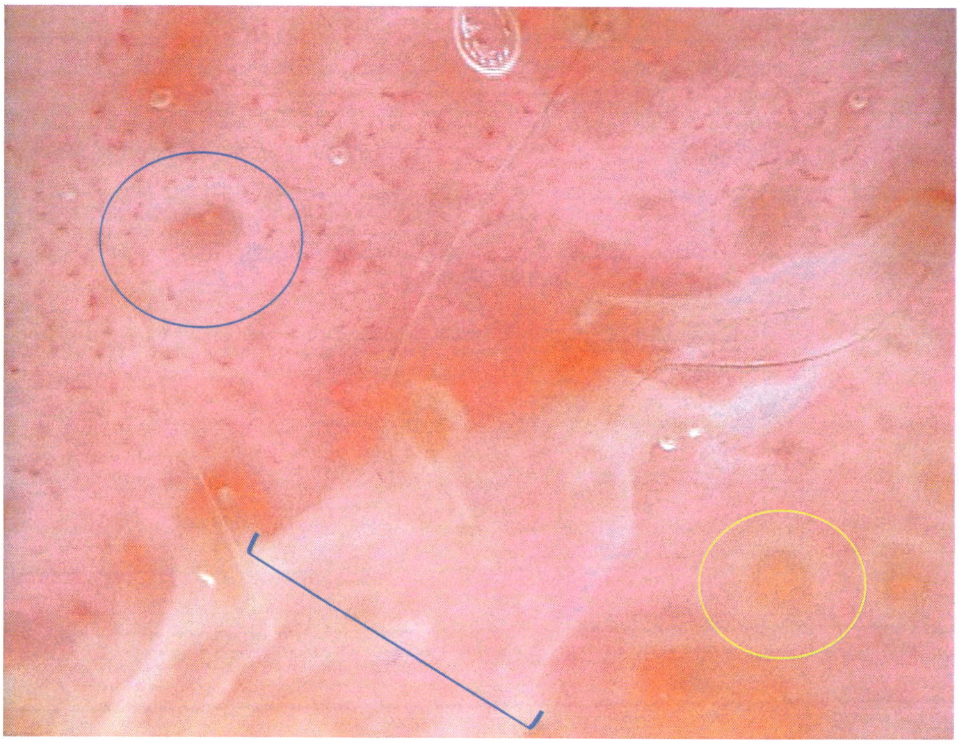

Fig. 32.4 Dotted vessels with a whitish halo, white lamellar structures, and large yellow dots in pemphigus vulgaris. Dotted vessels are aligned in linear or circular (*blue ring*) shapes. These groups of dotted vessels are surrounded by a whitish halo. White lamellar structures (*blue bracket*) correspond to a partly detached epidermis overlying the erosion. Some authors call these lamellar structures *waves hitting a shore* because of their white longitudinal appearance overlying a different colored (usually erythematous) area. Large yellow dots (*yellow ring*) with a whitish halo (fried-egg sign) represent another characteristic feature of pemphigus of the scalp [19]. These yellow dots appear to correspond to follicular openings covered by residues of detached epidermis (×70)

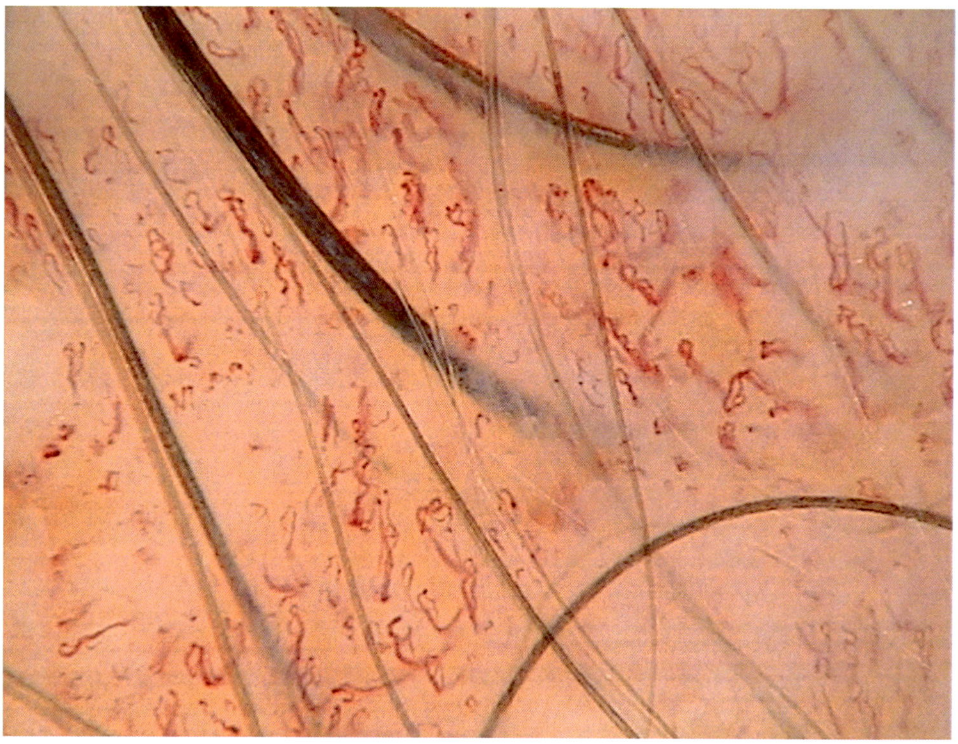

Fig. 32.5 Elongated blood vessels in pemphigus vulgaris. Considerably elongated helical and serpentine-like blood vessels are a common finding in early lesions of both pemphigus vulgaris and pemphigus foliaceus. This vascular pattern is not specific for pemphigus. Our experience shows that similar elongated serpentine-like blood vessels may be observed in cutaneous T-cell lymphoma, scalp lesions in the course of inflammatory bowel disease, and other multisystem disorders involving the scalp. The area in this image is partly covered by a whitish epidermal veil [28] (×70)

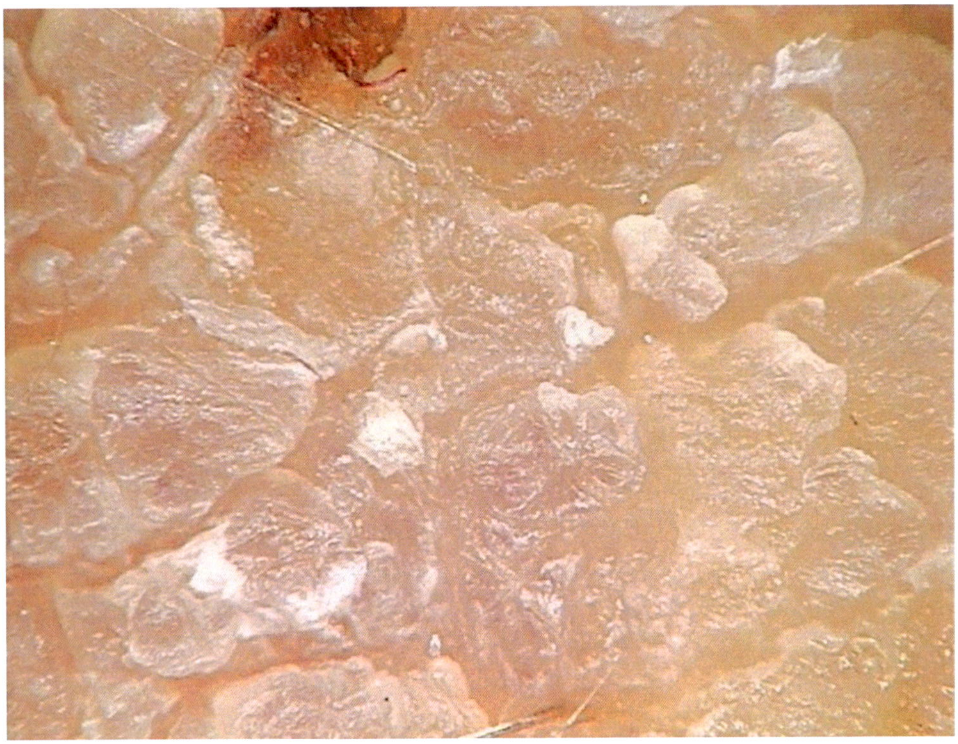

Fig. 32.6 Polygonal white lamellar structures in pemphigus foliaceus. Large white thick polygonal scales with protruding edges correspond to partly detaching elements of the epidermis. Brownish crusts are visible at the top of the image [28] (×70)

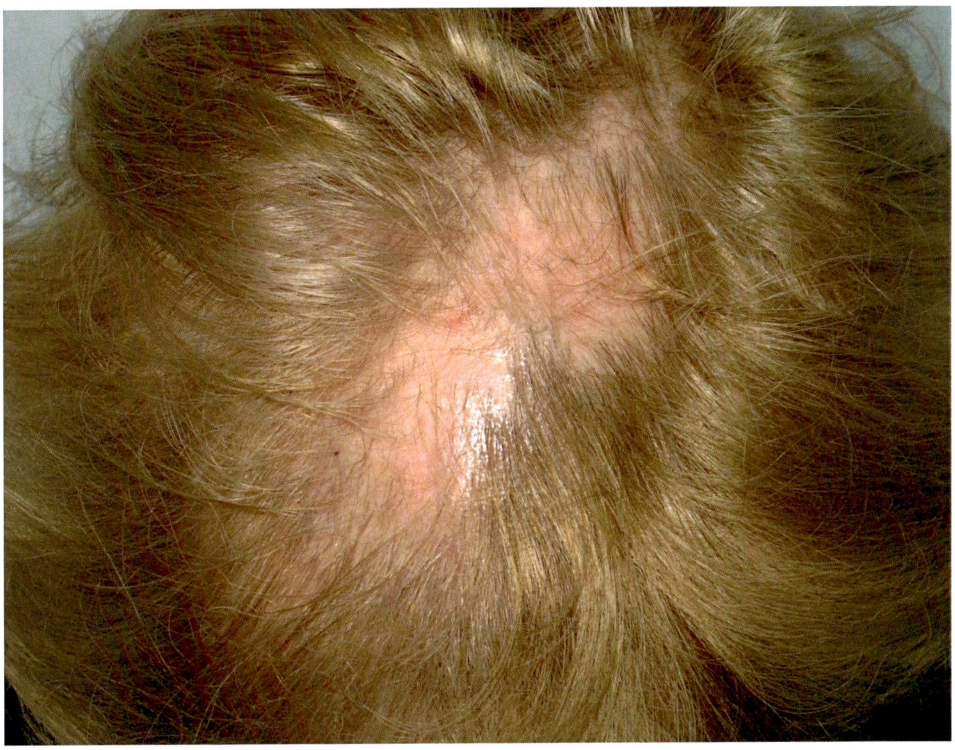

Fig. 32.7 Cicatricial alopecia in a patient with Brunsting-Perry type pemphigoid. Brunsting-Perry type pemphigoid is an immunologically heterogenous condition [13–15]. In this condition, cicatricial alopecia is a frequent finding. Scalp lesions may be observed in patients with various clinical and immunologic variants of pemphigoid. Blisters, erosions, and scarring are typical clinical manifestations of scalp involvement during the course of pemphigoid

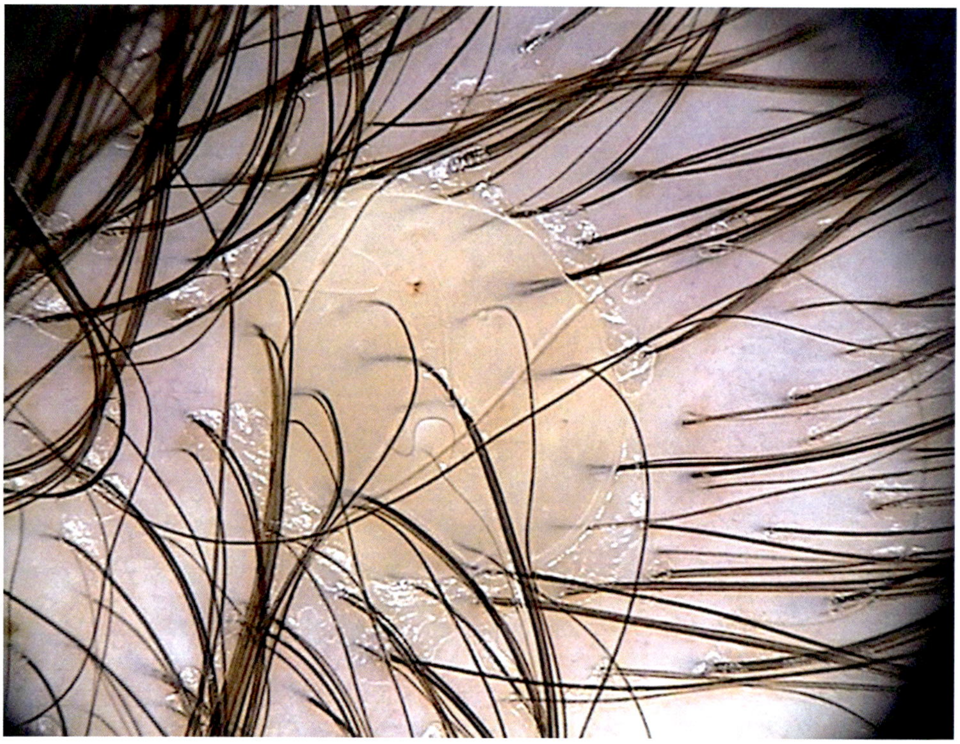

Fig. 32.8 A blister in bullous pemphigoid. In bullous pemphigoid, blisters are visible as areas of sharply demarcated creamy white circular or oval structures. Hair shafts emerge from the midpart of the blister. This type of lesion usually heals without scarring [28] (×20)

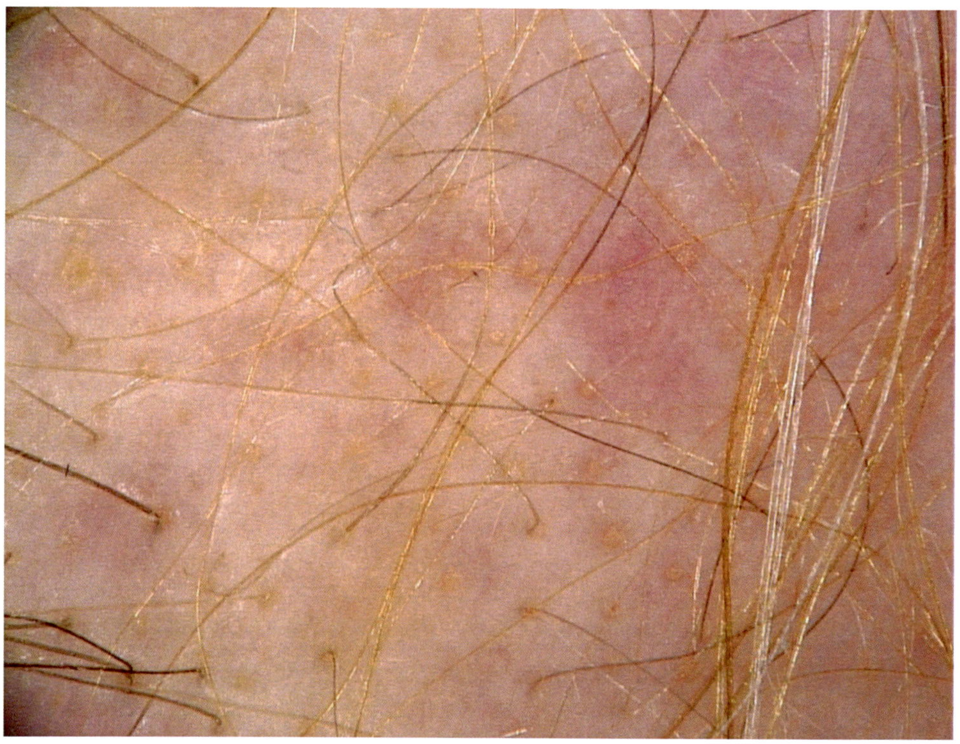

Fig. 32.9 Large yellow dots with a whitish halo (fried-egg sign) in pemphigoid. Large yellow dots with a whitish halo (fried-egg sign) may be observed in both pemphigus and pemphigoid. They most probably correspond to follicular openings covered by residues of detached epidermis. Sebum in the follicular infundibulum gives the detached epidermal portion, which covers the follicular opening, a yellowish color, whereas the perifollicular portion of the detached epidermis appears white [28] (×20)

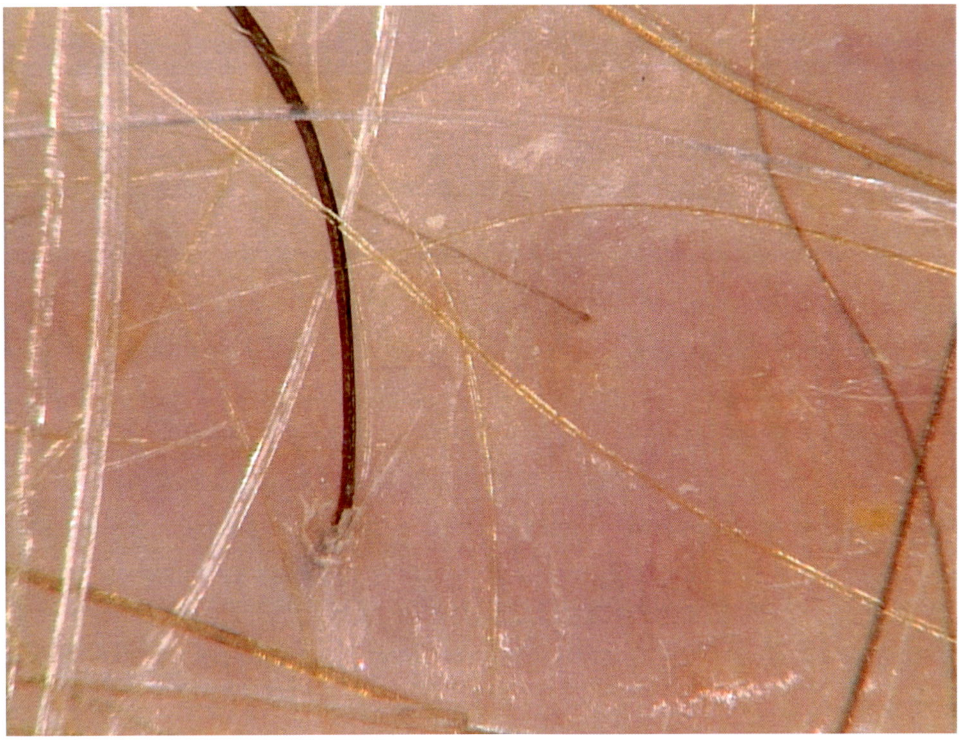

Fig. 32.10 Cicatricial alopecia in the course of pemphigoid. This image shows an erythematous area with a significantly decreased number of follicular openings. Large yellow dots are present (*bottom right*). Subtle parallel folds indicate scarring. Mild perifollicular scaling surrounds the terminal hair in the *middle* of the image [28] (×70)

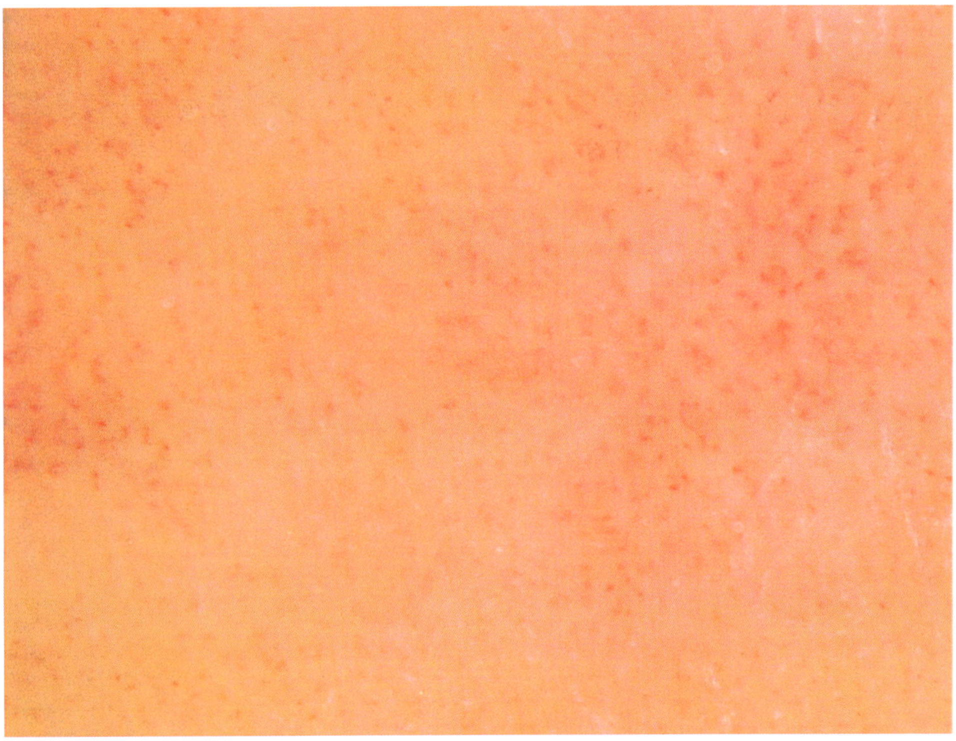

Fig. 32.11 Dermatitis herpetiformis. Dermatitis herpetiformis (Duhring's disease) is characterized by clusters of multiple blood vessels (dotted, comma, or linear) that are regularly distributed and form linear and circular structures. This pattern of blood vessel distribution may lead to the misdiagnosis of psoriasis [28] (×50)

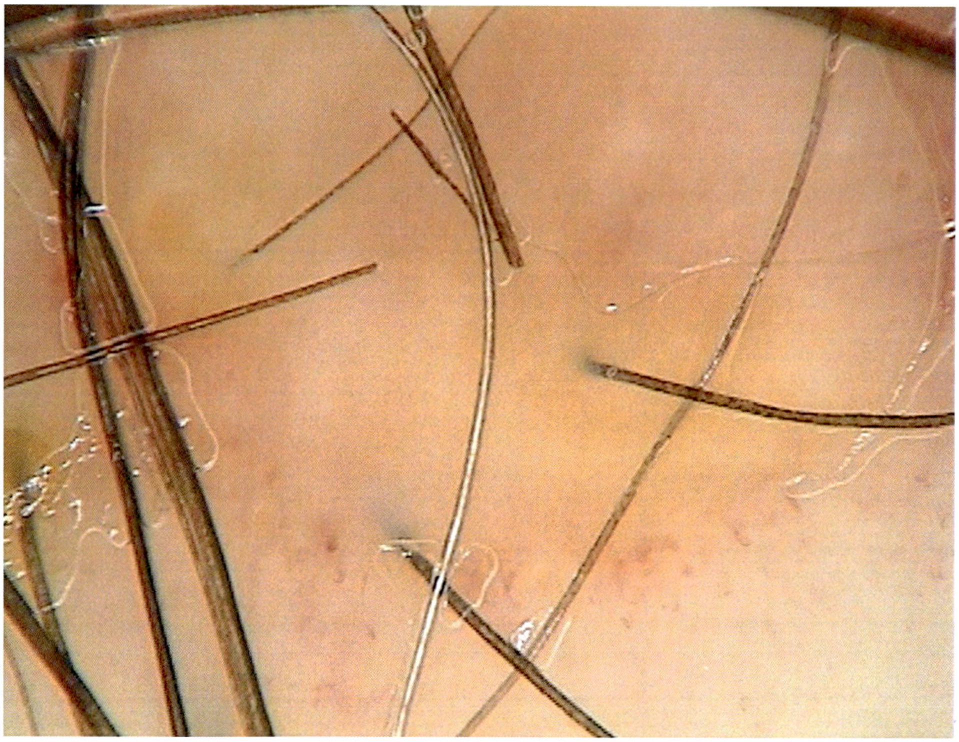

Fig. 32.12 Epidermal detachment: differential diagnosis. Epidermal detachment always appears as white or creamy white areas, usually well demarcated. This image shows a vesicle in a patient with herpes zoster. Hairs emerge from the midpart of the vesicle. Crown-like vessels at the periphery of this vesicle also are present in other diseases with formation of vesicles or blisters [28] (×70)

References

1. Bystryn JC, Rudolph JL. Pemphigus. Lancet. 2005;366(9479): 61–73.
2. Arya SR, Valand AG, Krishna K. A clinico-pathological study of 70 cases of pemphigus. Indian J Dermatol Venereol Leprol. 1999;65(4):168–71.
3. Esmaili N, Chams-Davatchi C, Valikhani M, Daneshpazhooh M, Balighi K, Hallaji Z, et al. Pemphigus vulgaris in Iran: a clinical study of 140 cases. Int J Dermatol. 2007;46(11):1166–70.
4. Salmanpour R, Shahkar H, Namazi MR, Rahman-Shenas MR. Epidemiology of pemphigus in south-western Iran: a 10-year retrospective study (1991–2000). Int J Dermatol. 2006; 45(2):103–5.
5. Chams-Davatchi C, Valikhani M, Daneshpazhooh M, Esmaili N, Balighi K, Hallaji Z, et al. Pemphigus: analysis of 1209 cases. Int J Dermatol. 2005;44(6):470–6.
6. Veraitch O, Ohyama M, Yamagami J, Amagai M. Alopecia as a rare but distinct manifestation of pemphigus vulgaris. J Eur Acad Dermatol Venereol. 2011. doi:10.1111/j.1468-3083.2011.04363.x.
7. Sar-Pomian M, Kolacinska-Strasz Z, Labecka H, Krainska-Wojcik T, Olszewska M. Scalp lesions in pemphigus. Przegl Dermatol. 2010;97:14–20.
8. Lapiere K, Caers S, Lambert J. A case of long-lasting localized pemphigus vulgaris of the scalp. Dermatology. 2004; 209(2):162–3.
9. Rackett SC, Rothe MJ, Hoss DM, Grin-Jorgensen CM, Grant-Kels JM. Treatment-resistant pemphigus vegetans of the scalp. Int J Dermatol. 1995;34(12):865–6.
10. Wilson CL, Dean D, Wojnarowska F. Pemphigus and the terminal hair follicle. J Cutan Pathol. 1991;18(6):428–31.
11. Ioannides D, Hytiroglou P, Phelps RG, Bystryn JC. Regional variation in the expression of pemphigus foliaceus, pemphigus erythematosus, and pemphigus vulgaris antigens in human skin. J Invest Dermatol. 1991;96(2):159–61.
12. Ball S, Walkden V, Wojnarowska F. Cicatricial pemphigoid rarely involves the scalp. Australas J Dermatol. 1998;39(4):258–60.
13. Fukuda S, Tsuruta D, Uchiyama M, Mitsuhashi Y, Kobayashi H, Ishikawa T, et al. Brunsting-Perry type pemphigoid with IgG autoantibodies to laminin-332, BP230 and desmoplakins I/II. Br J Dermatol. 2011;165(2):433–5.
14. Minato H, Ishii N, Fukuda S, Wakasa T, Wakasa K, Sogame R, et al. Heterogeneity of Brunsting-Perry type pemphigoid: a case showing blister formation at the lamina lucida, immune deposition beneath the lamina densa and autoantibodies against the 290-kD polypeptide along the lamina densa. J Dermatol. 2011;38(9): 887–92.
15. Kneisel A, Hertl M. Autoimmune bullous skin diseases. Part 1: clinical manifestations. J Dtsch Dermatol Ges. 2011;9(10):844–956; quiz 857.
16. Miteva M, Murrell DF, Tosti A. Hair loss in autoimmune cutaneous bullous disorders. Dermatol Clin. 2011;29(3):503–9, xi.
17. Rose C, Brocker EB, Zillikens D. Clinical, histological and immunpathological findings in 32 patients with dermatitis herpetiformis Duhring. J Dtsch Dermatol Ges. 2010;8(4):265–70, 271.
18. Gul U, Soylu S, Heper AO. An unusual case of dermatitis herpetiformis presenting with initial scalp localization. Indian J Dermatol Venereol Leprol. 2009;75(6):620–2.
19. Kurzeja M, Rakowska A, Olszewska M, Rudnicka L.Trichoscopy (dermoscopy of the scalp) in autoimmune bullous skin diseases. Abstract CD. 21st Congres of the European Academy of Dermatology and Venereology, Prague 27-30.09.2012.
20. Koch PJ, Mahoney MG, Cotsarelis G, Rothenberger K, Lavker RM, Stanley JR. Desmoglein 3 anchors telogen hair in the follicle. J Cell Sci. 1998;111(Pt 17):2529–37.
21. Schaerer L, Trueb RM. Direct immunofluorescence of plucked hair in pemphigus. Arch Dermatol. 2003;139(2):228–9.
22. Kurzeja M, Rakowska A, Rudnicka L, Olszewska M. Criteria for diagnosing pemphigus vulgaris and pemphigus foliaceus by reflectance confocal microscopy. Skin Res Technol. 2012 Aug;18(3)339–46. doi:10.1111/j.1600-0846.2011.00574.x.

23. Delmonte S, Semino MT, Parodi A, Rebora A. Normal anagen effluvium: a sign of pemphigus vulgaris. Br J Dermatol. 2000;142(6):1244–5.
24. Koslu A, Topal IO, Ekmekci TR. Trichogram findings in pemphigus patients. Indian J Dermatol Venereol Leprol. 2009;75(3):303–4.
25. Saijyo S, Tagami H. Tufted hair folliculitis developing in a recalcitrant lesion of pemphigus vulgaris. J Am Acad Dermatol. 1998;38(5 Pt 2):857–9.
26. Petronić-Rosić V, Krunić A, Mijusković M, Vesić S. Tufted hair folliculitis: a pattern of scarring alopecia? J Am Acad Dermatol. 1999;41(1):112–4.
27. Jappe U, Schroder K, Zillikens D, Petzoldt D. Tufted hair folliculitis associated with pemphigus vulgaris. J Eur Acad Dermatol Venereol. 2003;17(2):223–6.
28. Kurzeja M Application of reflectance confocal microscopy in diagnosing pemphigus vulgaris and pemphigus foliaceus. PhD Thesis, Medical University of Warsaw, Warsaw 2013.

Part XI

Trichoscopy in Children

Trichoscopy in Children

33

Mariya Miteva and Antonella Tosti

Abstract

This chapter reviews the role of trichoscopy in the diagnosis of hair and scalp disorders in children. We discuss features observed in the normal scalp, in infectious diseases that commonly affect children, and in alopecia areata, and highlight the role of trichoscopy in a rapid noninvasive diagnosis.

Keywords

African American • Alopecia areata • Children • Aplasia cutis congenita • Congenital triangular alopecia • Dirty dots • Hair casts • Pediculosis • Tinea capitis • Trichotillomania

The normal scalp of children often shows *dirty dots*. Fu et al. [1] identified dirty dots as a normal finding on the scalp in 10 of 19 healthy children. Dirty dots represent nonmicrobial environmental particles easily removed by shampooing.

Dermoscopy of tinea capitis shows two typical features: *comma hairs* and *corkscrew hairs*. Comma hairs are slightly curved, fractured hair shafts; they have been described as the dermoscopic marker of tinea capitis in white children with *Microsporum canis* infection [2, 3]. Hughes et al. [4] reported corkscrew hairs as an additional dermoscopic finding in children with *Trichophyton* or *Microsporum* infection. Broken and dystrophic hairs also are seen [4].

Dermoscopy is a very fast method for diagnosing pediculosis capitis, as it shows nits and parasites. Dermoscopy also allows differentiation between nits containing nymphs and empty nits of hatched parasites and nits from pseudo-nits [5].

Hair casts may be idiopathic in children [6]. They are seen in young girls as diffuse small 3–7-mm white cylindric casts that slide along the hair shafts. These children usually seek help for severe dandruff or pediculosis. Hair casts often may be seen in African American children with traction alopecia; they are a sign that traction is ongoing [7].

In alopecia areata, in our experience, yellow dots are uncommonly seen in prepubertal children. Usually, dermoscopy shows only broken and exclamation mark hairs. Clustered short vellus hairs and circle hairs may be the predominant feature in some patients.

Dermoscopy is a helpful tool for recognizing congenital triangular alopecia in atypical locations (other than the frontotemporal scalp) and in adults. Dermoscopic features include normal follicular openings with vellus hairs surrounded by normal terminal hair [8].

Trichotillomania may be very difficult to distinguish from alopecia areata with dermoscopy [9], as it also shows broken hairs and yellow dots [10, 11]. In the authors' experience, only two features allow differentiation between the two disorders: the presence of exclamation mark hairs (characteristic of alopecia areata) and the presence of coiled hairs (characteristic of trichotillomania).

Scarring alopecia is uncommon in children. However, dermoscopy is very useful in distinguishing small patches of alopecia areata from scars.

Dermoscopy has been shown to help in distinguishing aplasia cutis congenita from sebaceous nevus [12]. In sebaceous nevus, dermoscopy reveals bright yellow dots unassociated with hair follicles. Aplasia cutis congenita shows complete lack of skin appendages and translucent appearance [12].

M. Miteva • A. Tosti (✉)
Department of Dermatology and Cutaneous Surgery, University of Miami Health System, University of Miami L. Miller School of Medicine, 1600 NW 10th Ave., RSMB, Room 2023A, Miami 33136, FL, USA
e-mail: atosti@med.miami.edu

L. Rudnicka et al. (eds.), *Atlas of Trichoscopy*,
DOI 10.1007/978-1-4471-4486-1_33,

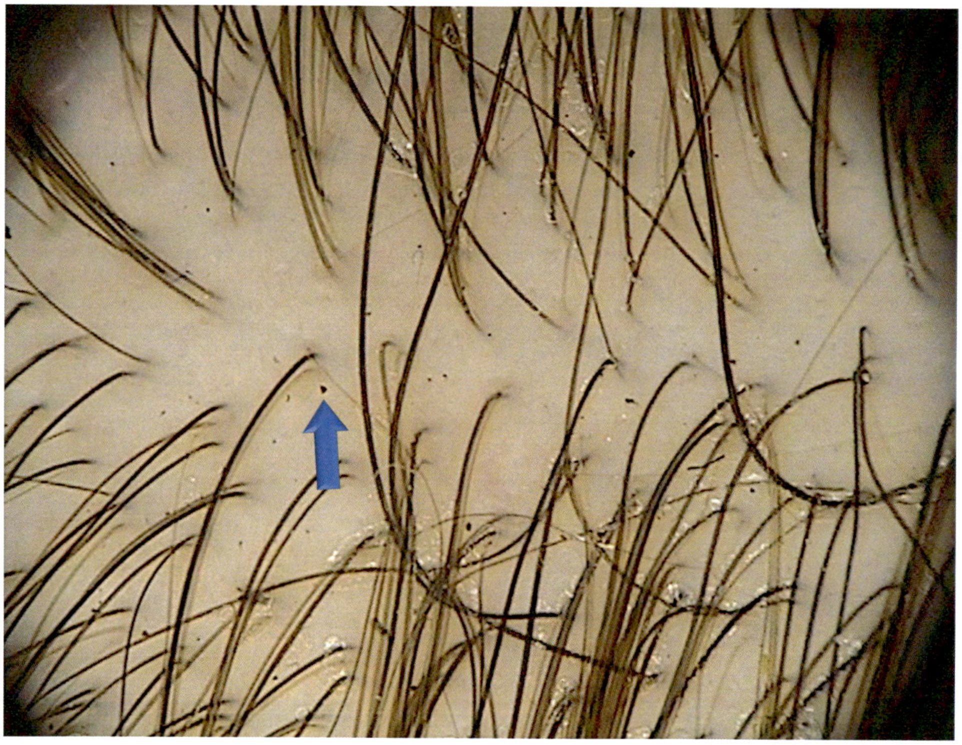

Fig. 33.1 Normal scalp in children. Note the presence of small irregular black particles (dirty dots; *arrow*)

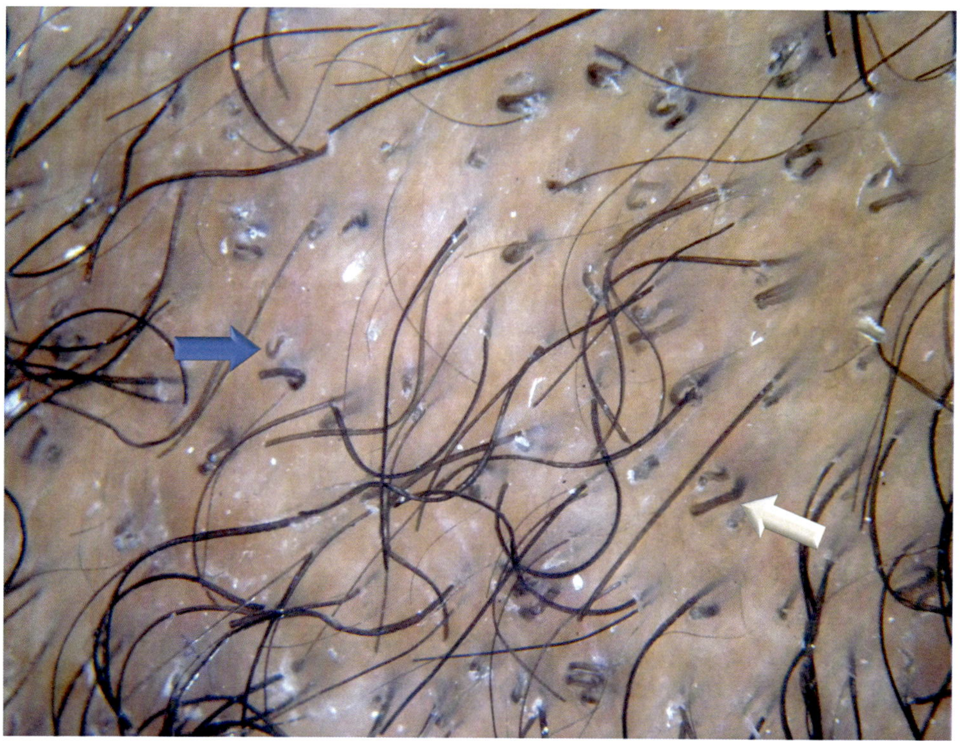

Fig. 33.2 Tinea capitis. Note the presence of many comma hairs (*blue arrow*) and broken hairs (*white arrow*)

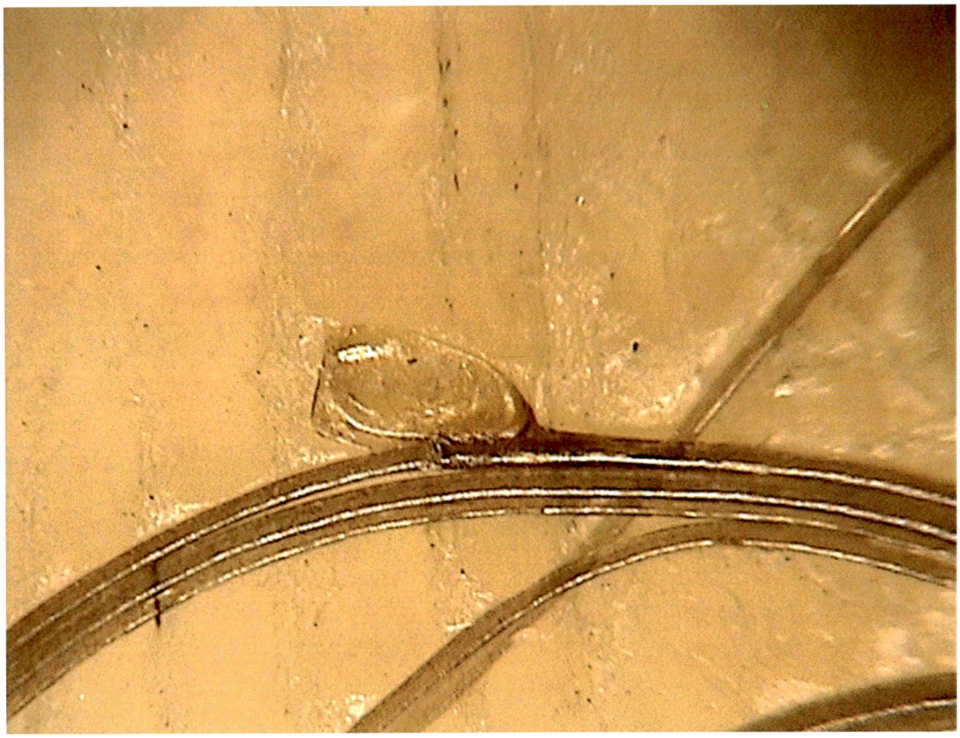

Fig. 33.3 **Pediculosis**. The image shows an empty nit in a child with pediculosis

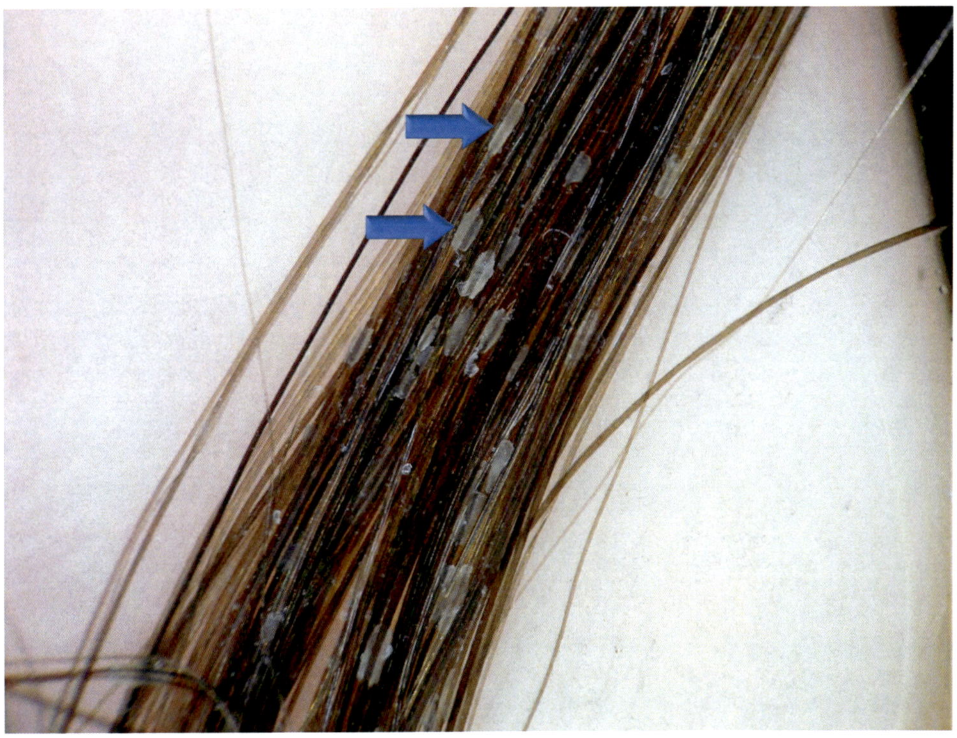

Fig. 33.4 Idiopathic hair casts (*arrows*) in a young Caucasian girl

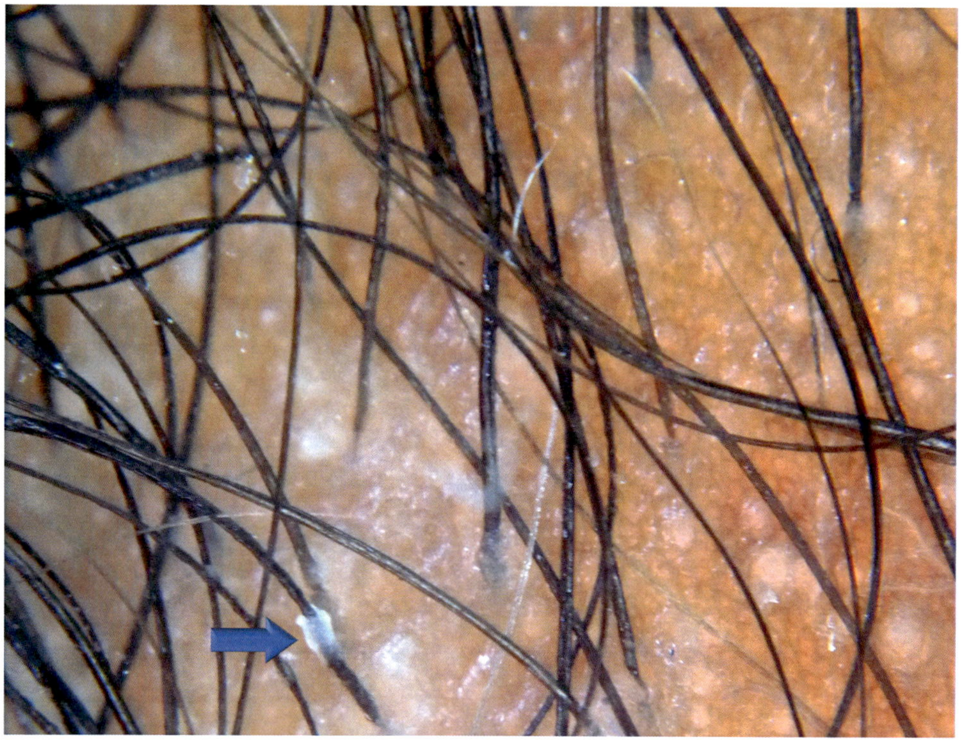

Fig. 33.5 Idiopathic hair casts (*arrow*) in an African American child with traction alopecia

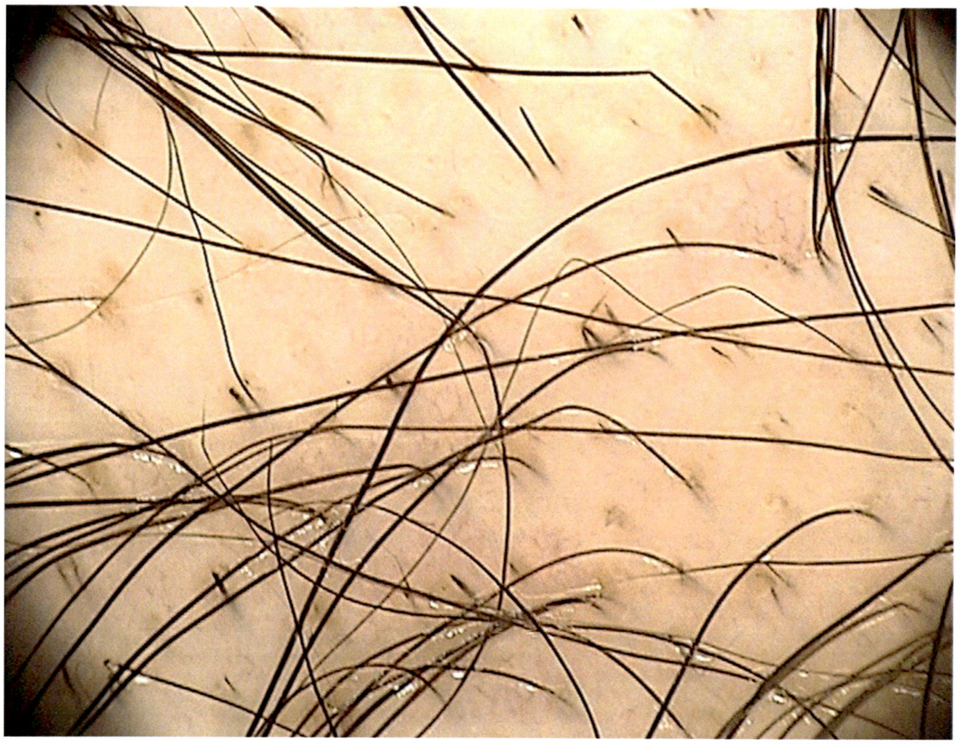

Fig. 33.6 Trichoscopy in a child with active alopecia areata. Note the presence of many broken hairs

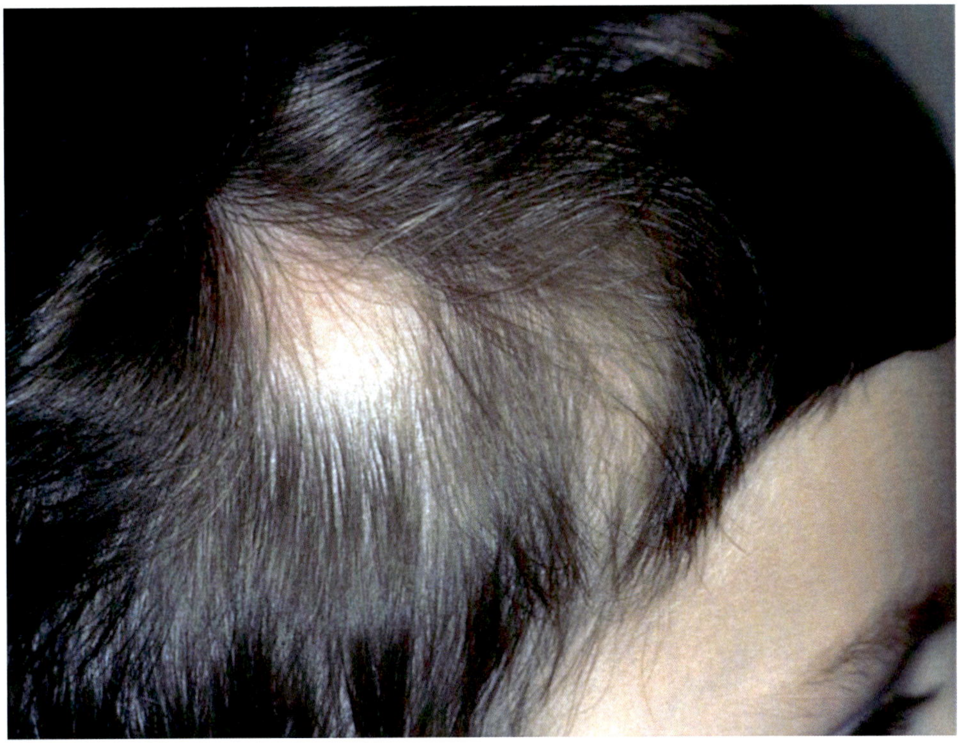

Fig. 33.7 Congenital triangular alopecia. Trichoscopy is a helpful tool for recognizing congenital triangular alopecia in atypical locations. This clinical image shows a boy with congenital triangular alopecia in an atypical location

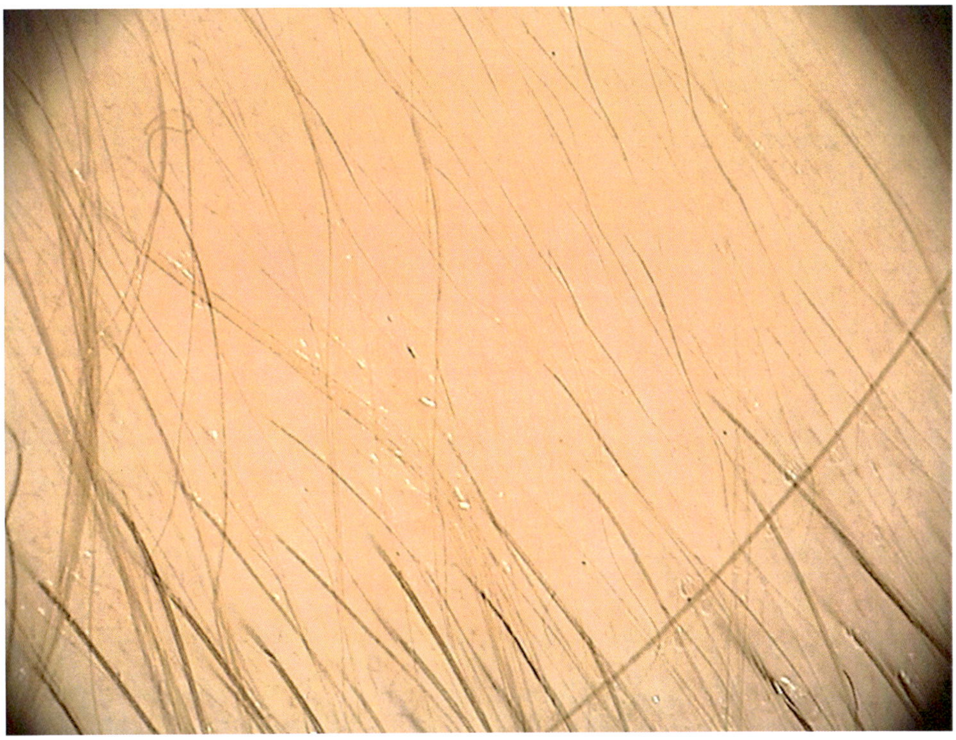

Fig. 33.8 Congenital triangular alopecia. Trichoscopy shows that the patch contains multiple vellus hairs

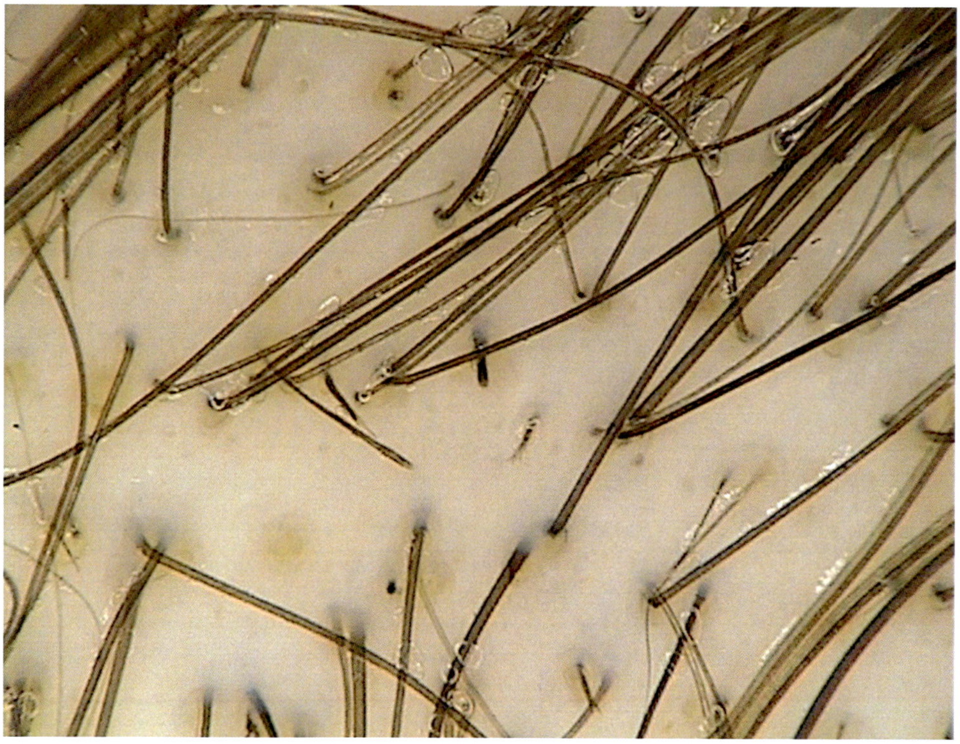

Fig. 33.9 Trichotillomania. Note the presence of yellow dots and broken hairs in this trichoscopic image from a child with trichotillomania

References

1. Fu JM, Starace M, Tosti A. A new dermoscopic finding in healthy children. Arch Dermatol. 2009;145(5):596–7.
2. Tangjaturonrusamee C, Piraccini BM, Vincenzi C, Starace M, Tosti A. Tinea capitis mimicking folliculitis decalvans. Mycoses. 2011;54(1):87–8.
3. Slowinska M, Rudnicka L, Schwartz RA, Kowalska-Oledzka E, Rakowska A, Sicinska J, et al. Comma hairs: a dermatoscopic marker for tinea capitis: a rapid diagnostic method. J Am Acad Dermatol. 2008;59(5 Suppl):S77–9.
4. Hughes R, Chiaverini C, Bahadoran P, Lacour JP. Corkscrew hair: a new dermoscopic sign for diagnosis of tinea capitis in black children. Arch Dermatol. 2011;147(3):355–6.
5. Bakos RM, Bakos L. Dermoscopy for diagnosis of pediculosis capitis. J Am Acad Dermatol. 2007;57(4):727–8.
6. Taieb A, Surleve-Bazeille JE, Maleville J. Hair casts. A clinical and morphologic study. Arch Dermatol. 1985;121(8):1009–13.
7. Tosti A, Miteva M, Torres F, Vincenzi C, Romanelli P. Hair casts are a dermoscopic clue for the diagnosis of traction alopecia. Br J Dermatol. 2010;163(6):1353–5.
8. Iorizzo M, Pazzaglia M, Starace M, Militello G, Tosti A. Videodermoscopy: a useful tool for diagnosing congenital triangular alopecia. Pediatr Dermatol. 2008;25(6):652–4.
9. Inui S, Nakajima T, Itami S. Coudability hairs: a revisited sign of alopecia areata assessed by trichoscopy. Clin Exp Dermatol. 2010;35(4):361–5.
10. Inui S, Nakajima T, Nakagawa K, Itami S. Clinical significance of dermoscopy in alopecia areata: analysis of 300 cases. Int J Dermatol. 2008;47(7):688–93.
11. Abraham LS, Torres FN, Azulay-Abulafia L. Dermoscopic clues to distinguish trichotillomania from patchy alopecia areata. An Bras Dermatol. 2010;85(5):723–6.
12. Neri I, Savoia F, Giacomini F, Raone B, Aprile S, Patrizi A. Usefulness of dermatoscopy for the early diagnosis of sebaceous naevus and differentiation from aplasia cutis congenita. Clin Exp Dermatol. 2009;34(5):e50–2.

Part XII

Precancerous Scalp Lesions and Scalp Tumors

Benign Melanocytic Tumors

34

Iris Zalaudek, Elvira Moscarella, Alexandre Abramavicus, Giuseppe Albertini, and Giuseppe Argenziano

Abstract

Common scalp nevi in children and teenagers are classically pigmented, whereas most scalp nevi in adults are usually nodular and nonpigmented with a smooth or papillomatous, occasionally keratotic, surface. Scalp nevi have no documented risk for malignant transformation.

Keywords

Basal cell carcinoma • Blue nevus • Dermoscopy • Melanoma • Nevus • Nonmelanoma skin cancer (NMSC)

Scalp nevi in children and teenagers are known indicators for a higher total nevus count, which is the strongest risk factor for melanoma in adults [1]. Accordingly, teenagers with scalp nevi may benefit from regular total body skin examinations. Moreover, a subset of scalp nevi may reveal worrisome features on histopathology, although they have no documented risk for malignant transformation [2].

Common scalp nevi in children and teenagers are classically pigmented [3–5], whereas most scalp nevi in adults are usually nodular and nonpigmented with a smooth or papillomatous, occasionally keratotic, surface [6]. The age-related differences in scalp nevi between children and adults may mirror different stages in their evolution. Scalp nevi have no documented risk for malignant transformation; thus, they can be managed conservatively.

Blue nevi are common on the scalp and may develop at any age; however, once developed, they represent highly stable and persistent tumors. Importantly, their clinical and dermoscopic patterns may be indistinguishable from those of thick fast-growing melanoma, cutaneous metastases, and heavily pigmented basal cell carcinoma [7, 8].

Unlike blue nevi, advanced melanomas, metastases, and basal cell carcinoma are characterized by a history of change; consequently, the diagnosis of blue nevus should be confirmed by a "convincing" subjective history of an unchanged, stable lesion [9]. If such history is not available or is uncertain, immediate excision of any nodular tumor is recommended, regardless of the patient's age.

I. Zalaudek
Department of Dermatology, Medical University of Graz, Graz, Austria

E. Moscarella
Department of Dermatology, University of Modena and Reggio Emilia, Modena, Italy

A. Abramavicus
Department of Dermatology, Unit of Skin Tumors, São Paulo Hospital, São Paulo, Brazil

G. Albertini • G. Argenziano (✉)
Dermatology and Skin Cancer Unit, Arcispedale Santa Maria Nuova IRCCS, Reggio Emilia, Italy
e-mail: g.argenziano@gmail.com

L. Rudnicka et al. (eds.), *Atlas of Trichoscopy*,
DOI 10.1007/978-1-4471-4486-1_34, © Springer-Verlag London 2012

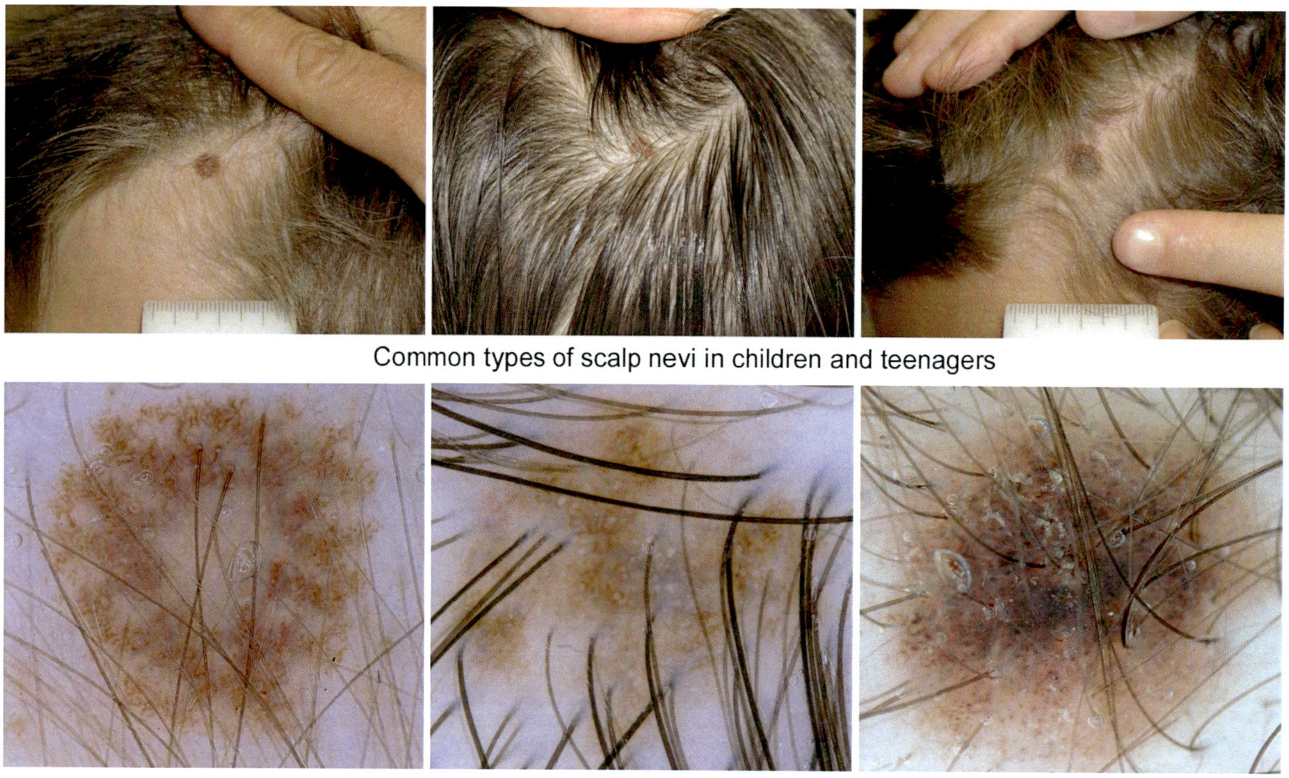

Fig. 34.1 Common scalp nevi in children and teenagers. Stereotypic clinical (*upper row*) and dermoscopic (*lower row*) appearance of common scalp nevi in children and teenagers. On dermoscopy, scalp nevi typically reveal a pigmented network with perifollicular hypopigmentation (*lower left and middle*) or a uniform globular pattern (*lower right*). Notably, peripherally located hypopigmented hair follicles may give rise to some border irregularity of the nevus

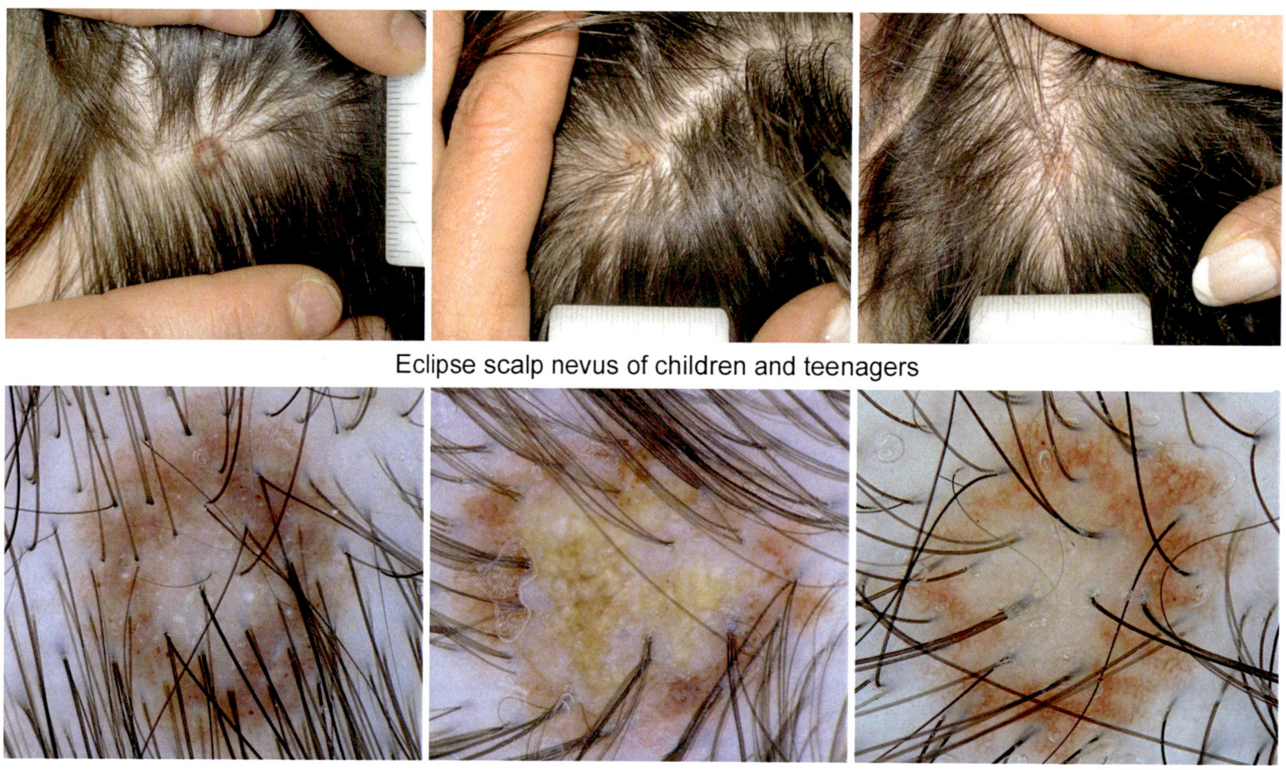

Fig. 34.2 Common scalp nevi with central hypopigmentation. Stereotypic clinical (*upper row*) and dermoscopic (*lower row*) appearance of common scalp nevi with central hypopigmentation, also called eclipse nevi. Dermoscopically, eclipse nevi show a central area of hypopigmentation, sometimes with a keratotic surface (*lower middle*), which is surrounded by a brown pigmented network of different color intensity

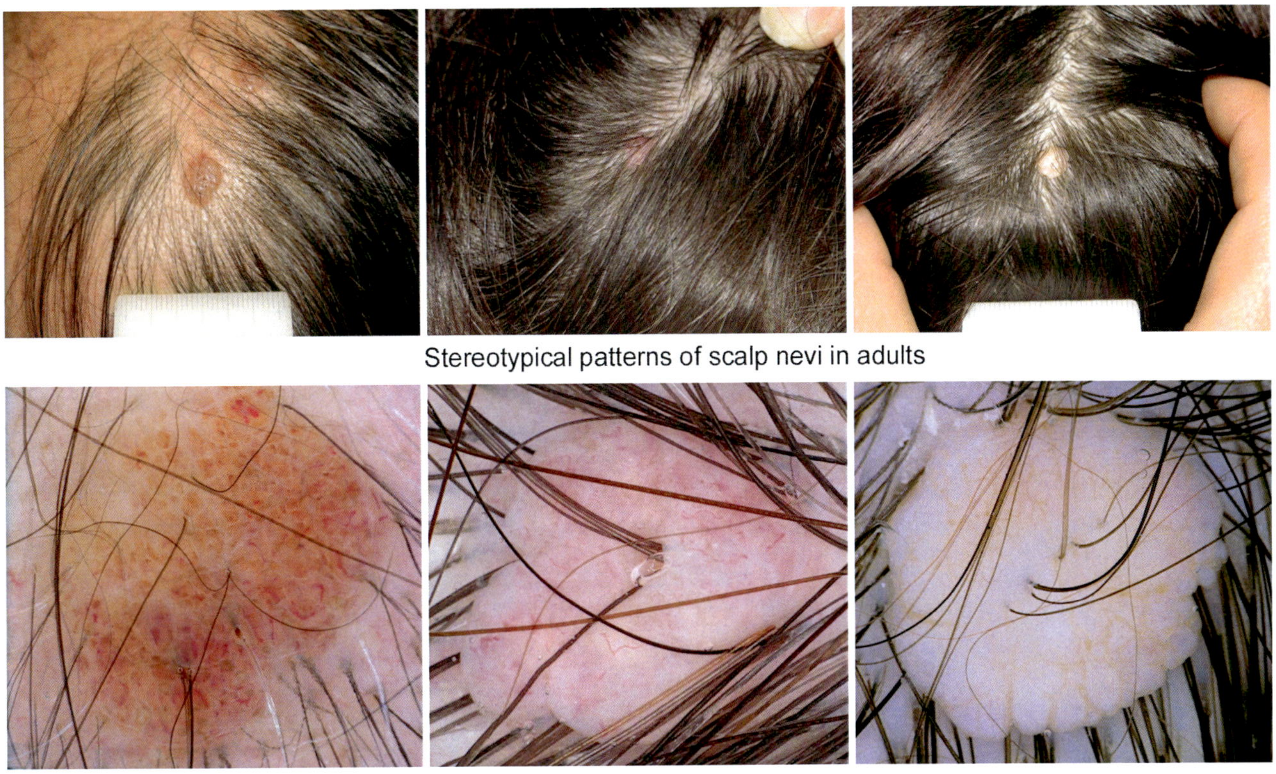

Fig. 34.3 **Scalp nevi in adults**. Stereotypic clinical (*upper row*) and dermoscopic (*lower row*) appearance of scalp nevi in adults. The nevi commonly exhibit a papillomatous surface and on dermoscopy show light brown, angulated globules; curved comma-shaped vessels (*lower left*) or elongated curved vessels of different lengths and diameters over a skin-colored background (*lower middle*); or no specific pigmented or vascular pattern (*lower right*)

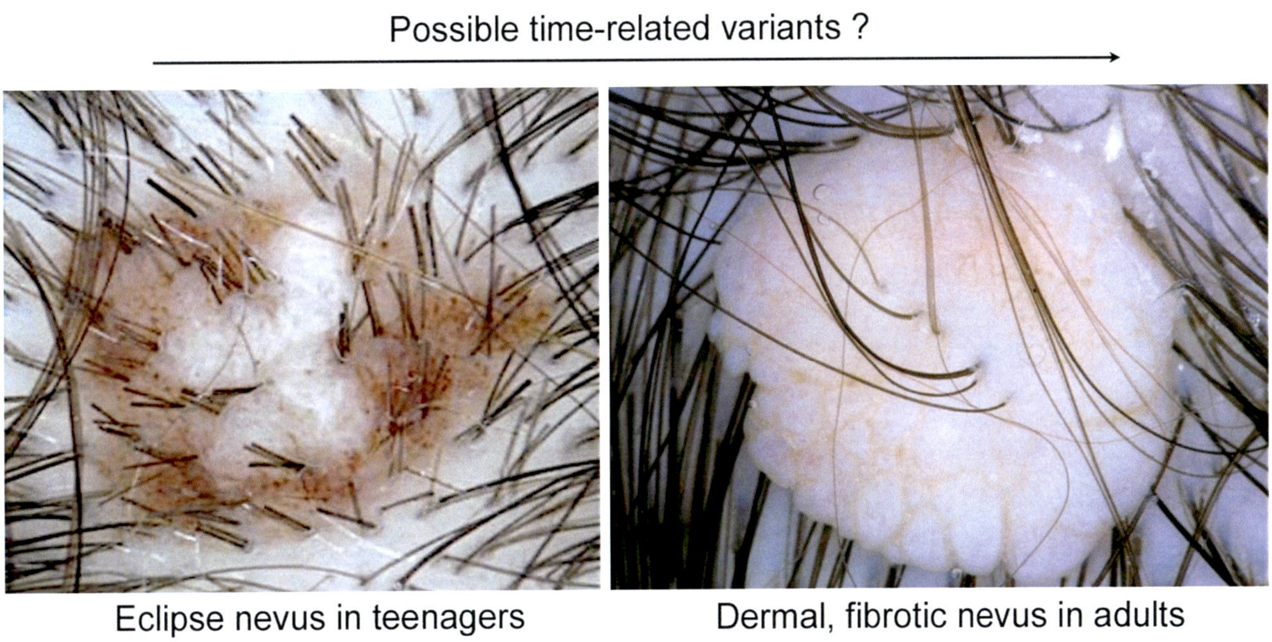

Fig. 34.4 **Eclipse nevi**. It has been hypothesized that eclipse nevi of youth may in time acquire the stereotypic appearance of a dermal nevus, as seen in adults

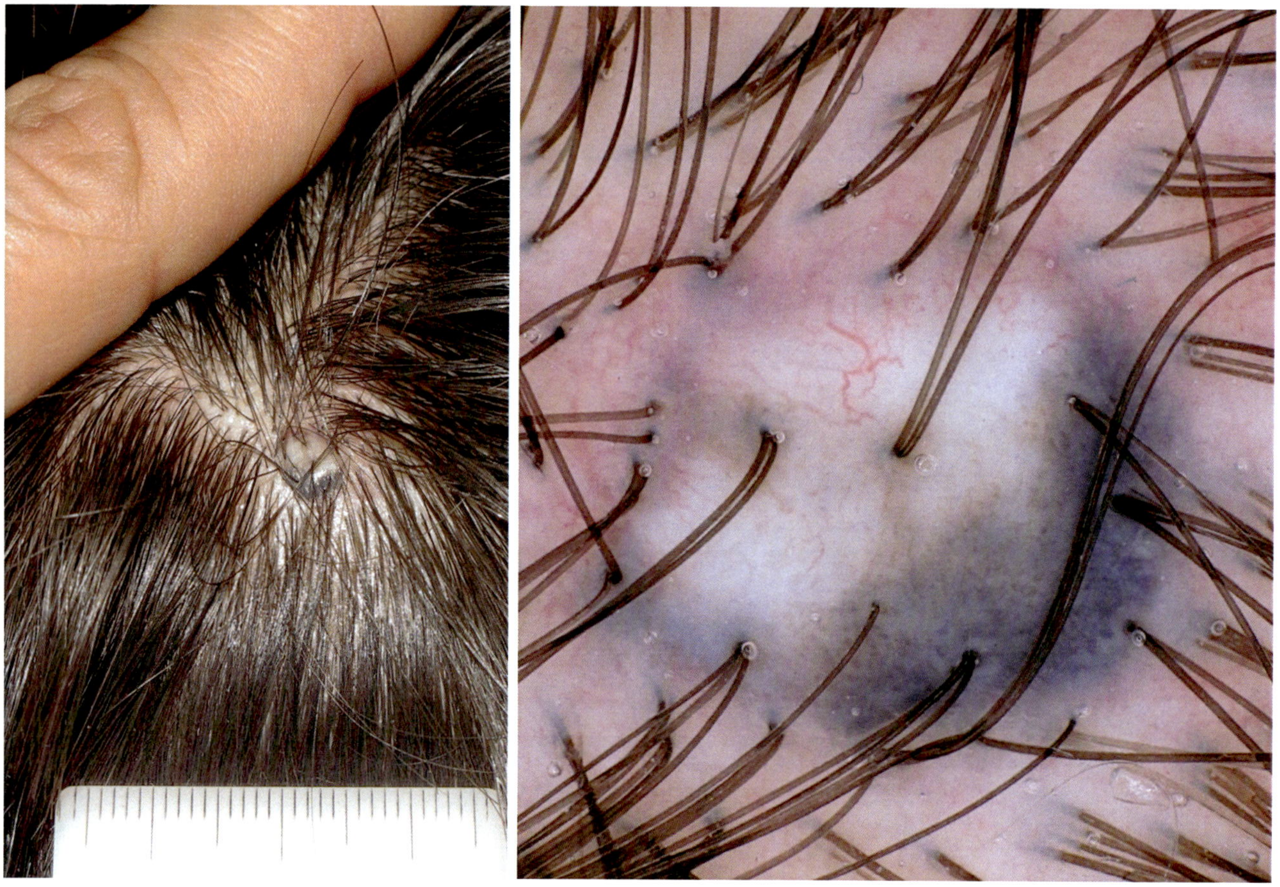

Fig. 34.5 Blue nevus of the scalp. Clinical (*left*) and dermoscopic (*right*) images of a blue nevus on the scalp. On dermoscopy, blue nevi present a structureless blue and white pigmentation, often associated with atypical linear vessels

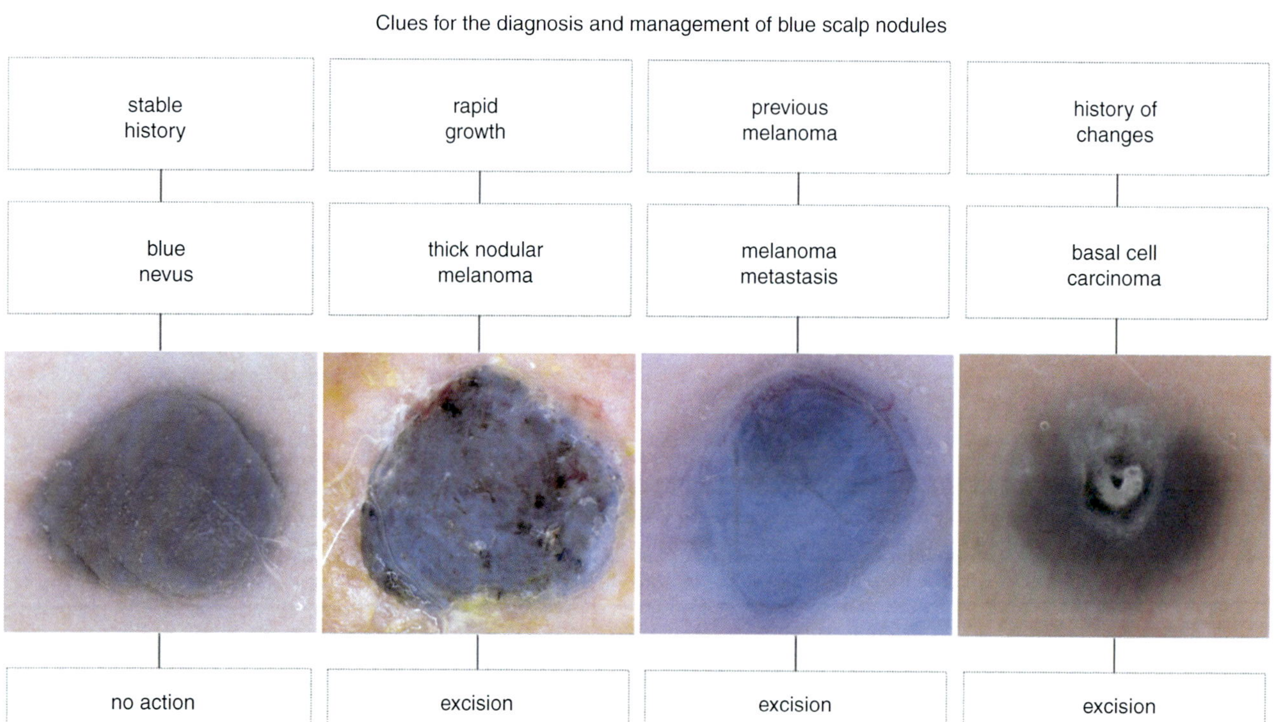

Fig. 34.6 Clues for the diagnosis and management of blue scalp nodules. Blue nevus, fast-growing melanoma, melanoma metastasis, and heavily pigmented basal cell carcinoma may reveal overlapping clinical and dermoscopic patterns. The history of a given lesion is an important clue for the diagnosis and management of blue nodules of the scalp

References

1. Gandini S, Sera F, Cattaruzza MS, Pasquini P, Abeni D, Boyle P, Melchi CF. Meta-analysis of risk factors for cutaneous melanoma: I Common and atypical naevi. Eur J Cancer. 2005;41(1):28–44.
2. Fabrizi G, Pagliarello C, Parente P, Massi G. Atypical nevi of the scalp in adolescents. J Cutan Pathol. 2007;34:365–9.
3. De Giorgi V, Sestini S, Grazzini M, et al. Prevalence and distribution of melanocytic naevi on the scalp: a prospective study. Br J Dermatol. 2010;162:345–9.
4. Kessides MC, Puttgen KB, Cohen BA. No biopsy needed for eclipse and cockade nevi found on the scalps of children. Arch Dermatol. 2009;145:1334–6.
5. Tcheung WJ, Bellet JS, Prose NS, et al. Clinical and dermoscopic features of 88 scalp nevi in 39 children. Br J Dermatol. 2011;165(1):137–43.
6. Stanganelli I, Argenziano G, Sera F, Blum A, Ozdemir F, Karaarslan IK, et al. Dermoscopy of scalp tumours: a multi-centre study conducted by the international dermoscopy society. J Eur Acad Dermatol Venereol. 2011. doi:10.1111/j.1468-3083.2011.04188.x.
7. Ferrara G, Soyer HP, Malvehy J, et al. The many faces of blue nevus: a clinicopathologic study. J Cutan Pathol. 2007;34:543–51.
8. Argenziano G, Longo C, Cameron A, Cavicchini S, Gourhant JY, Lallas A, et al. Blue-black rule: a simple dermoscopic clue to recognize pigmented nodular melanoma. Br J Dermatol. 2011. doi:10.1111/j.1365-2133.2011.10621.x.
9. Zalaudek I, Docimo G, Argenziano G. Using dermoscopic criteria and patient-related factors for the management of pigmented melanocytic nevi. Arch Dermatol. 2009;145:816–26.

Melanoma

35

Iris Zalaudek, Elvira Moscarella, Alexandre Abramavicus, Giuseppe Albertini, and Giuseppe Argenziano

Abstract

Primary scalp melanoma is referred to as the "invisible killer" because of its unnoticed growth and poorer prognosis compared with thickness-matched melanomas of the trunk. Accordingly, scalp dermoscopy should be performed routinely during dermatologic visits.

Keywords

Algorithm • "Blue" melanoma • Lentigo maligna • Melanoma • Pseudo-network • Seborrheic keratosis

Melanocytic tumors of the scalp differ epidemiologically, morphologically, and biologically from their counterparts on the trunk and therefore are assigned to the "special anatomic body sites" group of melanocytic skin tumors [1].

Primary scalp melanoma is referred to as the "invisible killer" because of its unnoticed growth and poorer prognosis compared with thickness-matched melanomas of the trunk [2]. Accordingly, the scalp should be examined routinely during dermatologic visits, whereby the use of dermoscopy should be considered standard of care in the diagnosis and management of scalp tumors [3–7].

I. Zalaudek
Department of Dermatology, Medical University of Graz, Graz, Austria

E. Moscarella
Department of Dermatology, University of Modena and Reggio Emilia, Modena, Italy

A. Abramavicus
Department of Dermatology, Unit of Skin Tumors, São Paulo Hospital, São Paulo, Brazil

G. Albertini
Dermatology and Skin Cancer Unit, Arcispedale Santa Maria Nuova IRCCS, Reggio Emilia, Italy

G. Argenziano (✉)
Dermatology and Skin Cancer Unit, Arcispedale Santa Maria Nuova IRCCS, Reggio Emilia, Italy
e-mail: g.argenziano@gmail.com

The prevailing dermoscopic patterns of scalp melanoma depend on the tumor type, growth rate, and thickness [3]. Thick, fast-growing, nodular melanoma often lacks specific dermoscopic patterns; yet, its diagnosis relies mostly on a history of rapid growth and the dermoscopic presence of different shades of blue and black [3, 8]. In contrast, thin scalp melanomas exhibit melanoma-specific criteria such as a brown-gray pseudo-network or an atypical network associated with areas of regression or diffuse hypopigmentation [3].

Because thick scalp melanoma may be a great masquerader that can mimic a wide range of benign skin tumors, a very low biopsy threshold is recommended for nodular tumors of the scalp. On the other hand, thin scalp melanoma may reveal overlapping features with regressing seborrheic keratosis and pigmented actinic keratosis. To avoid overlooking melanoma, biopsy is recommended for all flat scalp tumors showing regression, regardless of whether dermoscopic patterns suggestive of a melanocytic tumor are absent [3].

In conclusion, given the unfavorable prognosis of scalp melanoma, early detection and prompt treatment appear to be the best approach for improving survival. Based on the data extracted from the literature, an algorithm may be proposed for the management of pigmented scalp tumors. Particularly for adult men, scalp examinations should be performed during general dermatologic visits, whereby a low threshold is recommended for flat lesions showing regression or nodular tumors with blue color.

L. Rudnicka et al. (eds.), *Atlas of Trichoscopy*,
DOI 10.1007/978-1-4471-4486-1_35, © Springer-Verlag London 2012

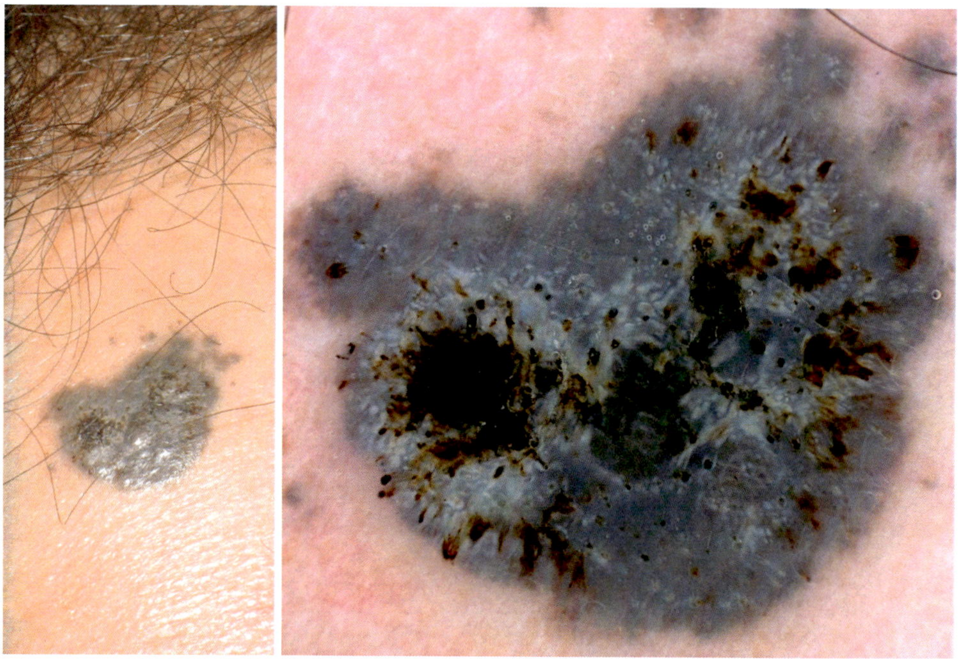

Fig. 35.1 Fast-growing melanoma. Shown are clinical (*left*) and dermoscopic (*right*) images of rapidly growing melanoma (thickness >2.5 mm). Dermoscopically structureless blue and white areas are seen. A clue favoring the diagnosis of advanced melanoma is the presence of irregular black blotches or dots, which are seen only exceptionally in blue nevus

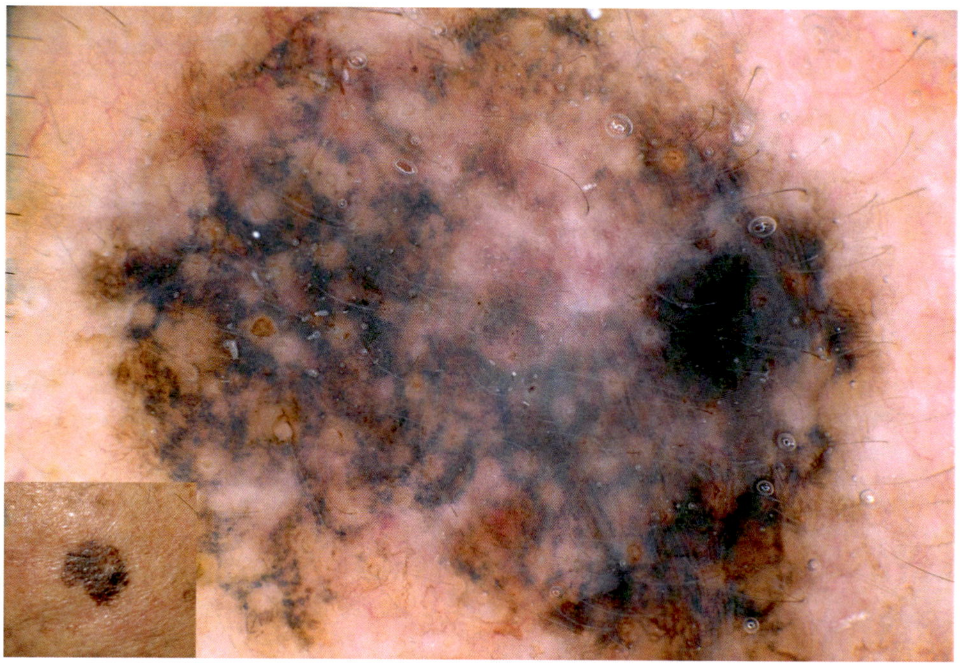

Fig. 35.2 Scalp melanoma, lentigo maligna type. Shown are clinical (*inset*) and dermoscopic images of thin scalp melanoma of the lentigo maligna type. Dermoscopy reveals a gray pseudo-network, gray pepper-like granules, structureless white areas, and some follicular openings filled with gray-black pigment

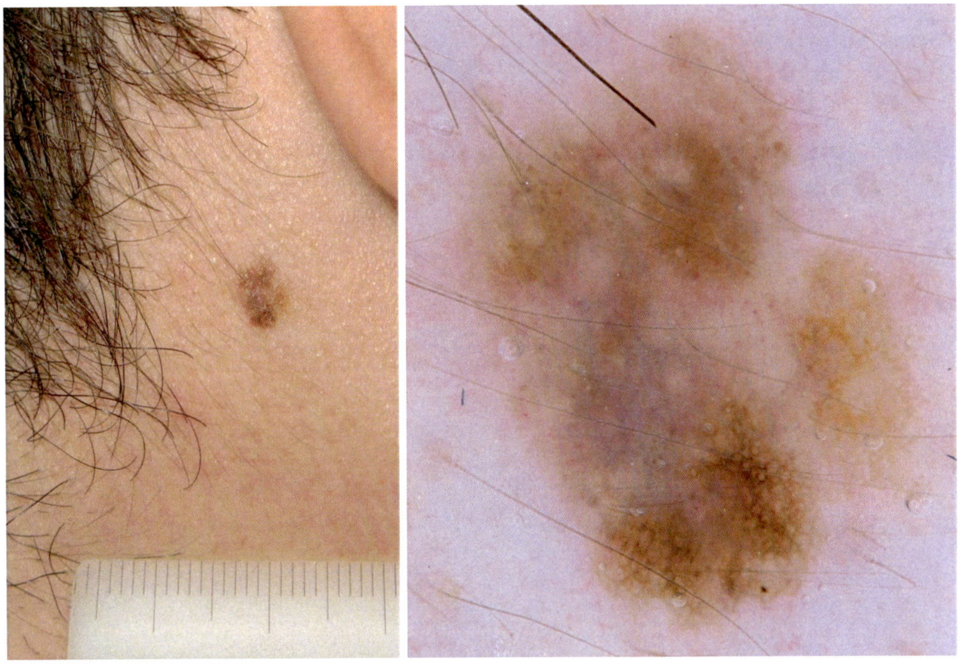

Fig. 35.3 Melanoma, superficial spreading type. Shown are clinical (*left*) and dermoscopic (*right*) examples of thin, slow-growing melanoma of the superficial spreading type. Dermoscopy reveals an atypical network, areas of regression (diffuse gray hue), and diffuse hypopigmentation. Note: some dotted vessels may be seen in correspondence to the hypopigmented areas

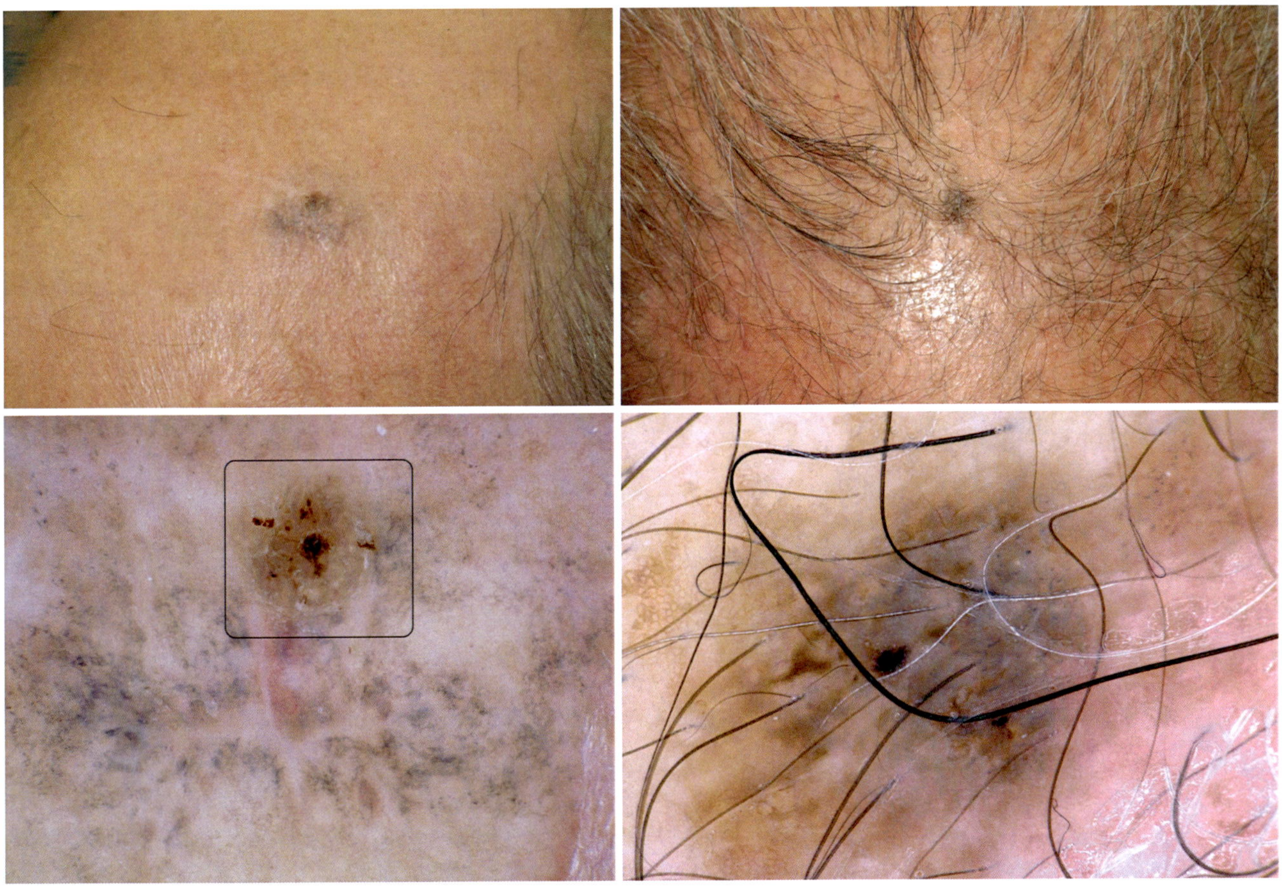

Fig. 35.4 Regressing melanoma and regressing seborrheic keratosis. Clinical and dermoscopic examples of nearly fully regressed melanoma (*left*) and regressing seborrheic keratosis (*right*). Dermoscopy of melanoma with extensive regression is typified by gray pepper-like granules (*lower left*). Importantly, in this case melanoma arose close to a preexisting seborrheic keratosis (*square*) and therefore was diagnosed as regressing seborrheic keratosis. Applying the rule to biopsy all lesions of the scalp showing regression prevented the clinician from missing this melanoma. Dermoscopy shows regressing seborrheic keratosis with diffuse gray areas, gray pepper-like granules, and thick brown-pigmented lines (*lower right*)

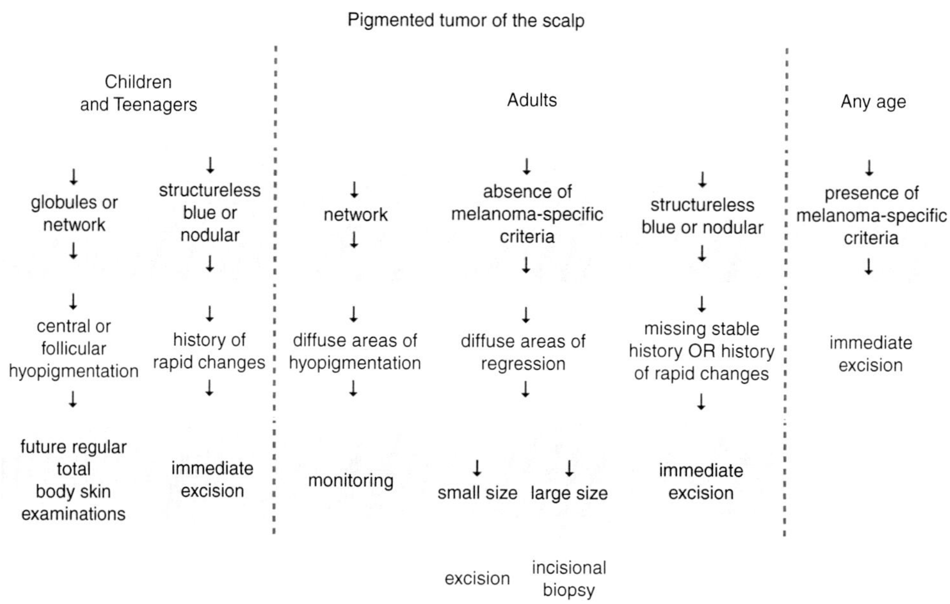

Fig. 35.5 Management recommendations for scalp tumors

References

1. Mason AR, Mohr MR, Koch LH, Hood AF. Nevi of special sites. Clin Lab Med. 2011;31(2):229–42.
2. Benmeir P, Baruchin A, Lusthaus S, Weinberg A, Ad-El D, Nahlieli O, et al. Melanoma of the scalp: the invisible killer. Plast Reconstr Surg. 1995;95(3):496–500.
3. Stanganelli I, Argenziano G, Sera F, Blum A, Ozdemir F, Karaarslan IK, et al. Dermoscopy of scalp tumours: a multi-centre study conducted by the international dermoscopy society. J Eur Acad Dermatol Venereol. 2011. doi:10.1111/j.1468-3083.2011.04188.x.
4. Aitken JF, Barbour A, Burmeister B, Taylor S, Walpole E, Australian Cancer Network, Smithers BM, Melanoma Guidelines Revision Working Party. Clinical practice guidelines for the management of melanoma in Australia and New Zealand. Sydney: Cancer Council Australia; Australian Cancer Network; Ministry of Health, New Zealand; 2008. p. 1–246.
5. Marsden JR, Newton-Bishop JA, Burrows L, Cook M, Corrie PG, Cox NH. Revised U.K. Guidelines for the management of cutaneous melanoma 2010. Br J Dermatol. 2010;163:238–56.
6. Argenziano G, Soyer HP, De Giorgi V, et al. Interactive atlas of dermoscopy. Milan: EDRA; 2000.
7. Zalaudek I, Leinweber B, Soyer HP, et al. Dermoscopic features of melanoma on the scalp. J Am Acad Dermatol. 2004;51: S88–90.
8. Argenziano G, Longo C, Cameron A, Cavicchini S, Gourhant JY, Lallas A, et al. Blue-black rule: a simple dermoscopic clue to recognize pigmented nodular melanoma. Br J Dermatol. 2011. doi:10.1111/j.1365-2133.2011.10621.x.

Nonmelanoma Skin Cancer

36

Iris Zalaudek, Elvira Moscarella, Alexandre Abramavicus,
Giuseppe Albertini, and Giuseppe Argenziano

Abstract

Clinically, nonmelanoma skin cancer classically appears nonpigmented so is also referred to as "white skin cancer." Dermoscopically, however, nonmelanoma skin cancers represent "red skin cancer," as their diagnosis is based primarily on vascular patterns and additional dermoscopic clues.

Keywords

Actinic keratosis • Basal cell carcinoma • Intraepithelial carcinoma • Nonmelanoma skin cancer (NMSC) • Squamous cell carcinoma

The scalp represents a unique anatomic region with a high concentration of pilosebaceous follicles and a rich vascular and lymphatic supply. Scalp tumors account for approximately 2 % of all skin tumors that may derive from different cell types of the pilosebaceous unit, from the interfollicular epidermis and dermis or as cutaneous metastases from other tumors [1].

The group of nonmelanoma skin cancers (NMSCs) includes basal cell carcinoma (BCC) and various forms of keratinocyte neoplasia, such as actinic keratosis (AK), intraepithelial carcinoma (IEC), and invasive squamous cell carcinoma (SCC). NMSCs are much more common than melanoma and rarely develop metastases. However, because of their high incidence, locally aggressive growth pattern (i.e., cancerization field), and tendency to recur after treatment, the morbidity and costs related to these cancers are very high.

The most important risk factors for scalp NMSC are male gender, age over 60 years, androgenetic alopecia, signs of chronic sun damage, and a personal history of skin cancer [2, 3].

Clinically, NMSC classically appears nonpigmented so is also referred to as "white skin cancer." Dermoscopically, however, NMSCs represent "red skin cancer," as their diagnosis is based mostly on vascular patterns and additional dermoscopic clues [4]. Although pigmented variants of NMSC do exist, they are less frequent compared with nonpigmented types.

AK is the most common neoplasm within the continuum of SCC. Once it develops, AK may follow one of the following pathways: regression, persistence, or progression to invasive SCC. The actual risk of an individual AK progressing to invasive SCC varies from 0.1 to 20 % [5].

Although it may be difficult clinically to differentiate grade I or II AK from IEC or early SCC [6], dermoscopy allows reliable differentiation between these different stages of progression within the continuum of keratinocytic cancer

I. Zalaudek
Department of Dermatology, Medical University of Graz, Graz, Austria

E. Moscarella
Department of Dermatology, University of Modena and Reggio Emilia, Modena, Italy

A. Abramavicus
Department of Dermatology, Unit of Skin Tumors, São Paulo Hospital, São Paulo, Brazil

G. Albertini • G. Argenziano (✉)
Dermatology and Skin Cancer Unit, Arcispedale Santa Maria Nuova IRCCS, Reggio Emilia, Italy
e-mail: g.argenziano@gmail.com

L. Rudnicka et al. (eds.), *Atlas of Trichoscopy*,
DOI 10.1007/978-1-4471-4486-1_36, © Springer-Verlag London 2012

[5]. Although pigmented forms of SCC are uncommon, they represent a major pitfall in the diagnosis of melanoma [7].

Because of specific vascular patterns and clues, invasive SCC can be diagnosed confidently with dermoscopy [4].

In BCC, the prevailing vascular and pigmented dermoscopic features are influenced by the tumor type and tumor volume [4].

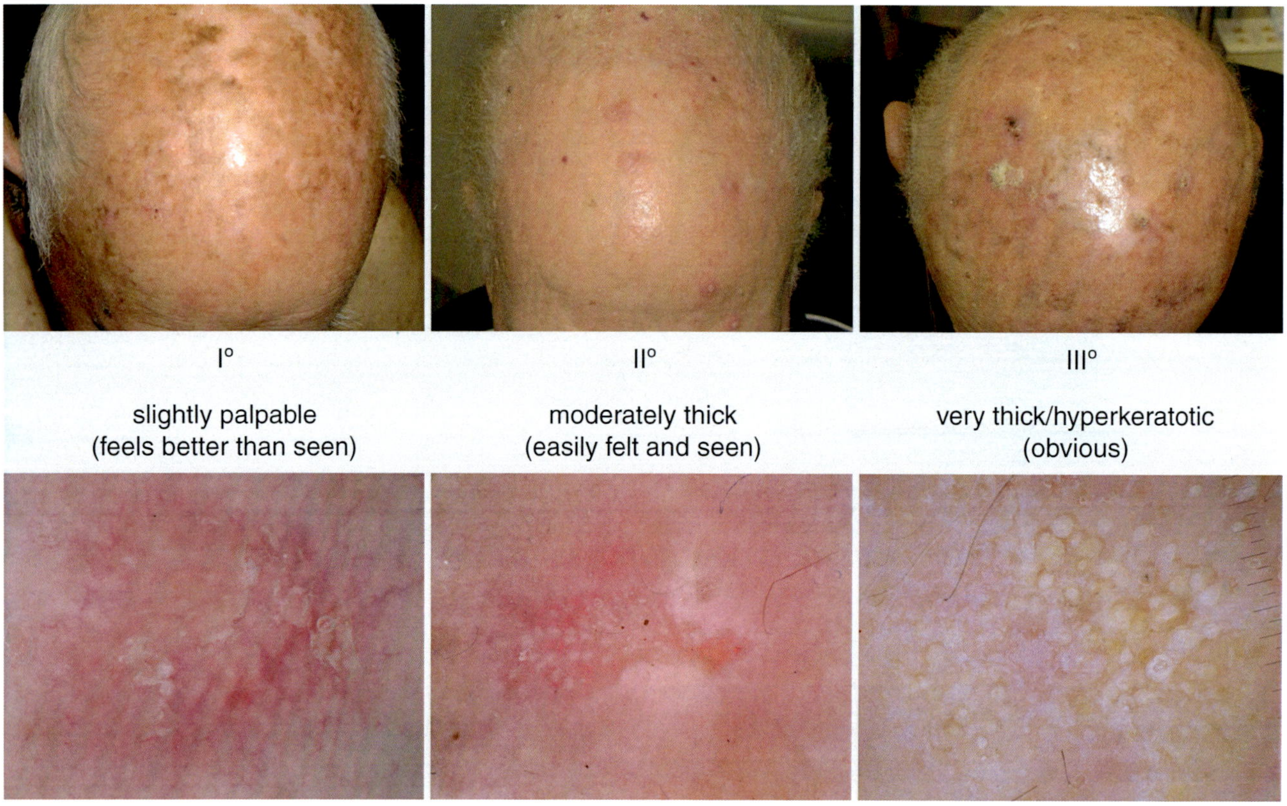

Fig. 36.1 Clinical grading of nonpigmented AKs and their dermoscopic patterns. Based on clinical visibility and palpability, nonpigmented AKs may be classified into three different grades, whereby grade III AKs are thought to carry the highest risk for progression into invasive SCC [8]. *Lower row:* Dermoscopy of grade I AK (*left*) shows diffuse erythema and surface scales; grade II AK (*middle*) shows white-red structureless areas and evident white follicular openings; grade III AK (*right*) shows a structureless white background intermingled with evident yellow keratotic hair follicles of different diameter

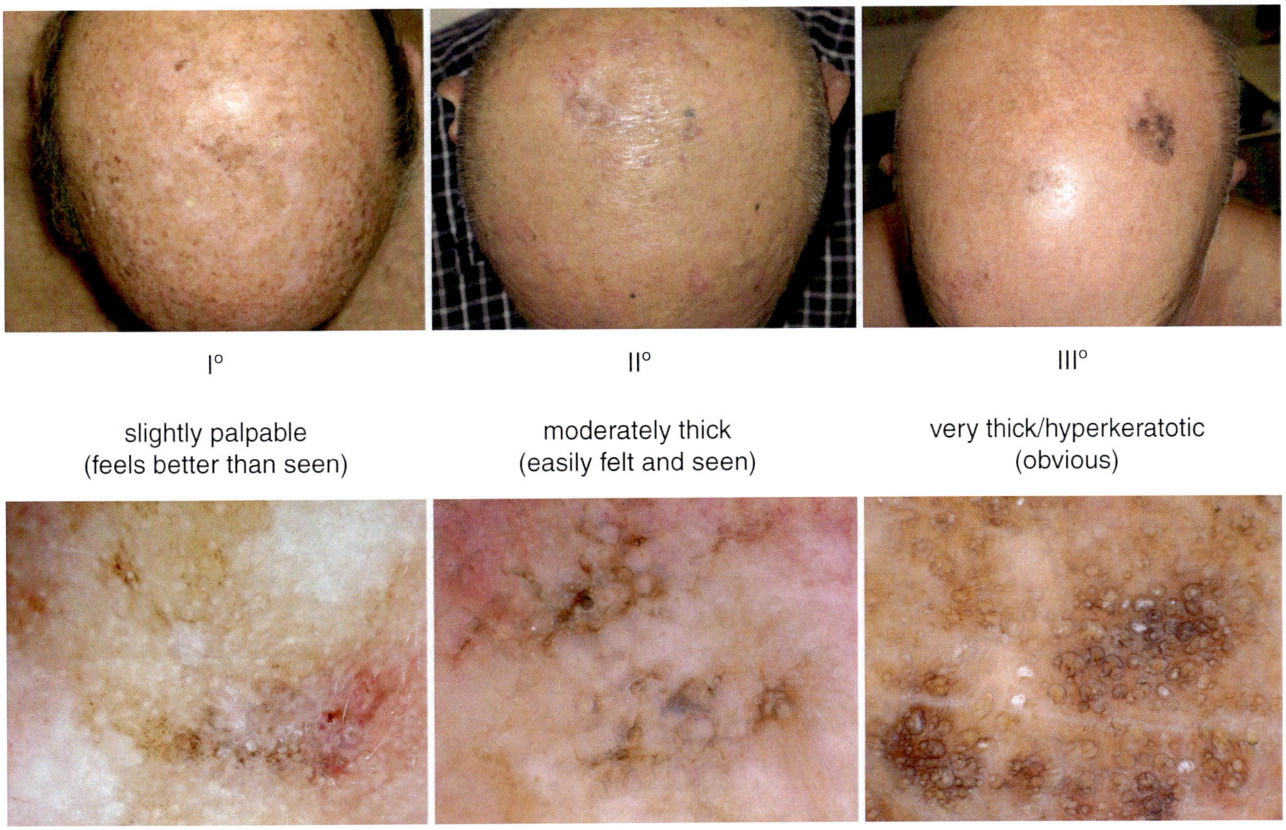

Fig. 36.2 Clinical grading of pigmented AKs and their dermoscopic patterns. *Lower row*: Dermoscopy of grade I AK (*left*) reveals diffuse brown areas intermingled with small white hair follicles; grade II AK (*middle*) shows thick superficial brown-gray lines surrounding targetoid follicular openings; grade III AK (*right*) shows a structureless brown-gray background intermingled with evident brown keratotic hair follicles of different diameter

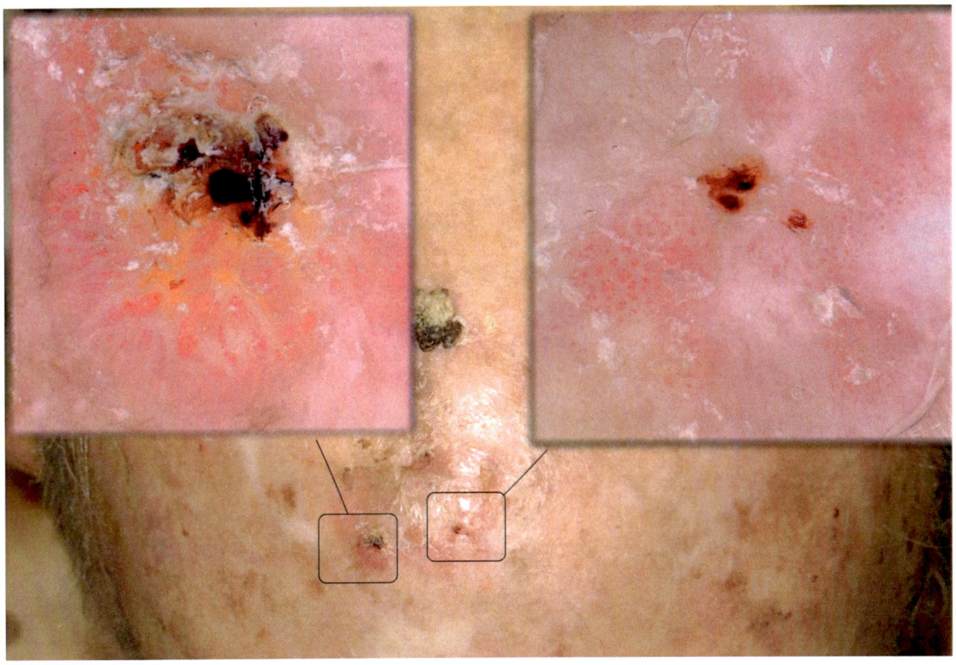

Fig. 36.3 Clinical and dermoscopic images of different stages of progression of SCC. IEC (*right*) shows grouped large dotted and coiled (glomerular) vessels, small red-brown erosions, and diffuse scales, whereas early invasive SCC (*left*) displays a central white to yellow amorphous, partially hemorrhagic crust surrounded by large coiled (glomerular) and elongated helical vessels. Note that the vessels are surrounded by a white halo, which is a hallmark of all keratinizing tumors

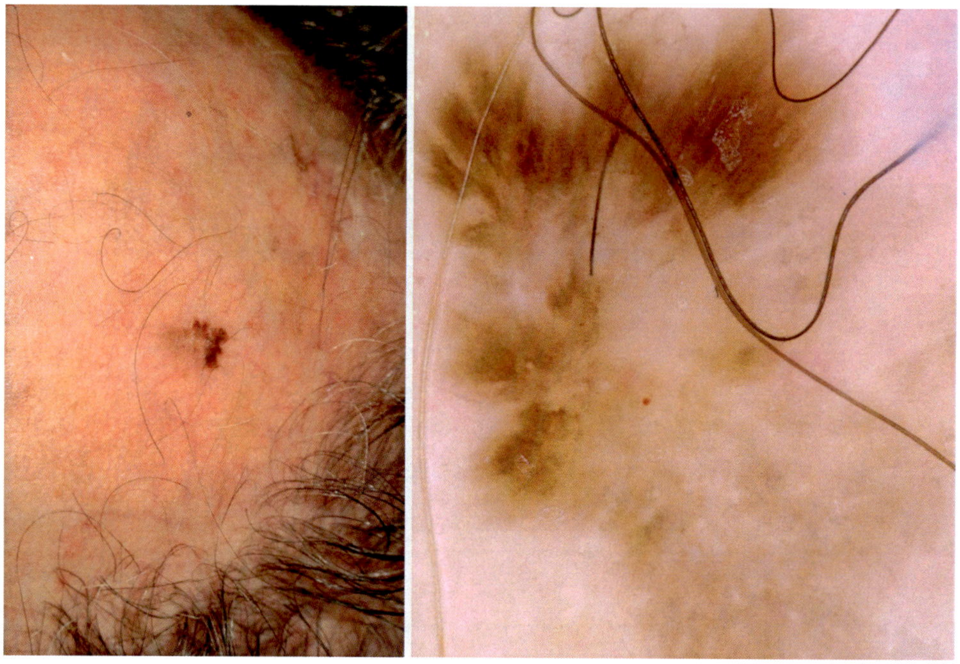

Fig. 36.4 **Pigmented intraepidermal carcinoma**. The clinical image (*left*) shows a pigmented intraepidermal carcinoma mimicking scalp melanoma. On dermoscopy (*right*), peripherally arranged fine brown lines may be seen arising from a nonpigmented center

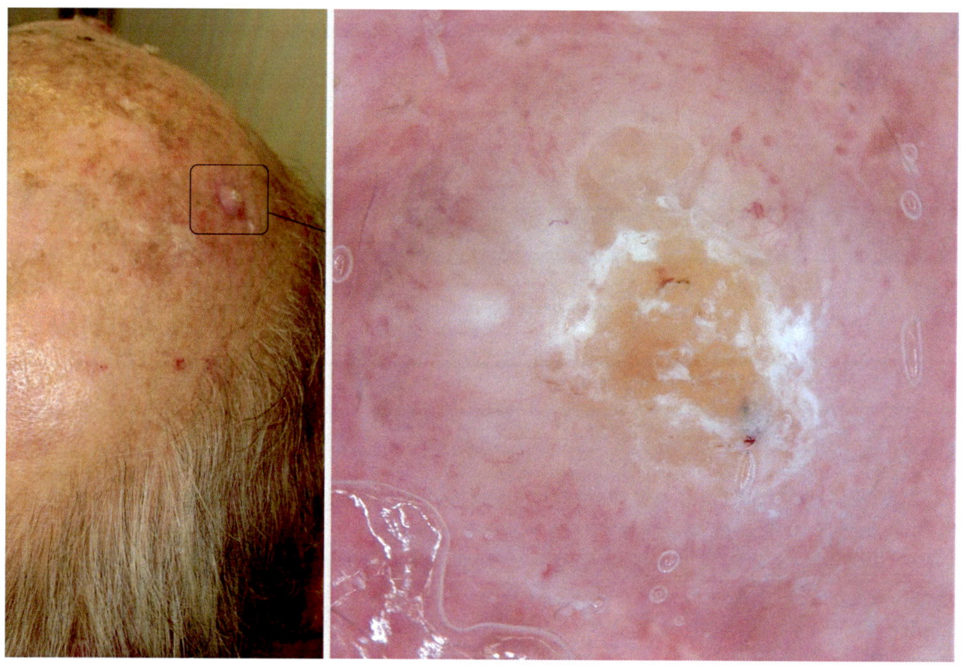

Fig. 36.5 **Invasive SCC**. The stereotypic clinical (*left*) and dermoscopic (*right*) images show invasive SCC. Dermoscopy reveals keratin-filled hair follicular openings, which appear as opaque, yellowish, variable, large, and roundish structures, over a white background. Also visible are polymorphous vessels composed of linear irregular, dotted, and coiled vessels in a radial arrangement

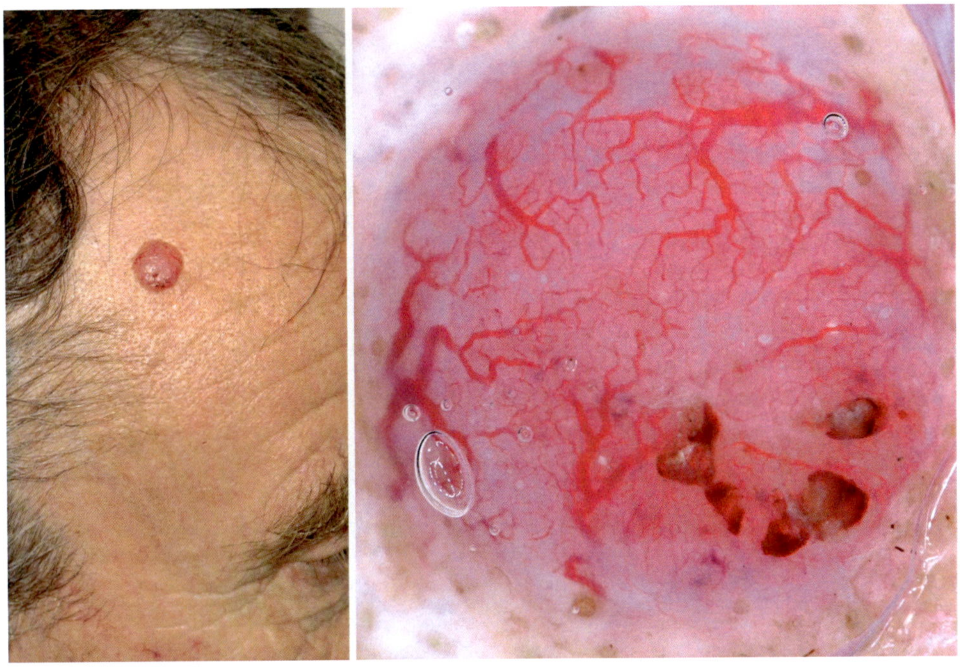

Fig. 36.6 **Nodular nonpigmented BCC.** The stereotypic clinical (*left*) and dermoscopic (*right*) images show nodular nonpigmented BCC. The dermoscopic hallmarks of BCC—sharply focused, dull red branching and arborizing vessels often associated with ulceration—are evident in the picture

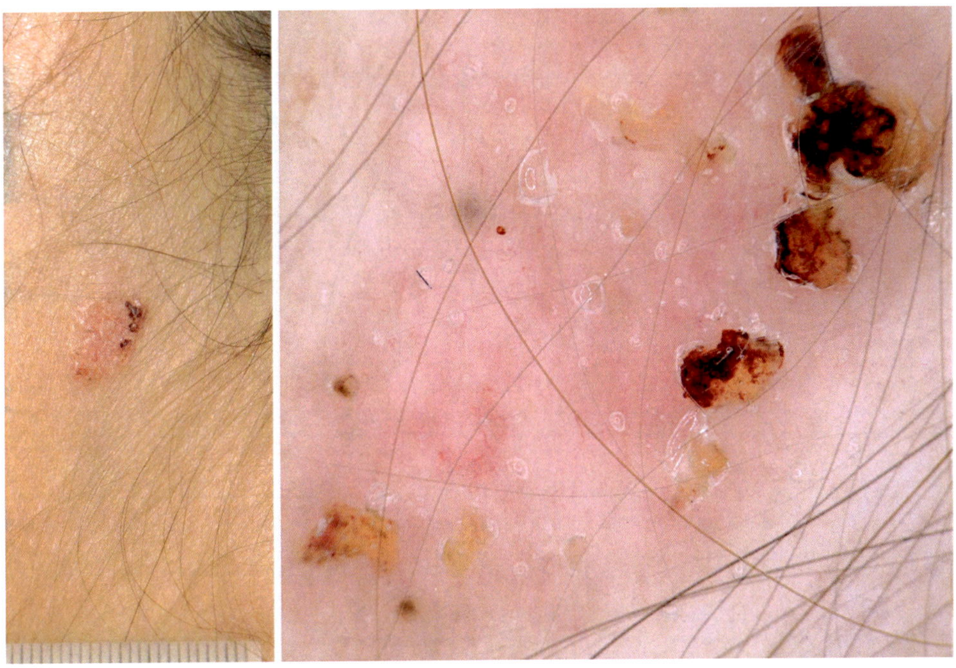

Fig. 36.7 **Stereotypic appearance of nonpigmented superficial BCC.** In contrast to nodular BCC, superficial BCC lacks evident arborizing vessels but shows a white-red structureless area (*right*). The key to diagnosis is the presence of small, often peripherally located erosions, which already are seen clinically (*left*)

References

1. Tosti A, Pazzaglia M, Piraccini BM. Chapter 18: Scalp tumors. In: Blume-Peytavi U, Tosti A, Whiting DA, Trueb R, editors. Hair growth and disorders. Berlin: Springer; 2008. p. 380–7.
2. Gandini S, Sera F, Cattaruzza MS, Pasquini P. Meta-analysis of risk factors for cutaneous melanoma: III. Family history, actinic damage and phenotypic factors. Eur J Cancer. 2005;41:2040–59.
3. Stanganelli I, Argenziano G, Sera F, Blum A, Ozdemir F, Karaarslan IK, et al. Dermoscopy of scalp tumours: a multi-centre study conducted by the international dermoscopy society. J Eur Acad Dermatol Venereol. 2011. doi:10.1111/j.1468-3083.2011.04188.x.
4. Zalaudek I, Kreusch J, Giacomel J, Ferrara G, Catricalà C, Argenziano G. How to diagnose nonpigmented skin tumors: a review of vascular structures seen with dermoscopy: part II. Nonmelanocytic skin tumors. J Am Acad Dermatol. 2010;63(3): 377–86; quiz 387–8.
5. Zalaudek I, Giacomel J, Schmid K, Bondino S, Rosendahl C, Cavicchini S, et al. Dermatoscopy of facial actinic keratosis, intraepidermal carcinoma, and invasive squamous cell carcinoma: a progression model. J Am Acad Dermatol. 2012;66:589–97. Epub 2011 Aug 11.
6. Rowert-Huber J, Patel MJ, Forschner T, Ulrich C, Eberle J, Kerl H, et al. Actinic keratosis is an early in situ squamous cell carcinoma: a proposal for reclassification. Br J Dermatol. 2007;156 Suppl 3:8–12.
7. Zalaudek I, Ferrara G, Leinweber B, Mercogliano A, D'Ambrosio A, Argenziano G. Pitfalls in the clinical and dermoscopic diagnosis of pigmented actinic keratosis. J Am Acad Dermatol. 2005;53(6): 1071–4.
8. De Giorgi V, Sestini S, Grazzini M, et al. Prevalence and distribution of melanocytic naevi on the scalp: a prospective study. Br J Dermatol. 2010;162:345–9.

Vascular Tumors

37

Iris Zalaudek, Elvira Moscarella, Alexandre Abramavicus, Giuseppe Albertini, and Giuseppe Argenziano

Abstract

Dermoscopy of scalp hemangiomas shows well-defined red and purple globules. Pyogenic granulomas show large structureless red globules, white intersecting lines, and linear vessels. Early angiosarcoma begins as ill-defined areas with an indurated border, whereas advanced lesions may be elevated, nodular, or occasionally ulcerated and reddish purple.

Keywords

Angiosarcoma • Pyogenic granuloma • Vascular tumor

Hemangiomas and pyogenic granulomas are benign vascular tumors frequently encountered on the scalp. However, although both lesions are benign and carry no risk of malignant transformation, biopsy and histopathologic diagnosis are always mandatory in suspected cases of pyogenic granuloma, regardless of the patient's age [1]. This is because amelanotic melanoma is virtually impossible to differentiate.

Angiosarcoma is an uncommon malignant neoplasm characterized by rapidly proliferating, extensively infiltrating anaplastic cells derived from blood vessels and lining irregular blood-filled spaces. Angiosarcoma is potentially lethal and has a high tendency to recur [2, 3]. Whereas early lesions begin as ill-defined areas with an indurated border, advanced lesions may be elevated, nodular, or occasionally ulcerated. On dermoscopy, angiosarcoma reveals the typical colors of vascular tumors, namely red and purple [4].

I. Zalaudek
Department of Dermatology, Medical University of Graz, Graz, Austria

E. Moscarella
Department of Dermatology, University of Modena and Reggio Emilia, Modena, Italy

A. Abramavicus
Department of Dermatology, Unit of Skin Tumors, São Paulo Hospital, São Paulo, Brazil

G. Albertini • G. Argenziano (✉)
Dermatology and Skin Cancer Unit, Arcispedale Santa Maria Nuova IRCCS, Reggio Emilia, Italy
e-mail: g.argenziano@gmail.com

L. Rudnicka et al. (eds.), *Atlas of Trichoscopy*,
DOI 10.1007/978-1-4471-4486-1_37, © Springer-Verlag London 2012

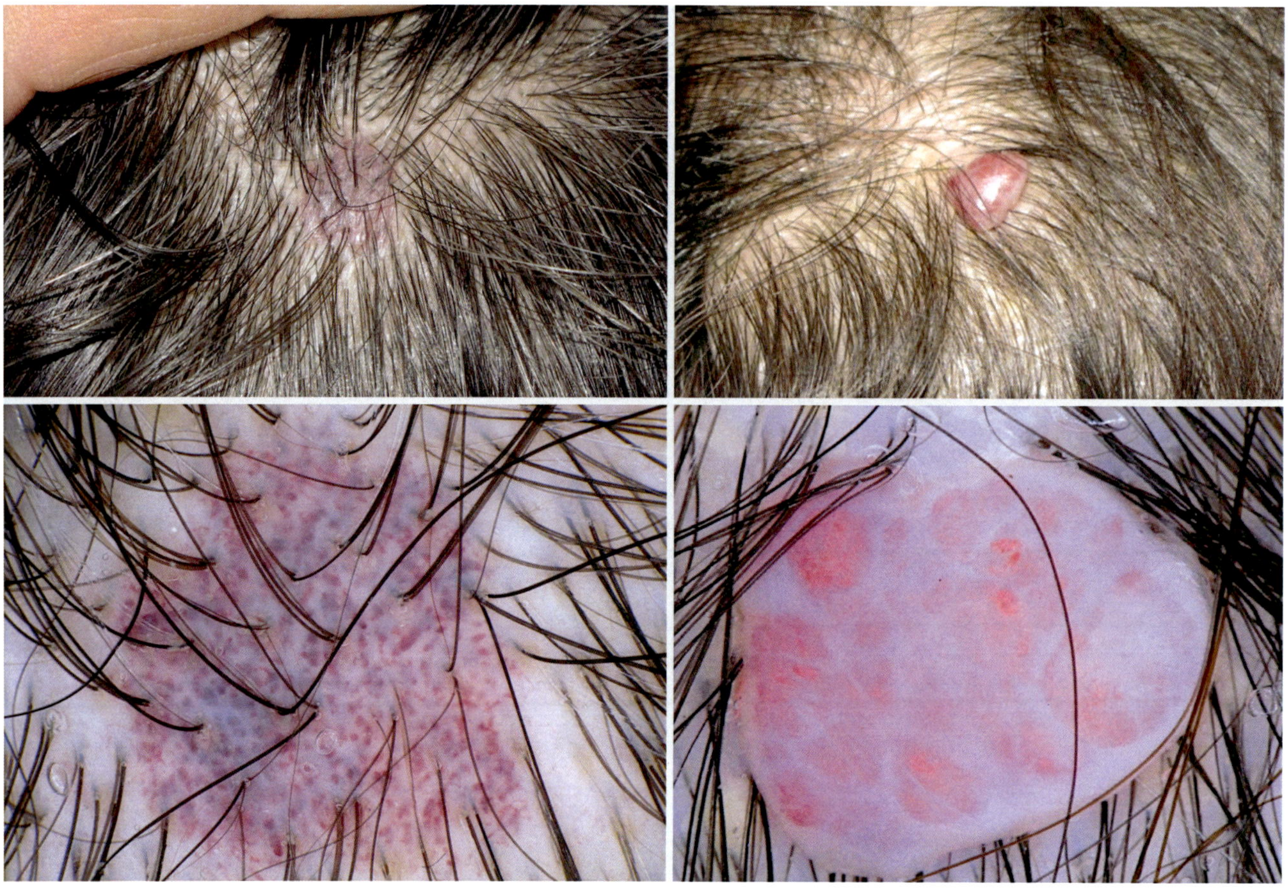

Fig. 37.1 **Clinical and dermoscopic features of benign vascular tumors**. *Left*: Hemangioma of the scalp shows the same patterns as on the trunk, namely well-defined red and purple globules. *Right*: Pyogenic granuloma showing large structureless red globules, white intersecting lines, and linear vessels. Because the same patterns may be seen in amelanotic melanoma, histopathologic examination is mandatory in all cases of pyogenic granuloma

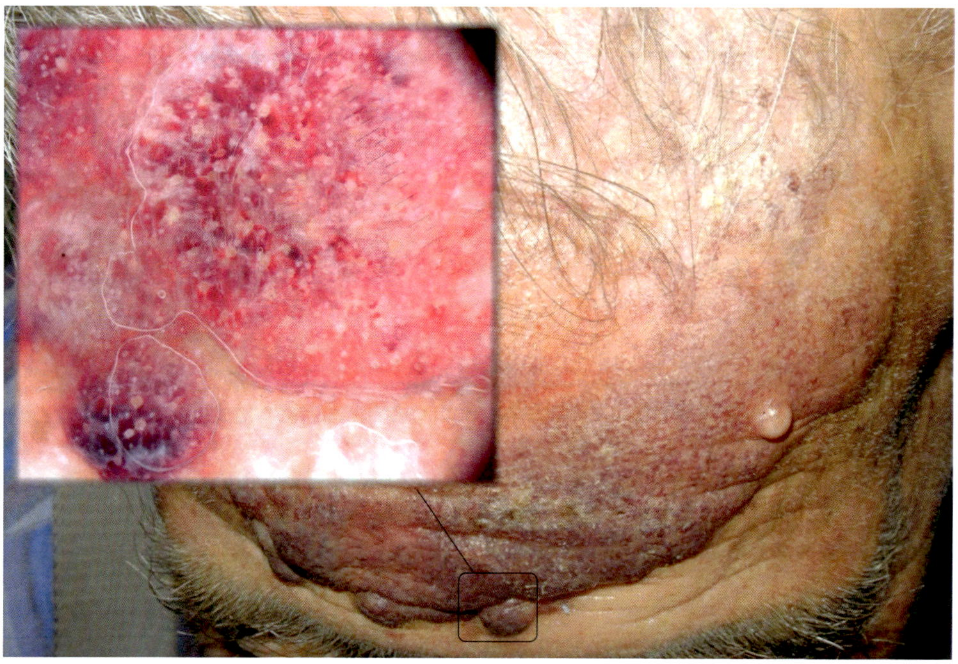

Fig. 37.2 **Clinical and dermoscopic patterns of advanced angiosarcoma**. Dermoscopy (*inset*) reveals a structureless red-purple area, which seems to be intermingled with white to yellow follicular openings

References

1. Zaballos P, Carulla M, Ozdemir F, Zalaudek I, Bañuls J, Llambrich A, et al. Dermoscopy of pyogenic granuloma: a morphological study. Br J Dermatol. 2010;163(6):1229–37.
2. Albores-Saavedra J, Schwartz AM, Henson DE, Kostun L, Hart A, Angeles-Albores D, Chablé Montero F. Cutaneous angiosarcoma. Analysis of 434 cases from the Surveillance, Epidemiology, and End Results Program, 1973–2007. Ann Diagn Pathol. 2011;15(2):93–7.
3. Guadagnolo BA, Zagars GK, Araujo D, Ravi V, Shellenberger TD, Sturgis EM. Outcomes after definitive treatment for cutaneous angiosarcoma of the face and scalp. Head Neck. 2011;33(5):661–7.
4. De Giorgi V, Grazzini M, Rossari S, Gori A, Verdelli A, Cervadoro E, Lotti T. Dermoscopy pattern of cutaneous angiosarcoma. Eur J Dermatol. 2011;21(1):113–4.

Part XIII

Trichoscopy in Asian Patients

Trichoscopy in Asian Patients

38

Shigeki Inui

Abstract

Compared with Caucasian patients, few racial differences in trichoscopy exist among Asian patients. These differences include a greater mean hair diameter and a higher thin hair ratio in healthy individuals. In alopecia areata, black dots and regrowing vellus hairs may be seen easily, but yellow dots may be difficult to detect. In androgenetic alopecia, the peripilar sign is detected less commonly. There is a masking effect by normal skin of color in contrast to Caucasian skin.

Keywords

Alopecia areata • Androgenetic alopecia • Asian skin • Black dots • Indian phototype Japanese phototype • Vitiligo • Yellow dots

In contrast to the normal female Caucasian population, among normal Asian females, there are few racial differences in hair density due to extreme interindividual variations, but the mean hair diameter is greater and the thin hair ratio higher (12.9 %) [1]. Although there are no reports comparing hair indexes in normal male subjects, a similar tendency may be expected. Moreover, Asian skin and hair color result in different appearances on trichoscopy. This chapter discusses the differences in trichoscopic findings in Asian hair loss patients.

Characteristic trichoscopic features of alopecia areata in Asians are black dots, tapering (exclamation mark) hairs, broken hairs, yellow dots, and short vellus hairs [2]. Black dots, which are remnants of exclamation mark or broken hairs, provide a sensitive marker for disease activity and severity; however, this finding may not be readily seen in patients with blond hair. Because of a darker shade of interfollicular skin, regrowing white short vellus hairs are observed more frequently in Asians than in Caucasians; therefore, the presence of multiple short vellus hairs is a sensitive diagnostic marker for alopecia areata that is specific for Asian patients [3]. In contrast, yellow dots are somewhat difficult to detect compared with Caucasian patients or Asian patients with vitiligo [4], because of interference with skin color. There is a masking effect in normal skin of color in contrast to Caucasian skin.

When treated with contact immunotherapy, 6 % of Asian patients develop pigmented contact dermatitis due to therapeutic contactants [5]. Reticular and/or globular pigmentation–sparing orifices and eccrine pores are seen on trichoscopy.

Hair diameter diversity, the peripilar sign, and yellow dots are trichoscopically observed in Asian patients with androgenetic alopecia. The peripilar sign is seen in all cases of androgenetic alopecia in Caucasians [6], but in Asian patients this feature is observed in only 66 % of cases (33/50) and is attributed to the discrepancy in interference with skin color [7].

Although the trichoscopic images shown here were obtained mainly from Japanese patients, recent results from India show results similar to ours [8]. Because skin and hair color influence trichoscopic features, it is of interest to study trichoscopic characteristics in Asians with hair diseases.

S. Inui
Department of Regenerative Dermatology, Osaka University School of Medicine 2-2 G2, Yamadaoka Suita-shi, Osaka 5650871, Japan
e-mail: inui@r-derma.med.osaka-u.ac.jp

L. Rudnicka et al. (eds.), *Atlas of Trichoscopy*,
DOI 10.1007/978-1-4471-4486-1_38, © Springer-Verlag London 2012

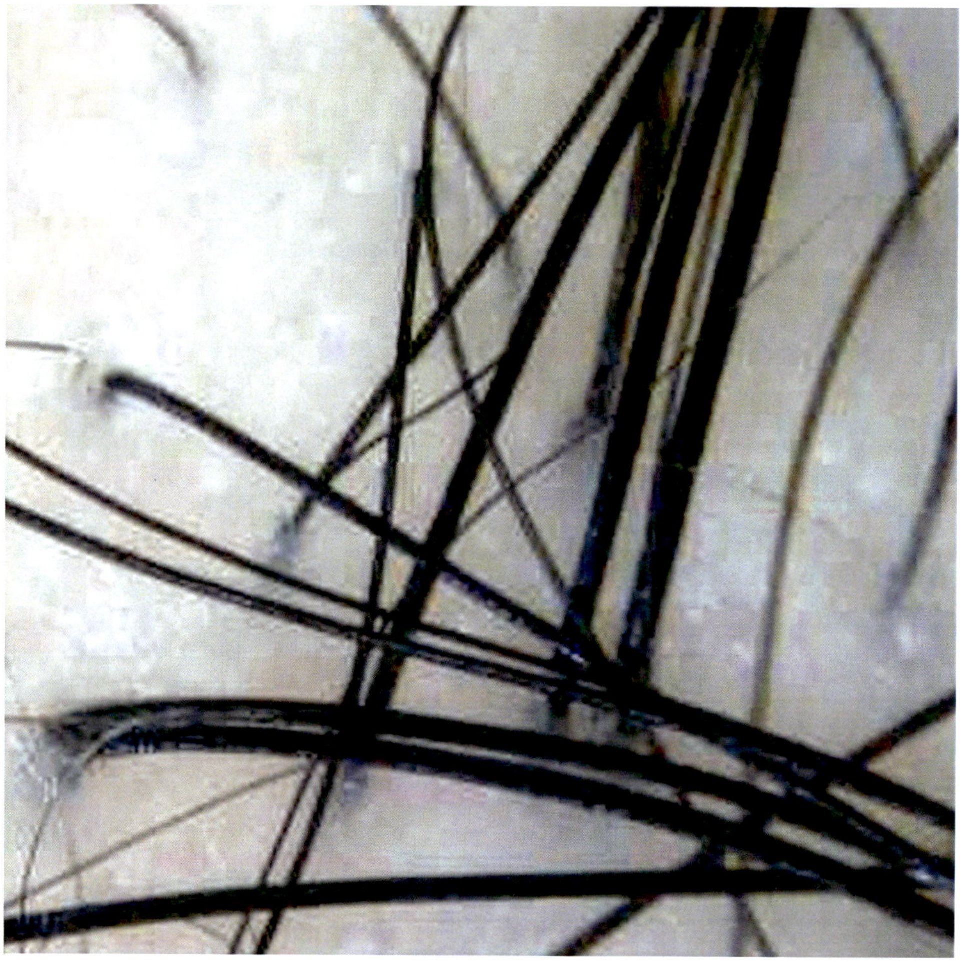

Fig. 38.1 Trichoscopy in the normal vertex scalp of a 20-year-old Japanese woman. Normal scalp hairs in Asian females have a greater mean hair diameter and higher thin hair ratio (12.9 %) than those in Caucasian females [1]. Because of the higher thin hair ratio, the threshold of hair diameter diversity should be 20 % for detecting vellus hair transformation. This picture was taken using the DermLite II Pro dermatoscope (3Gen, LCC, San Juan Capistrano, CA; ×10)

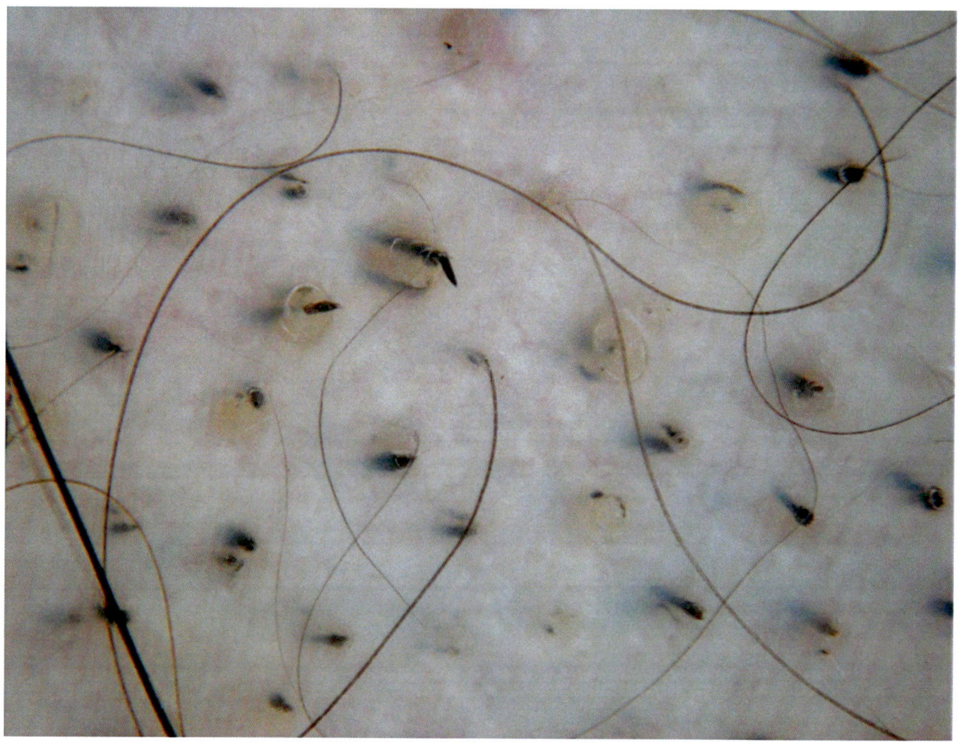

Fig. 38.2 Black dots, broken hairs, and yellow dots on the scalp of a 50-year-old Japanese woman with rapidly exacerbating alopecia areata. This picture was taken using the DermLite II Pro (×10)

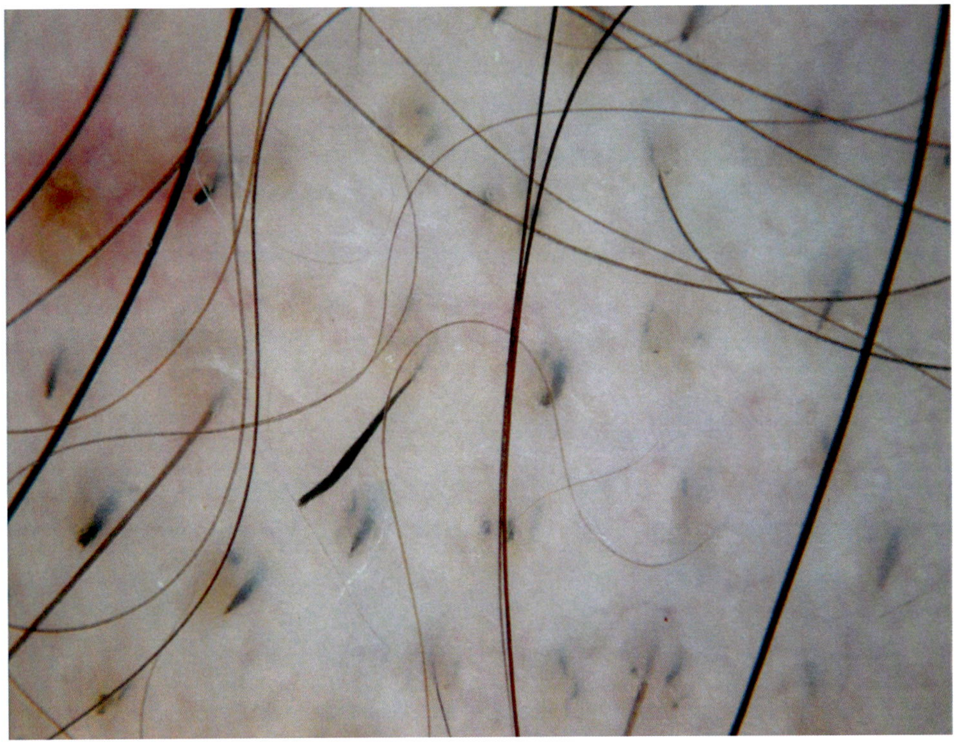

Fig. 38.3 **Tapering (exclamation mark) hairs and multiple black and yellow dots on the scalp of a 50-year-old Japanese woman with rapidly exacerbating alopecia areata**. This picture was taken using the DermLite II Pro (×10)

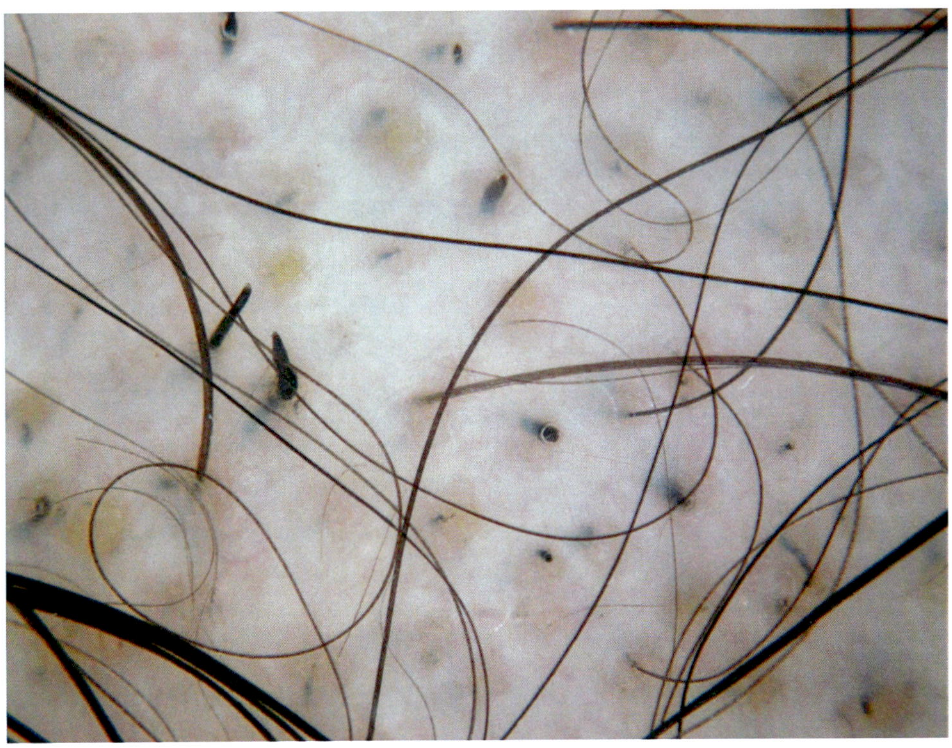

Fig. 38.4 **Broken hairs on the scalp of a 50-year-old Japanese woman with rapidly exacerbating alopecia areata**. Black and yellow dots also are visible. This picture was taken using the DermLite II Pro (×10)

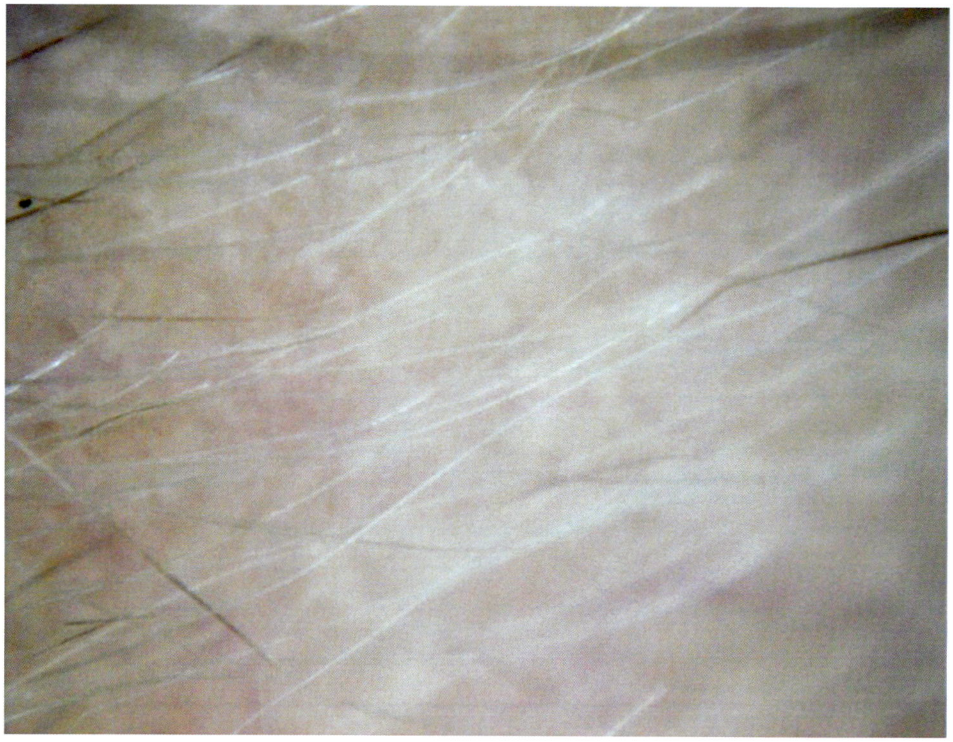

Fig. 38.5 Short vellus hairs on the scalp of an 8-year-old Japanese girl with remitting alopecia areata. This picture was taken using the DermLite II Pro (×10)

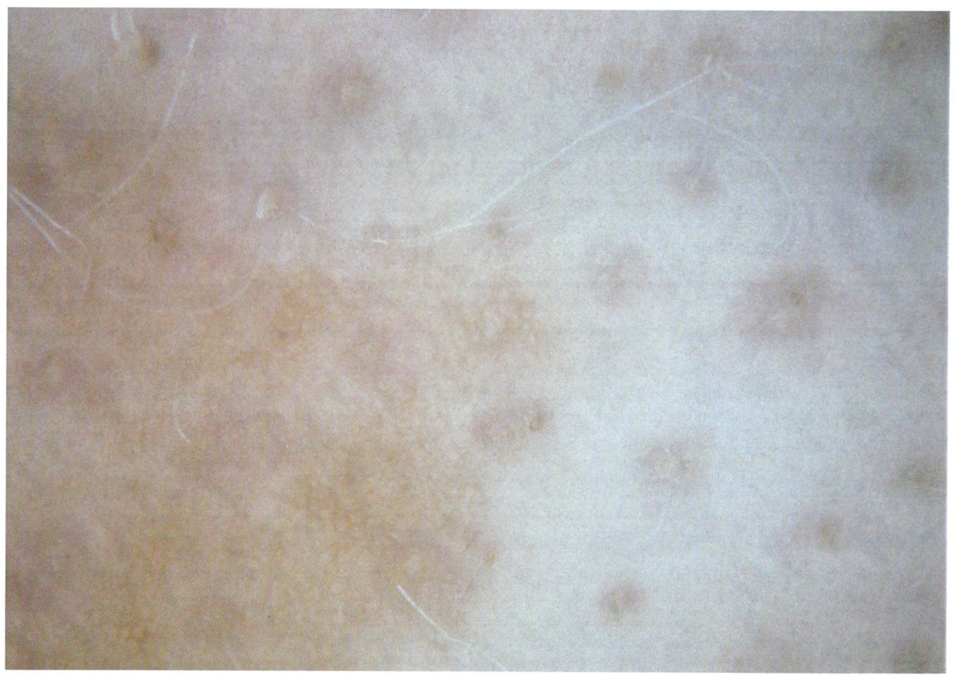

Fig. 38.6 Masking of yellow dots by normal skin color in a 13-year old Japanese girl with alopecia areata and vitiligo. On the right, numerous yellow dots are seen on hypopigmented, vitiligous skin, whereas on the left, yellow dots are masked by the slightly tanned, normal skin color. This picture was taken using the DermLite II Pro (×10)

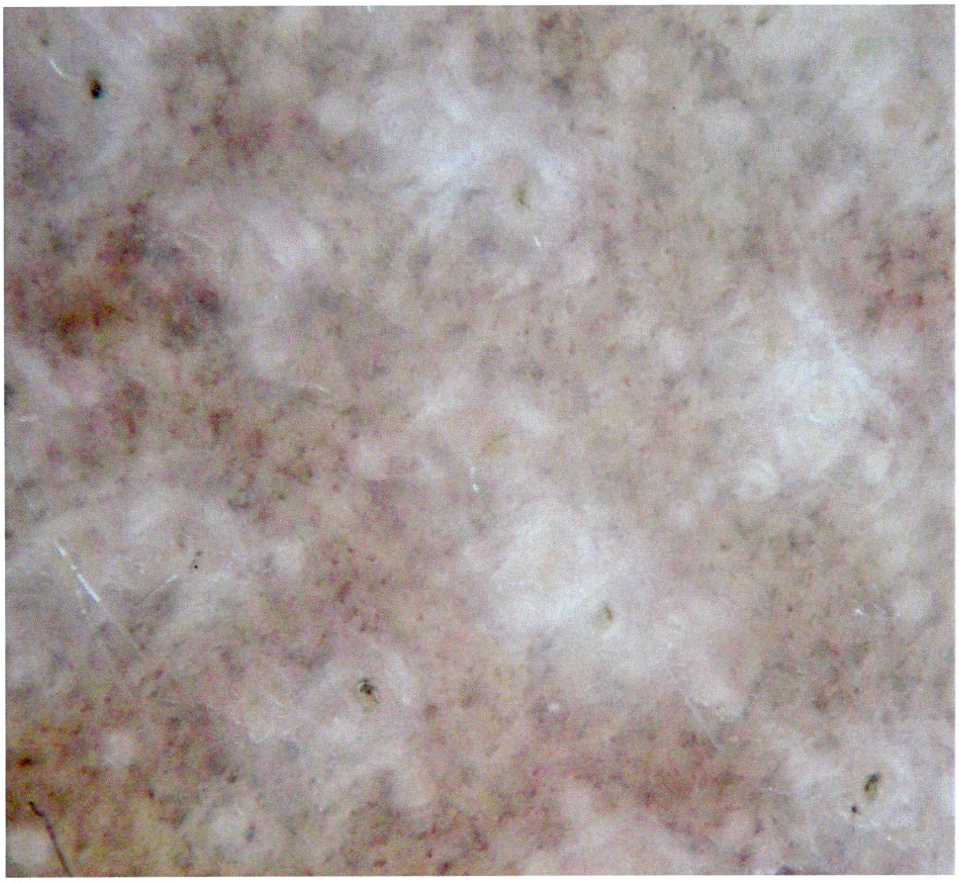

Fig. 38.7 Pigmented contact dermatitis in a patient with alopecia areata treated with contact immunotherapy. This trichoscopic image shows reticular and granular slate-colored pigmentations on the scalp. Broken hairs, yellow dots, and eccrine pores also are observed. This picture was taken using the DermLite II Pro (×10)

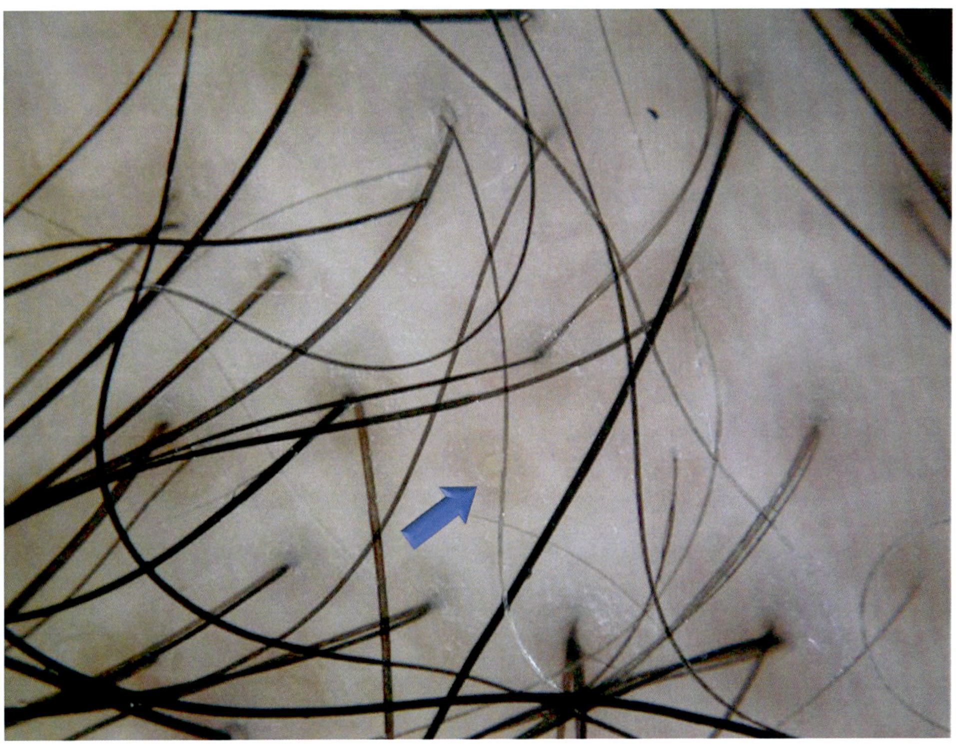

Fig. 38.8 Trichoscopy in an Asian patient with androgenetic alopecia. Hair diameter diversity, the peripilar sign, and a yellow dot (*arrow*) are seen in a 42-year-old Japanese man with androgenetic alopecia. This picture was taken using the DermLite II Pro (×10)

References

1. Tajima M, Hamada C, Arai T, Miyazawa M, Shibata R, Ishino A. Characteristic features of Japanese women's hair with aging and with progressing hair loss. J Dermatol Sci. 2007;45(2):93–103.
2. Inui S, Nakajima T, Nakagawa K, Itami S. Clinical significance of dermoscopy in alopecia areata: analysis of 300 cases. Int J Dermatol. 2008;47(7):688–93.
3. Karadağ Köse O, Göleç AT. Clinical evaluation of alopecias using a handheld dermatoscope. J Am Acad Dermatol. 2012;67:206–14. Epub 2011 Oct 22.
4. Ross EK, Vincenzi C, Tosti A. Videodermoscopy in the evaluation of hair and scalp disorders. J Am Acad Dermatol. 2006;55(5):799–806.
5. Inui S, Nakajima T, Itami S. Coudability hairs: a revisited sign of alopecia areata assessed by trichoscopy. Clin Exp Dermatol. 2010;35(4):361–5.
6. Deloche C, de Lacharriere O, Misciali C, Piraccini BM, Vincenzi C, Bastien P, et al. Histological features of peripilar signs associated with androgenetic alopecia. Arch Dermatol Res. 2004;295(10):422–8.
7. Inui S, Nakajima T, Itami S. Scalp dermoscopy of androgenetic alopecia in Asian people. J Dermatol. 2009;36(2):82–5.
8. Mane M, Nath AK, Thappa DM. Utility of dermoscopy in alopecia areata. Indian J Dermatol. 2011;56(4):407–11.

Part XIV

Trichoscopy in Patients with Dark Skin Phototypes

Trichoscopy in Patients with Dark Skin Phototypes

39

Bruna Duque-Estrada and Leonardo Spagnol Abraham

Abstract

Trichoscopy of patients with dark skin phototypes has demonstrated unique characteristics due to the contrast of the melanocytic network and the follicular units. Dermatologists should be aware of the distinctive patterns of these skin phototypes.

Keywords

African American patients • Alopecia areata • Androgenetic alopecia • Black skin • Brazilian patients • Eyebrows • Central centrifugal cicatricial alopecia • Discoid lupus erythematosus Folliculitis decalvans • Frontal fibrosing alopecia • Hairstyling • Lichen planopilaris

Trichoscopy of patients with dark skin phototypes has demonstrated unique characteristics due to the contrast of the melanocytic network, the follicular units and the eccrine ducts. Physicians should be aware of the distinctive patterns of these skin phototypes.

Examination of the normal scalp in skin phototypes IV, V, and VI shows a perifollicular pigmented network (honeycomb pattern). This network consists of hyperchromic lines composed of melanocytes in the rete ridge system, in contrast to hypochromic areas formed by fewer melanocytes localized in the suprapapillary epidermis [1]. Pinpoint white dots regularly distributed among follicular units, which correspond to eccrine pores of the scalp, also may be appreciated [2, 3].

In androgenetic alopecia, when follicular miniaturization progresses, the pigmented network becomes evident [4]. Pinpoint white dots may be confused with miniaturized empty follicular ostia (kenogen hairs), and differentiation is possible only with confocal microscopy [3].

Inside alopecic patches of alopecia areata, yellow dots are poorly observed and dystrophic hairs, mainly exclamation mark hairs, are the most important features for diagnosis [5–7].

Almost 100 % of African American patients have a history of hairdressing associated with traction of the scalp for many years through the use of elastic bands, plaits, or extensions. The scalp periphery is the site of predilection for traction alopecia, and trichoscopy shows several vellus hairs, a pigmented network, and pinpoint white dots [8].

Central centrifugal cicatricial alopecia also affects primarily African American patients and represents an important cause of scarring hair loss in this group. Alopecia begins near the vertex or midscalp and slowly progresses centrifugally. Absence of follicular ostia, perifollicular scaling, pinpoint white dots, and vellus hairs may be observed, although dermoscopic findings are not specific for the disease.

Trichoscopy may reveal signs of inflammation and follicular destruction in many forms of primary cicatricial alopecia. Classic lichen planopilaris in dark-skinned patients shows pinpoint white dots inside the honeycomb pigmented network (as interfollicular epidermis is commonly unaffected by the inflammatory process), forming a "starry sky" pattern. A variable degree of slight erythema, as well as perifollicular scaling, is visible [2]. A peculiar round perifollicular distribution of blue-gray dots—the "target pattern"—may

B. Duque-Estrada (✉)
Department of Dermatology, Instituto de Dermatologia
Prof. Rubem David Azulayl, Rua Santa Luzia, 206 – Centro,
Rio de Janeiro 20.020-020, Brazil
e-mail: bruna.pinto@uol.com.br

L.S. Abraham
Department of Hair Diseases, Instituto de Dermatologia
Prof. Rubem David Azulay, Rio de Janeiro, Brazil

L. Rudnicka et al. (eds.), *Atlas of Trichoscopy*,
DOI 10.1007/978-1-4471-4486-1_39, © Springer-Verlag London 2012

be observed and represents histopathologic melanophages located predominantly around hair follicles [9].

In frontal fibrosing alopecia, a clinical variant of lichen planopilaris that affects the hairline and eyebrows, trichoscopy shows a pigmented network, pinpoint white dots, perifollicular scaling, and perifollicular erythema.

In African American patients with chronic cutaneous lupus erythematosus (discoid lupus erythematosus), round and polycyclic red dots, a sign of early lesions, are difficult to observe but have been seen in a few patients with phototype IV [10]. Classic tortuous vessels, a hyperpigmented network, and areas of hypopigmentation are observed. Blue-gray dots in a speckled distribution pattern along the alopecic patch, as well as chrysalis structures, also are seen often [9].

The trichoscopic pattern of folliculitis decalvans is usually monomorphic, with multiple arborizing red vessels, a diffuse deep erythema, tufted folliculitis, and a variable degree of pustular lesions, depending on the intensity of the inflammatory process [1, 5]. Severe scaling, crusting, and chrysalis structures very often are observed in this type of alopecia.

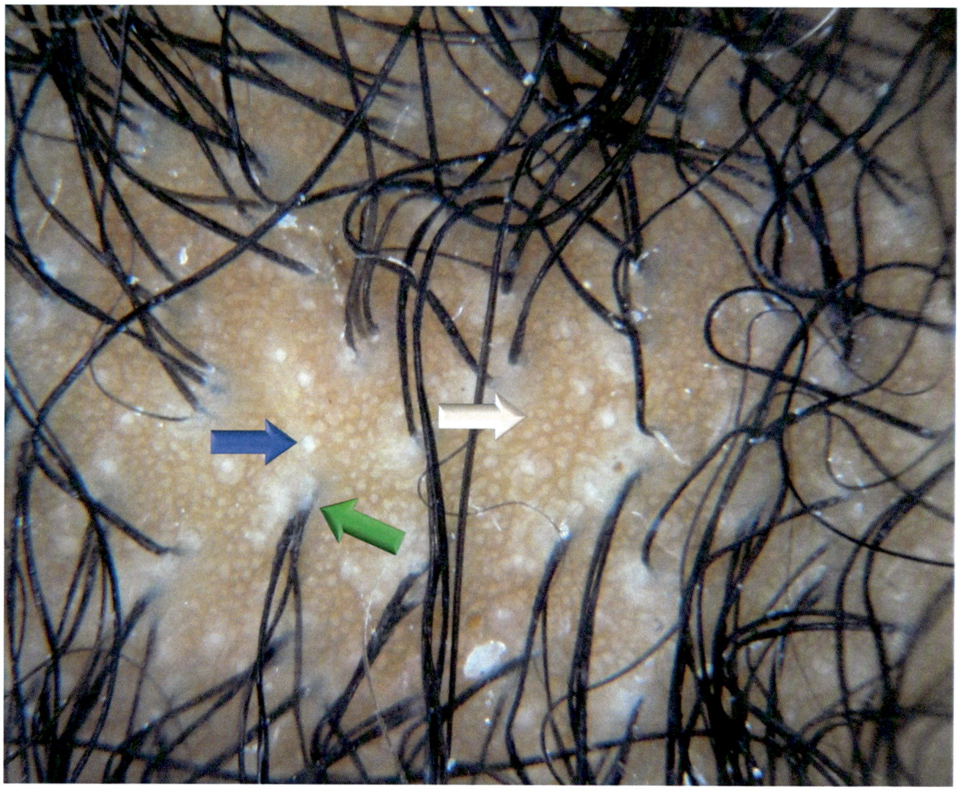

Fig. 39.1 Normal scalp. Normal scalp in a child with Fitzpatrick phototype VI showing pinpoint white dots (*blue arrow*) and a regular perifollicular pigmented network in a honeycomb pattern (*white arrow*). A white halo (*green arrow*), which corresponds to the normal follicular epithelium, can be identified

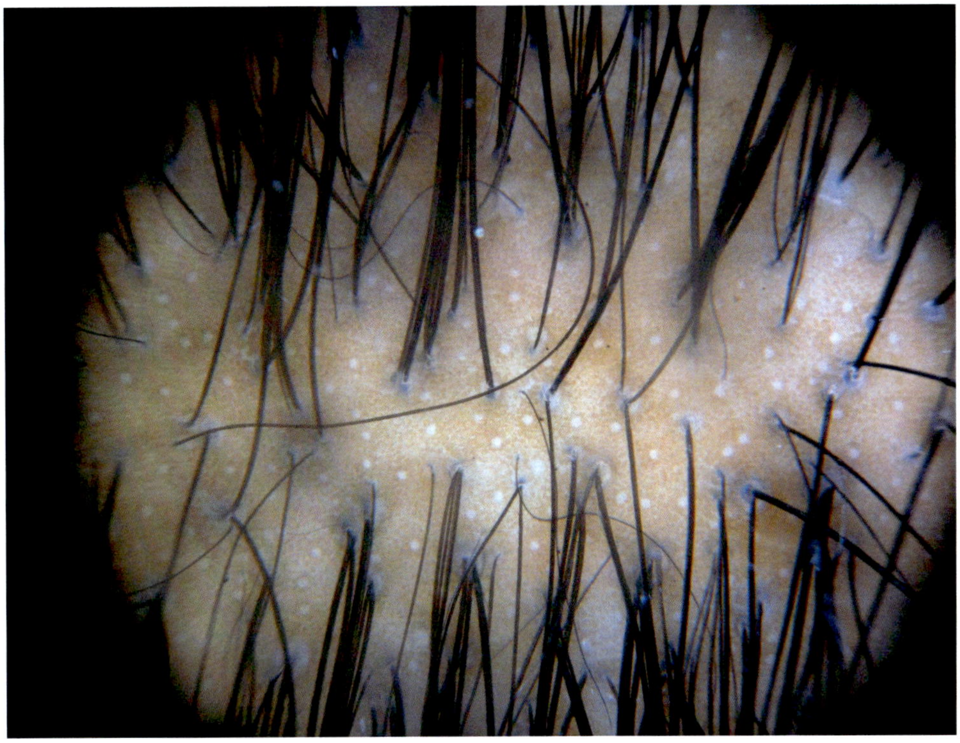

Fig. 39.2 Androgenetic alopecia. Diameter diversity of more than 20 % of the hair is the most important diagnostic feature. A pigmented network and white dots are observed on the scalp of dark-skinned patients and in the photodamaged scalp of patients with long-lasting alopecia

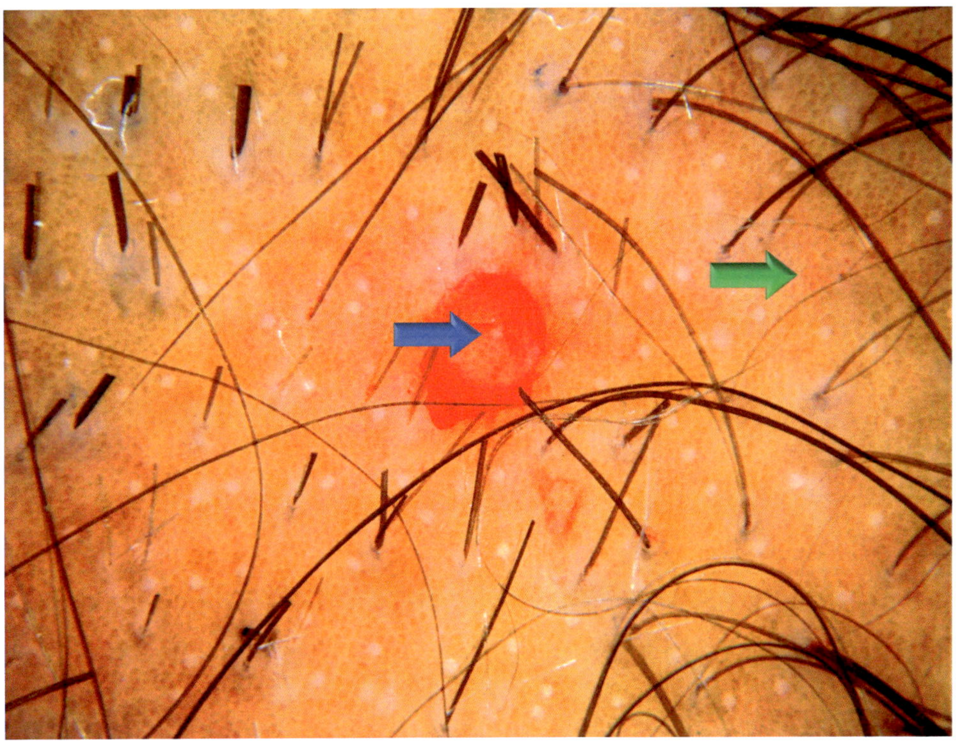

Fig. 39.3 Androgenetic alopecia. Trichoscopy of a 35-year-old woman with shaved hairs shows pinpoint white dots inside a 1-mm micropunch mark (*blue arrow*) and miniaturized hair follicles. Note that differentiation between follicles and eccrine pores is very difficult. Capillary vessels also are difficult to visualize in this skin phototype (*green arrow*)

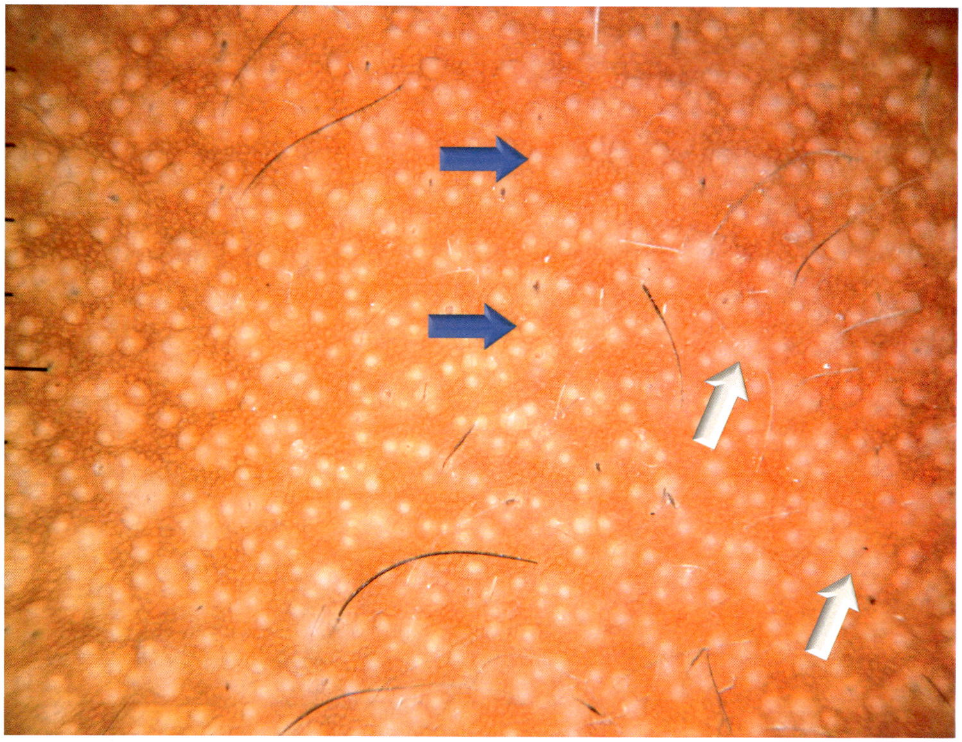

Fig. 39.4 Alopecia areata. Exclamation mark hairs and black dots are important markers of disease activity. Two types of white dots are observed inside the alopecic patches: isolated pinpoint white dots between the follicular units (*blue arrows*) and white dots in groups of two or three surrounded by a white circular halo (*white arrows*), which represent empty follicular units

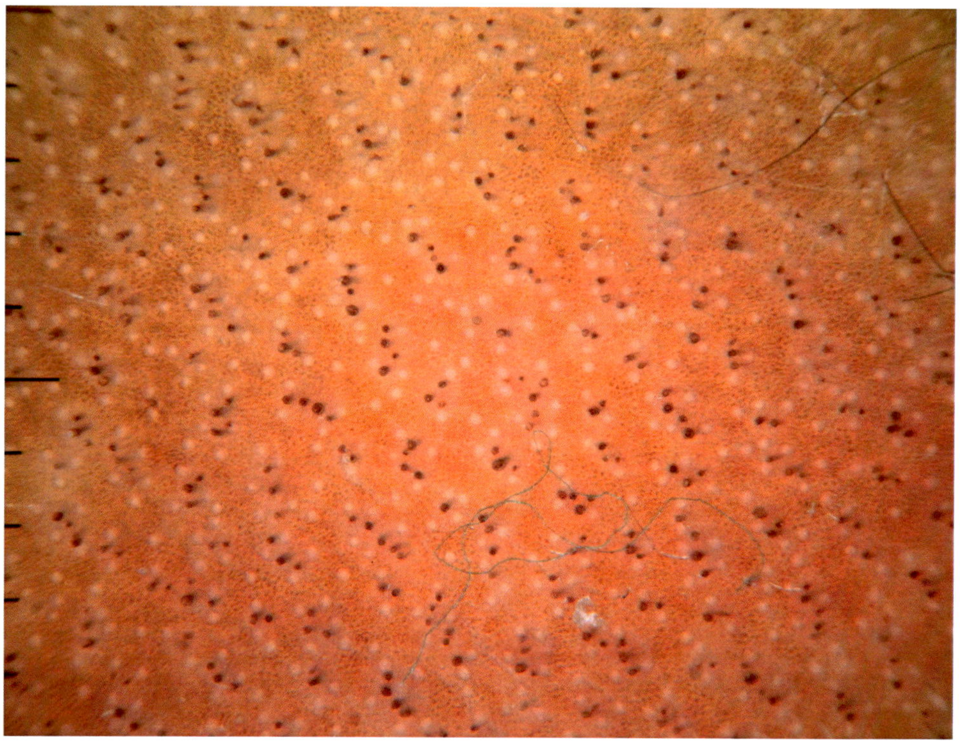

Fig. 39.5 Alopecia areata after anthralin therapy. Shown is a dermoscopic image from a 12-year-old boy with alopecia areata treated with anthralin. The medication has the capacity to pigment follicular units. The pigmented points must be differentiated from true black dots, as no fractured hairs are observed. Pinpoint white dots are seen clearly between the pigment go inside the follicular opening

Fig. 39.6 Yellow dots in a speckled pattern in alopecia areata. The diminished contrast of pigmented scalp and the yellowish color of the dots make this finding difficult to observe

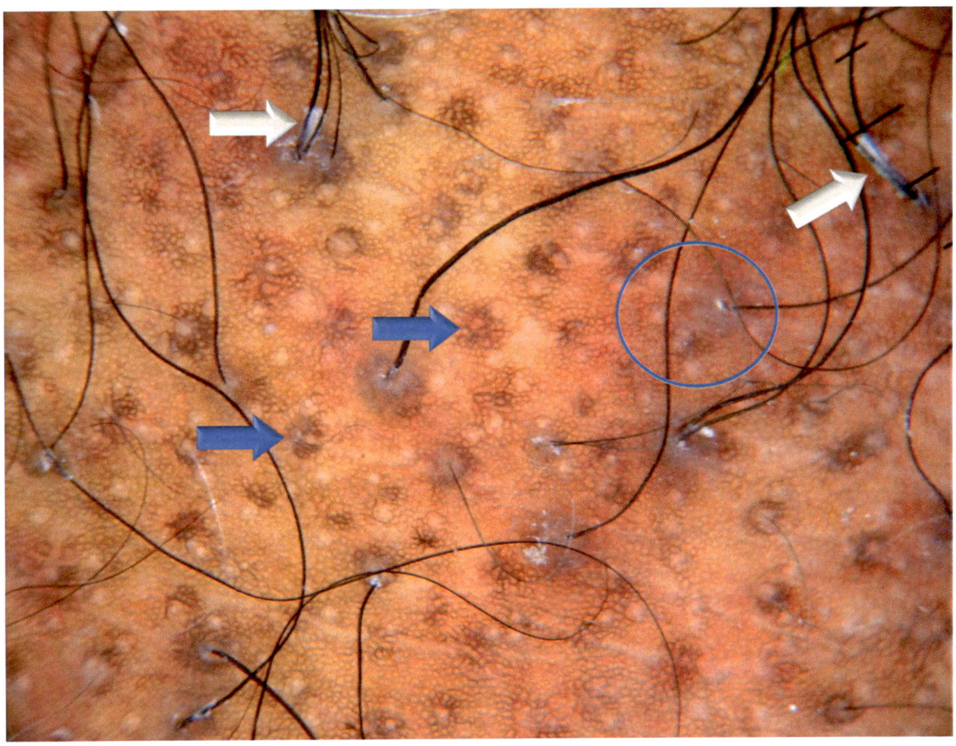

Fig. 39.7 Traction alopecia in a 70-year-old woman. Fractured hair shafts, erythema (*circle*), hair casts (*white arrows*), and pustules are seen. Late-stage traction alopecia may reveal vellus hair shafts associated with a cicatricial pattern—loss of follicular ostia (*blue arrows*). A variable degree of perifollicular hyperpigmentation also is observed in all types of alopecia manifesting in dark-skinned patients

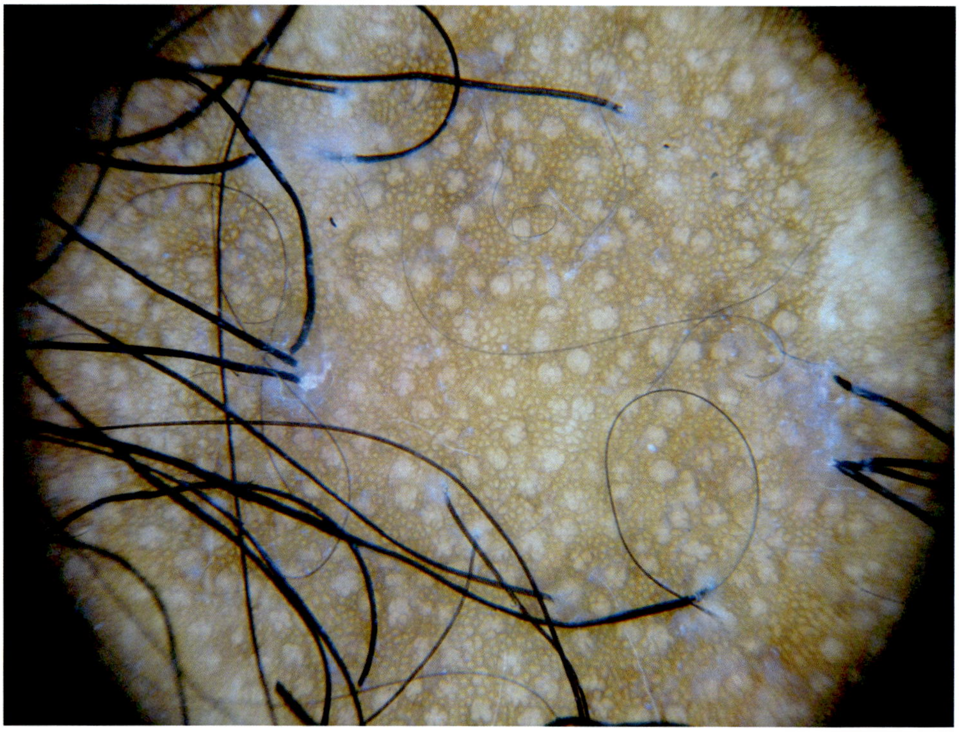

Fig. 39.8 Central centrifugal cicatricial alopecia. Trichoscopic findings are very similar to those found in traction alopecia and lichen planopilaris: absence of follicular ostia, perifollicular scaling, pinpoint white dots, and vellus hairs. We believe there is no specific or diagnostic finding of central centrifugal cicatricial alopecia on trichoscopy

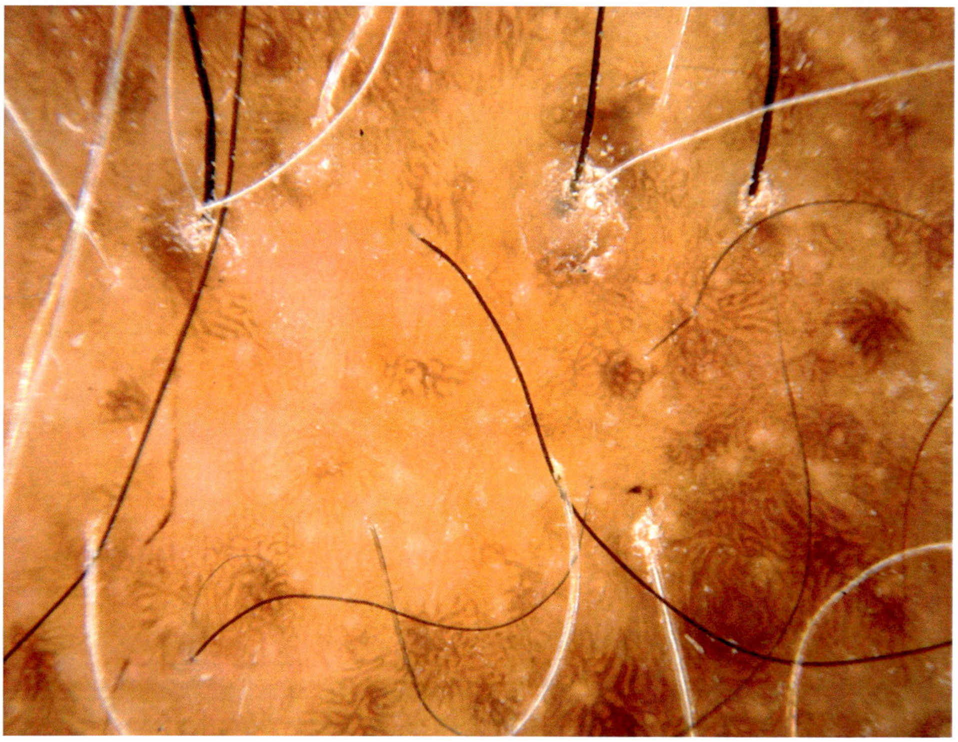

Fig. 39.9 Classic lichen planopilaris. Dermoscopy reveals an intact honeycomb pigmented network associated with perifollicular scaling. Signs of acute inflammation rarely are observed in this skin phototype

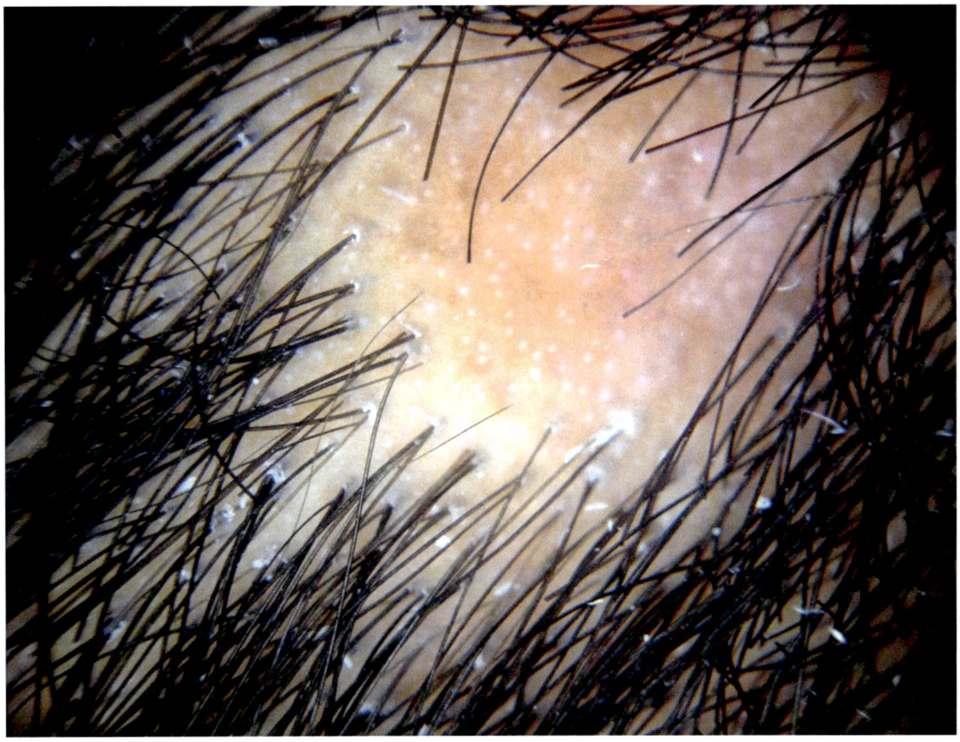

Fig. 39.10 Lichen planopilaris, acute phase. A diffuse erythema associated with the pigmented network may be observed

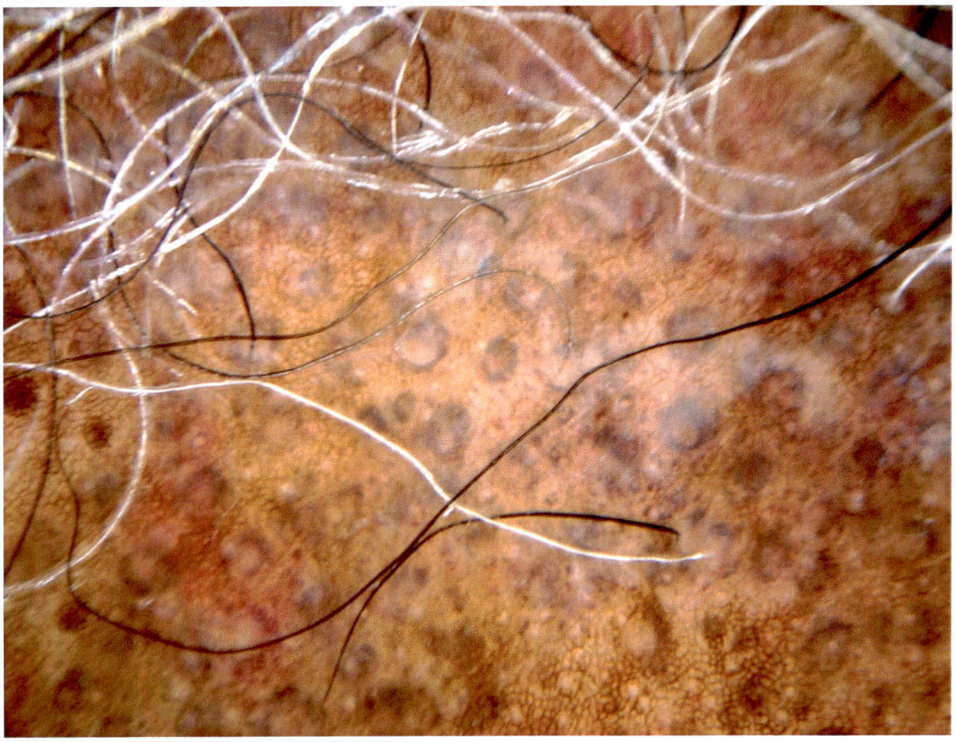

Fig. 39.11 Lichen planopilaris. Lichen planopilaris usually affects the perifollicular epidermis, sparing the interfollicular epidermis. We believe the reminiscent pigmented network associated with target blue-gray dots in a perifollicular distribution (target pattern) may help in differentiating lichen planopilaris from other scarring alopecias, such as discoid lupus erythematosus of the scalp

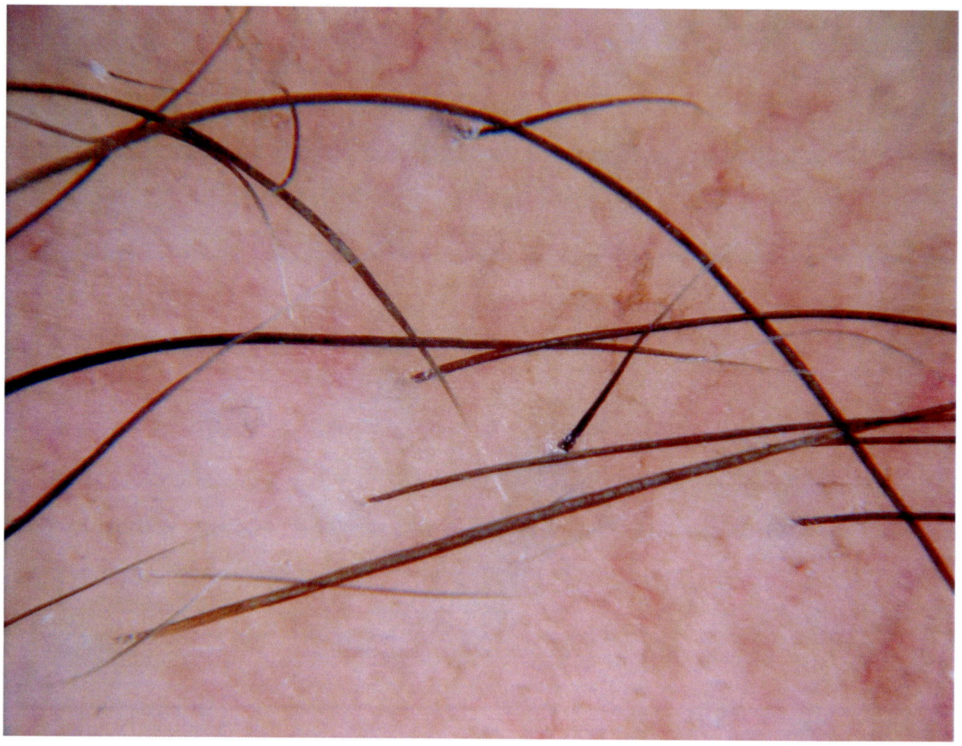

Fig. 39.12 **Eyebrow area in frontal fibrosing alopecia**. Trichoscopy of frontal fibrosing alopecia shows perifollicular desquamation and erythema. This image of the eyebrows of a patient with frontal fibrosing alopecia exhibits the same pattern observed on the scalp

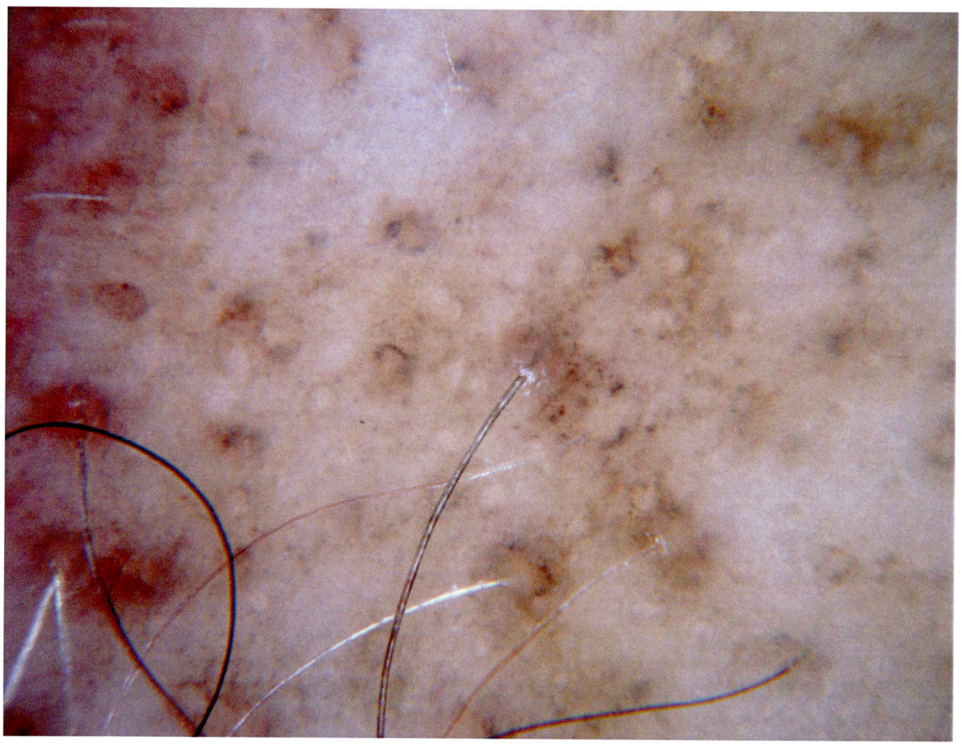

Fig. 39.13 **Discoid lupus erythematosus**. In discoid lupus erythematosus, scalp atrophy manifests as a diffuse white area and is well-appreciated in dark-skinned patients, who lose the pigmented network inside the plaques. In late stages, a pigmented network might be seen at the periphery of the plaque of discoid lupus erythematosus. Hyperkeratotic follicular plugging is well-observed. Blue-gray dots in a speckled distribution pattern along the alopecic patch represent pigment incontinence in the papillary dermis of follicular and interfollicular epidermis

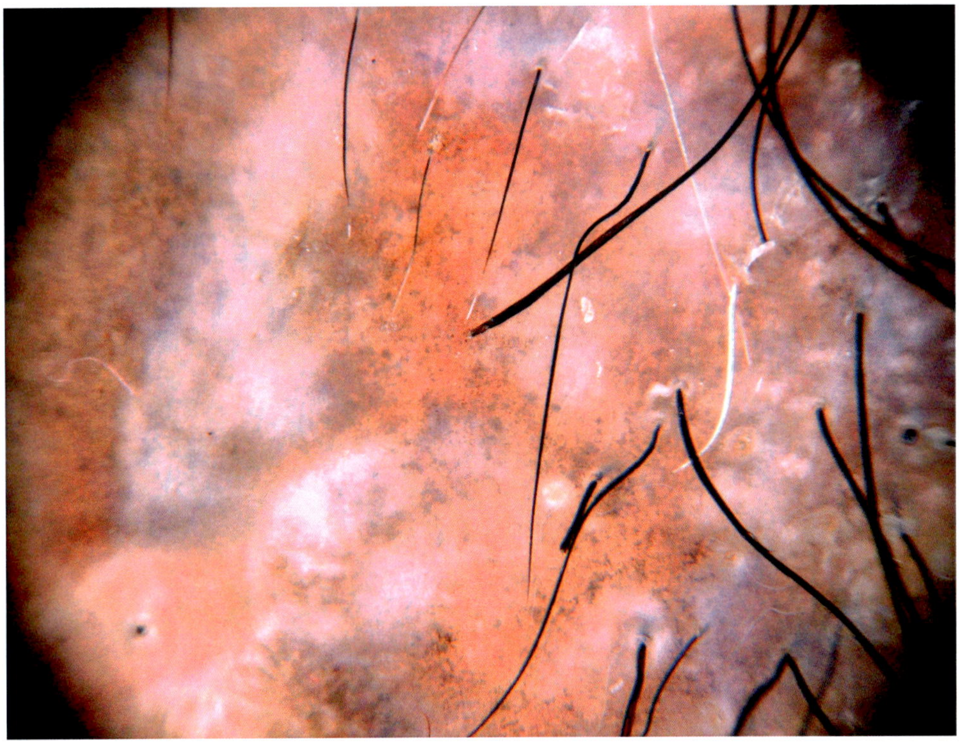

Fig. 39.14 Discoid lupus erythematosus. In discoid lupus erythematosus of the scalp, chrysalis structures represent birefringent collagen bundles and appear as shiny, bright white, linear streaks in the alopecic areas. These structures represent fibrosis and are best observed with polarized light dermoscopy. The chrysalis structures are probably the most important hallmark of cicatricial alopecias

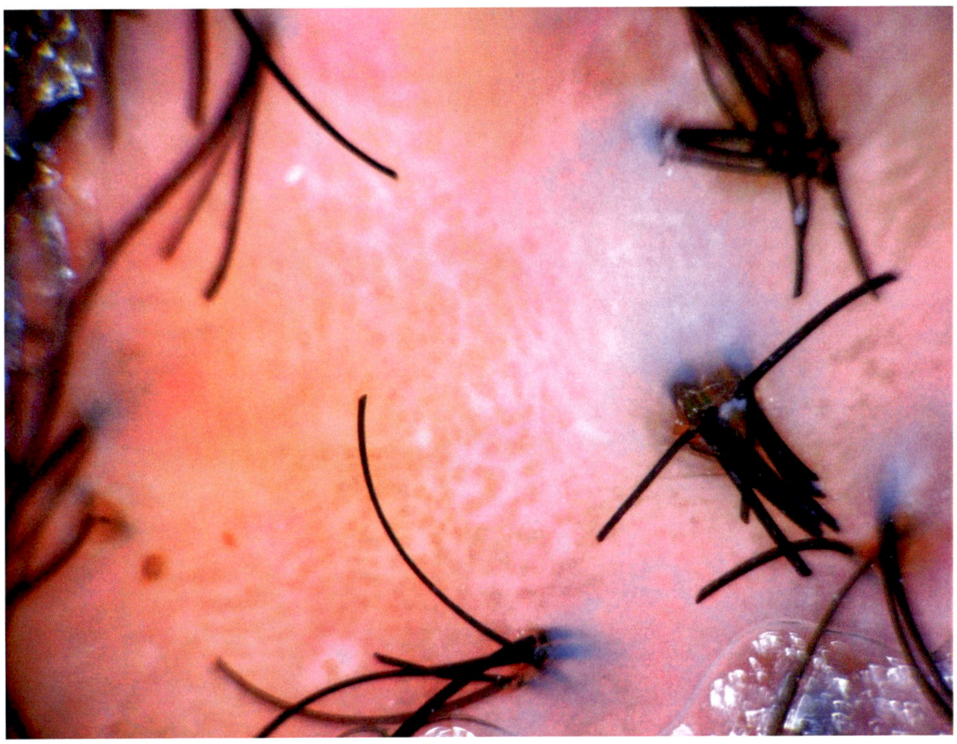

Fig. 39.15 Folliculitis decalvans. Folliculitis decalvans demonstrates a monomorphic pattern of several hair shafts emerging from the scalp (tufted hairs) and is associated with linear vessels, pustules, and chrysalis structures

References

1. Ross EK, Vincenzi C, Tosti A. Videodermoscopy in the evaluation of hair and scalp disorders. J Am Acad Dermatol. 2006;55: 799–806.
2. Abraham LS, Pineiro-Maceira J, Duque-Estrada B, Barcaui CB, Sodre CT. Pinpoint white dots in the scalp: dermoscopic and histopathological correlation. J Am Acad Dermatol. 2010;63:721–2.
3. Ardigò M, Torres F, Abraham LS, Piñeiro-Maceira J, Cameli N, Berardesca E, Tosti A. Reflectance confocal microscopy can differentiate dermoscopic white dots of the scalp between sweat gland ducts or follicular infundibulum. Br J Dermatol. 2011;164(5):1122–4.
4. de Lacharrière O, Deloche C, Misciali C, et al. Hair diameter diversity: a clinical sign reflecting the follicle miniaturization. Arch Dermatol. 2001;137:641–6.
5. Karadağ Köse O, Güleç AT. Clinical evaluation of alopecias using a handheld dermatoscope. J Am Acad Dermatol. 2012;67:206–14. Epub 2011 Oct 22.
6. Inui S, Nakajima T, Nakagawa K, Itami S. Clinical significance of dermoscopy in alopecia areata: analysis of 300 cases. Int J Dermatol. 2008;47:688–93.
7. de Moura LH, Duque-Estrada B, Abraham LS, Barcaui CB, Sodre CT. Dermoscopy findings of alopecia areata in an African-American patient. J Dermatol Case Rep. 2008;272(4): 52–4.
8. Tosti A, Duque-Estrada B. Hair loss. In: Micali G, Lacarruba F, editors. Dermatoscopy in clinical practice beyond pigmented lesions. London: Informa Healthcare; 2010. p. 31–44.
9. Duque-Estrada B, Tamler C, Sodré CT, Barcaui CB, Pereira FB. Dermoscopy patterns of cicatricial alopecia resulting from discoid lupus erythematosus and lichen planopilaris. An Bras Dermatol. 2010;85:179–83.
10. Tosti A, Torres F, Misciali C, Vincenzi C, Starace M, Miteva M, Romanelli P. Follicular red dots: a novel dermoscopic pattern observed in scalp discoid lupus erythematosus. Arch Dermatol. 2009;145:1406–9.

Part XV

Algorithms in Trichoscopy

Algorithms in Trichoscopy

40

Adriana Rakowska, Lidia Rudnicka,
Malgorzata Olszewska, and Alfredo Rossi

Abstract

Algorithms and diagnostic criteria are useful for the practical differential diagnosis of hair loss by trichoscopy. Currently, three trichoscopic algorithms are available: the first trichoscopic algorithm by Inui, the 3-A system for differential diagnosis of hair loss, and the Videodermoscopy Scalp Psoriasis Severity Index (VSCAPSI) for evaluation of scalp psoriasis. The only cause of hair loss for which specific diagnostic criteria were established is androgenetic alopecia.

Keywords

Algorithm • Alopecia areata • Androgenetic alopecia • Cicatricial alopecia • Clinical trials Folliculitis decalvans • Diagnosis • Lichen planopilaris • Lupus • Monitoring • Noncicatricial alopecia • Psoriasis • Telogen effluvium • Tinea capitis • Trichotillomania • Videodermoscopy

Algorithms and diagnostic criteria are useful for the differential diagnosis of hair loss by trichoscopy. The first algorithm, created in 2011 by Inui [1], is a two-step method of evaluating trichoscopic results. In the first step, noncicatricial alopecia is differentiated from cicatricial alopecia based on the presence or absence of (empty) hair follicles. In the second step, both types of hair loss are categorized based on the presence or absence of specific trichoscopic findings [1].

We have proposed another approach to the differential diagnosis of hair loss by trichoscopy [2]. In this method, called the *3-A system* (for *three-algorithm system*), the first step is based on clinical evaluation and the second on trichoscopic results. First, hair loss is clinically categorized as diffuse, focal noncicatricial, or cicatricial alopecia. A simplified algorithm was generated for each of these three clinical situations. These algorithms allow the differential diagnosis of most common diseases, such as androgenetic alopecia, alopecia areata, telogen effluvium, tinea capitis, discoid lupus erythematosus, lichen planopilaris, folliculitis decalvans, dissecting cellulitis, and trichotillomania. They do not include rare diseases that must be diagnosed based on trichoscopic pattern analysis and/or histopathology.

The only cause of hair loss for which specific diagnostic criteria have been established is female androgenetic alopecia [3]. These criteria are based on trichoscopy performed with high-magnification digital dermoscopy. The major criteria are (1) yellow dots in the frontal area, (2) lower average hair thickness in the frontal than in the occipital area, and (3) more than 10 % of thin hairs in the frontal area. Minor criteria relate to an increased frontal-to-occipital ratio of (1) follicular units with one hair, (2) vellus hairs, and (3) the peripilar sign. Fulfillment of two major criteria or one major

A. Rakowska
Department of Dermatology, CSK MSW, Warsaw, Poland

L. Rudnicka (✉)
Faculty of Health Sciences, Medical University of Warsaw, Poland

Department of Dermatology, CSK MSW, Woloska 137, Warsaw, 02-502, Poland
e-mail: lidia.rudnicka@euderm.eu

M. Olszewska
Department of Dermatology, Medical University of Warsaw, Warsaw, Poland

A. Rossi
Medicina Interna e Specialità Mediche Sapienza, University of Rome, Policlinico Umberto I Roma, Rome, Italy

L. Rudnicka et al. (eds.), *Atlas of Trichoscopy*,
DOI 10.1007/978-1-4471-4486-1_40, © Springer-Verlag London 2012

criterion and two minor criteria allows the trichoscopic diagnosis of androgenetic alopecia with 98 % specificity [3].

Simplified criteria for androgenetic alopecia are (1) thickness heterogeneity of long terminal hair shafts in the frontal area (>20 % of thin hairs) and (2) twice as many follicular units with one hair in the frontal than the occipital area. These criteria, developed for low-magnification examinations [3, 4], are helpful in clinical practice, but their sensitivity and specificity need to be evaluated.

It must be emphasized that the sole presence of yellow or black dots is not a differentiating criterion, because both trichoscopic features may be present in multiple diseases [3, 5–7].

Rossi et al. [8] created the Videodermoscopy Scalp Psoriasis Severity Index (VSCAPSI) for evaluating and monitoring scalp psoriasis. This index is based on a combination of clinical and trichoscopic (videodermoscopic) observations. The scalp is divided into four areas (left, right, front, and back). In each area, the vascular pattern, erythema, and desquamation (scaling) is assessed separately. The final calculated score may range from 0 to 11, with higher values corresponding to more severe scalp psoriasis. This method is most useful for evaluating moderately severe scalp psoriasis.

The 3-A system and VSCAPSI are examples of combining clinical evaluation with trichoscopy in the differential diagnosis and scoring of hair and scalp diseases. They also reflect how trichoscopy is being incorporated into the diagnostic process as a vital, but not the sole, diagnostic procedure.

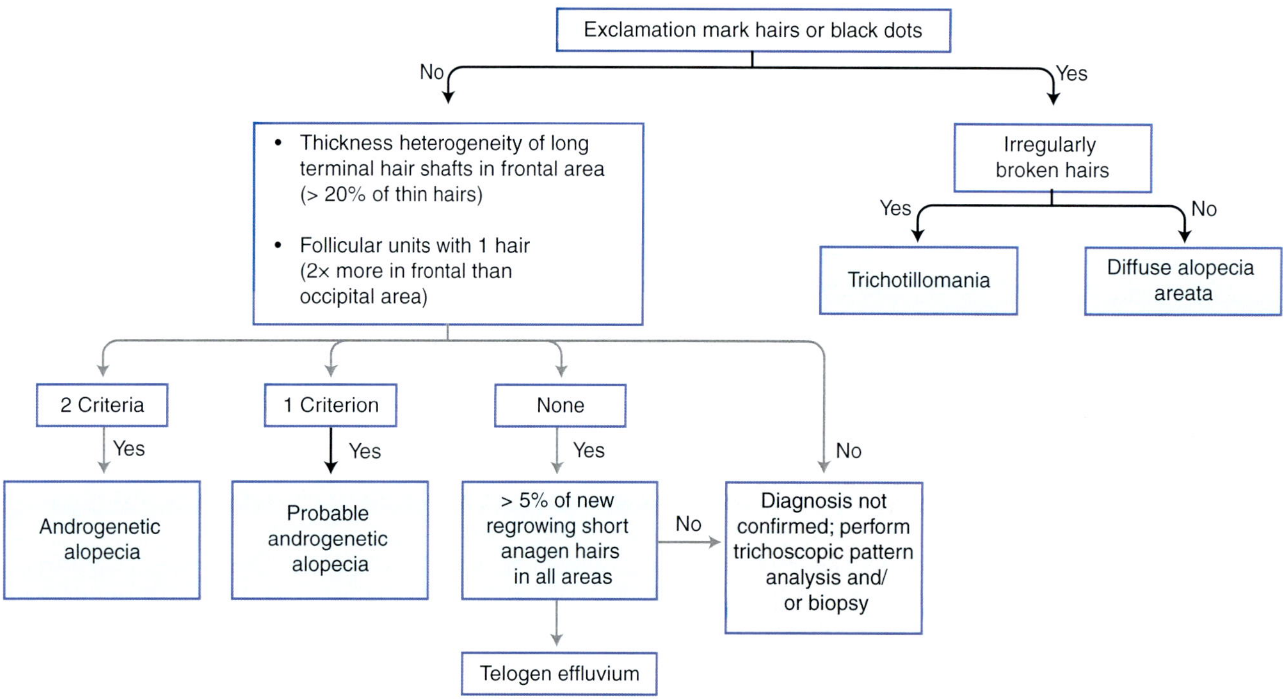

Fig. 40.1 Algorithm for the trichoscopic differential diagnosis of diffuse noncicatricial alopecia (chart I of the 3-A system)

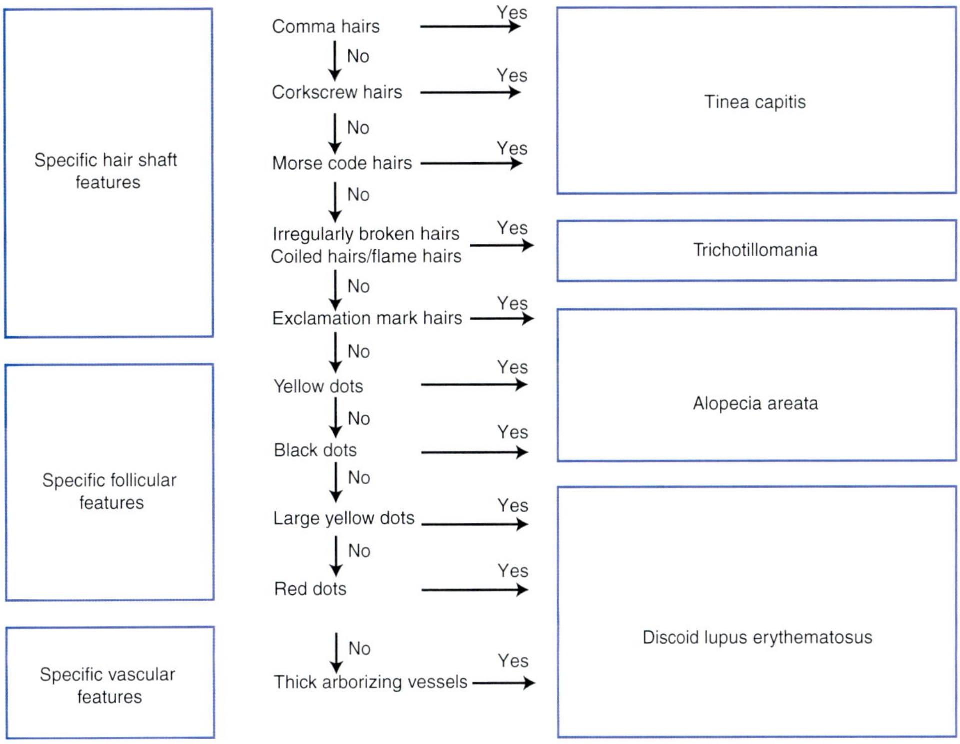

Fig. 40.2 Algorithm for the trichoscopic differential diagnosis of focal noncicatricial alopecia (chart II of the 3-A system)

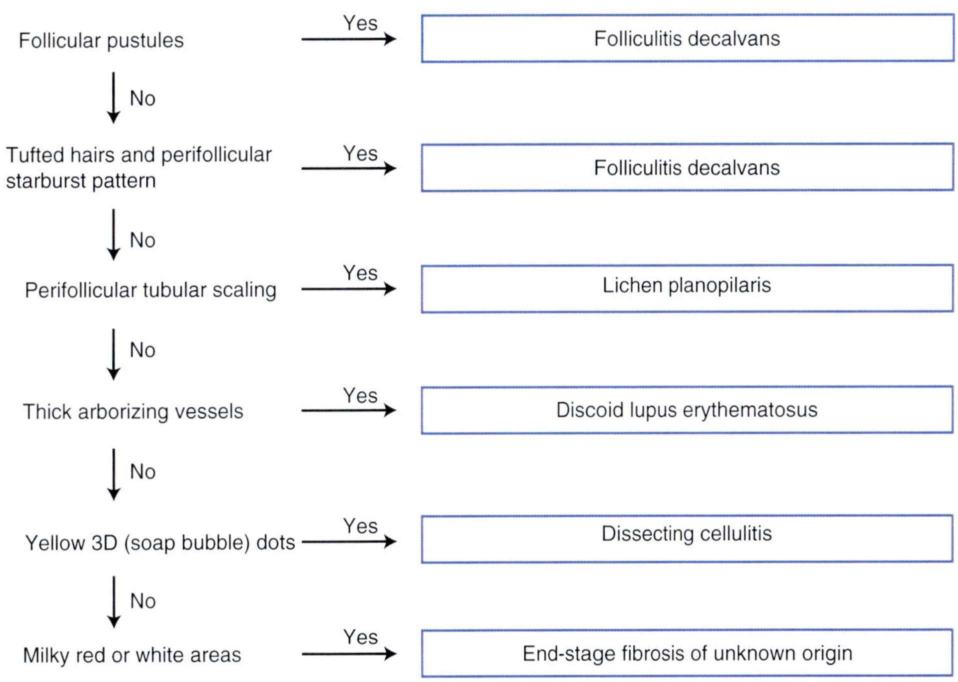

Fig. 40.3 Algorithm for trichoscopy differential diagnosis of cicatricial alopecia (chart III of the 3A-system). *3D* three-dimensional

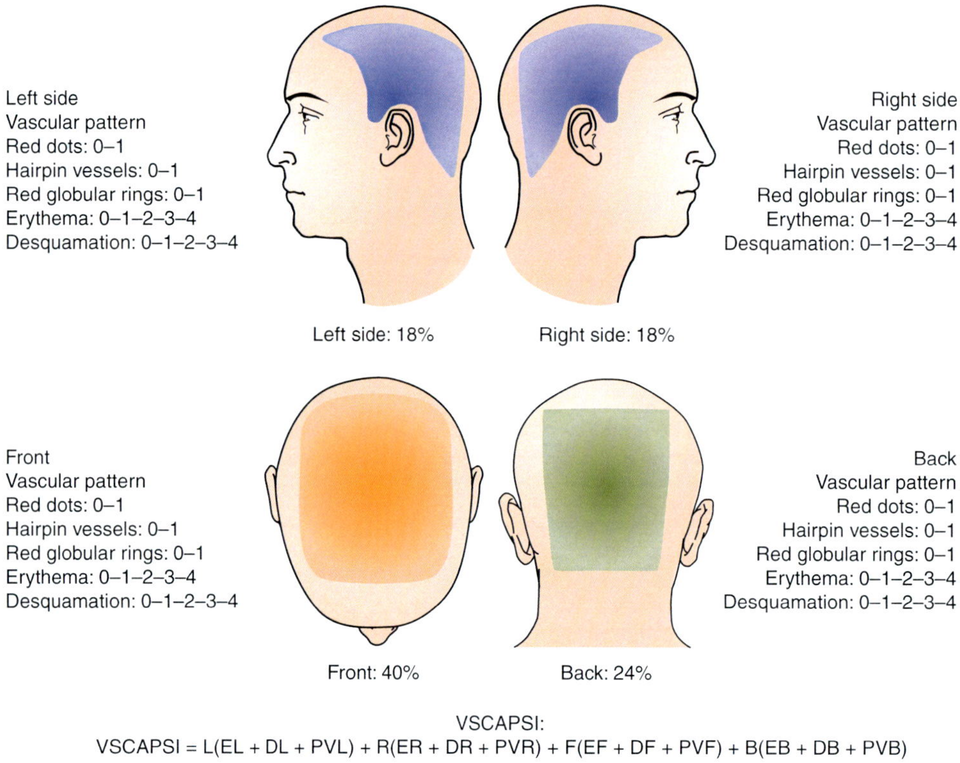

Fig. 40.4 The Videodermoscopy Scalp Psoriasis Severity Index (VSCAPSI). The VSCAPSI divides the scalp into four areas: the left side (L, 18 % of the scalp surface), right side (R, 18 %), front (F, 40 %), and back (B, 24 %). In each area, the presence and morphology of vascular patterns (PV) and the severity of the erythema (E) and desquamation (D) is assessed. Scalp psoriasis presents three vascular patterns: red dots, hairpin vessels, and red globular rings. In each field of view, it is possible to observe none, one, two, or all three vascular patterns, scored 0, 1, 2, and 3, respectively. Erythema is scored 0–4 depending on severity. Similarly, desquamation (scaling) is scored 0–4, depending on severity. The VSCAPSI score is calculated based on the following formula: VSCAPSI = L(EL + DL + PVL) + R(ER + DR + PVR) + F(EF + DF + PVF) + B(EB + DB + PVB). Scores range from a minimum of 0.0 to a maximum of 11.0. The VSCAPSI score is 0 in a patient with no scalp psoriasis and (theoretically) 11 in the most severe form of the condition. The VSCAPSI is especially useful for evaluating scalp psoriasis of moderate severity (*Adapted from* Rossi et al. [8], *with permission*)

References

1. Inui S. Trichoscopy for common hair loss diseases: algorithmic method for diagnosis. J Dermatol. 2011;38(1):71–5.
2. Rudnicka L, Rakowska A. Three trichoscopy algorithms for clinical practice. J Dermatol Case Rep. 2012 (submitted).
3. Rakowska A, Slowinska M, Kowalska-Oledzka E, Olszewska M, Rudnicka L. Dermoscopy in female androgenic alopecia: method standardization and diagnostic criteria. Int J Trichol. 2009;1(2):123–30.
4. de Lacharriere O, Deloche C, Misciali C, Piraccini BM, Vincenzi C, Bastien P, et al. Hair diameter diversity: a clinical sign reflecting the follicle miniaturization. Arch Dermatol. 2001;137(5):641–6.
5. Kowalska-Oledzka E, Rakowska A, Slowinska M, Olszewska M, Rudnicka L. Black dots are not specific for alopecia areata. J Clin Exp Dermatol. 2012;37:615–9. Epub 2012 Jun 8.
6. Miteva M, Tosti A. Hair and scalp dermatoscopy. J Am Acad Dermatol. 2012 Nov;67(5):1040–8.
7. Rudnicka L, Olszewska M, Rakowska A, Slowinska M. Trichoscopy update 2011. J Dermatol Case Rep. 2011;5(4):82–8.
8. Rossi A, Mandel VD, Garelli V, Mari E, Fortuna MC, Carlesimo M, et al. Videodermoscopy scalp psoriasis severity index (VSCAPSI): a useful tool for evaluation of scalp psoriasis. Eur J Dermatol. 2011;21(4):546–51.

Part XVI

Monitoring Therapy with Trichoscopy

Monitoring Hair and Scalp Diseases

41

Lidia Rudnicka, Adriana Rakowska, and Ana Maria Costa Pinheiro

Abstract

Monitoring disease activity and treatment efficacy with trichoscopy is a new field of exploration. Available data show that the method may be useful in monitoring tinea capitis, scalp psoriasis, alopecia areata, androgenetic alopecia, telogen effluvium, and other hair and scalp diseases, making trichoscopy a helpful tool beyond clinical practice. This technique also may be applied in research and clinical trials.

Keywords

Alopecia areata • Androgenetic alopecia • Clinical trials • Management • Monitoring Psoriasis • Research • Telogen effluvium • Tinea capitis • Therapy • Treatment

Trichoscopy serves mainly as an aid in the differential diagnosis of hair and scalp diseases, but it also may be used as a tool to assess disease activity and to monitor treatment efficacy. Distinct diseases show different features of disease activity.

Trichoscopy was first used in 2005 to monitor treatment efficacy in female androgenetic alopecia [1]. Olszewska and Rudnicka [1] used a digital videodermoscope to evaluate the efficacy of dutasteride therapy by measuring hair shaft thickness before and during therapy. Six months after therapy began, a significant increase in average hair shaft thickness was observed. Other parameters that may be used in monitoring androgenetic alopecia include the proportion of thin hairs, proportion of follicular units with one hair, average number of yellow dots per field of view, proportion of follicular units with brown perifollicular discoloration (the peripilar sign), and proportion of follicular units with one or three hairs [2–5].

In alopecia areata, increased disease activity is characterized by the presence of black dots, micro–exclamation mark hairs, broken hairs, monilethrix-like hairs, and trichorrhexis nodosa. In inactive disease, trichoscopy shows regularly distributed yellow dots [4–6]. Yellow dots may not be present in children or in patients with extremely longstanding, clinically inactive disease [5]. In a recent study, trichoscopy was used to evaluate diphenylcyclopropenone treatment efficacy in 20 patients with alopecia areata [7]. The authors showed that after 24 weeks of therapy, trichoscopy revealed the disappearance or a significant reduction in features of active disease, such as exclamation mark hairs and black dots. Simultaneously, features of hair regrowth, such as the presence of upright regrowing hairs, was observed [7].

In trichotillomania, active disease is characterized by the presence of multiple broken hairs, which differ in shape and length. Black dots may be present. These features are not visible after a few months of successful therapy [4].

In telogen effluvium, the active regrowing phase is characterized by the presence of multiple upright regrowing hairs [8].

Active tinea capitis is characterized by the presence of comma and/or corkscrew hairs. These hair shaft abnormalities disappear after successful therapy [9].

L. Rudnicka (✉)
Faculty of Health Sciences, Medical University of Warsaw, Poland

Department of Dermatology, CSK MSW, Woloska 137, Warsaw 02-502, Poland
e-mail: lidia.rudnicka@euderm.eu

A. Rakowska
Department of Dermatology, CSK MSW, Warsaw, Poland

A.M.C. Pinheiro
Department of Internal Medicine, Hospital Universitario de Brasilia, Brasilia, Brazil

L. Rudnicka et al. (eds.), *Atlas of Trichoscopy*,
DOI 10.1007/978-1-4471-4486-1_41, © Springer-Verlag London 2012

Active diseases in the spectrum of primary cicatricial alopecia (e.g., lichen planopilaris, central centrifugal alopecia, discoid lupus erythematosus, folliculitis decalvans, dissecting cellulitis) show disease-specific trichoscopic features. In the inactive disease phase, a white or milky red area is seen as the sole, common manifestation of these diseases.

Monitoring of inflammatory scalp diseases, such as psoriasis, is more complex. A digital videodermoscopy system, the Videodermoscopy Scalp Psoriasis Severity Index (VSCAPSI), was developed to precisely assess the severity of scalp psoriasis. For details, see Chap. 40.

A simplified method for determining the success of psoriasis therapy is to look for the disappearance of scaling and fading of dotted/coiled blood vessels.

As the aforementioned examples show, trichoscopy may serve as an effective tool in monitoring disease activity and treatment efficacy in clinical practice, as well as in research and clinical trials. The usual interval between consecutive examinations is 2–6 months.

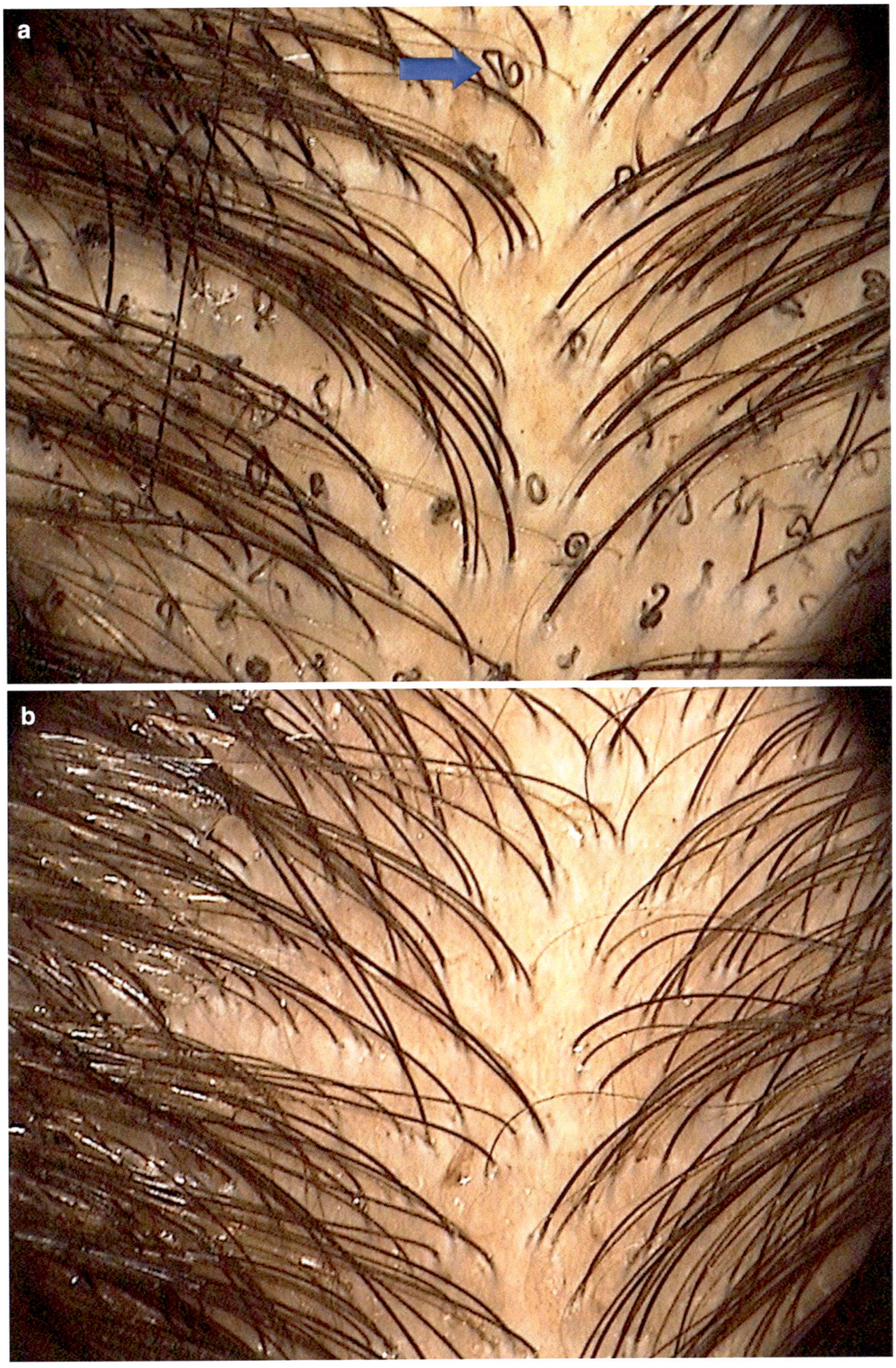

Fig. 41.1 **Monitoring treatment efficacy in tinea capitis**. Active tinea capitis is characterized by the presence of comma and/or corkscrew hairs and/or Morse code hairs. Vazquez-Lopez et al. [9] described the case of a 5-year-old dark-skinned girl with tinea capitis due to *Trichophyton violaceum* infection. In that patient trichoscopy showed multiple corkscrew hairs. After 3 months of successful therapy, all corkscrew hairs disappeared and trichoscopy was within the normal range. This image shows a similar comparison of active tinea capitis with (**a**) multiple corkscrew hairs (*arrow*) and (**b**) normal trichoscopy in the same patient (×20)

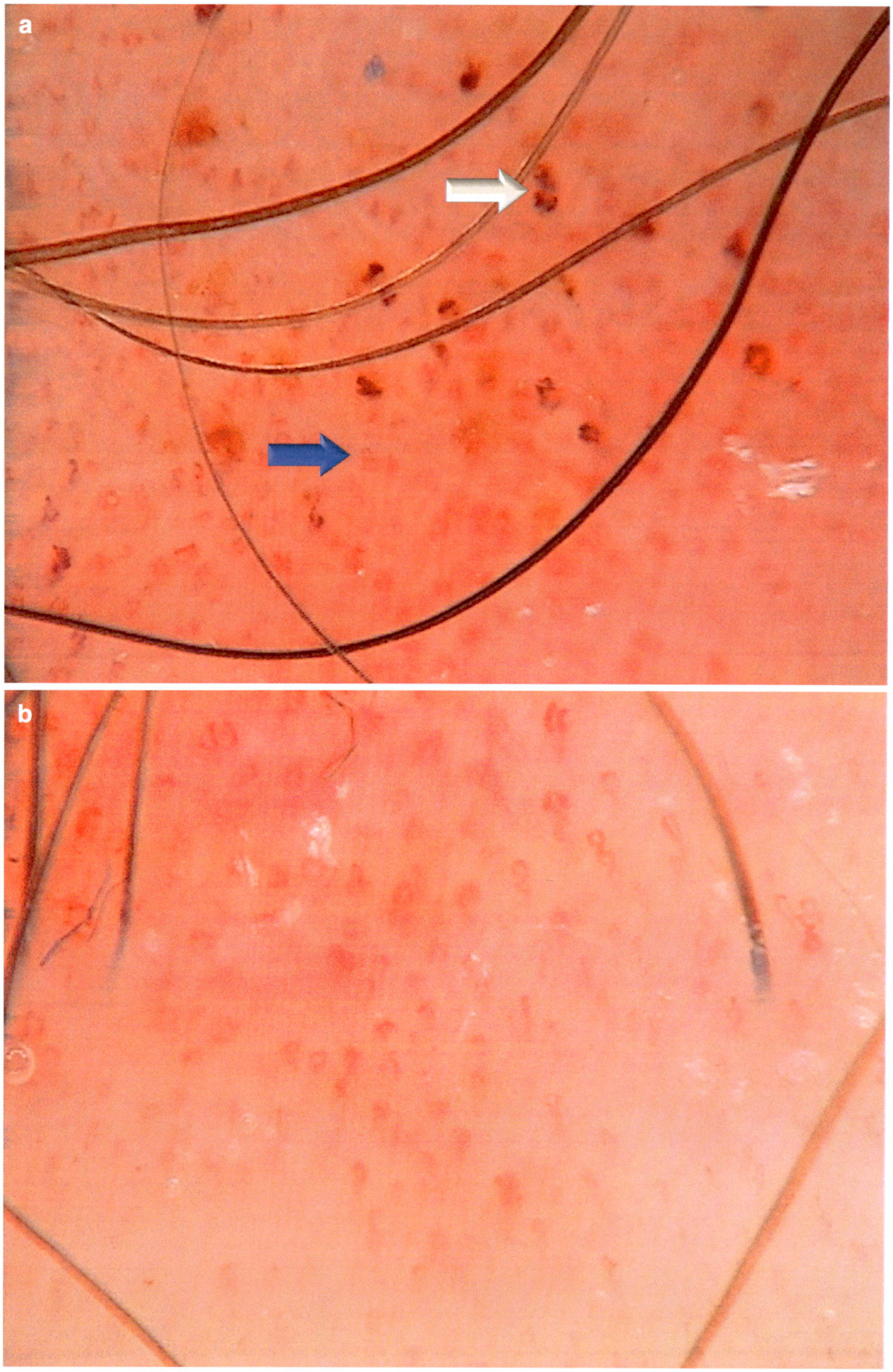

Fig. 41.2 Monitoring treatment efficacy in psoriasis. Shown are trichoscopic images of scalp psoriasis (periauricular area) in a 39-year-old patient (**a**) before and (**b**) 2 months after introduction of combined therapy with ustekinumab (systemic) and calcipotriol/betamethasone (topical). In the active disease phase, trichoscopy shows multiple glomerular (coiled) vessels (*blue arrow*) arranged in lines or rings. Blood extravasations (*white arrow*), which are common in scalp psoriasis, correspond to splinter hemorrhages observed in nails [10] and are a marker of active disease. After 2 months of therapy, the hemorrhages are no longer visible and blood vessels are fading. In patients with intense scaling, blood vessels may not be visible. The disappearance of scaling and fading of vascular structures may be almost simultaneous (×70)

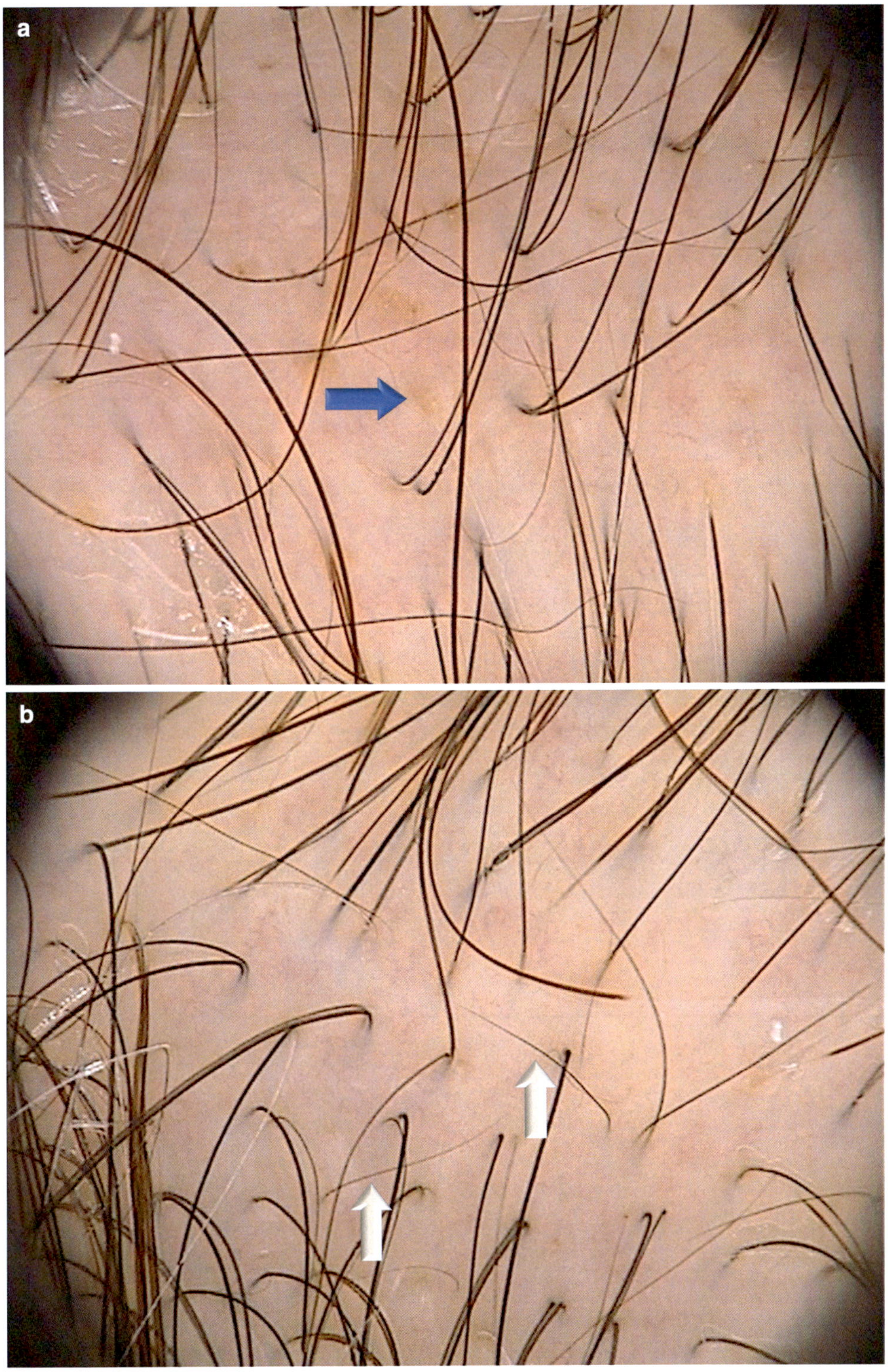

Fig. 41.3 Monitoring treatment efficacy in telogen effluvium. Shown are trichoscopic images from a 26-year-old woman with telogen effluvium in the course of iron deficiency (**a**) before and (**b**) after 2 months of iron supplementation. The most striking difference is the presence of upright regrowing hairs (*white arrows*), a trichoscopic feature of hair regrowth. Other differences include a decrease in the proportion of follicular units with only one hair and the disappearance of empty follicular openings (*blue arrow*). The presence of some hair shaft thickness heterogeneity in both images indicates coexisting androgenetic alopecia (×20)

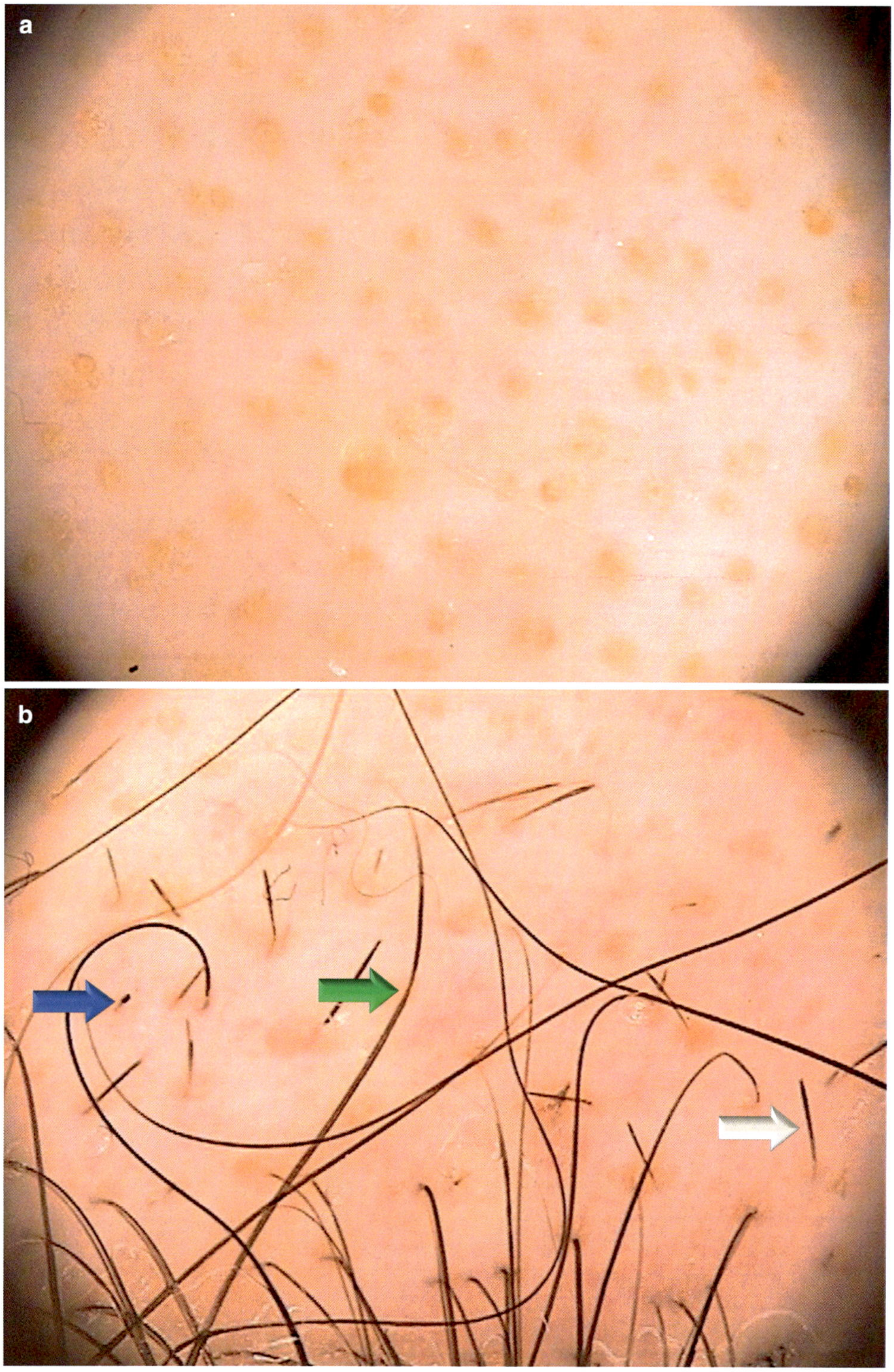

Fig. 41.4 Monitoring treatment efficacy in alopecia areata. Shown are trichoscopic images of alopecia areata in a 36-year-old woman (**a**) before and (**b**) 2 months after triamcinolone therapy. Although some hair regrowth is visible, black dots (*blue arrow*), micro–exclamation mark hairs (*white arrow*), and Pohl-Pinkus constrictions (*green arrow*) are markers of high disease activity and are negative prognostic trichoscopic features, indicating that this patient requires a change in treatment modality (×20)

References

1. Olszewska M, Rudnicka L. Effective treatment of female androgenic alopecia with dutasteride. J Drugs Dermatol. 2005;4(5):637–40.
2. Rakowska A, Slowinska M, Kowalska-Oledzka E, Olszewska M, Rudnicka L. Dermoscopy in female androgenic alopecia: method standardization and diagnostic criteria. Int J Trichol. 2009;1(2):123–30.
3. Ross EK, Vincenzi C, Tosti A. Videodermoscopy in the evaluation of hair and scalp disorders. J Am Acad Dermatol. 2006;55(5):799–806.
4. Rudnicka L, Olszewska M, Rakowska A, Slowinska M. Trichoscopy update 2011. J Dermatol Case Rep. 2011;5(4):82–8.
5. Miteva M, Tosti A. Hair and scalp dermatoscopy. J Am Acad Dermatol. 2012;67(5):1040–8.
6. Inui S, Nakajima T, Nakagawa K, Itami S. Clinical significance of dermoscopy in alopecia areata: analysis of 300 cases. Int J Dermatol. 2008;47(7):688–93.
7. Ganzetti G, Campanati A, Simonetti O, Cataldi I, Giuliodori K, Offidani AM. Videocapillaroscopic pattern of alopecia areata before and after diphenylciclopropenone treatment. Int J Immunopathol Pharmacol. 2011;24(4):1087–91.
8. Inui S. Trichoscopy for common hair loss diseases: algorithmic method for diagnosis. J Dermatol. 2011;38(1):71–5.
9. Vazquez-Lopez F, Palacios-Garcia L, Argenziano G. Dermoscopic corkscrew hairs dissolve after successful therapy of Trichophyton violaceum tinea capitis: a case report. Australas J Dermatol. 2012;53(2):118–9. doi:10.1111/j.1440-0960.2011.00850.x.
10. Baran R. The burden of nail psoriasis: an introduction. Dermatology. 2010;221 Suppl 1:1–5.

Part XVII

Trichoscopy Report

Trichoscopy Report

42

Lidia Rudnicka and Malgorzata Olszewska

Abstract

The results of trichoscopy should be presented in a form that allows effective communication between dermatologists. In clinical practice, we use two types of reporting forms: a short form and a full trichoscopy report. The short form serves mainly diagnostic purposes, whereas the full trichoscopy report is used to monitor treatment efficacy in clinical trials and research.

Keywords

Clinical trials • Dermoscope • Examination • Form • Report • Research • Results

Trichoscopy is a diagnostic method in dermatology and should serve dermatologists in their therapeutic decision-making process. It may be performed in the office by the treating dermatologist or as a service to other colleagues. In the latter case, the trichoscopic results should be presented in a form that allows effective communication between dermatologists.

Unlike skin cancer dermoscopy, in which each lesion requires a separate description [1], in hair and scalp diseases a general overview usually is sufficient.

In clinical practice, we use two types of reporting forms of reports: a short form and a full trichoscopy report.

A short report may be generated based on trichoscopy performed with a handheld dermoscope or digital (video) dermoscope. It usually contains the following elements:

1. Relevant information about the patient (e.g., name, age)
2. Date of the examination
3. Short anamnesis and clinical description of the hair/scalp condition
4. Imaging equipment and magnification used
5. Description of trichoscopic findings
   (a) In diffuse hair loss: the frontal, occipital, and temporal areas
   (b) In focal hair loss: the hairless lesion, hair-bearing margin, and healthy-appearing area of the scalp
6. Clinical conclusion (diagnosis or differential diagnosis, disease activity, other clinically relevant information)

In 2009, a full trichoscopy report form was proposed [2]. The report is based on trichoscopic results obtained by digital dermoscopes and serves mainly in the quantitative monitoring of treatment efficacy. The full report requires software that assists in performing measurements, particularly measurement of hair shaft thickness (*see* Fig. 2.8 for details). Although this report provides very precise information about trichoscopic results, it is very time consuming and difficult to generate for every patient in a busy clinical practice. Thus, we use this type of report only in selected patients, in clinical trials, and for research purposes.

The full trichoscopic report is based on separate descriptions of findings in the frontal and occipital areas and in one temporal area. The frontal area is defined as approximately 2 cm from the frontal hairline and 2 cm from the midline. The occipital area is 2 cm lateral from the protuberans occipitalis [3]. The report includes numeric values for the following measurable features: average number of terminal hairs in one field of view; percentage of thin hairs

L. Rudnicka (✉)
Faculty of Health Sciences, Medical University of Warsaw, Poland

Department of Dermatology, CSK MSW, Woloska 137, Warsaw 02-502, Poland
e-mail: lidia.rudnicka@euderm.eu

M. Olszewska
Department of Dermatology, Medical University of Warsaw, Warsaw, Poland

L. Rudnicka et al. (eds.), *Atlas of Trichoscopy*,
DOI 10.1007/978-1-4471-4486-1_42, © Springer-Verlag London 2012

DERMATOLOGY SPECIALISTS

02392 Warsaw, Poland, Grojecka 186/309, www.euderm.pl

1 January 2013

TRICHOSCOPY REPORT

PATIENT'S NAME: xxxxxxx xxxxxx, **born** xx xx xxxx

CLINICAL: A 2-year history of focal, slowly progressing hair loss. Clinically a 2x2 cm, sharply demarcated hairless area. Moderate pruritus.

EQUIPMENT: Dermlite DL3® (magnification:10x)

TRICHOSCOPY: Mid-part of the lesion shows milky-red (strawberry ice cream color) areas, lacking follicular openings. In the hair-bearing margin, perifollicular scaling with a tendency to form white, tubular, scaly structures is visible. There are few elongated, linear blood vessels in concentric arrangement and discrete violaceous areas in interfollicular distribution. Hair and scalp is otherwise normal on trichoscopy.

CONCLUSIONS:
Lichen planopilaris. Features of moderate disease activity in the hair-bearing marigin of the lesion and cicatricial alopecia of recent onset in the central part of the lesion.

Signature

Xxxxxxx Xxxxxxx, MD

Fig. 42.1 Trichoscopy report, short form (sample)

DERMATOLOGY SPECIALISTS

02392 Warsaw, Poland, Grojecka 186/309, www.euderm.pl

1 January 2013

TRICHOSCOPY REPORT

PATIENT'S NAME: xxxxxxx xxxxxx, **born** xx xx xxxx (2nd follow-up trichoscopy)

	Frontal Area	Occipital area	Temporal areas
Average number of terminal hairs per FOV*	37.5	42.5	30.0
Proportion of thin (<0.03 mm) hairs	38%	29%	26%
Proportion of mid-thickness hairs 0,03-0,05 mm	31%	30%	39%
Proportion of thick (>0,05 mm) hairs	31%	41%	37%
Average hair shaft thickness (mm)	0.048	0.058	0.052
Proportion of follicular units with brown perifollicular discoloration (peripilar sign)	83%	13%	23%
Proportion of follicular units with 3 or more hairs	30%	80%	50%
Proportion of follicular units with 2 hairs	40%	20%	40%
Proportion of follicular units with 1 hair	30%	0%	10%
Average number of yellow dots per FOV*	2.5	0.5	0.3
Average number of upright regrowing hairs per FOV*	0	0	0
Scaling (0-4)	0	0	0
Other anbormalities (black dots, broken hairs, fibrotic white dots etc)	No	No	No

* VOD = field of view in 70-fold magnification, corresponding to $9mm^2$

EQUIPMENT: FotoFinder Dermoscope II® (magnification: 70x)

CONCLUSION:

Female androgenetic alopecia. Hair thinning, peripilar sign and yellow dots predominantly in the frontal area. Compared to previous examination (6 months ago), an increase in average hair shaft thickness and in proportion of follicular units with 3 or more hairs is observed in all areas.

Signature

Xxxxxxx Xxxxxxx, MD

Fig. 42.2 Full trichoscopy report (sample)

(<0.03 mm); percentage of medium-sized hairs (0.03–0.05 mm); percentage of thick hairs (>0.05 mm); average hair shaft thickness; proportion of follicular units with one, two, and three or more hairs; number of yellow dots per field of view; and proportion of follicular units with brown perifollicular discoloration (the peripilar sign). Other parameters included in this report are specific features of diseases, such as hair shaft structure abnormalities, the predominant type of blood vessels, and abnormalities in the perifollicular and interfollicular areas.

Normal values were established for fields of view at a 20-fold and 70-fold magnification, equivalent to approximately 1 cm^2 and 9 mm^2, respectively. The field of view may differ among devices from different manufacturers; therefore, the same type of device should be used to monitor treatment efficacy in a particular patient.

The full trichoscopy report is most useful for evaluating diffuse hair loss and for global assessment of the hair's condition. It has limited value in monitoring focal noncicatricial or cicatricial alopecia. In such cases, the short trichoscopy report is more applicable.

References

1. Malvehy J, Puig S, Argenziano G, Marghoob AA, Soyer HP. Dermoscopy report: proposal for standardization. Results of a consensus meeting of the International Dermoscopy Society. J Am Acad Dermatol. 2007;57(1):84–95.
2. Rakowska A. Trichoscopy (hair and scalp videodermoscopy) in the healthy female. Method standardization and norms for measurable parameters. J Dermatol Case Rep. 2009;3(1):14–9.
3. Hillmann K, Blume-Peytavi U. Diagnosis of hair disorders. Semin Cutan Med Surg. 2009;28(1):33–8.

Part XVIII

Lymphoproliferative Disorders

Systemic Lymphoproliferative Diseases

43

Ralph M. Trüeb

Abstract
Trichoscopic examination of the scalp may be helpful in the diagnosis and differential diagnosis of alopecic and nonalopecic conditions related to systemic lymphoproliferative diseases, particularly follicular mucinosis, folliculotropic mycosis fungoides, and multiple myeloma with monoclonal dysproteinemia.

Keywords
Alopecia mucinosa • Follicular filiform spicules • Follicular mucinosis • Lymphoma • Lymphoproliferative diseases • Monoclonal gammopathy • Multiple myeloma • Mycosis fungoides

Dermoscopy is a noninvasive diagnostic tool that permits recognition of morphologic structures not visible to the naked eye. While the general dermatologist is familiar with dermoscopy as a diagnostic aid, primarily for the differentiation of pigmented skin lesions, dermatologists involved in the management of hair loss have discovered dermoscopy of hair and scalp or trichoscopy as a valuable tool in the differential diagnosis of the alopecias. It is the objective of this chapter to review dermoscopic findings of the scalp related to systemic lymphoproliferative diseases.

Follicular mucinosis is an uncommon condition affecting the pilosebaceous unit, presenting clinically as grouped follicular papules or plaques with associated hair loss (alopecia mucinosa), most commonly on the face, neck, and scalp. The term is used in pathology to describe mucinous infiltration with cystic mucinous changes in the epithelium of hair follicles. It may be primary (idiopathic) or secondary to cutaneous T cell lymphoma (mycosis fungoides). Accumulating experience shows that patient age, distribution of lesions, and duration or extent of disease do not reliably distinguish between benign primary follicular mucinosis and secondary follicular mucinosis associated with cutaneous lymphoma. More recently, it has been suggested that individuals with follicular mucinosis demonstrating a clonal T cell receptor gene rearrangement may be at higher risk for the development of lymphoma. Therefore, continued long-term follow-up of patients with clonal primary follicular mucinosis is necessary [1]. Follicular mucin may be seen on dermoscopy as follicular plugs of amorphous material in dilated follicular ostia.

Folliculotropic mycosis fungoides represents another cutaneous lymphoproliferative disorder affecting the pilosebaceous unit. Histopathologic examination demonstrates an infiltration of atypical lymphocytes predominantly around the follicles, while Alcian blue stain fails to show mucinosis. The morphologic spectrum of clinical presentation is distinct from conventional mycosis fungoides, which is at least partially the result of the disease's ability to simulate a variety of inflammatory conditions afflicting the follicular unit. The disease course seems more aggressive and shows a poorer outcome [2].

Folliculotropic mycosis fungoides shows distinct clinical features, with predominant head and facial involvement. The morphologic spectrum of lesions is broad and includes erythematous papules and plaques with follicular prominence, with or without alopecic patches, and comedonal, acneiform, or cystic lesions that may be visualized on dermoscopy.

R.M. Trüeb
Center for Dermatology and Hair Diseases,
Bahnofplatz 1A, Wallisellen, CH-8304, Switzerland
e-mail: r.trueeb@derma-haarcenter.ch, ralph.trueeb@bluewin.ch

L. Rudnicka et al. (eds.), *Atlas of Trichoscopy*,
DOI 10.1007/978-1-4471-4486-1_43, © Springer-Verlag London 2012

Follicular filiform spicules represent yet another rare follicular phenomenon associated with lymphoproliferative disease. Patients with multiple myeloma and monoclonal gammopathy may present with multiple horn-like filiform spicules in the follicular orifices of the face, particularly on the nose and ears [3]. Histopathologic studies reveal follicular plugs of compact homogeneous eosinophilic material filling the intercellular spaces surrounding the keratinocytes. Biochemical investigations demonstrate that skin matter from spicules is made up of monoclonal dysprotein with electrophoretic characteristics identical to those found in patient serum [4]. The predominance of lesions in cold-exposed body regions, the morphologic identification of the follicular dysprotein deposits as cryogel in a patient with cryoglobulinemia, and the laboratory findings concerning the temperature and pH dependence of the precipitation of the dysprotein led to the hypothesis that the horny spicules represent a paraneoplastic manifestation directly related to the cryoglobulin [5, 6]. The follicular filiform spicules also may be visualized on dermoscopy of the scalp. The material visualized by dermoscopy represents monoclonal paraprotein casts.

In summary, dermoscopic examination of the scalp may be helpful in the diagnosis and differential diagnosis of alopecic or nonalopecic conditions related to systemic lymphoproliferative diseases, particularly follicular mucinosis, folliculotropic mycosis fungoides, and multiple myeloma with monoclonal dysproteinemia.

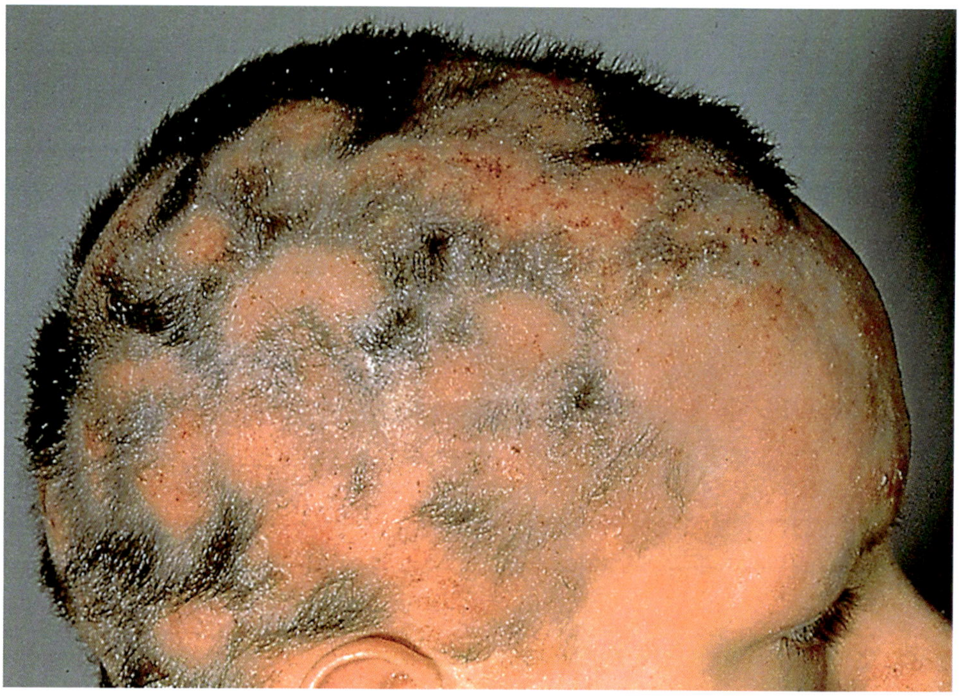

Fig. 43.1 **Follicular mucinosis (alopecia mucinosa)**. Clinical presentation. Plaques associated with hair loss (*Reproduced from* Trüeb RM [7], *with permission*)

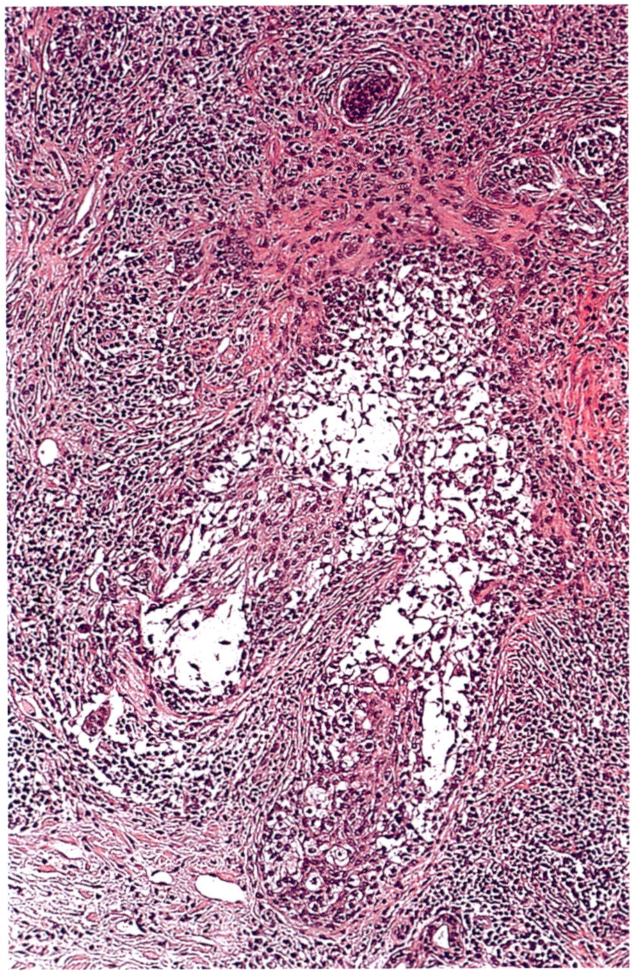

Fig. 43.2 Follicular mucinosis. Histopathology shows mucinous infiltration with cystic mucinous changes in the follicular epithelium (*Reproduced from* Trüeb RM [7], *with permission*)

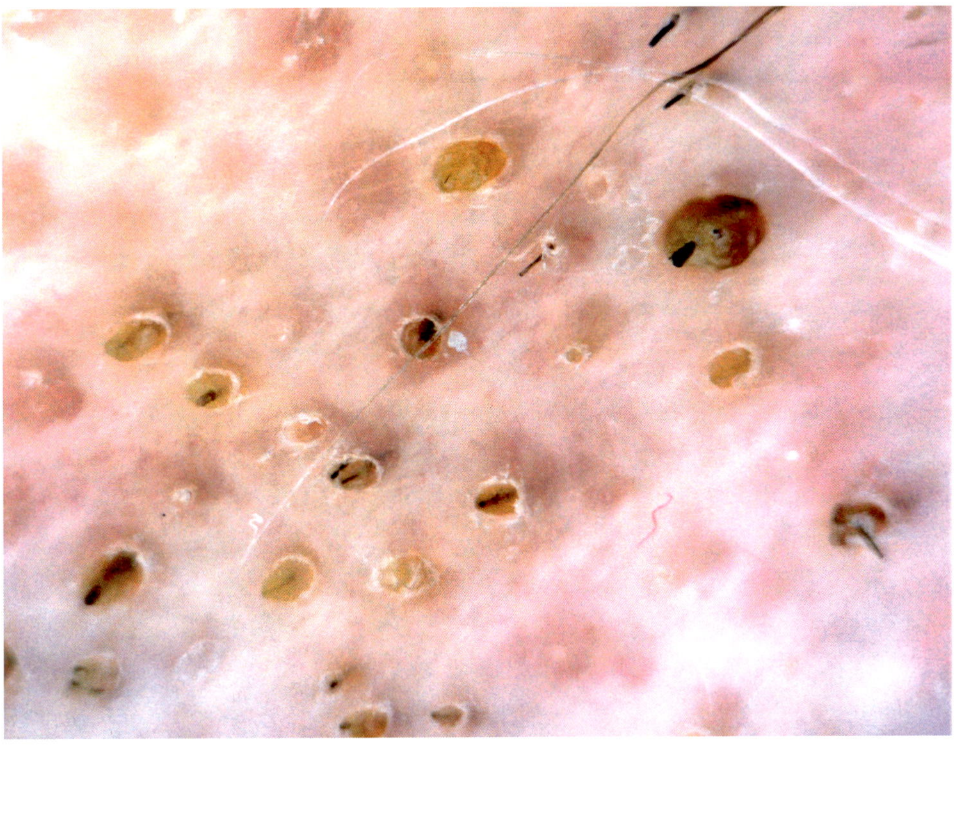

Fig. 43.3 Follicular mucinosis. Trichoscopy shows dilated follicular ostia with follicular plugs of amorphous material

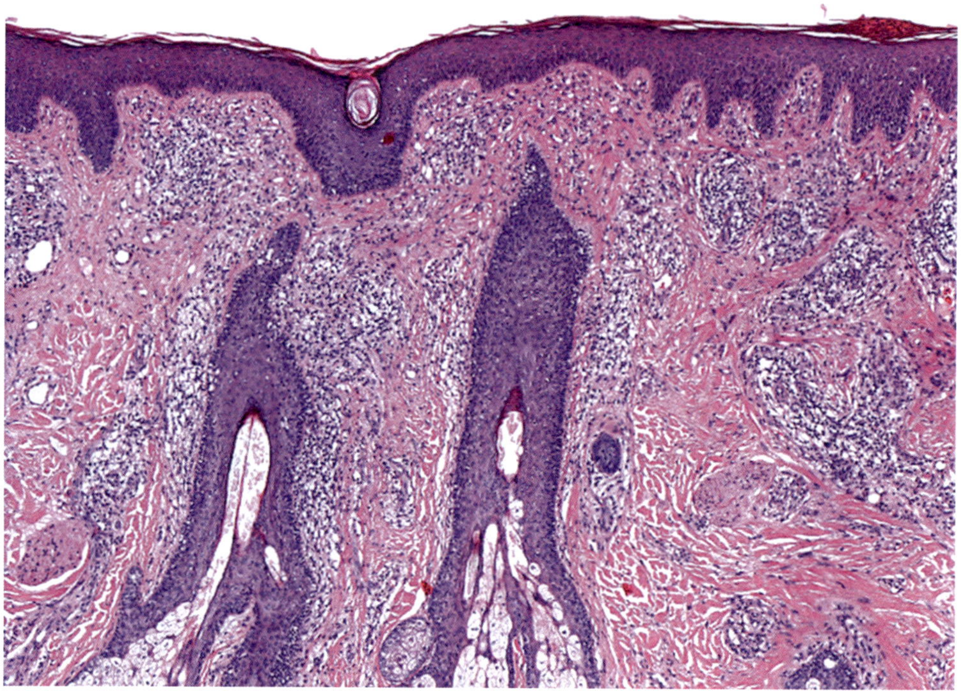

Fig. 43.4 Folliculotropic mycosis fungoides. Histopathology shows perifollicular infiltration with atypical lymphocytes (*Courtesy of* Professor Werner Kempf, MD, kempf und pfalz histologische diagnostik, Zurich, Switzerland)

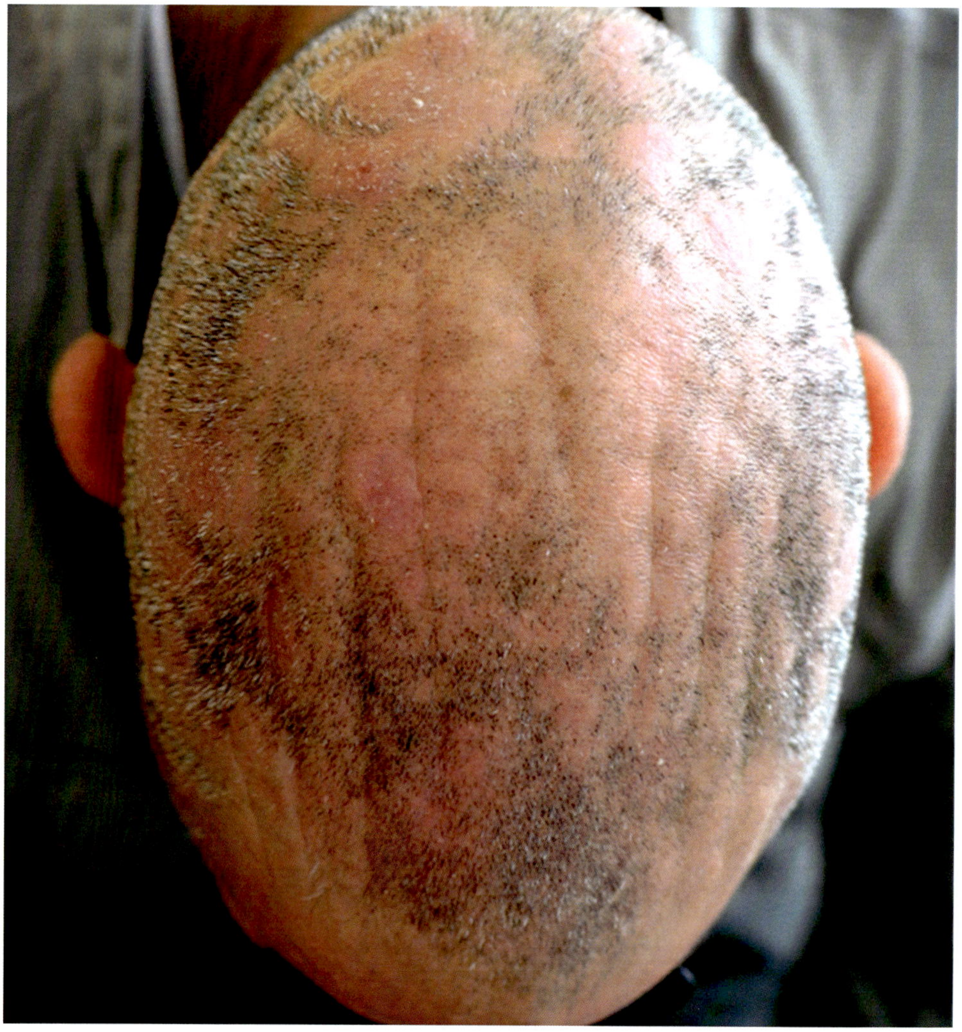

Fig. 43.5 Folliculotropic mycosis fungoides, clinical presentation. Erythematous plaques and focal alopecia are seen

Fig. 43.6 Folliculotropic mycosis fungoides. Trichoscopy shows comedonal lesions within alopecic patches

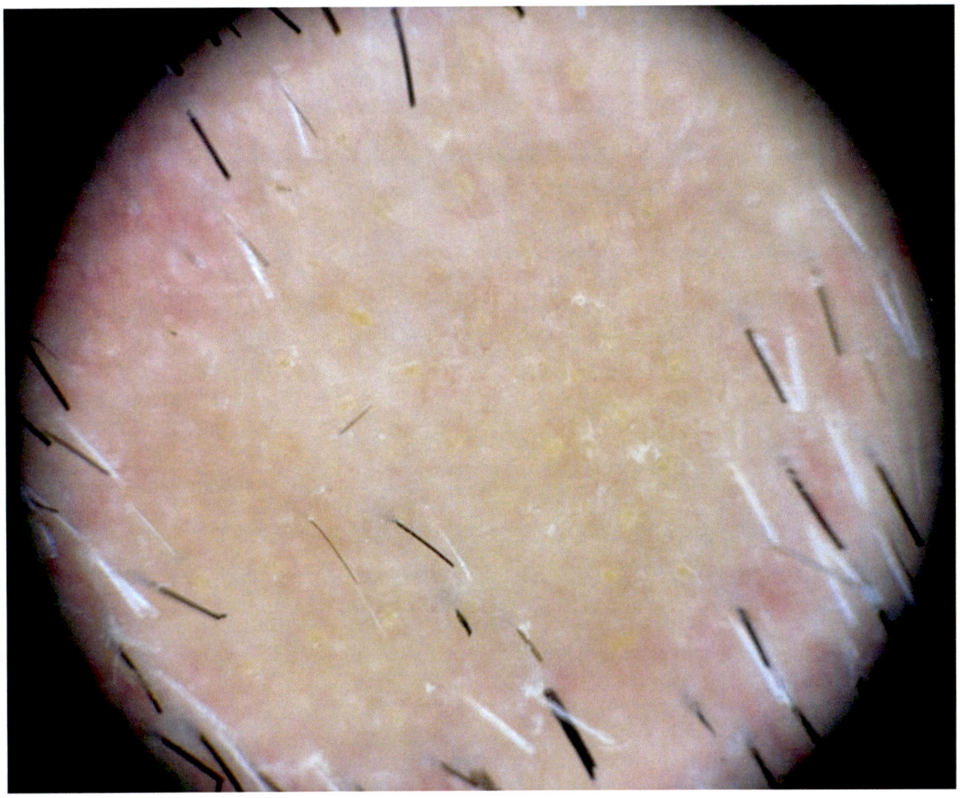

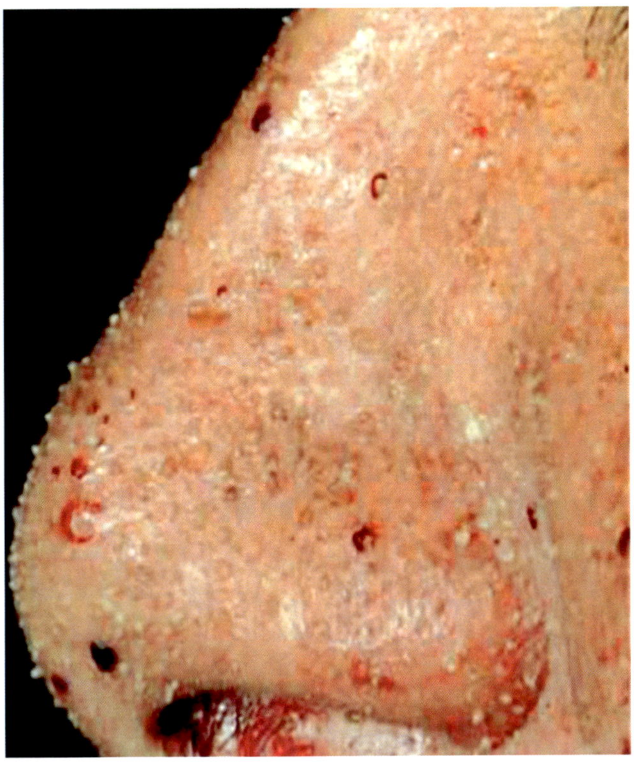

Fig. 43.7 Follicular filiform spicules. Shown is the clinical presentation of follicular filiform spicules on the nose of a patent with monoclonal gammopathy diagnosed with multiple myeloma (*Courtesy of* Lisa Weibel, MD, Department of Dermatology, University Hospital of Zurich, Switzerland)

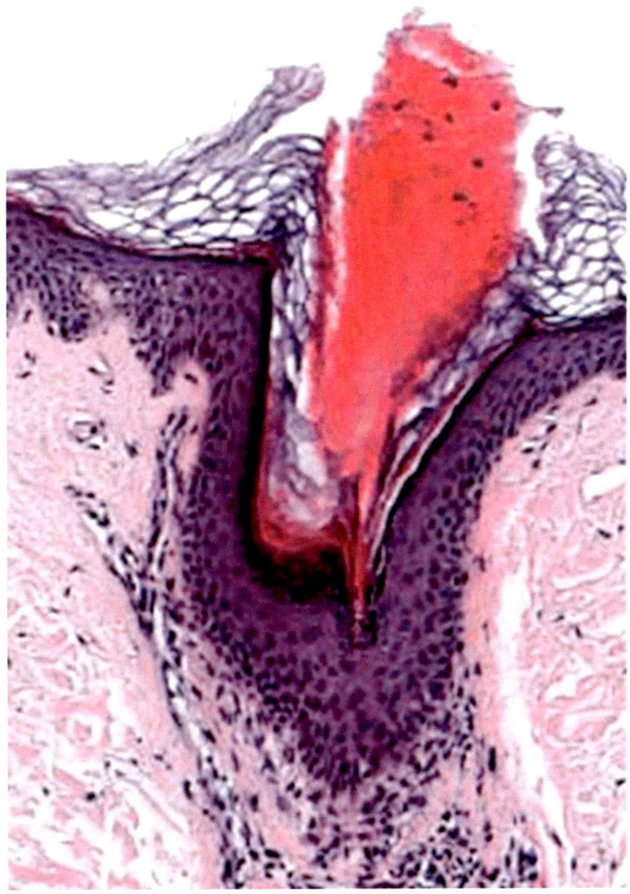

Fig. 43.8 Follicular filiform spicule. Histopathology shows a follicular plug of compact homogenous eosinophilic material in a patent with monoclonal gammopathy diagnosed with multiple myeloma

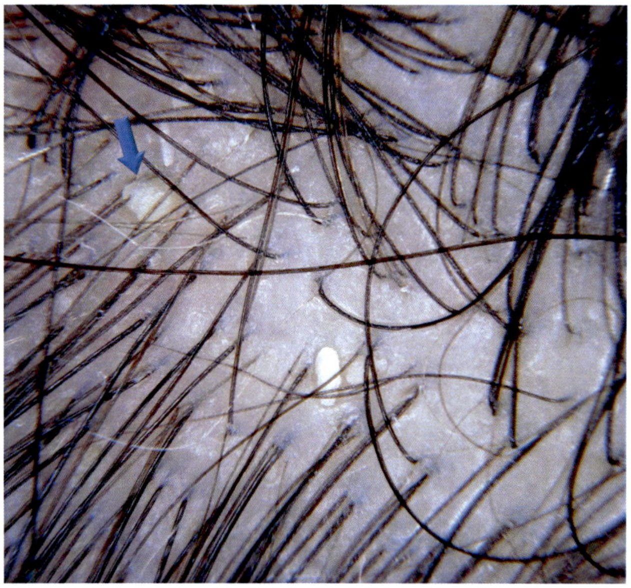

Fig. 43.9 Follicular filiform spicules. Trichoscopy shows follicular filiform spicules (*arrow*) on the scalp of a patent with monoclonal gammopathy diagnosed with multiple myeloma (*Courtesy of* Lisa Weibel, MD, Department of Dermatology, University Hospital of Zurich, Switzerland)

References

1. Brown HA, Gibson LE, Pujol RM, Lust JA, Pittelkow MR. Primary follicular mucinosis: long-term follow-up of patients younger than 40 years with and without clonal T-cell receptor gene rearrangement. J Am Acad Dermatol. 2002;47(6):856–62.
2. Gerami P, Rosen S, Kuzel T, Boone SL, Guitart J. Folliculotropic mycosis fungoides: an aggressive variant of cutaneous T-cell lymphoma. Arch Dermatol. 2008;144(6):738–46.
3. Weibel L, Berger M, Regenass S, Kamarashev J, Hafner J, French LE. Follicular spicules of the nose and ears—quiz case. Arch Dermatol. 2009;145(4):479–84.
4. Satta R, Casu G, Dore F, Longinotti M, Cottoni F. Follicular spicules and multiple ulcers: cutaneous manifestations of multiple myeloma. J Am Acad Dermatol. 2003;49(4):736–40.
5. Requena L, Sarasa JL, Ortiz Masllorens F, Martín L, Piqué E, Olivares M, et al. Follicular spicules of the nose: a peculiar cutaneous manifestation of multiple myeloma with cryoglobulinemia. J Am Acad Dermatol. 1995;32:834–9.
6. Bork K, Böckers M, Pfeifle J. Pathogenesis of paraneoplastic follicular hyperkeratotic spicules in multiple myeloma. Follicular and epidermal accumulation of IgG dysprotein and cryoglobulin. Arch Dermatol. 1990;126(4):509–13.
7. Trüeb RM. Haare. Praxis der Trichologie. Darmstadt: Steinkopff; 2003.

Part XIX

Trichoscopy in General Medicine

Trichoscopy in General Medicine 44

Lidia Rudnicka, Adriana Rakowska,
Malgorzata Olszewska, Joanna Czuwara,
Monika Slowinska, Justyna Sicinska,
Elzbieta Szymanska, and Ewa Ring

Abstract

Hair loss and scalp lesions may accompany several systemic disorders, such as metabolic abnormalities, endocrine conditions, autoimmune diseases, nutritional deficiencies, internal malignancy, and hematologic diseases. Hair problems may be the initial complaint causing patients to seek medical assistance. Thus, when performing trichoscopy, dermatologists should maintain a high index of suspicion when patients present with unexplained trichologic complaints.

Keywords

Addison's disease • Alopecia mucinosa • Amicrobial pustulosis • Autoimmune disease Crohn's disease • Cutaneous T-cell lymphoma • Dermatomyositis • Follicular mucinosis • Hyperbilirubinemia • Hormones • Hypothyroidism • Langerhans cell histiocytosis Lymphoma • Monoclonal gammopathy • Multicentric reticulohistiocytosis • Multiple myeloma • Mycosis fungoides • Sarcoidosis • Systemic lupus erythematosus • Systemic sclerosis • Vessels • Xeroderma pigmentosum

Several systemic diseases may be accompanied by hair loss, which may be the initial complaint causing patients to seek medical assistance. Thus, dermatologists should maintain a high index of suspicion when patients present with unexplained trichologic complaints.

Hair and scalp abnormalities may be associated with metabolic abnormalities, endocrine conditions, immune and autoimmune diseases, nutritional deficiencies, internal malignancy, or hematologic diseases. Hepatic and renal insufficiency also may affect hair growth and the appearance of scalp skin.

Diseases of the thyroid gland are the most common cause of hair problems in clinical practice. Hypothyroidism is associated with decreased sebaceous activity and a reduced hair growth rate, resulting in fragile, fine, brittle hair of decreased density. Occasionally, diffuse, gradually progressing alopecia may be the only clinical manifestation of thyroid insufficiency [1–3]. In hyperthyroidism, the hair also may be fine and brittle, with a tendency toward early graying [2, 4]. Autoimmune thyroid diseases are believed to be associated with an increased tendency to develop alopecia areata [5].

Hyperprolactinemia may be associated with androgenetic alopecia and telogen effluvium [2].

In pituitary failure, the scalp hair is thin and dry. Typically, patients experience a loss of axillary and pubic hair. Loss of the lateral part of the eyebrows is common in pituitary failure and several other endocrine and nonendocrine diseases. Loss of the lateral one third of the eyebrow, called the *Hertoghe sign*, is associated most commonly with hypothyroidism [6].

L. Rudnicka (✉)
Faculty of Health Sciences, Medical University of Warsaw, Poland

Department of Dermatology, CSK MSW, Woloska 137, Warsaw 02-502, Poland
e-mail: lidia.rudnicka@euderm.eu

A. Rakowska • J. Czuwara • M. Slowinska • J. Sicinska
E. Szymanska • E. Ring
Department of Dermatology, CSK MSW, Warsaw, Poland

M. Olszewska
Department of Dermatology, Medical University of Warsaw, Warsaw, Poland

L. Rudnicka et al. (eds.), *Atlas of Trichoscopy*,
DOI 10.1007/978-1-4471-4486-1_44, © Springer-Verlag London 2012

Increased ovarian production of androgens and testicular androgenic deficiency both may cause reduced hair growth and increased hair loss. In Addison's disease (chronic adrenal insufficiency), darkening of the hair may be observed. In parathyroid gland dysfunction, the hair usually is thick, but focal or diffuse alopecia may develop [2].

Alopecia in patients with malnutrition may be associated with iron, zinc, biotin, vitamin D_3, or protein deficiency [3]. Selenium deficiency may result in early hair graying [7].

In systemic connective tissue diseases, such as systemic sclerosis, systemic lupus erythematosus, and dermatomyositis, diffuse hair thinning is observed but hair loss is rare. In systemic lupus erythematosus, focal alopecia may result from a concomitant discoid (cutaneous) lupus erythematosus lesion [8, 9].

Diffuse or focal hair loss may be associated with lymphoproliferative disorders, particularly follicular mucinosis [10]. Hyperkeratotic or filiform follicular spicules may be the first manifestation of multiple myeloma, or of its progression or relapse [11].

Hair loss also may develop in the course of other malignant disorders.

A specific clinical type of scalp abnormality with hair loss is cutis verticis gyrata. The secondary form of this condition may be associated with diverse inflammatory and malignant diseases [12].

For most of these conditions, trichoscopic data from peer-reviewed literature are not yet available. Thus, this chapter focuses on presentations of representative cases from our clinical practice.

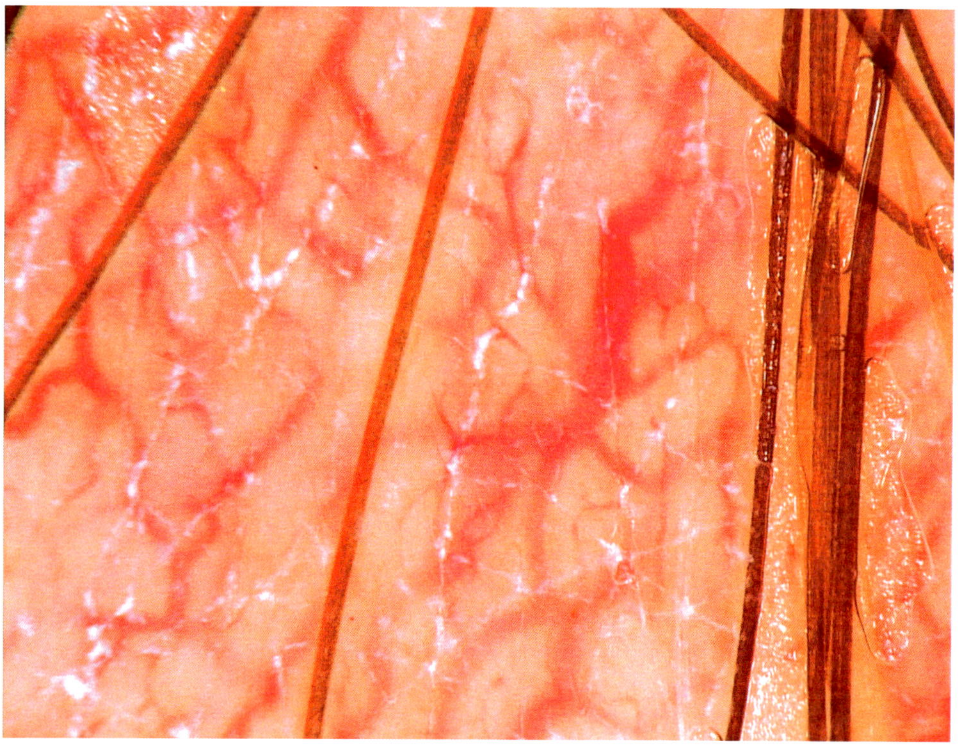

Fig. 44.1 **Longstanding systemic sclerosis (anti-topoisomerase I positive) in a 43-year-old woman**. Multiple thick arborizing vessels, corresponding to telangiectasia, also were observed on the patient's face. This image shows that thick arborizing vessels, which previously were associated only with skin tumors, also may be present on the scalp of patients with noncancerous diseases. Thick arborizing vessels in basal cell carcinoma differ from the vessels in this image by being concentrically located and associated with skin lesions and by their bright red color and "in focus" appearance. Occasionally, extremely elongated blood vessels forming bizarre structures are observed in systemic sclerosis. Our experience shows that vascular abnormalities on the scalp increase in number with disease duration and severity. They are not observed in systemic sclerosis of recent onset (×70)

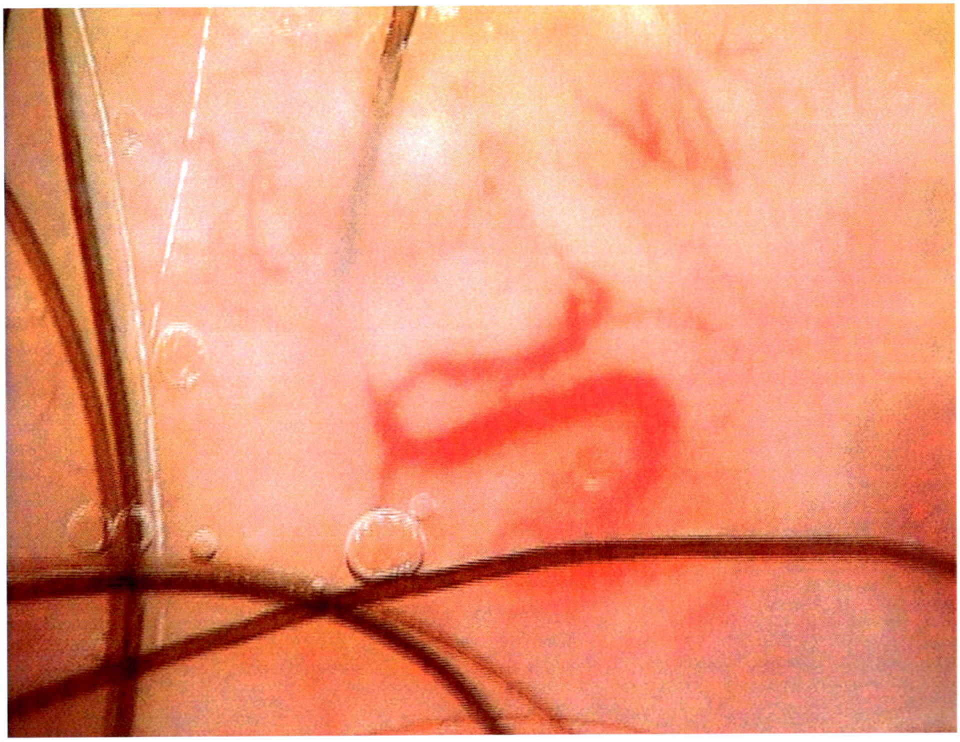

Fig. 44.2 Dermatomyositis in a 47-year-old patient. Trichoscopy shows irregularly enlarged, giant capillaries, comparable with R (Raynaud) capillaries on capillaroscopy. Some of these vessels have a root-like appearance. The patient also demonstrated thick arborizing vessels and extravasations on trichoscopy (×70)

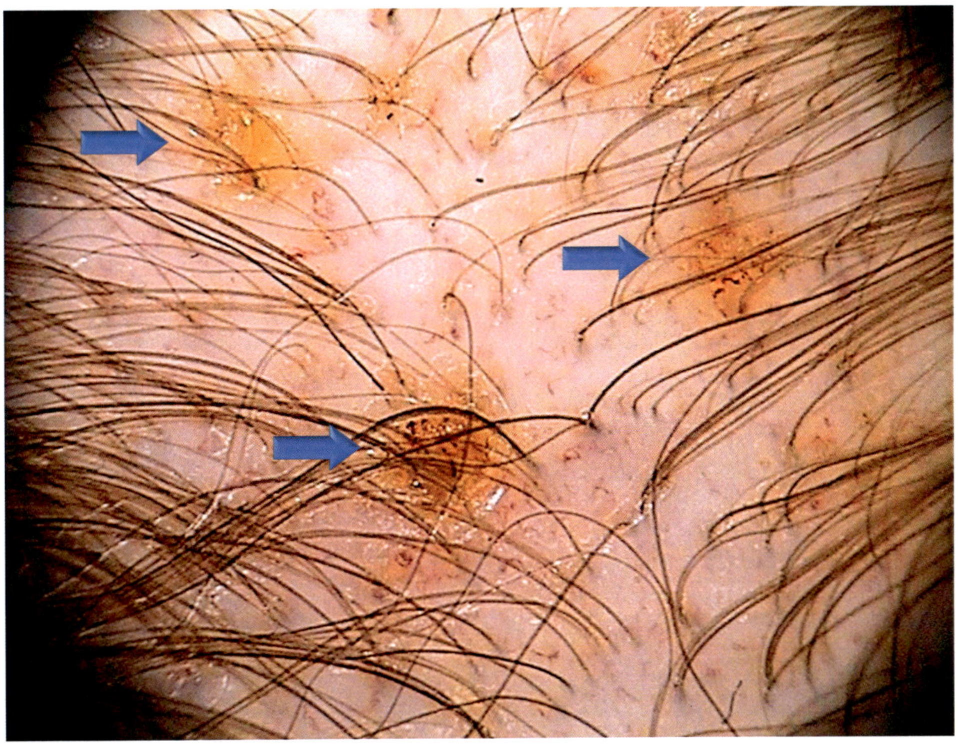

Fig. 44.3 Amicrobial pustulosis in a 39-year-old patient with systemic lupus erythematosus treated with low-dose prednisone and rituximab infusions (2×1,000 mg every 6 months). Trichoscopy shows multiple yellow, pustule-like structures with a translucent overlying epidermis (*arrows*) and small extravasations within the lesions. Histopathology showed subcorneal, spongiform neutrophilic pustules, consistent with the diagnosis of amicrobial pustulosis. Amicrobial pustulosis is a rare entity characterized by relapsing pustular lesions mainly involving the scalp and cutaneous folds. The disease typically occurs in the context of an autoimmune disorder and is classified within the spectrum of neutrophilic dermatoses. The image also shows multiple short linear vessels and comma vessels (×20)

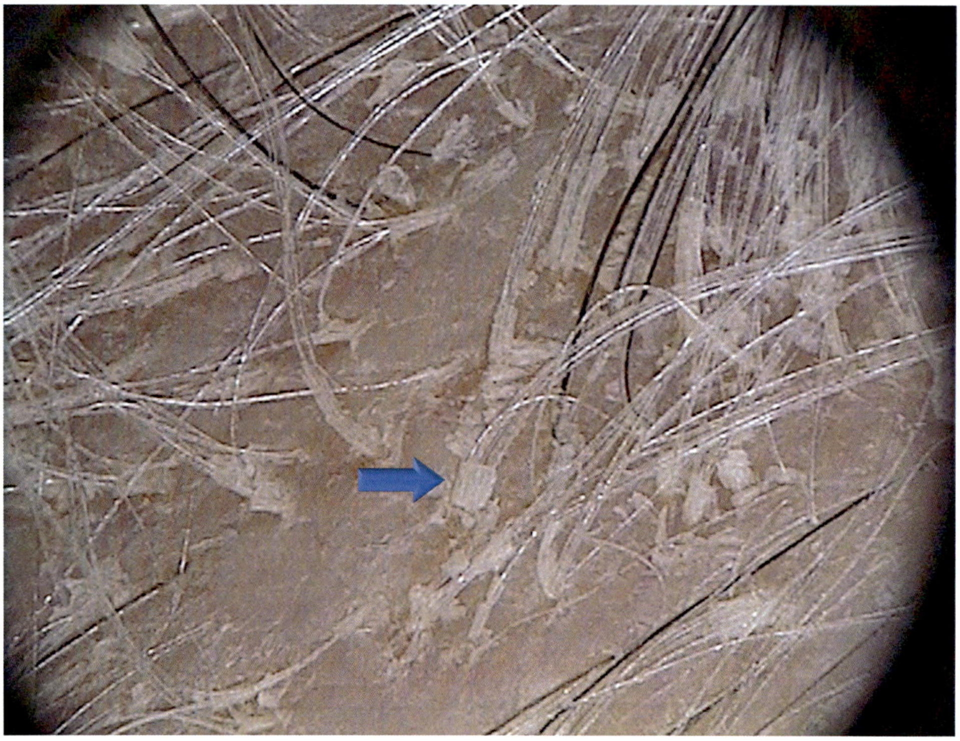

Fig. 44.4 Newly diagnosed multiple myeloma in a 75-year-old woman. On dry trichoscopy, whitish rhomboidal follicular spicules with a soft/wet appearance (*arrow*) are observed emerging from the follicular openings together with hair shafts. There is no abnormal scaling between follicular units. Follicular spicules, a typical dermatologic observation in multiple myeloma [11, 13], are seen most frequently on the nose. It has been shown that follicular spicules contain monoclonal protein with electrophoretic characteristics identical to those found in the patient's serum [13]. Follicular spicules observed on trichoscopy may be the first indicator of multiple myeloma. However, differential diagnosis with benign perifollicular hyperkeratosis may be difficult for a less-experienced trichoscopist. For more detailed information about trichoscopy in lymphoproliferative disorders, see Chapter 43 (dry trichoscopy, ×20)

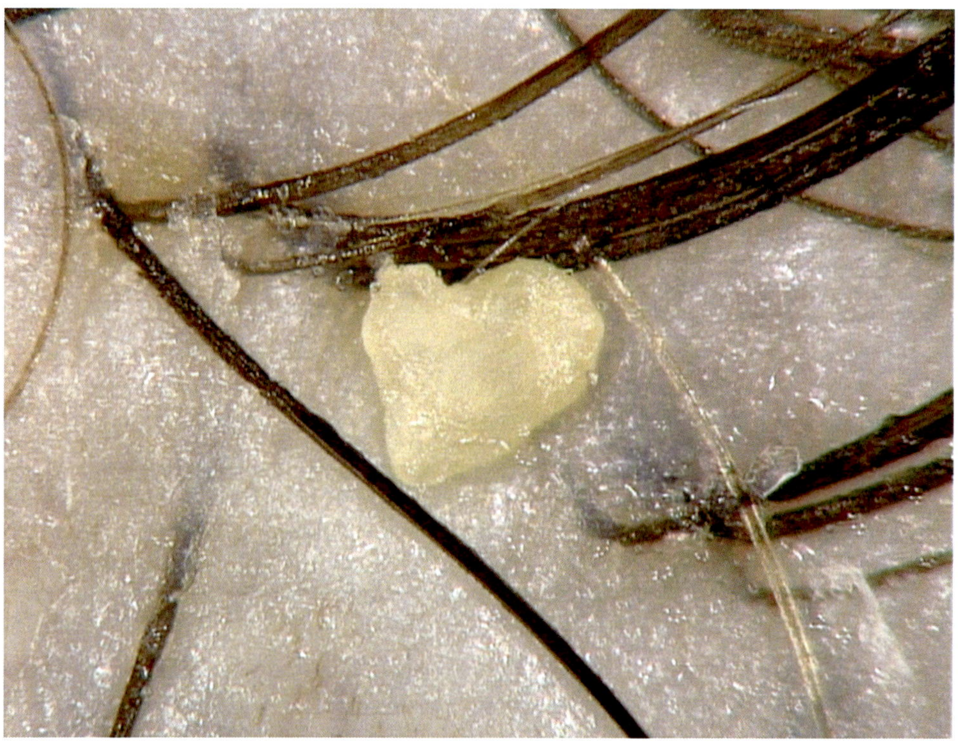

Fig. 44.5 Multiple myeloma in a 79-year-old patient. In this patient, trichoscopy showed follicular spicules as well as aggregates containing monoclonal protein. These structures were detached from the follicular openings and appeared dry and firm, with a tendency to form polygonal structures (dry trichoscopy, ×70)

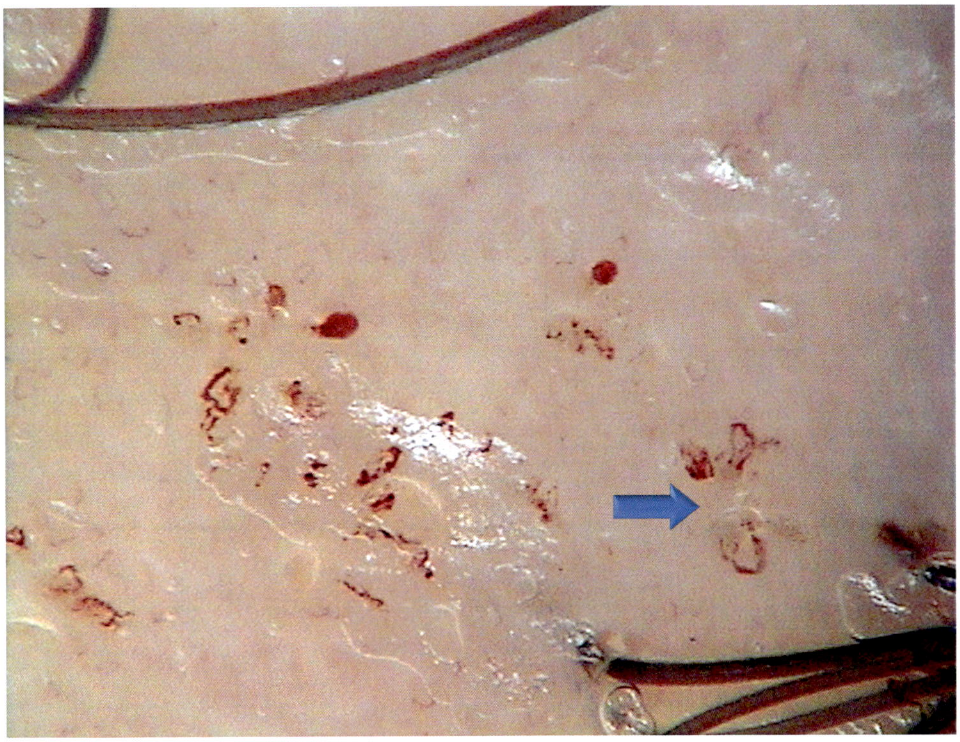

Fig. 44.6 Sézary syndrome, cutaneous T-cell lymphoma, in a 47-year-old man. The patient had a 2-year history of Sézary syndrome and alopecia in the course of the disease. Trichoscopy shows a decreased number of follicular openings and an atypical vascular pattern. Elongated looped vessels form concentric (flower-like) structures. The open parts of the loops are directed toward the inside, which differentiates this pattern from the concentric loops in lichen planopilaris. These concentric loops ("vascular flowers," *arrow*) also may be observed in other types of cutaneous T-cell lymphoma (×70)

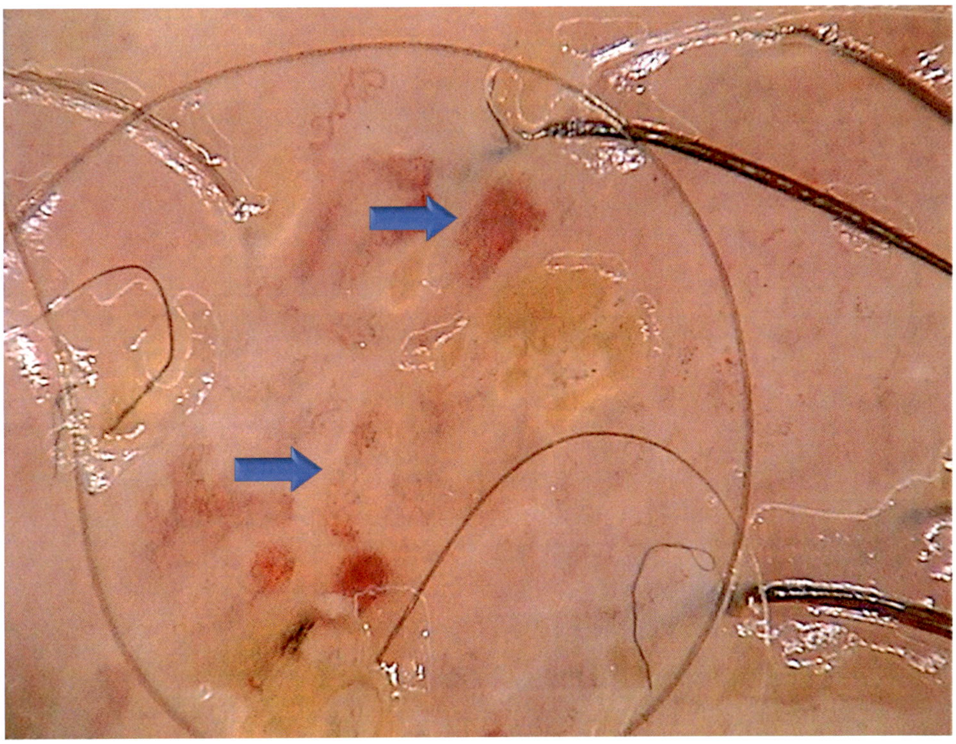

Fig. 44.7 Recently diagnosed mycosis fungoides, cutaneous T-cell lymphoma, in a 66-year-old man. Trichoscopy shows characteristic orange-yellow patchy areas [14]. The vascular pattern consists of granular, relatively well-margined, milky red areas (*arrows*) surrounded by normal-appearing skin. Within some of these areas, serpentine-like blood vessels are visible. These vascular structures must be differentiated from the milky red areas seen in amelanotic melanoma [15] (×70)

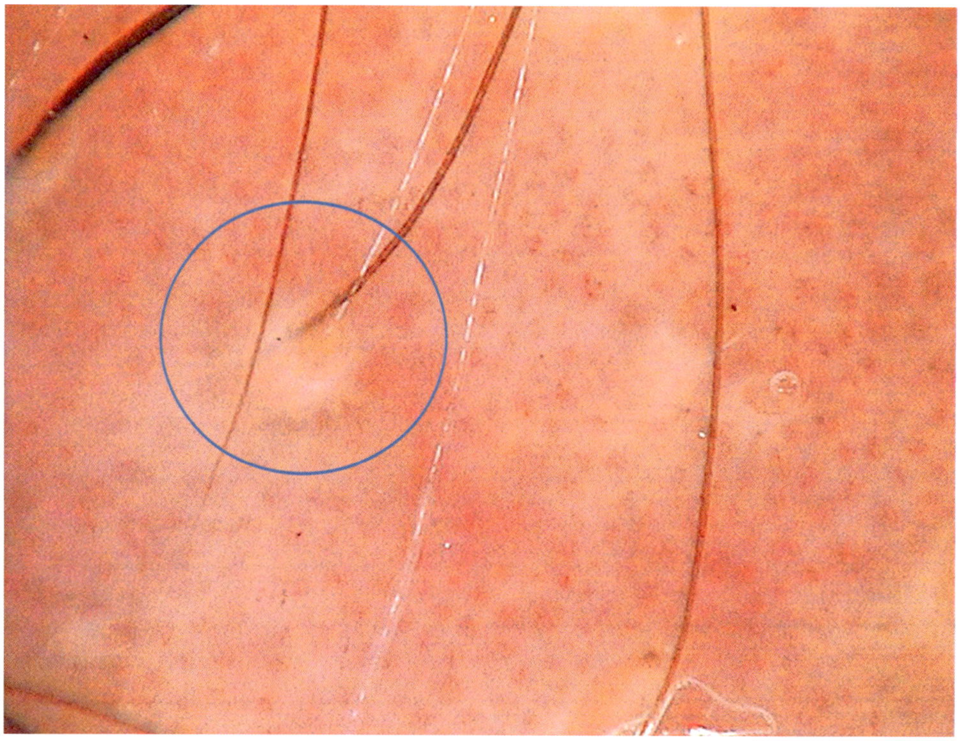

Fig. 44.8 **Cutaneous T-cell lymphoma: mycosis fungoides.** The image shows granular milky red areas in a perifollicular arrangement (*blue ring*). Within some of these areas, dotted vessels are visible. Normal-appearing skin surrounds the granular milky red areas. The number of follicular units is significantly decreased (×20)

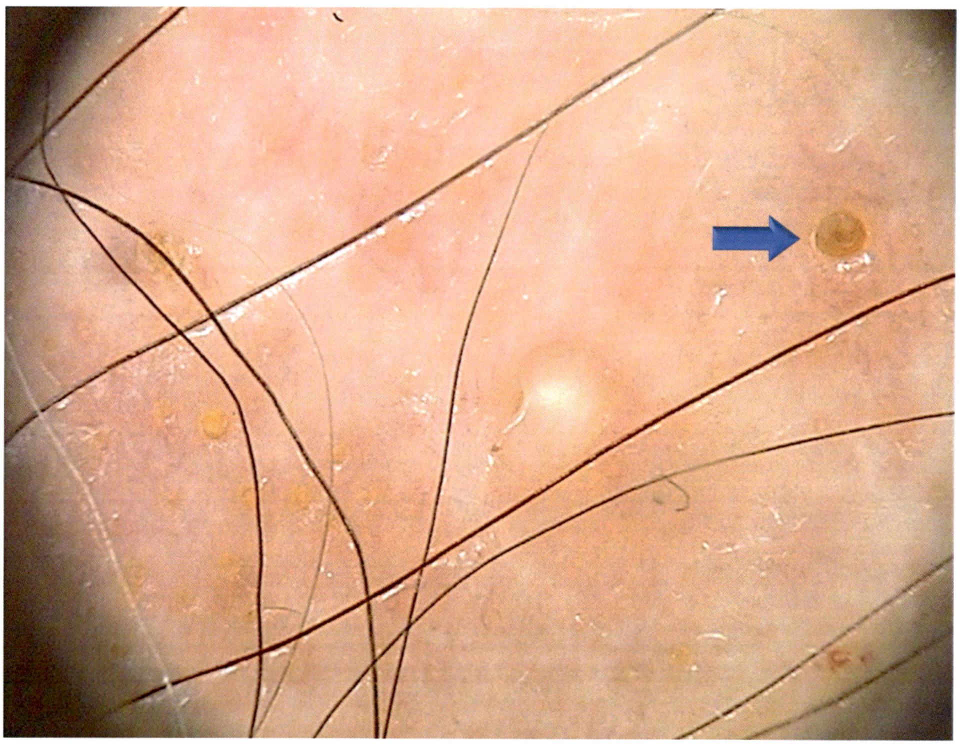

Fig. 44.9 **Alopecia mucinosa.** This 67-year-old woman with alopecia mucinosa (follicular mucinosis) presented with focal alopecia and acneiform lesions in the vertex area. Trichoscopy shows empty follicular openings with follicular plugs (*arrow*), which consist of yellow-brown material (×20)

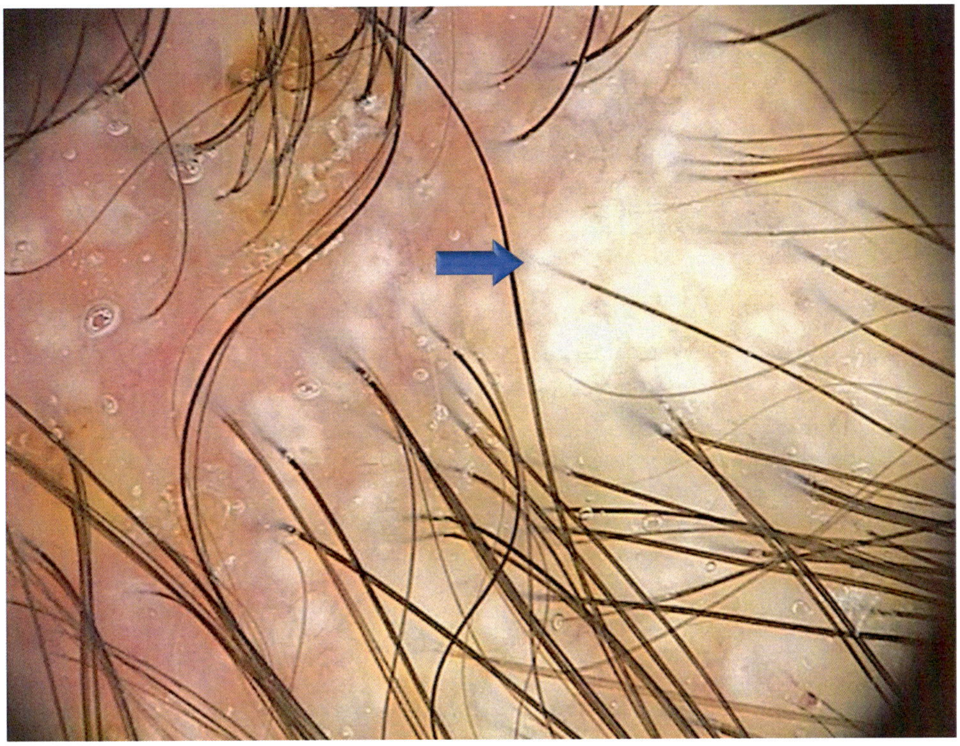

Fig. 44.10 **Langerhans cell histiocytosis**. This image is from a 31-year-old man with scalp involvement in the course of Langerhans cell histiocytosis. Acute generalized Langerhans cell histiocytosis is exceptionally rare in adults. Those affected by the disease present with a characteristic erythematous or brownish red, discrete, scaly, papular or papulopustular eruption. The scalp frequently is involved; other sites of predilection are the groins, axillae, chest, and back [16, 17]. Trichoscopy shows cotton wool–like, cloudy structures (*arrow*) in a perifollicular distribution. These structures correspond to perifollicular Langerhans cell infiltrates, accompanied by interstitial edema in the upper dermis. Erythema, observed on trichoscopy, corresponds to prominently dilated dermal capillary vessels. The hair shafts are not affected by the disease (×20)

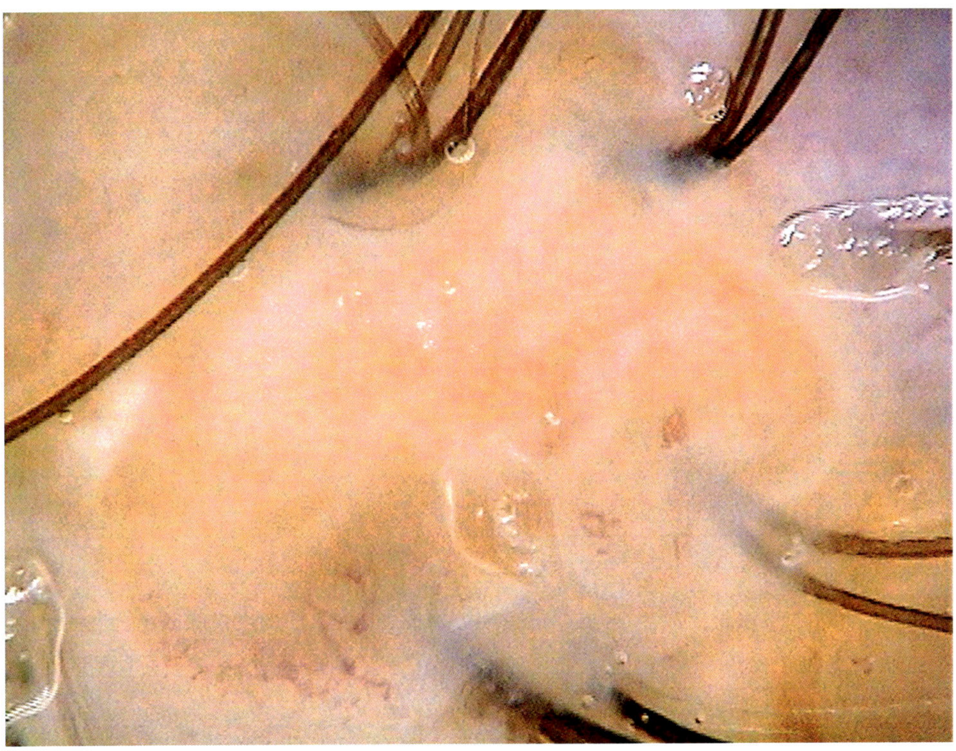

Fig. 44.11 **Multicentric reticulohistiocytosis of recent onset in a 48-year-old woman**. Multicentric reticulohistiocytosis is classified as a non-Langerhans histiocytosis frequently coexisting with destructive seronegative ulcerative polyarthritis and synovitis [18]. Clinically, it manifests as small reddish brown and orange macules, papules, and nodules on the dorsal surface of the hands, nail folds, face, oral mucous membranes, neck, and scalp. In 15–30 % of patients, a malignancy or an autoimmune disease may develop simultaneously or shortly after the onset of multicentric reticulohistiocytosis [18, 19]. Trichoscopy shows orange-brown skin discoloration in a whirl-like arrangement on a whitish background (×50)

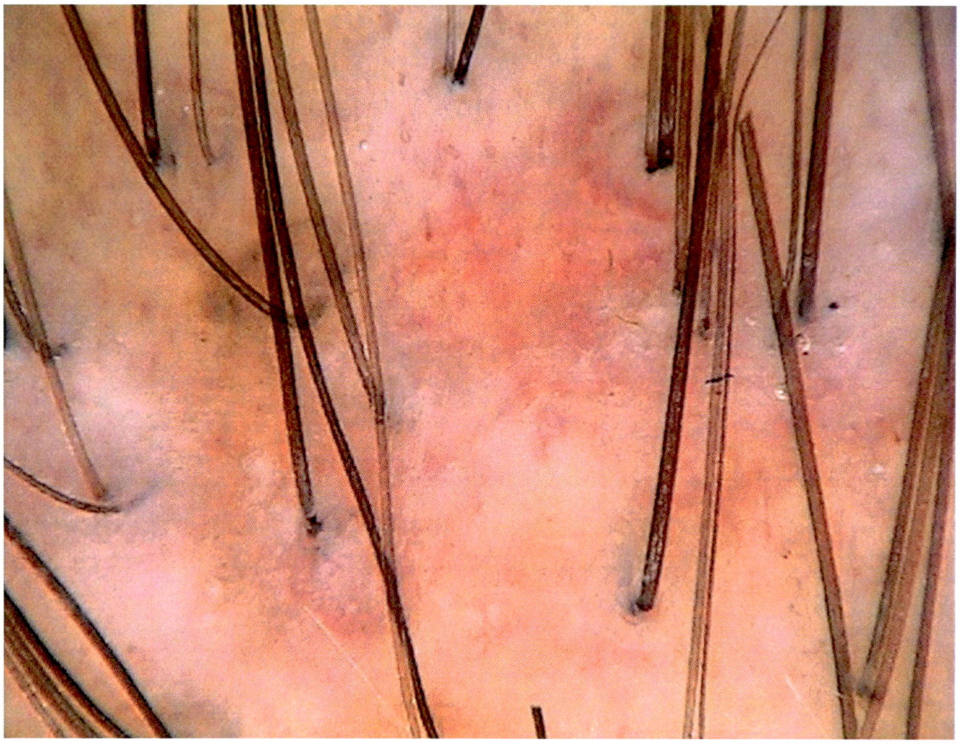

Fig. 44.12 **Noncarcinomatous skin changes in a 28-year-old man with xeroderma pigmentosum and a history of multiple basal and squamous cell carcinomas**. Xeroderma pigmentosum is a rare autosomal recessive disease characterized by a 1000-fold increased risk of developing cutaneous malignancies [20, 21]. The most characteristic clinical finding is generalized poikiloderma associated with skin atrophy, telangiectasias, spotted hyperpigmentation, and hypopigmentation. Dermoscopy is used for early skin cancer detection in these patients [20–22]; however, dermoscopy of noncarcinomatous skin lesions in xeroderma pigmentosum appears not to have been described yet. Trichoscopy of noncarcinomatous scalp skin in our patient revealed a mixture of white, red, and brownish areas. Depending on the scalp area, these areas were distributed in a macular or whirly manner. A wide range of vascular structures were observed. Thick arborizing vessels were most common in the noncarcinomatous skin of this patient (×70)

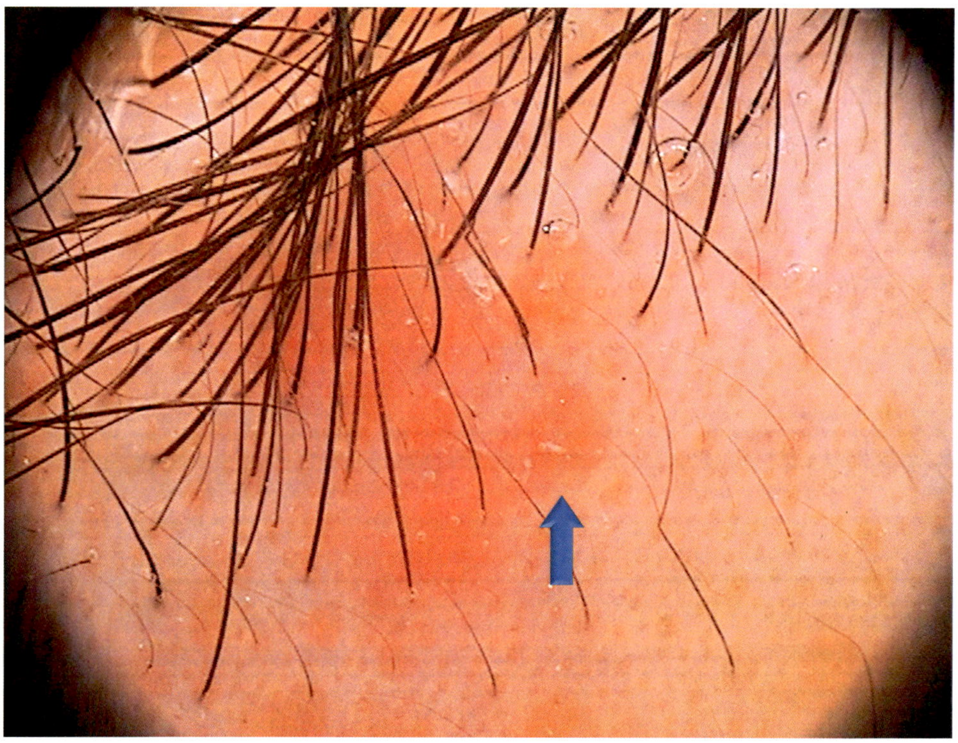

Fig. 44.13 **Cutaneous sarcoidosis in a 39-year-old patient**. Trichoscopy shows relatively sharply demarcated, semi-translucent orange areas (*arrow*) in an interfollicular distribution. The orange macules vary in size and tend to merge into larger polycyclic areas. This presentation corresponds to the previously described "apple-jelly sign" of sarcoidosis [23–25] (×20)

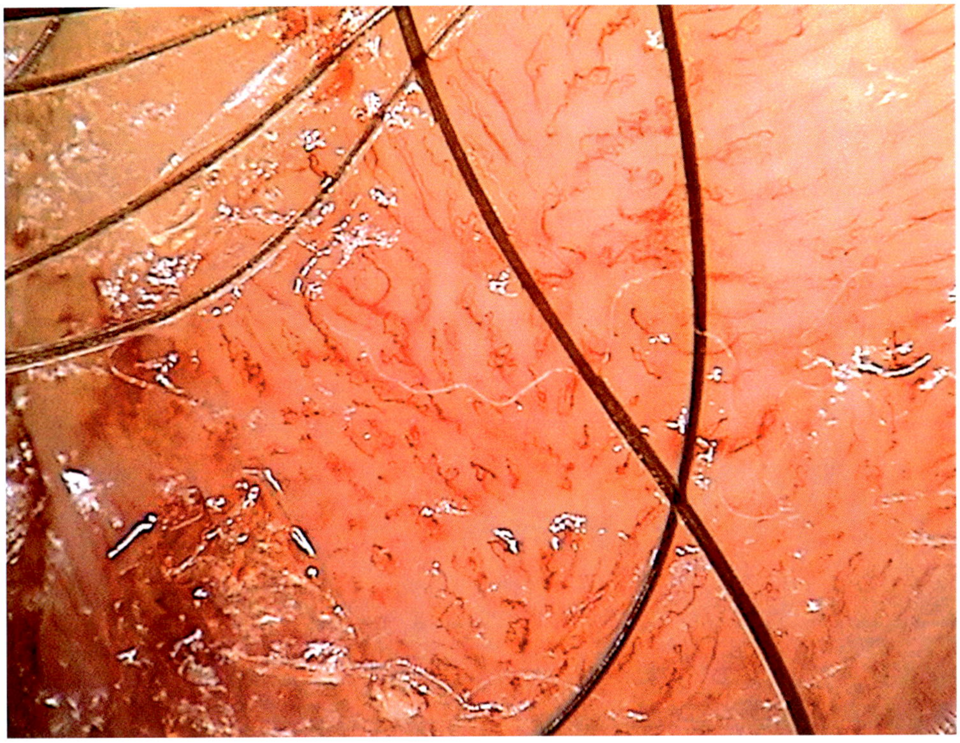

Fig. 44.14 **Alopecia in the course of Crohn's disease**. This 21-year-old woman developed transient alopecia and psoriasis in the course of Crohn's disease treated with infliximab. This type of alopecia recently was described as a novel type of noncicatricial alopecia [26, 27]. Trichoscopy shows multiple elongated, linear, and serpentine-like vessels aligned in a regular parallel distribution (×50)

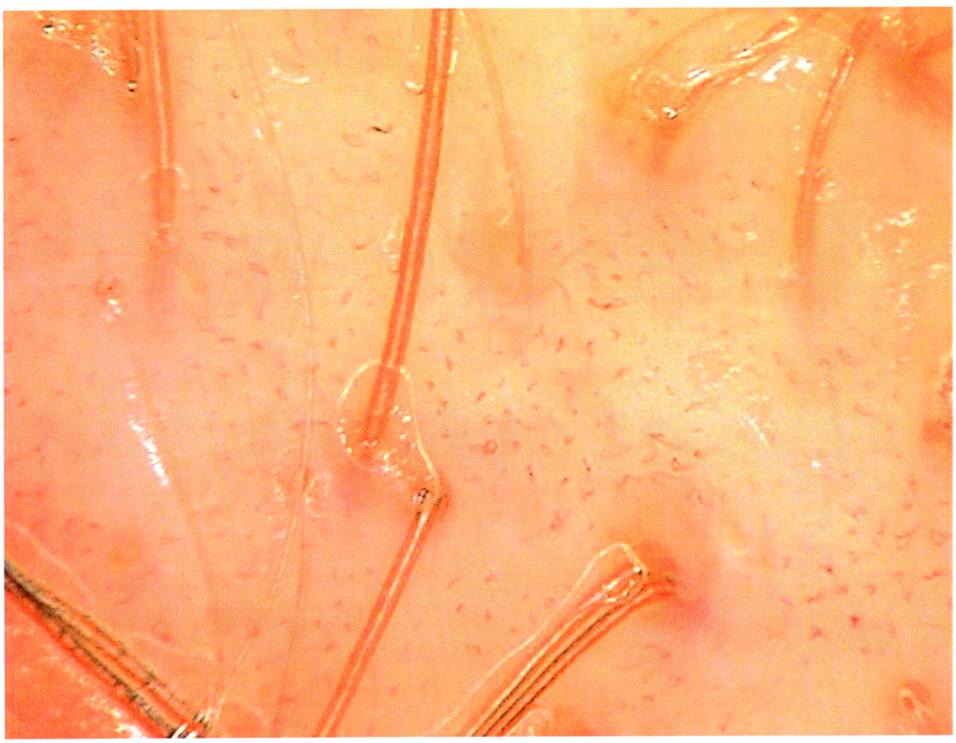

Fig. 44.15 **Hyperbilirubinemia**. This image is from a 16-year-old boy with hyperbilirubinemia in the course of Gilbert syndrome. The diagnosis was established after trichoscopy, which revealed a yellow background color. The patient had no other clinical symptoms of jaundice (×70)

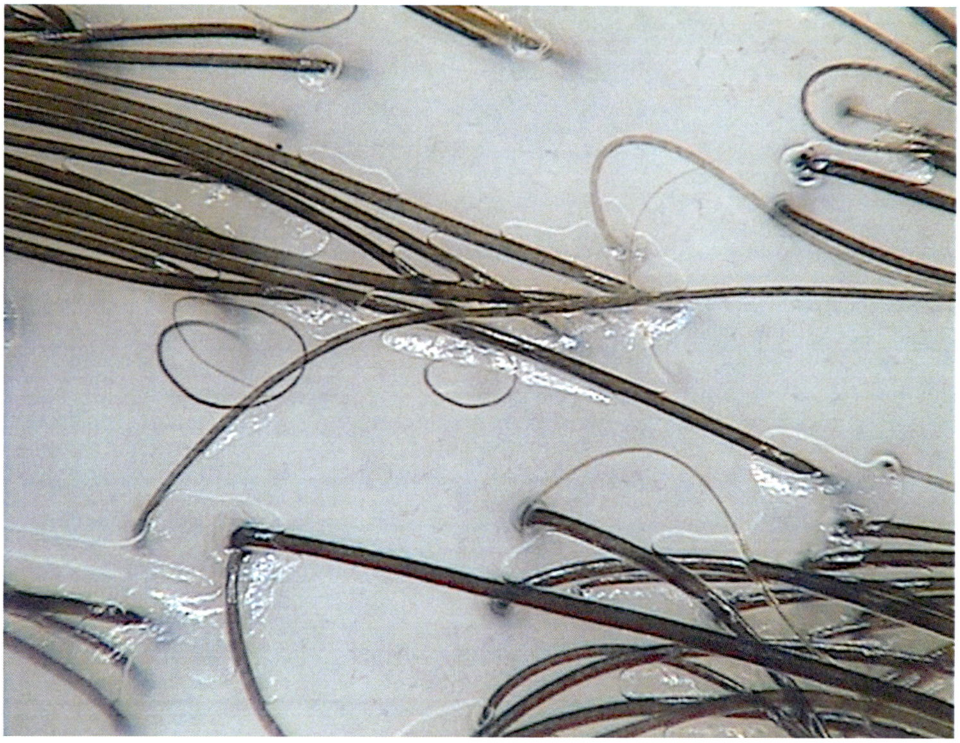

Fig. 44.16 Hypothyroidism. Shown is a trichoscopic image from a 45-year-old woman with longstanding hypothyroidism in the course of Hashimoto's disease. Our preliminary data show that in hypothyroidism, hair shaft thickness is not altered, but the number of follicular units with three hairs is significantly decreased [1]. The most characteristic trichoscopic features of hypothyroidism include a decreased number of blood vessels and the presence of extensive areas lacking blood vessels. These avascular areas usually are uniformly white, lacking the pink tone of normal skin (×70)

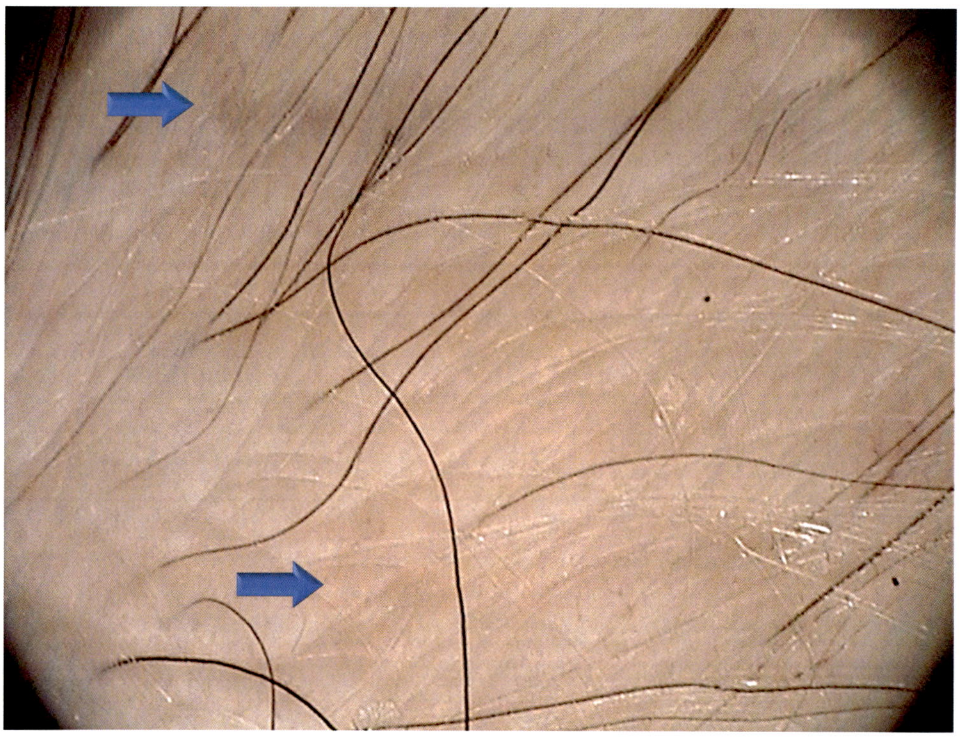

Fig. 44.17 Addison's disease (primary adrenocortical insufficiency) in a 49-year-old female patient. Trichoscopy shows diffuse, slightly violaceous skin discoloration with discrete, irregular brown areas (*arrows*). In this gray-haired patient, the disease onset was associated with a partial regain of hair pigmentation. The corresponding manifestation on trichoscopy was the presence of groups of pigmented hairs, usually in co-localization with interfollicular brown areas (×20)

References

1. Olszewska M, Warszawik O, Rakowska A, Slowinska M, Rudnicka L. Methods of hair loss evaluation in patients with endocrine disorders. Endokrynol Pol. 2010;61(4):406–11.
2. Trueb RM. Hormones and hair growth. Hautarzt. 2010;61(6): 487–95.
3. Camacho-Martinez FM. Hair loss in women. Semin Cutan Med Surg. 2009;28(1):19–32.
4. Redondo P, Guzman M, Marquina M, Pretel M, Aguado L, Lloret P, et al. Repigmentation of gray hair after thyroid hormone treatment. Actas Dermosifiliogr. 2007;98(9):603–10.
5. Kasumagic-Halilovic E. Thyroid autoimmunity in patients with alopecia areata. Acta Dermatovenerol Croat. 2008;16(3):123–5.
6. Kumar KV, Prusty P. Visual vignette. The Hertoghe sign. Endocr Pract. 2011;17(4):666.
7. Daniells S, Hardy G. Hair loss in long-term or home parenteral nutrition: are micronutrient deficiencies to blame? Curr Opin Clin Nutr Metab Care. 2010;13(6):690–7.
8. Trueb RM. Involvement of scalp and nails in lupus erythematosus. Lupus. 2010;19(9):1078–86.
9. Gong Y, Ye Y, Zhao Y, Caulloo S, Chen X, Zhang B, et al. Severe diffuse non-scarring hair loss in systemic lupus erythematosus—clinical and histopathological analysis of four cases. J Eur Acad Dermatol Venereol. 2011. doi:10.1111/j.1468-3083.2011.04388.x.
10. LeBoit PE. Alopecia mucinosa, inflammatory disease or mycosis fungoides: must we choose? And are there other choices? Am J Dermatopathol. 2004;26(2):167–70.
11. Tay LK, Lim FL, Ng HJ, Lee HY, Pang SM, Thirumoorthy T. Cutaneous follicular hyperkeratotic spicules—the first clinical sign of multiple myeloma progression or relapse. Int J Dermatol. 2010; 49(8):934–6.
12. Rahman A, Mahmood A. Cutis verticis gyrata secondary to infiltrating ductal carcinoma breast. J Coll Physicians Surg Pak. 2012;22(2):120–2.
13. Satta R, Casu G, Dore F, Longinotti M, Cottoni F. Follicular spicules and multiple ulcers: cutaneous manifestations of multiple myeloma. J Am Acad Dermatol. 2003;49(4):736–40.
14. Lallas A, Apalla Z, Lefaki I, Tzellos T, Karatolias A, Sotiriou E, et al. Dermoscopy of early stage mycosis fungoides. J Eur Acad Dermatol Venereol. 2012. doi:10.1111/j.1468-3083.2012.04499.x.
15. Zalaudek I, Kreusch J, Giacomel J, Ferrara G, Catricala C, Argenziano G. How to diagnose nonpigmented skin tumors: a review of vascular structures seen with dermoscopy: part I. Melanocytic skin tumors. J Am Acad Dermatol. 2010;63(3):361–74; quiz 75–6.
16. Wright TS. Cutaneous manifestations of malignancy. Curr Opin Pediatr. 2011;23(4):407–11.
17. Fogo A, du Vivier A. The cutaneous manifestations of haematological malignancy. Clin Med. 2009;9(4):366–70.
18. Kaul A, Tolat SN, Belgaumkar V, Mhaske CB. Multicentric reticulohistiocytosis. Indian J Dermatol Venereol Leprol. 2010; 76(4):404–7.
19. Ben Abdelghani K, Mahmoud I, Chatelus E, Sordet C, Gottenberg JE, Sibilia J. Multicentric reticulohistiocytosis: an autoimmune systemic disease? Case report of an association with erosive rheumatoid arthritis and systemic Sjogren syndrome. Joint Bone Spine. 2010;77(3):274–6.
20. Green WH, Wang SQ, Cognetta Jr AB. Total-body cutaneous examination, total-body photography, and dermoscopy in the care of a patient with xeroderma pigmentosum and multiple melanomas. Arch Dermatol. 2009;145(8):910–5.
21. Malvehy J, Puig S, Marti-Laborda RM. Dermoscopy of skin lesions in two patients with xeroderma pigmentosum. Br J Dermatol. 2005;152(2):271–8.
22. Segura S, Puig S, Carrera C, Lecha M, Borges V, Malvehy J. Non-invasive management of non-melanoma skin cancer in patients with cancer predisposition genodermatosis: a role for confocal microscopy and photodynamic therapy. J Eur Acad Dermatol Venereol. 2011;25(7):819–27.
23. Vazquez-Lopez F, Palacios-Garcia L, Gomez-Diez S, Argenziano G. Dermoscopy for discriminating between lichenoid sarcoidosis and lichen planus. Arch Dermatol. 2011;147(9):1130.
24. Pellicano R, Tiodorovic-Zivkovic D, Gourhant JY, Catricala C, Ferrara G, Caldarola G, et al. Dermoscopy of cutaneous sarcoidosis. Dermatology. 2010;221(1):51–4.
25. Torres F, Tosti A, Misciali C, Lorenzi S. Trichoscopy as a clue to the diagnosis of scalp sarcoidosis. Int J Dermatol. 2011;50(3):358–61.
26. Doyle LA, Sperling LC, Baksh S, Lackey J, Thomas B, Vleugels RA, et al. Psoriatic alopecia/alopecia areata-like reactions secondary to anti-tumor necrosis factor-alpha therapy: a novel cause of noncicatricial alopecia. Am J Dermatopathol. 2011;33(2):161–6.
27. Medkour F, Babai S, Chanteloup E, Buffard V, Delchier JC, Le-Louet H. Development of diffuse psoriasis with alopecia during treatment of Crohn's disease with infliximab. Gastroenterol Clin Biol. 2010;34(2):140–1.

Index

L. Rudnicka et al. (eds.), *Atlas of Trichoscopy*,
DOI 10.1007/978-1-4471-4486-1, © Springer-Verlag London 2012

E

M

N

O

P

FSC
www.fsc.org
MIX
Papier | Fördert gute Waldnutzung
FSC® C083411

Zeitfracht Medien GmbH
Ferdinand-Jühlke-Straße 7
99095 Erfurt, Deutschland
produktsicherheit@kolibri360.de